Bisher Abdullah, MD

Review of

Pediatric Gastrointestinal Disease and Nutrition

Review of

Pediatric Gastrointestinal Disease and Nutrition

JEANNIE HUANG, MD, MPH
Assistant Professor in Residence
Department of Pediatrics
University of California, San Diego
San Diego, California

W. ALLAN WALKER, MD
Conrad Taff Professor of Nutrition and Pediatrics
Director, Division of Nutrition
Harvard Medical School
Director, Mucosal Immunology Laboratory
Combined Program in Pediatric Gastroenterology and Nutrition
Massachusetts General Hospital
Boston, Massachusetts

2005
BC Decker Inc
Hamilton • London

BC Decker Inc
P.O. Box 620, L.C.D. 1
Hamilton, Ontario L8N 3K7
Tel: 905-522-7017; 800-568-7281
Fax: 905-522-7839; 888-311-4987
E-mail: info@bcdecker.com
www.bcdecker.com

03 04 05 06 / WPC / 9 8 7 6 5 4 3 2 1

ISBN 1-55009-300-2

Printed in the United States

Sales and Distribution

United States
BC Decker Inc
P.O. Box 785
Lewiston, NY 14092-0785
Tel: 905-522-7017; 800-568-7281
Fax: 905-522-7839; 888-311-4987
E-mail: info@bcdecker.com
www.bcdecker.com

Canada
BC Decker Inc
20 Hughson Street South
P.O. Box 620, LCD 1
Hamilton, Ontario L8N 3K7
Tel: 905-522-7017; 800-568-7281
Fax: 905-522-7839; 888-311-4987
E-mail: info@bcdecker.com
www.bcdecker.com

Foreign Rights
John Scott & Company
International Publishers' Agency
P.O. Box 878
Kimberton, PA 19442
Tel: 610-827-1640
Fax: 610-827-1671
E-mail: jsco@voicenet.com

Japan
Igaku-Shoin Ltd.
Foreign Publications Department
3-24-17 Hongo
Bunkyo-ku, Tokyo, Japan 113-8719
Tel: 3 3817 5680
Fax: 3 3815 6776
E-mail: fd@igaku-shoin.co.jp

UK, Europe, Scandinavia, Middle East
Elsevier Science
Customer Service Department
Foots Cray High Street
Sidcup, Kent
DA14 5HP, UK
Tel: 44 (0) 208 308 5760
Fax: 44 (0) 181 308 5702
E-mail: cservice@harcourt.com

Singapore, Malaysia, Thailand, Philippines, Indonesia, Vietnam, Pacific Rim, Korea
Elsevier Science Asia
583 Orchard Road
#09/01, Forum
Singapore 238884
Tel: 65-737-3593
Fax: 65-753-2145

Australia, New Zealand
Elsevier Science Australia
Customer Service Department
STM Division
Locked Bag 16
St. Peters, New South Wales, 2044
Australia
Tel: 61 02 9517-8999
Fax: 61 02 9517-2249
E-mail: stmp@harcourt.com.au
www.harcourt.com.au

Mexico and Central America
ETM SA de CV
Calle de Tula 59
Colonia Condesa
06140 Mexico DF, Mexico
Tel: 52-5-5553-6657
Fax: 52-5-5211-8468
E-mail:
editoresdetextosmex@prodigy.net.mx

Brazil
Tecmedd Importadora E Distribuidora
De Livros Ltda.
Avenida Maurílio Biagi, 2850
City Ribeirão, Ribeirão Preto – SP –
Brasil
CEP: 14021-000
Tel: 0800 992236
Fax: (16) 3993-9000
E-mail: tecmedd@tecmedd.com.br

India, Bangladesh, Pakistan, Sri Lanka
Elsevier Health Sciences Division
Customer Service Department
17A/1, Main Ring Road
Lajpat Nagar IV
New Delhi – 110024, India
Tel: 91 11 2644 7160-64
Fax: 91 11 2644 7156
E-mail: esindia@vsnl.net

PREFACE

As the field of pediatric gastroenterology has developed from an obscure subspecialty to an essential component of every major academic pediatric program throughout the world, so too must the literature develop to cover more extensively the pathophysiologic basis of gastrointestinal disease in children of all ages. The fourth edition of *Pediatric Gastrointestinal Disease: Pathophysiology* was conceived to fill the void that existed, and with this review book, we have attempted to provide a useful companion text, one with which students and practitioners of pediatric medicine can test their proficiency in the field.

This review is organized, much like the parent text, into sections that establish a comprehensive approach to pediatric gastroenterology. Although it was conceived as a companion text, it also functions as a stand-alone review, with each section consisting of synopses of various topics followed by questions and answers. To aid in the true acquisition of knowledge, questions are provided in numerous formats: true or false, multiple choice, choose the best answer, and mix and match. This review should prove an indispensable aid to the student preparing for board examinations.

As with the parent text, we hope and expect that the collective approach of this review will be beneficial to all physicians, and physicians-to-be, in dealing with gastrointestinal problems in children.

JSH, WAW
January, 2005

DEDICATION

I would like to dedicate this review textbook to my husband Nathaniel Chuang and son Ethan for their patience and encouragement during its inception and development. Also, I wish to thank my parents, Song and Ann Huang, and my sister Susan for their unwavering faith in me all these years.

Jeannie Huang

To all my former trainees and current faculty members in the field of pediatric gastroenterology.

W. Allan Walker

CONTENTS

SECTION 4
RESEARCH METHODOLOGY

SECTION 5 NUTRITIONAL PRINCIPLES OF THERAPY

PHYSIOLOGY AND PATHOPHYSIOLOGY

MOTILITY DISORDERS

SYNOPSIS

ANATOMY

1. Muscle at small intestine (SI), colon: 2 perpendicularly oriented layers of smooth muscle in tunica muscularis (thick inner circular layer and thinner outer longitudinal layer). Longitudinal layer is continuous in SI, but concentrated into 3 bands (taeniae) at colon.
2. Nerves and ganglia: submucosa (Meissner plexus), and between circular and longitudinal layers (Auerbach plexus).
3. Interstitial cells of Cajal, which are C-kit receptor positive, are the pacemakers of intestinal motility.
4. Contraction of gut smooth muscle depends on actin and myosin filaments—modulated by intracellular free Ca^{2+}.

REGULATION OF INTESTINAL MOTOR ACTIVITY

1. Neurohumoral mechanisms: intestinal smooth muscle innervated by neurons in enteric nervous system (ENS). Somatostatin and enkephalins modulate background excitability of intrinsic neural network and smooth muscle cells. Acetylcholine (ACh) action on smooth muscle excitatory via muscarinic receptors; norepinephrine direct inhibition on smooth muscle.
2. Myogenic mechanisms: 3 types of membrane electrical potential: resting potential, slow wave potential, and action or spike potential. Not well understood in colon.

    a. Resting potential: intracellular high K, low Na. Maintained via Na,K-adenosinetriphosphatase (ATPase).
    b. Slow wave potential: frequency = 8–11 cycles/min (SI); > 20 cycles/min in colon associated with prolonged tonic contractions. There is a delay in onset of the slow wave with distance from mouth such that slow wave appears to propagate aborally. Length of each frequency plateau becomes shorter in more caudal bowel.
    c. Action or spike potential: one-to-one association with contraction. Spike activity occurs only during depolarized phase of slow wave. In the presence of inhibitory background, partial depolarization usually insufficient to cause spike. In proximal bowel, where longest slow wave frequency plateaus occur, contractions migrate over long distances (propulsion rapid). At terminal SI, frequency plateaus shortest, and contractions migrate only short distances (Figure 1).
3. During depolarization: intracellular calcium concentration rises, calcium binds to calmodulin, and calmodulin binds to caldesmon, which then exposes the myosin-binding domain of actin. The calcium–calmodulin complex also activates myosin light-chain kinase. These events lead to myosin binding with actin and muscle contraction.
4. Maximum contraction frequency governed by slow wave frequency: 11–12 cycles/min in duodenum; 7–8 cycles/min in terminal ileum.
5. Specializations in smooth muscle for continuous contraction: gastrointestinal (GI) sphincters have increased numbers of mitochondria and smooth endoplasmic reticulum (ER); initiation of contraction is

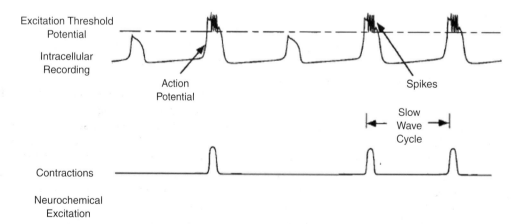

FIGURE 1 Illustration of regulation of rhythmic phasic contractions by slow waves and spikes. The resting potential of smooth muscle cells is negative with respect to the extracellular fluid potential. The depolarization during spontaneous slow waves does not exceed the excitation threshold; therefore, no contractions occur. The release of acetylcholine by neurochemical excitation depolarizes the plateau phase of the slow waves beyond the excitation threshold; spikes are superimposed on the plateau phase and the cell contracts. Adapted with permission from Sarna SK. In vivo myoelectric activity: methods, analysis and interpretation. In: Wood JD, editor. Handbook of physiology, section 6: the gastrointestinal system. Vol. 1. Motility and circulation. Bethesda (MD): The American Physiological Society; 1989. p. 817–63.

slower but contraction duration longer; prolonged cycling of myosin cross-bridges.

ENTERIC NERVOUS SYSTEM

1. Neural crest cells give rise to vagal and sacral segments. Vagal outnumber sacral neural crest cells (20%).
2. Migration of vagal neural crest cells occurs craniocaudally—cells at rectum at 12 weeks. Mutations in *RET*, endothelin B, glial cell-derived neurotrophic factor, and endothelin 3 result in abnormal migration, survival, proliferation, and differentiation of ganglion cells (Hirschsprung disease).
3. Neurotransmitters: excitatory: ACh, tachykinins such as substance P; inhibitory: nitric oxide (NO), vasoactive intestinal polypeptide, pituitary adenylyl cyclase–activating peptide (PACAP).
4. 5-hydroxytryptamine (5-HT) receptors 95% in gut. 5-HT1 receptors relax GI smooth muscle, while 5-HT2, 5-HT3, and 5-HT4 receptors are involved in contraction.
5. Enterochromaffin cells have important sensory functions. Enterochromaffin cells are pressure sensors, initiating the peristaltic reflex in response to pressure on mucosa by food after a meal by releasing 5-HT. 5-HT3 is predominant receptor type on extrinsic afferent nerves. Blockade of 5-HT3 receptors on these nerves provides relief of nausea.
6. Intrinsic primary afferent neurons are contained entirely in gut wall (cell bodies and connections). Slow-adapting neurons fire for the duration of the mechanical stimulus with discharge frequency proportional to the stimulus intensity. Fast-adapting units signal the onset of a mechanical stimulus with a brief discharge followed by cease of firing.
7. Intestinofugal neurons: cell bodies in ENS and projections outside the gut. Intestinofugal neurons mediate enteroenteric inhibitory reflexes.
8. Autonomic neurons: cell bodies in brain or dorsal root ganglia.
9. Mast cells: sense antigens, secrete histamine, which increases secretion, and initiate motor activity to expel noxious substances.
10. Reflexes mediated by the ENS include peristalsis and rectoanal inhibitory reflex (RAIR). Peristalsis: migrating contraction proximal to a bolus with relaxation distal to the bolus resulting in propulsion. RAIR: reflex relaxation of internal anal sphincter in response to rectal dilatation by stool, balloon, or air during manometry. Reflex is absent in Hirschsprung disease. NO is putative inhibitory transmitter.
11. ENS has adaptive ability. ENS neuronal regeneration after injury occurs; neurotrophins (eg, nerve growth factor, neurotrophin 3, and brain-derived neurotrophic factor) are involved. Inflammation alters ENS responses.
12. Propagated peristalsis may be interrupted by gut transection and anastomosis.

HORMONAL REGULATION OF GI MOTILITY

1. Cholecystokinin released by duodenal enteroendocrine cells causes reflex delay of gastric emptying via paracrine stimulation of vagal afferents.
2. During fasting, another group of duodenal endocrine cells releases motilin—the physiologic stimulus for the interdigestive migrating motor complex (MMC).

NORMAL MOTILITY: TYPES OF CONTRACTIONS

1. Phasic: brief. Can be propagated or nonpropagated. Nonpropagated phasic contractions are also called segmenting contractions and serve to mix intestinal contents for maximal exposure of mucosa to luminal contents.
2. Tonic: prolonged contractions typical of GI sphincters. Gastric fundus and colon also exhibit tonic contractions; function may be used to reduce luminal diameter.
3. Ultrapropulsive contractions: giant migrating contractions. Include esophageal phase of swallowing and high-amplitude propagating contractions responsible for mass movements in the colon.

PATTERNS OF CONTRACTIONS

ESOPHAGUS

1. High-amplitude peristaltic contractions. Swallowing induces primary peristalsis originating at pharynx. Secondary peristalsis originates in body of esophagus, stimulated by wall distention.
2. Lower esophageal sphincter (LES) tonically contracted. Vagal-mediated transient relaxation occurs during swallowing, vomiting, burping. Transient LES relaxation occurs spontaneously and is primary mechanism for gastroesophageal reflux.

STOMACH

1. Two functionally discrete regions.
2. Fundus (receptacle) relaxes to receive food; mediated by vagal efferents.
3. Gastric sieving: antral contractions propel food toward a closed pylorus, passing particles < 1 mm (delivery to duodenum). Solid meal gastric emptying thus delayed (in contrast liquids are usually unimpeded).
4. Motility abnormalities may be result of damage to muscle, nerve, or interstitial cells of Cajal (ICC). Impaired fundic relaxation is prominent feature of neuropathy. Absence of antral contraction in response to meal typical in postviral gastroparesis.

SMALL INTESTINE

1. Intestinal (myenteric or peristaltic) reflex: Distending bolus initiates contraction above and relaxation below point of stimulation (via myenteric plexus). Intestinal inhibitory reflex: inhibition of intestinal contractions at all adjacent loci during marked distention of bowel (via sympathetic nerves and ENS).

2. MMC: recurrent band of contraction propagating from LES to ileocecal (IC) junction (some initiated at jejunum, do not involve stomach or duodenum) to sweep intestines clear of undigested food, sloughed enterocytes, and bacteria. Four phases: cycle lasts about 100 min.
   - Phase I: only slow waves, no spikes (10–15 min)
   - Phase II: irregular spiking, contractile activity begins, more intense (50–80 minutes)
   - Phase III: 1 spike, and contraction per slow wave (3–5 minutes). Originates at antrum (70%) or duodenum (30%). Regularity linked with motilin.
   - Phase IV: spike activity subsides rapidly
3. Fed pattern: ingestion of meal interrupts MMC, initiates irregular myoelectric spike and associated contractions. Disruption proportional to amount ingested. Intraluminal fat associated with isolated contractile activity; carbohydrate, protein produce more sequential contractions. Two-thirds of meal transit intestine before return of MMC.
4. There is a direct relationship between SI transit time and absorption. Usual absorption complete within 100 cm of intestine. Ileal transit slower than jejunal. Ileal brake: presence of lipid or protein in ileum slows transit.
5. Giant migrating contractions: long, high-amplitude contractions occur 1–2/h at ileum, rare at jejunum. Can be provoked by intravenous opiates and ACh or by irritants—bile acids, short-chain fatty acids.
6. Migrating action potential complexes (MAPCs): cluster of aborally propulsive migrating contractions.
7. Repetitive bursts of action potentials (RBAPs): occur in response to invasive bacterial enteritis.
8. Functional significance of MAPC, RBAP unknown.
9. Vomiting: preceded by disruption of slow wave frequency and retrograde propagation of giant intestinal contraction from mid SI to antrum, then series of phasic contractions at all gut levels.
10. Functional abdominal pain (FAP): greater frequency of discrete clustered contractions, with abdominal discomfort, than in control subjects. Pain also associated with prolonged high-pressure contractions at ileum (normal interdigestive and postprandial ileal motility).

COLON

1. Transit through colon 10 times slower than through SI (1–3 days). Especially slow at ascending and sigmoid colon. Cycles of 3–6 contractions/min occur independent of small bowel MMCs—appear to have role in fecal continence.
2. Contractions in oral direction more frequent at cecum and ascending colon.
3. Sigmoid colon specialized to obstruct flow of feces, greater frequency of retrograde peristaltic activity.
4. At transverse, descending colon, colonic MMCs usually in aboral but occasionally orad direction.
5. Mass movement: giant migrating contractions. More common during waking hours. Occur only 1–2 times a day, often before defecation. Gastrocolic reflex: sensation not isolated to stomach, motility not limited to colon.

6. Defecation: In infant: reflex response. In older child, adult: controlled act. Rectum can accommodate gradual increase in volume, but rapid rectal distention elicits sensation of rectal fullness, contraction of the external anal sphincter (EAS), puborectal muscle and relaxation of the internal anal sphincter (IAS). EAS response mediated through spinal reflex (absent in patients with low spinal injury), relaxation of IAS mediated by enteric nervous plexus.
7. Currarino triad: associated with a triad of anorectal malformation, sacral bony abnormality, and presacral mass.

INTESTINAL PSEUDO-OBSTRUCTION

1. Clinical syndrome characterized by GI obstruction in absence of mechanical blockage.
2. Most common cause: transient postoperative ileus (Table 1). After surgery, contractile activity returns to stomach in 3–4 h, to SI 5–7 h, to proximal colon in 1–2 d, distal colon 2–3 d. Colon most affected with delayed transit 6–7 d.
3. Absence of ICC identified in chronic constipation, intestinal pseudo-obstruction, hypertrophic pyloric stenosis, inflammatory bowel disease, diabetes dysmotility, and paraneoplastic syndrome. Unknown if causative or secondary phenomenon.
4. Myopathy manifests as reduction of amplitude of contractions while preserving normal temporal and spatial coordination.
5. Neuropathy manifests as disordered motility, producing uncoordinated GI contractions with normal amplitude (Figure 2).

TABLE 1   CAUSES OF ACUTE OR TRANSIENT INTESTINAL PSEUDO-OBSTRUCTION

1. Unrelieved mechanical obstruction
2. Postoperative ileus
3. Drug toxicity
   a. Anticholinergic agents
   b. Phenothiazines
   c. Tricyclic antidepressants
   d. Narcotics
   e. Verapamil
   f. Cyclosporine
   g. Clonidine
   h. Ganglionic blockers
   i. Antiparkinsonian medications (benztropine, trihexyphenidyl)
4. Electrolyte imbalance
   a. Hypokalemia
5. Post-traumatic shock
   a. Fracture of femur or pelvis
   b. CNS or spinal cord injury
6. Intra-abdominal inflammation (eg, cholecystitis, pancreatitis, appendicitis, urinary tract infection)
7. Extra-abdominal inflammation (eg, septicemia, pneumonia, meningitis)
8. Miscellaneous causes
   a. Irradiation
   b. Chemotherapy
   c. Congestive heart failure, myocardial infarction

CNS = central nervous system.

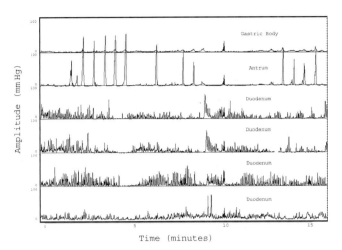

FIGURE 2 Fasting antroduodenal manometry in visceral neuropathy: contraction amplitudes are normal, but motility is disorganized, and normal patterns are absent.

QUESTIONS

MATCH THE FOLLOWING TO THEIR CHARACTERISTICS:
a. Interstitial cells of Cajal
b. Meissner plexus
c. Auerbach plexus
d. Small intestine
e. Colon

1. Between circular and longitudinal muscle layers
2. Taeniae longitudinal muscle
3. Pacemaker cells of the gut
4. Continuous longitudinal muscle layer
5. Submucosal location

MULTIPLE CHOICE:
6. The following are true about the migrating motor complex (MMC), except:
   a. There are 4 phases
   b. Cycles last about 100 min
   c. All originate from the lower esophageal sphincter
   d. The MMC travels from the lower esophageal sphincter to the ileocolic junction
   e. Feeding interrupts the MMC

7. What is the most common cause of transient intestinal pseudo-obstruction?
   a. Postoperative ileus
   b. Electrolyte imbalance
   c. Mechanical obstruction
   d. Post-traumatic shock
   e. Intra-abdominal inflammation (eg, cholecystitis, pancreatitis, appendicitis, urinary tract infection)

8. Currarino triad includes all of the following except:
   a. Hirschsprung disease
   b. Anorectal malformation
   c. Sacral bony abnormality
   d. Presacral mass
   e. None of the above

TRUE OR FALSE:
9. All migrating contractions travel in a caudal direction.
10. Functional abdominal pain or irritable bowel syndrome is associated with motility abnormalities.
11. Giant migrating contractions are provoked by opiates.
12. The enteric nervous system is primarily derived from sacral neural crest cells.
13. Gastroesophageal reflux is caused by low tone at the lower esophageal sphincter

CHOOSE THE BEST ANSWER:
14. Specializations in smooth muscles allowing for prolonged contractions include all of the following except:
    a. Increased mitochondria
    b. More smooth endoplasmic reticulum
    c. Prolonged cycling of myosin cross-bridges
    d. Reduced number of peroxisomes
    e. All of the above are specializations allowing prolonged contraction

---

BILE FORMATION AND CHOLESTASIS

SYNOPSIS

BILE
1. Secretion is key means by which liver controls cholesterol balance, toxin excretion, and lipid- or fat-soluble vitamin digestion and absorption in the gut.
2. Composed of bile acids, cholesterol, phospholipids, heavy metals, and detoxified metabolites. Bile acids and phospholipids combine in 1:2 ratio in bile to make mixed micelles, which allow excretion of cholesterol.
3. Biliary proteins: albumin, immunoglobulin M, G, and A, and hepatocellular enzymes such as alkaline phosphatase and γ-glutamyltransferase (GGT) (Figure 1).
4. Bile is major excretory route for copper, iron, manganese, and zinc.

BILE FLOW
1. Anatomic: hepatocytes are polarized cells with basolateral (contact with portal blood for secretion and uptake) and apical surfaces (excretion).
2. Bile acid–dependent bile flow increases as the bile acid pool expands. Osmotic diffusion of water and electrolytes or bicarbonate into bile is determined by the concentration of bile acids and bile acid flux. Bile acids unincorporated into micelles have stronger osmotic properties, resulting in higher bile flow rates (such as ursodeoxycholate) (Figure 2).
3. Solutes pass from basolateral to apical surface by a variety of methods: binding proteins, diffusion, and trafficking along cytoskeleton.
4. Newly formed bile flows from pericentral region, toward periportal hepatocytes and into bile ductules of portal triads.

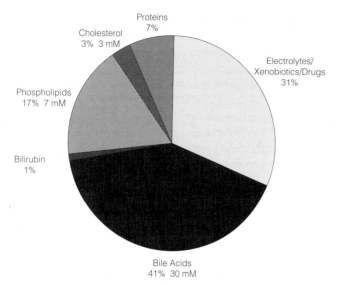

Proteins 7%
Cholesterol 3% 3 mM
Phospholipids 17% 7 mM
Bilirubin 1%
Electrolytes/Xenobiotics/Drugs 31%
Bile Acids 41% 30 mM

FIGURE 1 Human bile composition. Bile is predominantly water, with only 3 to 5% of its weight determined by solid solutes. Bile acids are the major solute of bile, and their micelle partners, cholesterol and phospholipids, contribute significantly to the solute composition as well. Xenobiotics, electrolytes, and proteins make up over a third of the biliary solute load, whereas conjugated bilirubin is the smallest component. Adapted from Vlahcevic ZR, Heuman DM, Hylemon PB. Physiology and pathophysiology of enterohepatic circulation of bile acids. In: Zakim D, Boyer J, editors. Hepatology: a textbook of liver disease. 3rd ed. Philadelphia: WB Saunders; 1996. p. 381.

5. As bile flows through biliary tree, it is modified by secretions of cholangiocytes.
6. Bile is stored in gallbladder until meal activates duodenal release of cholecystokinin, causing gallbladder contraction.
7. Normal adult liver secretes 600–800 cc bile/d.

BILE ACID ENTEROHEPATIC CIRCULATION
1. Bile acids pass through small intestine where modified by bacteria (dehydroxylation and deconjugation), then

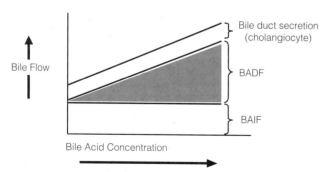

Bile Flow
Bile duct secretion (cholangiocyte)
BADF
BAIF
Bile Acid Concentration

FIGURE 2 Bile flow determinants. Bile flow is primarily bile acid dependent (BADF) in humans, increasing as the bile acid pool size expands. Bile acid–independent flow (BAIF) remains relatively constant and is determined by glutathione, glutathione conjugates, and bicarbonate, among other solutes. Cholangiocytes secrete water and bicarbonate into bile and can contribute up to 40% of total bile flow, depending on the state of feeding.

are almost entirely reabsorbed in the terminal ileum and transported back to the liver via the portal vein.
2. Occurs 8–10 times/d, twice at each meal.
3. Highly efficient: loss of only 5% of circulating bile acids/d (this loss compensated by hepatic bile acid synthesis to maintain bile acid pool).
4. Less efficient in infants and small children than in adults.

CANALICULAR MEMBRANE TRANSPORTERS
1. Bile salt export pump: primary adenosine triphosphate (ATP)–dependent transporter responsible for bile acid export into bile. Mutations associated with progressive familial intrahepatic cholestasis (PFIC2): clinical syndrome of progressive intrahepatic cholestasis and cirrhosis liver failure, pruritus, low GGT levels, normal serum cholesterol, and coarse appearance of canalicular bile on electron microscopy.
2. Multidrug resistance protein 2 (MDR2): responsible for the majority of bile salt–independent bile flow. Mutations lead to reduced bile acid independent flow and Dubin-Johnson syndrome.
3. Multidrug resistance protein 3 (MDR3): responsible for phospholipids secretion into bile. Mutations result in PFIC3, with elevated GGT with biliary tree damage. Cholestasis of pregnancy identified in heterozygous carriers of MDR3 mutations. Possible role in gallstone formation.
4. Familial intrahepatic cholestasis 1 (FIC1): mutations associated with PFIC1. Mutations result in reduction of hydrophobic bile salts in bile. Patients with benign recurrent intrahepatic cholestatis (BRIC) have FIC1 mutations. BRIC patients have normal liver function, life expectancy with intermittent jaundice, and pruritus.
5. ABCG5 and ABCG8: ATP-binding cassette proteins that are biliary cholesterol transporters. When mutated, produce accumulated serum plant sterols (sitosterolemia) and cholesterol gallstones.

TOTAL PARENTERAL NUTRITION–ASSOCIATED CHOLESTASIS
1. Contributing factors: total parenteral nutrition components, hydrophobic bile acids, prematurity, sepsis, and poor bowel function.
2. Molecular explanation unclear.

SEPSIS-ASSOCIATED CHOLESTASIS
1. Basolateral transporters are down-regulated in sepsis.
2. Leads to decreased import of bile acids from systemic circulation into the hepatocyte and into bile.
3. Bile flow is reduced, leading to cholestasis and conjugated hyperbilirubinemia.
4. With treatment of infection, cholestasis typically resolves.

DISORDERS OF BILE ACID SYNTHESIS
1. Atypical and hepatotoxic bile acids accumulate in the liver, leading to cholestasis, liver dysfunction, and end-stage liver failure if not treated.

2. Cholestasis results from decrease in primary bile acids that stimulate bile flow.

CYSTIC FIBROSIS
1. Cholangiocytes lining the bile ducts secrete chloride and water into bile via the cystic fibrosis transmembrane regulator transporter.
2. Found on luminal side of cholangiocytes.
3. Thick viscous secretions result in cholestasis secondary to bile duct plugs: cause obstruction, focal biliary fibrosis, and focal biliary cirrhosis.

QUESTIONS

TRUE OR FALSE:
1. Bile flow is primarily dependent on bile acid flow.
2. Bile acid–independent bile flow increases in response to cholecystokinin.
3. The apical surface of hepatocytes is in contact with portal blood.
4. Bile acid enterohepatic circulation results in the loss of 15% of circulating bile acids each day.

MATCH THE FOLLOWING AFFECTED PROTEINS TO THE CORRESPONDING DISEASE (MAY BE MORE THAN ONE):
a. PFIC1
b. PFIC2
c. PFIC3
d. BRIC
e. Dubin-Johnson syndrome
f. Sitosterolemia
g. Cholestasis of pregnancy

5. Bile salt export pump
6. Multidrug resistance protein 2
7. Multidrug resistance protein 3
8. Familial intrahepatic cholestasis 1
9. ABCG5

NORMAL HEPATOCYTE FUNCTION AND MECHANISMS OF DYSFUNCTION

SYNOPSIS

LIVER
1. Largest organ in the body, weighs 2–2.5% of total body weight.
2. Hepatocytes make up 60% of total liver cells. Other 40% are Kupffer cells, lymphocytes, endothelial cells, and stellate cells (fat storage or Ito cells, which store vitamin A).
3. At basolateral membrane, hepatocytes exchange metabolites with blood.
4. At apical membrane, hepatocytes secrete bile, waste products, cholesterol, and phospholipids.

5. Two models of hepatic organization (Figure 1):
   a. Lobules: have central vein, portal area (hepatic arteriole, portal venule, bile ductule, nerves, and lymphatics), and liver plates.
   b. Acinus: arranged around axis with hepatic arteriole, portal venule, and bile ductule. Zone 1 hepatocytes are periportal, receive blood rich in oxygen and nutrients, and specialize in oxidative metabolism. Zone 3 hepatocytes receive blood lower in nutrients and oxygen and detoxify drugs.
6. Blood flow: liver is the first organ to receive the nutrient-enriched blood from the gut. 80% of liver blood supply from the portal vein (intestines).
7. Hepatocyte carbohydrate metabolism: ability to fast relies on ability of hepatocytes to store glycogen and synthesize glucose from amino acids, glycerol, and glycogen degradation. Glucose entry or exit from hepatocytes occurs via glucose transporter 2.
8. Hepatocyte protein metabolism: all proteins in plasma except the immunoglobulin G are synthesized by hepatocytes. Most prominent is albumin. Other than factor VIII, all of the coagulation factors are synthesized in the liver (factors II, VII, IX, and X dependent on vitamin K).
9. Hepatocytes are the main cells responsible for deamination of amino acids in their conversion into energy or for synthesis of carbohydrates (CHO) and lipids.
10. Hepatocytes: responsible for converting ammonia into urea for excretion by kidneys.
11. Hepatocyte lipid metabolism: fatty acid oxidation, synthesis of cholesterol, phospholipids, lipoproteins, lipids from excess CHO and proteins. Triacylglycerol (TAG) broken down in liver into glycerol and 3 fatty

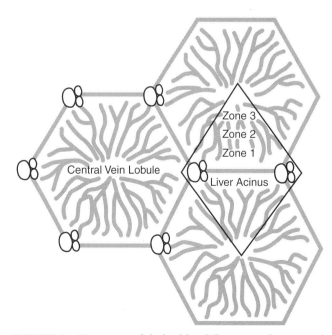

FIGURE 1 Hepatocyte lobule: blood flow goes from portal triads toward the central vein. Bile is collected in the opposite direction into the portal ducts. Sinusoids and hepatic cords are arranged as trabeculae between portal and central vein areas.

acid molecules, then broken down into acetyl coenzyme A, converted to acetoacetate (ketone), and transported to other parts of the body. Uptake of cholesterol and lipoproteins via specific receptors.

12. Liver stores large amounts of vitamins including vitamins A, D, B_{12}. Hepatocytes contain large amounts of apoferritin. When excess iron available, combines with apoferritin to form ferritin.

13. Liver excretes calcium via bile.

14. Many drugs metabolized and excreted by the liver, as well as hormones (eg, thyroxine, estrogen, and cortisol).

LIVER REGENERATION

1. Growth factors: hepatic growth factor, epidermal growth factor, and transforming growth factor-α.

2. Highest concentrations of liver-related growth factors are seen during acute liver failure and after major hepatic resection.

APOPTOSIS

1. Common pathway of cell death during liver disease.

2. Plays a role in various hepatic diseases: ischemia–reperfusion, viral hepatitis, autoimmune hepatitis, toxic injury.

3. Fas ligand (FasL) binding of Fas receptor mediates cell death.

4. Ursodeoxycholate has antiapoptotic actions.

5. Other proapoptosis molecules: caspase-8, Bid, and caspase-3, -6, -7, and -9.

6. Bcl-2: inhibits apoptosis in the liver.

QUESTIONS

TRUE OR FALSE:

1. The liver comprises up to 2.5% of total body weight.

2. Hepatocytes comprise 85% of the liver.

3. Eighty percent of the liver's blood flow is derived from the hepatic artery.

CHOOSE THE BEST ANSWER:

4. The liver does all of the following except:
   a. Synthesize glucose
   b. Produce immunoglobulins
   c. Synthesize most of the coagulation factors
   d. Metabolize and excrete thyroxine
   e. Is the major organ of fatty acid oxidation

5. The following molecules lead to apoptosis in the liver except:
   a. FasL
   b. Caspase-8
   c. Caspase-9
   d. Bid
   e. Bcl-2

MATCH THE TERMS TO THEIR LOCATIONS:

6. Liver lobule
7. Liver acinus

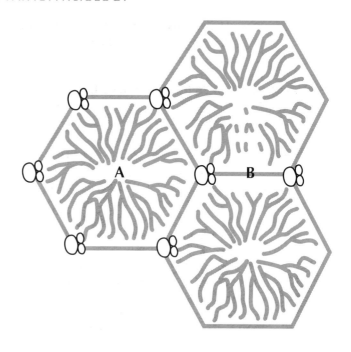

DRUG-INDUCED BOWEL INJURY

SYNOPSIS

PILL ESOPHAGITIS

1. Swallowed tablet or capsule lodges in esophagus and releases contents: concentrations of active ingredients can be very high and cause damage to the mucosa.

2. Incidence: 1/10,000 per yr.

3. Risk factors: swallowing without water, supine position, larger pills, gelatinous capsules, and certain sustained release formulations. Patients with esophageal functional or anatomic abnormalities that delay esophageal emptying considered at risk.

4. Most frequent medications (90% of cases): antibiotics, potassium chloride, nonsteroidal anti-inflammatory drugs (NSAIDs), and quinidine. Also alendronate and pamidronate.

5. Symptoms: acute-onset retrosternal pain, continuous or worsened by swallowing (dysphagia). Long-standing injury can lead to stricture or hemorrhage.

6. Endoscopic diagnosis.

7. Symptoms usually subside with discontinuation of drug therapy. May require total parenteral nutrition (TPN) or surgery.

CHEMOTHERAPY-INDUCED ORAL AND ESOPHAGEAL MUCOSITIS

1. Anticancer drugs affect tissue turnover, resulting in ulceration and inflammation throughout the gastrointestinal (GI) system. Oral lesions accompany esophageal changes.

2. Causative agents: methotrexate, vinca alkaloids, dactinomycin, doxorubicin, bleomycin, cytosine arabinoside, and 5-fluorouracil (5-FU).

3. Treatment supportive. Uncomplicated lesions usually heal within 2 wks. In methotrexate dosing, can be prevented via folinic acid rescue.

NSAID-INDUCED GASTRODUODENAL ULCER

1. NSAIDs (nonselective): most common cause of drug-induced mucosal injury of stomach and duodenum.
2. Mechanism: inhibition of cyclooxygenase (COX) in GI mucosa, reducing mucosa-protective prostaglandins.
3. Risk factors: advanced age, history of ulcer, use of concurrent corticosteroids, higher NSAID doses, multiple NSAID use, anticoagulant use, and serious systemic disorder.
4. Rank order of NSAIDs: low-risk: ibuprofen and diclofenac; high risk: ketoprofen and azapropazone. Data not standardized by equivalent dosing.
5. COX-2 inhibitors: beneficial in adult studies in minimizing risk of mucosal damage.
6. Pharmacologic approaches to counteract ulcerogenic effects: misoprostol, proton pump inhibitors (PPIs), and H_2 receptor antagonists.
7. *Helicobacter pylori* infection and NSAID use: major and independent risk factors for gastroduodenal mucosal injury.

PROSTAGLANDIN E_1-INDUCED ANTRAL HYPERPLASIA

1. Antral mucosal hyperplasia without evidence of pyloric stenosis: reported in neonates with congenital heart disease receiving prostaglandin E_1 (PGE_1) to continue patency of the ductus arteriosus.
2. Patients receiving the drug > 120 h may be at greater risk. May improve with drug withdrawal. Surgery may be necessary.

ERYTHROMYCIN-INDUCED INFANTILE HYPERTROPHIC PYLORIC STENOSIS

1. Systemic erythromycin within the first 2 weeks of life: 7–10-fold increased risk of pyloric stenosis.
2. Mechanism not understood. Possible association with maternal use of erythromycin late in pregnancy or in lactation period. No other macrolide associations.

NEUTROPENIC ENTEROCOLITIS: TYPHLITIS AND ILEOCECAL SYNDROME

1. Severe inflammation leading to bowel necrosis can be seen in cecum, ascending colon, terminal ileum of leukemia patients receiving chemotherapy.
2. Symptoms: pain at right lower quadrant abdomen, fever, diarrhea with or without blood, and nausea or vomiting. May lead to intestinal perforation, peritonitis, or sepsis.
3. Treatment: similar as for other forms of necrotizing enterocolitis; antibiotics, antifungals, NPO status, surgical resection as needed, or nutritional support (ie, TPN).

CHEMOTHERAPY-INDUCED INTESTINAL MUCOSITIS

1. Most common agent: methotrexate.
2. Symptoms: abdominal pain, diarrhea, vomiting, melena, and protein-losing enteropathy.

DRUG-INDUCED INTESTINAL HYPOMOTILITY

1. Intestinal motility reduced by drugs with anticholinergic properties.
2. Vincristine damages nerve tissues: leads to adynamic ileus (usually within 2–3 d of therapy); worse if receiving itraconazole concomitantly.

DEXAMETHASONE-INDUCED INTESTINAL PERFORATION IN PREMATURE INFANTS

1. Perforation: at small bowel.
2. Concurrent use of indomethacin: increased risk.

ANTIBIOTIC-ASSOCIATED DIARRHEA

1. Antibiotics responsible for one-quarter of cases of drug-induced diarrhea. 70–80% unrelated to *Clostridium difficile*. Subsides with discontinuation.
2. *C. difficile* infection: a nosocomial illness; causes 20% of antibiotic-associated diarrhea. Usually occurs 4–18 d after first dose of offending agent. Changes in normal gut flora, acquisition and colonization of bacteria, and toxin production.
3. Most common antibiotics: ampicillin, amoxicillin, cephalosporins, lincomycin, and clindamycin. 60% of neonates and infants asymptomatically colonized by *C. difficile*.
4. Pseudomembranous enterocolitis mainly affects large intestine, rarely small intestine. *C. difficile* is most common cause, often induced by preceding antibiotic therapy. Other causes: ischemia, verotoxin-producing *Escherichia coli*, and drugs such as chlorpropamide, gold, and NSAIDs.
5. Symptoms of *C. difficile* infections: profuse watery or mucoid diarrhea with or without blood, abdominal pain, and fever.
6. Treatment: mild cases: supportive care and antibiotic cessation; severe symptoms: therapy with oral metronidazole or vancomycin for 1–2 weeks. Relapse in 40–60%: additional metronidazole or vancomycin or probiotics.

NSAID-INDUCED INTESTINAL INJURY

1. Small intestinal and colonic lesions: small intestinal perforation associated with slow-release NSAIDs well documented in adults. Preterm neonates more susceptible to adverse effects of NSAIDs, especially perforation.
2. Strictures at small intestine and colon: in adults after prolonged NSAID use. Multiple thin, web-like diaphragms pathognomonic in adults.

NSAID ENTEROPATHY

1. Disturbance of small intestinal function: associated with NSAID use in absence of macroscopic pathology; pathogenesis unknown.
2. Clinical scenarios: iron-deficiency anemia, protein-losing enteropathy, and mild lipid malabsorption. Fecal calprotectin may be used as a diagnostic test (high in this condition).

COLITIS

1. Chronic use (> 6 mo) of NSAIDs (eg, mefenamic and flufenamic acids) may cause colitis.
2. Mechanism unknown.

QUESTIONS

MATCH THE DRUG WITH THE ASSOCIATED BOWEL INJURY:

a. Bowel perforation
b. Antral hyperplasia
c. Pill esophagitis
d. Adynamic ileus
e. Colitis
f. *Clostridium difficile* infection
g. Mucositis
h. Infantile hypertrophic pyloric stenosis
i. Multiple thin, web-like diaphragms in the intestine

1. Erythromycin
2. Prostaglandin E_1
3. Methotrexate
4. Dexamethasone
5. Amoxicillin
6. Potassium chloride
7. Vincristine
8. Mefenamic acid
9. NSAIDs
10. Alendronate
11. Cephalosporins

RADIATION ENTERITIS

GASTROINTESTINAL DAMAGE FROM RADIATION EXPOSURE

1. Significant factor: phase of cell cycle. Sensitivity to radiation therapy most pronounced in mitotic and G2 phases. Resistance most pronounced in synthesis phase.
2. Phases of cell cycle:
   a. G1: brief period after mitosis without deoxyribonucleic acid (DNA) synthesis
   b. S: DNA synthesis
   c. G2: no DNA synthesis
   d. Mitosis: cell division
3. Tissue perfusion modifies radiation sensitivity. Hypoxic cells are particularly resistant to radiation therapy.
4. Radiation most severe in rapidly dividing cells: enterocytes, hematopoietic, and tumor cells.
5. Replacement of cells: 4–6 d for small intestine, colon, and rectum. Earliest impact of radiation on gut occurs in crypts where cells dividing most rapidly.
6. Accepted radiation dose unit: 1 Gy (100 rad).

RADIATION THERAPY SIDE EFFECTS

1. Initially: capillary endothelial swelling, capillary leakage, lymphatic leakage, and edema.
2. Recovery phase: vascular or connective tissue changes; can progress to obliterative endoarteritis and endophlebitis leading to intestinal ischemia, ulcerations, and necrosis. Strictures caused by progressive fibrosis.

PATHOPHYSIOLOGY

1. E-selectin and intercellular adhesion molecule 1 (ICAM-1) involved in mediating leukocyte sequestration in irradiated bowel. Nuclear factor κ-B implicated in inducing transcription of E-selectin and ICAM-1 in irradiated endothelium. Platelet adherence to vascular wall and abnormal endothelial cell proliferation lead to occlusion.
2. Up-regulation of CD31 on endothelial cells plays role in platelet adherence.
3. Transmembrane glycoprotein thrombomodulin located on luminal surface of endothelial cells is important in maintaining thrombohemorrhagic balance. Radiation causes local thrombomodulin deficiency.
4. Matrix metalloproteinases (MMPs)-2 and -9 increased after radiation therapy in human rectal mucosa. MMPs regulate equilibrium between extracellular matrix synthesis, and breakdown.
5. Immediately after radiation less inducible nitric oxide; tissue less responsive to exogenous 5-hydroxytryptamine (5-HT). Radiation-induced apoptosis: increased *TP53*. *BCL2* is protective especially at colon, while *BCLW* is protective at small intestine.
6. After radiation, increased transforming growth factor (TGF)-β-1, which is a fibrogenic and proinflammatory cytokine.
7. Fibroblast growth factors enhance survival of epithelial cells after radiation induction.

EFFECTS OF RADIATION ON MOTILITY

Radiation of gut does not affect normal migrating motor complexes. Storage function of irradiated gut is decreased.

MICROSCOPIC ABNORMALITIES IN RADIATION-DAMAGED BOWEL

1. Reduced mitotic activity followed by a reduction in villus size; presence of apoptotic cells at crypts; hyperemia, edema, and inflammatory infiltration.
2. On electron microscopy: reduced microvilli, disrupted tight junctions, and dilated endoplasmic reticulum.
3. Late effects: subintimal fibrosis, vascular changes, ischemic bowel, infarction, atrophy, and fibrosis.

CLINICAL FINDINGS IN CHILDREN

1. Acute enteritis: vomiting, diarrhea, weight loss, and intestinal hemorrhage (rare).
2. Chronic enteritis: bowel obstruction (complete or partial), vomiting, diarrhea, abdominal pain, and abdominal distention.
3. Late effects of enteritis: bowel obstruction (complete or partial) and esophageal obstruction (dysphagia, vomiting, or substernal pain).

MECHANISMS

1. Acute radiation enteritis: interruption of enterocyte replacement; villous atrophy, disaccharidase deficiency, steatorrhea, and occasional mucosal ulceration.
2. Chronic radiation enteritis: mainly vascular obliteration, obliterative endoarteritis and endophlebitis, intestinal

ischemia, diffuse chronic mucosal inflammation, villous atrophy, progressive fibrosis, secondary disaccharidase deficiency, protein losing enteropathy, and small bowel bacterial overgrowth (SBBO) and vitamin B_{12} deficiency.

3. Late effects of radiation: degeneration of vessel walls, subintimal fibrosis, ischemic bowel with infarction, submucosal and muscular atrophy or fibrosis, ongoing perivascular inflammation, and stricture or small bowel obstruction.

FACTORS INFLUENCING OCCURRENCE AND SEVERITY

1. Dose and fractionation.
2. Tumor size and extent.
3. Volume of normal bowel treated.
4. Concomitant chemotherapy.
5. Radiation intracavitary implants.
6. Individual patient variables: prior abdominal or pelvic surgery, hypertension, diabetes mellitus, pelvic inflammatory disease, and inadequate nutrition; can decrease vascular flow to the bowel wall and impair bowel motility, increasing the chance of radiation injury.
7. Higher daily and total dose delivered to normal bowel and greater volume of normal bowel treated, the greater the risk of radiation enteritis.

ACUTE RADIATION ENTERITIS

1. Early clinical symptoms: within 8 weeks considered acute. Diarrhea, sometimes bloody; occasional nausea, vomiting, and abdominal pain. Can resemble acute ulcerative colitis. Thoracic radiation can cause acute radiation esophagitis: mild substernal burning to dysphagia.
2. Diagnosis: no investigation for minor symptoms, unless reduction in dose considered. Endoscopy: see histology. Hydrogen breath testing can detect disaccharide intolerance, but many patients receive antibiotics, which negates usefulness of test.
3. Treatment: usually self-limited: resolves without nutritional support. For severe symptoms, radiation therapy must be stopped or decreased, or intervals must be increased. Symptoms usually abate 2 weeks after cessation. If lactose-intolerant, decrease lactose. Nausea or emesis: 5-HT3 antagonist, which may also inhibit serotonin-mediated small intestine (SI) dysmotility. Nausea, vomiting, and diarrhea: nonsteroidal anti-inflammatory drugs (NSAIDs); cholestyramine can improve diarrhea in adults after pelvic radiation. Severe symptoms: elemental feeds or total parenteral nutrition (TPN). Severe rectal bleeding: laser therapy. Radiation proctitis: rectal sucralfate enemas. Hemorrhagic gastrointestinal lesions: argon plasma coagulation.
4. Prophylaxis: place prone for pelvis radiation therapy to decrease exposure to SI if possible. In adults, elemental diet or TPN can diminish diarrhea and improve nitrogen balance during acute phase. NSAIDs given prophylactically may ameliorate acute radiation enteritis.

CHRONIC RADIATION ENTERITIS

1. Background: 11% of children develop delayed intestinal syndrome with vomiting or diarrhea and distended abdomen. Intestinal lesions (adhesions, fibrosis) usually appear up to 6 mo after completion of radiation therapy. In delayed damage, bowel involvement almost always more extensive than suspected. Development of acute radiation enteritis does not predict those patients who will ultimately develop chronic radiation damage. Patients with no clinical history of acute symptoms may present years later (up to 20 y) with chronic radiation intestinal damage.
2. Predisposing factors for injury: dose, previous abdominal surgery, thin body habitus, elderly age, female sex, vascular disease, and chemotherapy.
3. Diagnosis: radiograph to detect strictures and dilatation, but involvement cannot be localized radiologically. Isotope labeling of white blood cells to detect inflammation or abscesses. Endoscopy rarely helpful (areas out of reach). Fecal fat studies for malabsorption. Shilling test to assess vitamin B_{12} absorption. D-xylose breath test to detect SBBO. Occasional arteriography to show arterial stenosis after radiation.
4. Treatment: supportive. Obstruction: surgery. Diet for children: gluten-free, lactose-free, and low in fiber and fat. Undernourished: low-fat diet with medium-chain triglycerides, essential fatty acids, and pancreatic enzyme supplements; fat-soluble vitamins if malabsorption. Enteritis of terminal ileum and watery diarrhea: cholestyramine. SBBO: antibiotics. SI inflammation or proctocolitis: sulfasalazine with prednisone; antiinflammatory agents, and short-chain fatty acid enemas. Severe bleeding: trace by endoscopy and treat locally.

VERY LATE EFFECTS

1. Usually 6 m to 5 yr after radiation, but up to 29 yr afterwards. Frequency depends on dose delivered.
2. Enteritis fibrosis without inflammatory infiltrate common in late radiation. Diffuse fibrosis of muscularis propria and submucosa can present with stenosis.
3. Villous atrophy.
4. Secondary malignancies rare.

QUESTIONS

CHOOSE THE BEST ANSWER:

1. The radiation-sensitive phases of the cell cycle are:
   a. G1.
   b. S.
   c. G2.
   d. Mitosis.

2. The following are treatments for radiation enteritis except:
   a. Nonsteroidal antiinflammatory drugs.
   b. 5-HT3 antagonist.
   c. Gluten-free diet.
   d. Rectal sucralfate enemas.
   e. Diet low in fiber and fat.
   f. All of the above are used to treat radiation enteritis.

3. When do clinical signs of acute radiation enteritis begin?
   a. Immediately after initial radiation.
   b. After 1–2 weeks.
   c. After 1 month.
   d. At 1–2 months.
   e. All of the above.

4. The following affect the risk of developing radiation enteritis except:
   a. Gender.
   b. Tumor size and extent.
   c. Concomitant chemotherapy.
   d. History of abdominal surgery.
   e. Nutritional status.
   f. All of the above affect the risk of developing radiation enteritis.

TRUE OR FALSE:

5. Hypoxic cells are radiation-resistant.
6. Chronic radiation enteritis can occur years later and in the absence of a history of acute radiation enteritis.

ANSWERS

MOTILITY DISORDERS
1. c.
2. e.
3. a.
4. d.
5. b.
6. c.
7. a.
8. a.
9. False.
10. True.
11. True.
12. False. Vagal.
13. False. Primarily secondary to transient lower esophageal sphincter relaxation.
14. d.

BILE FORMATION AND CHOLESTASIS
1. True.
2. False.
3. False. The basolateral surface is in contact.
4. False. 5%.
5. b.
6. e.
7. c and g.
8. a and d.
9. f.

NORMAL HEPATOCYTE FUNCTION AND MECHANISMS OF DYSFUNCTION
1. True.
2. False. 60%.
3. False. Portal vein.
4. b.
5. e. Bcl-2 inhibits apoptosis.
6. a.
7. b.

DRUG-INDUCED BOWEL INJURY
1. h.
2. b.
3. g.
4. a.
5. f.
6. c.
7. d.
8. e.
9. i.
10. c.
11. f.

RADIATION ENTERITIS
1. c, d.
2. f.
3. e. Symptoms of acute enteritis occur within 8 weeks.
4. f.
5. True.
6. True.

CLINICAL PRESENTATION OF DISEASE

ACUTE DIARRHEA

SYNOPSIS

DEFINITION
Abrupt onset of increased stool fluid output > 10 cc/kg/d.

TABLE 1　　KNOWN CAUSES OF ACUTE DIARRHEA

INFECTIONS
Enteric infections, extraintestinal infections

DRUG-INDUCED
Antibiotic-associated, other drugs

FOOD ALLERGIES
Cow's milk protein allergy, soy protein allergy, multiple food allergies

DISORDERS OF DIGESTIVE OR ABSORPTIVE PROCESSES
Sucrase-isomaltase deficiency, late-onset hypolactasia

VITAMIN DEFICIENCIES
Niacin deficiency

INGESTION OF HEAVY METALS
Copper, tin, zinc

NORMAL PHYSIOLOGY
1. Small intestine (SI) absorbs large quantities of sodium, Cl, and HCO_3. Secretes H^+ ions and lesser amounts HCO_3 and Cl. Water passively follows the net transport of solutes.
2. Absorption occurs in mature epithelial cells lining middle and upper villi. Secretion occurs at crypts predominantly. Absorption occurs normally in excess of secretion with a net gain of water and electrolytes.

TABLE 2　　MAIN CAUSES OF ACUTE INFECTIOUS DIARRHEA

PATHOGEN IN DEVELOPED COUNTRIES	APPROXIMATE FREQUENCIES IN CASES OF SPORADIC DIARRHEA (%)
VIRUSES	
Rotavirus	25–40
Calicivirus	1–20
Norwalk-like virus	10
Astrovirus	4–9
Enteric-type adenovirus	2–4
BACTERIA	
Campylobacter jejuni	6–8
Salmonella	3–7
Escherichia coli	3–5
Enterotoxigenic	
Enteropathogenic	
Enteroaggregative	
Enteroinvasive	
Enterohemorragic	
Diffusely adherent	
Shigella	0–3
Yersinia enterocolitica	1–2
Clostridium difficile	0–2
Vibrio parahaemolyticus	0–1
Vibrio cholerae 01	Unknown
Vibrio cholerae non-01	Unknown
Aeromonas hydrophila	0–2
PARASITES	
Cryptosporidium	1–3
Giardia lamblia	1–3

ELECTROLYTE TRANSPORT
1. Entry of glucose and several amino acids coupled with Na (Figure 1). *SLC5A1* couples entry of glucose and galactose across brush border to Na. Dipeptide absorption not directly coupled to Na absorption.

TABLE 3　　ENDOGENOUS REGULATORS OF INTESTINAL WATER AND ELECTROLYTE TRANSPORT

SOURCE	STIMULATE ABSORPTION	STIMULATE SECRETION
Mucosal epithelial cells	Somatostatin	Serotonin Gastrin cholecystokinin Neurotensin Guanylin Nitric oxide
Lamina propria cells	?	Arachidonic acid metabolites Nitric oxide Several cytokines Bradykinin
Enteric neurons	Norepinephrine Neuropeptide Y	Acetylcholine Serotonin Vasoactive intestinal polypeptide Nitric oxide Substance P Purinergic agonists
Blood	Epinephrine Corticosteroids Mineralocorticosteroids	Vasoactive intestinal polypeptide Calcitonin Prostaglandins Atrial natriuretic peptide

2. Main transport of Na (with Cl also) occurs throughout the gastrointestinal (GI) tract, especially at SI. Mediated by 2 coupled antiports Na$^+$/H$^+$ cation exchanger (maintains intracellular pH) and Cl$^-$/HCO$_3$ anion exchanger. This is the transport process most responsible for intestinal Na and water absorption in the absence of intraluminal nutrients.

3. Cl and HCO$_3$ major anions secreted into gut, usually in crypts. Passive diffusion of cation (usually Na$^+$) and water follow.

PATHOGENESIS

1. In most acute-onset diarrhea, both secretory and osmotic mechanisms coexist (Table 4 and Figure 2).

2. *Vibrio cholerae* toxin loosens tight junctions between SI enterocytes, leading to fluid secretion into the lumen.

3. In rotavirus enteritis, selective invasion of mature enterocytes and serious disruption of absorption. Reduction of absorptive cells in gut unmasks secretion in the crypts and a secretory component is superimposed. Secretory nature augmented by rotavirus enterotoxin NSP4; causes Ca^{++}-dependent transepithelial Cl secretion.

TREATMENT

1. Rehydration.

2. Oral rehydration solution takes advantage of glucose-coupled Na influx in secretory diarrheas. Associated with fewer intravenous infusions, lower stool volume, and less emesis (World Health Organization).

3. Breastfed infants: continued breastfeeding promotes faster recovery and improved nutrition.

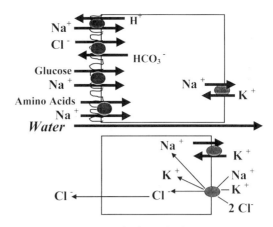

FIGURE 1 Main intestinal absorptive/secretory processes for electrolytes. In the villous cell (*top panel*), Na, K adenosine triphosphatase (ATPase) actively extrudes Na in exchange for K, thus maintaining the low intracellular Na concentration, which allows the "downhill" entry of the ionic pair Na-Cl and of the Na-coupled nutrients such as glucose and amino acids. It can also be seen that the entry of the ionic pair Na-Cl is in reality, across most of the intestinal tract, the result of a double antiport, Na being exchanged with H and Cl with HCO$_3$. In the crypt cell (*bottom panel*), the low Na cell concentration maintained by Na, K ATPase builds a Na gradient between the extracellular compartment and the cell. Energized by this gradient, a carrier in the basolateral membrane (lower part of the figure) couples the flow of one Na, two Cl, and one K from the serosal compartment into the crypt cell. As a result, Cl accumulates above its electrochemical equilibrium and under physiologic circumstances leaks into the lumen across a semipermeable apical membrane. Because absorptive activity in the villous cell quantitatively far exceeds the minor secretion from the crypts (as suggested in the figure by the arrows' sizes), the net result is absorption of electrolytes and nutrients. Water absorption then passively follows, mainly through the intercellular tight junctions.

TABLE 4   PATHOGENIC MECHANISMS AND LOCALIZATION OF THE MAIN INTESTINAL PATHOGENS

PREDOMINANT PATHOGENESIS*	SITE OF INFECTION	AGENT	CLINICAL FEATURES
Direct cytopathic effect	Proximal small intestine	*Rotavirus* Enteric-type adenovirus Calicivirus Norwalk-like virus EPEC *Giardia*	Copious watery diarrhea, vomiting, mild to severe dehydration; frequent lactose malabsorption, no hematochezia Course may be severe
Enterotoxigenicity	Small intestine	*Vibrio cholerae* ETEC Enteroaggregative *E. coli* *Klebsiella pneumoniae* *Citrobacter freundii* *Cryptosporidium*	Watery diarrhea (can be copious in cholera or ETEC), but usually mild course; no hematochezia
Invasiveness	Distal ileum and colon	*Salmonella* *Shigella* *Yersinia* *Campylobacter* Enteroinvasive *E. coli* *Amoeba*	Dysentery: very frequent stools, cramps, pain, fever, and often hematochezia with white blood cells in stools Variable dehydration Course may be protracted
Cytotoxicity	Colon	*Clostridium difficile* EHEC *Shigella*	Dysentery, abdominal cramps, fever, hematochezia EHEC or *Shigella* may be followed by hemolytic uremic syndrome

EHEC = enterohemorragic *Escherichia coli*; EPEC = enteropathogenic *Escherichia coli*; ETEC = enterotoxigenic *Escherichia coli*.
*Elaboration of various types of enterotoxins affecting ion transport has been demonstrated as an additional virulence factor for almost all of the bacterial pathogens.

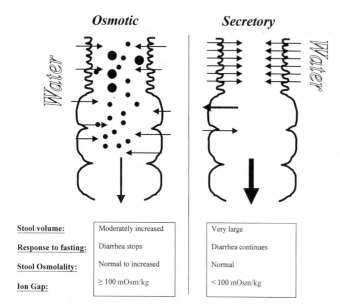

	Osmotic	**Secretory**
Stool volume:	Moderately increased	Very large
Response to fasting:	Diarrhea stops	Diarrhea continues
Stool Osmolality:	Normal to increased	Normal
Ion Gap:	≥ 100 mOsm/kg	< 100 mOsm/kg

FIGURE 2 Scheme of osmotic and secretory diarrhea. The left panel shows the situation in osmotically induced diarrhea. Undigested or unabsorbed substrates remain in the gut lumen and exert an osmotic force proportional to their concentration that drives fluid into the lumen. In the case of unabsorbed carbohydrates, colonic flora enzymes may partially digest them, thus further contributing to the osmotic load and water flow into the lumen. Secretory diarrhea (right panel) is characterized by a state of active secretion of anions by the enterocytes. In vivo, equivalent amounts of cations also passively follow, and the result is net secretion of water and electrolytes. The role of the colon varies according to the cause of the secretion. Ion Gap = Stool Osmolality − 2 × [Na$^+$ + K$^+$]

4. Formula-fed infants: rapid refeeding after oral rehydration therapy in first 4–6 hr well tolerated in > 3-month-old infants. Lactose intolerance not major problem in developed countries: 3%. If fecal pH decreases and > 0.5 to 1% reducing substances, lactose intolerance likely. Switch to soy.
5. Consider zinc in malnourished children with diarrhea (20 mg/d).
6. *Lactobacillus GG* or probiotics.

QUESTIONS

CHOOSE THE BEST ANSWER:
1. Acute diarrhea is defined as stool output greater than:
    a. 5 cc/kg/d
    b. 10 cc/kg/d
    c. 15 cc/kg/d
    d. 20 cc/kg/d
    e. 25 cc/kg/d

2. The main mechanism of sodium absorption in the intestine:
    a. Occurs at the intestinal crypt.
    b. Occurs throughout the gastrointestinal tract.
    c. Is not mediated by the Na$^+$/H$^+$ cation exchanger.
    d. Is not mediated by the Cl$^-$/HCO$_3$ anion exchanger.
    e. None of the above.

TRUE OR FALSE:
3. Secretion occurs at the tip of intestinal villi.
4. Dipeptide absorption is directly correlated with sodium absorption.
5. The main site of sodium absorption in the gut occurs at the colon.
6. In most forms of acute diarrhea, either a secretory or osmotic mechanism exists.
7. Breastfed infants should stop breastfeeding when they have acute diarrhea.
8. In secretory diarrhea, the ion gap is ≥ 100 mOsm/kg.

MATCH THE ENDOGENOUS REGULATOR WITH THE ACTION:
a. Secretion
b. Absorption
c. Neither
d. Both

9. Somatostatin
10. Serotonin
11. Corticosteroids
12. Nitric oxide
13. Neuropeptide Y

PERSISTENT DIARRHEA

SYNOPSIS

PERSISTENT DIARRHEA
1. Definition: episode that begins acutely and lasts for at least 14 days (World Health Organization).
2. Epidemiology: average prevalence in Asia, Latin America, and Africa is 10%.
3. Pathophysiology: osmotic diarrhea caused by nonabsorbed nutrients in the gastrointestinal (GI) tract associated with intestinal damage. Occurs when digestion or absorption impaired. Can have secretory component.

RISK FACTORS
1. Malnutrition: caloric, protein, and micronutrients (vitamin A, zinc).
2. Associated illness: pneumonia, urinary tract infection, anemia.
3. Prior illnesses: for example, measles.
4. Increased risk if not breastfed.
5. Decreased cell-mediated immunity: human immunodeficiency virus (HIV).

INTRACTABLE DIARRHEA SYNDROME
Heterogeneous conditions: extreme severity of persistent diarrhea. Result of a permanent defect in structure or function of intestine leading to progressive intestinal failure including structural enterocyte defects, immune-based disorders, multiple food intolerance, motility disorders, and short gut (Table 1 and Figure 1).

TABLE 1　　CAUSES OF PERSISTENT DIARRHEA

Infections
　　Bacterial: *Shigella, Salmonella, Yersinia enterocolitica, Escherichia coli, Clostridium difficile, Campylobacter jejuni, Vibrio cholerae, Mycobacterium avium* complex
　　Viral: rotavirus, adenovirus, astrovirus, torovirus, cytomegalovirus, HIV
　　Parasitic: *Cryptosporidium, Giardia, Entamoeba histolytica, Isospora, Strongyloides*
　　Postenteritis syndrome
　　Small bowel overgrowth
　　Tropical sprue
Diarrhea associated with exogenous substances: excessive intake of carbonated fluid, dietetic foods containing sorbitol, mannitol, or xylitol; excessive intake of antacids or laxatives containing lactulose or $Mg(OH)_2$; excessive intake of methylxanthine-containing drinks (cola, tea, coffee)
Abnormal digestive processes: cystic fibrosis, Shwachman-Diamond syndrome, isolated pancreatic enzyme pancreatitis, chronic pancreatitis, Pearson syndrome; trypsin/chymotrypsin, enterokinase deficiency
Disorders of bile acids: chronic cholestasis, use of bile acid sequestrants, primary bile acid malabsorption, terminal ileum resection
Carbohydrate malabsorption: congenital or acquired sucrase-isomaltase deficiency, congenital or acquired lactase deficiency, glucose-galactose malabsorption, fructose malabsorption
Immune-based disorders: food allergy, celiac disease, eosinophilic gastroenteritis, inflammatory bowel disease, autoimmune enteropathy, primary immunodeficiencies
Structural defects: microvillous inclusion disease, tufting enteropathy, phenotypic diarrhea, heparan-sulfate deficiency, $\alpha_2\beta_1$ and $\alpha_6\beta_4$ integrin deficiency, lymphangiectasia
Defects in electrolyte and metabolite transport: congenital chloride diarrhea, congenital sodium diarrhea, acrodermatitis enteropathica, selective folate deficiency, abetalipoproteinemia
Motility disorders: Hirschsprung disease, intestinal pseudo-obstruction (neurogenic and myophatic), thyrotoxicosis
Surgical causes: congenital or acquired short bowel (secondary to stenosis, segmental atresia, malrotation)
Neoplastic diseases: neuroendocrine hormone-producing tumors: VIPoma, APUDomas, mastocytosis

APUDoma = amineprecursor uptake and decarboxylation tumor; HIV = human immunodeficiency virus; VIPoma = vasoactive intestinal peptide-producing tumor.

1.　Electrolyte transport defects: congenital chloride diarrhea (mutation in *SLC26A3* gene): severe intestinal chloride malabsorption owing to defect in Cl/HCO_3 exchanger; congenital sodium diarrhea: secondary to defective Na/H exchanger.

2.　Structural enterocyte defects: microvillus inclusion disease, tufting enteropathy (abnormal laminin and heparin sulfate proteoglycan and integrins), and congenital heparin sulfate deficiency (severe enteric albumin loss in first weeks of life) result in net reduction of absorptive surface.

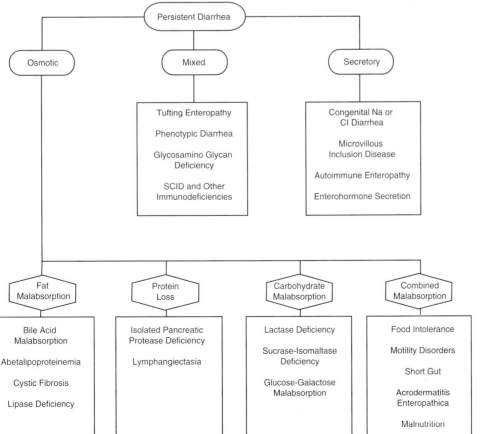

FIGURE 1 Scheme of specific etiologies of persistent diarrhea according to its pathophysiology. Assessment of the secretory, osmotic, or mixed mechanism of diarrhea and of predominant nutrient malabsorption may help identify the primary etiology, thereby directing the diagnostic workup through specific investigations. SCID = severe combined immunodeficiency.

3. Immune defects: phenotypic diarrhea characterized by immunodeficiency, facial abnormalities, woolly hair, and intractable diarrhea. Autoimmune disease as marked by the presence of antienterocyte immunoglobulin and cell mediated autoimmune response. Abnormal immune function: agammaglobulinemia, immunoglobulin A deficiency, acquired immunodeficiency syndrome, and combined immunodeficiency disorders can result in persistent diarrhea.
4. Allergy: cow's milk protein or multiple food allergies.
5. Motility disorders: including Hirschsprung disease, aganglionosis, and chronic intestinal pseudo-obstruction.
6. Short-gut syndrome: residual intestine insufficiency to carry on normal function. Small bowel bacterial overgrowth may be mechanism in diarrhea (blind loop).
7. Mitochondrial disease: GI symptoms may be initial manifestation.
8. Munchausen syndrome by proxy.

THERAPY
1. Rehydration.
2. Nutritional rehabilitation.
3. Treatment for infection.
4. Probiotics.
5. Proabsorptive agents: enkephalinase inhibitor racecadotril.
6. Antisecretory agents: somatostatin analogues.
7. Loperamide and chlorpromazine (but major side effects).
8. Growth hormone: trophic factor in short gut but also inhibits chloride secretion and promotes Na absorption.
9. Immunosuppression for autoimmune disease.

QUESTIONS

CHOOSE THE BEST ANSWER:
1. Persistent diarrhea is defined by diarrhea lasting more than:
   a. 1 week.
   b. 2 weeks.
   c. 10 days.
   d. 1 month.

2. The lowest prevalence of persistent diarrhea is:
   a. Latin America.
   b. Africa.
   c. Asia.
   d. North America.
   e. None of the above.

3. The following contribute to the persistent diarrhea of short gut syndrome:
   a. Lack of adequate absorptive surface area.
   b. Inadequate intestinal function.
   c. Poor motility.
   d. Small bowel bacterial overgrowth.
   e. All of the above.

TRUE OR FALSE:
4. Breastfeeding is associated with an increased risk of persistent diarrhea.
5. Measles is associated with an increased risk of persistent diarrhea.

PROTEIN-LOSING ENTEROPATHY

SYNOPSIS

BACKGROUND
Albumin is synthesized in the liver at a rate of 120–200 mg/kg/d in a normal adult—higher in first year of life. One-third of the body's albumin is intravascular. Exchangeable pool = 6–8 g/kg < 1 yr; 3–4 g/kg in older child. Malnutrition can decrease exchangeable pool to one-third normal size. 6–10% albumin degraded in 24-h period. Losses provoke moderate but limited increase in liver synthesis.

STUDY METHODS
a) Radiolabeled albumin used to measure gastrointestinal (GI) losses. Scintigraphy with technetium 99m-labeled albumin used to see site of protein loss in GI tract.
b) α-1 Antitrypsin (A1AT): not actively secreted, absorbed, or digested by GI tract. Concentration of stool A1AT correlates well with GI disorders. Spot samples agree with more prolonged collections. A1AT degraded at pH < 3, so does not account for gastric loss. Gross hematochezia alters results. Synthesis and secretion of A1AT may increase in response to inflammation.

CONGENITAL LYMPHANGIECTASIA (MILROY'S DISEASE)

PRIMARY INTESTINAL LYMPHANGIECTASIA
Diffuse or localized ectasia of the enteric lymphatics.
1. Onset: anytime in infancy or childhood: congenital lymphangiectasia (Milroy Disease).
2. Symptoms: GI: intermittent diarrhea or steatorrhea, nausea or vomiting, and abdominal pain (occasional). Chylous ascites may develop. Lymphedema may precede GI involvement. Reduced levels of immunoglobulin, lymphopenia, but not particularly susceptible to infections. Possible tetany with hypocalcemia.
3. Associations: Noonan syndrome, Klippel-Trénaunay-Weber syndrome.
4. Laboratory tests: low albumin, immunoglobulins, and lymphopenia; hypocalcemia may be present.
5. X-ray: barium may show thickened jejunal folds. Lymphoscintigraphy or lymphoangiography of Tc-99m colloid useful (scintigraphy more so).
6. Scattered white plaques seen on endoscopy (patients on high-fat diet).
7. Treatment: medium-chain triglycerides (MCT)–rich, low-fat, high-protein diet (usually permanently). Some

spontaneous remissions do occur. Some patients require calcium and water-soluble form of fat-soluble vitamin supplementation. Low γ-globulin levels do not need to be treated since antibodies will be generated. If refractory and localized, resection may be helpful. Total parenteral nutrition, antiplasmin, and octreotide helpful in some.

SECONDARY INTESTINAL LYMPHANGIECTASIA

Lymphatic obstruction, elevated lymphatic pressure.
1. Differential diagnosis: cardiac lesions (congestive heart failure or pericarditis) or status post Fontan procedure; inflammatory processes that cause retroperitoneal lymph node enlargement or fibrosis leading to mesenteric lymphatic obstruction; chemotherapy may directly damage lymphatic structures.
2. Treatment: steroids and heparin.

MÉNÉTRIER DISEASE

Marked protein-losing gastropathy with enlarged gastric folds at fundus and body stomach. Some cases associated with *Cytomegalovirus*.
1. Onset: age < 10 yr.
2. Abrupt presentation: vomiting, peripheral edema, and abdominal pain.
3. Laboratory tests: mild normochromic, normocytic anemia, eosinophilia, and hypoalbuminemia.
4. Diagnosis: excessive protein loss on ^{51}Cr albumin excretion. Upper gastrointestinal series shows thickened gastric folds in fundus and body with antral sparing.
5. Differential diagnosis: eosinophilic gastroenteropathy: usually involves the antrum with distinctive histology; gastric lymphomas and Zollinger-Ellison syndrome: very rare in childhood.
6. Prognosis: self-limited without recurrence or sequelae.
7. Treatment: if chronic, acid suppression, octreotide, or gastrectomy.

INFECTIONS AND SMALL BOWEL BACTERIAL OVERGROWTH

Protein loss may be extensive during *Salmonella*, *Shigella*, *Giardia* and other parasite, and *Clostridium difficile* infections or during small bowel bacterial overgrowth. *Helicobacter pylori* gastritis associated with excessive gastric protein loss.

OTHER ASSOCIATED CONDITIONS

1. Eosinophilic gastroenteritis and cow's milk or soy protein allergy.
2. Celiac disease.
3. Necrotizing enterocolitis.
4. Graft-versus-host disease.
5. Inflammatory bowel disease: fecal A1AT correlates with disease severity and small intestinal involvement but not with Crohn disease activity index.
6. Common variable immunodeficiency.
7. Vasculitic disorders: collagen vascular disease or Schönlein-Henoch purpura.
8. Cobalamin C deficiency.
9. Carbohydrate-deficient glycoprotein syndromes.

QUESTIONS

CHOOSE THE BEST ANSWER:
1. A 2-year-old male presents with recent onset of peripheral edema, nausea, vomiting, and intermittent diarrhea. Further investigations reveal an albumin of 2.0 g/dL. Barium study reveals thickened small intestinal folds. What should you do next?
   a. Put the patient on a low-fat diet and schedule an upper endoscopy.
   b. Put the patient on a high-fat diet and schedule an upper endoscopy.
   c. Put the patient on a low-fat diet and schedule a lower endoscopy.
   d. Put the patient on a high-fat diet and schedule a lower endoscopy.

2. Endoscopy of the above patient reveals scattered white plaques, and biopsies reveal dilated lacteals. Treatment for this condition will involve all of the following except:
   a. A low-fat diet.
   b. An MCT-rich diet.
   c. A high-protein diet.
   d. γ-globulin infusions.
   e. Calcium supplementation.

3. In which of the following protein-losing enteropathies would fecal α-1 antitrypsin (A1AT) not be reliable?
   a. Milroy disease.
   b. Small bowel bacterial overgrowth.
   c. Primary intestinal lymphangiectasia.
   d. Secondary intestinal lymphangiectasia.
   e. Ménétrier disease.

VOMITING

SYNOPSIS

VOMITING: TWO MEDULLARY CENTERS

1. Chemoreceptor trigger zone (CTZ): also known as area postrema, located on floor of fourth ventricle; contains specific receptors for many neuroactive compounds that cause vomiting.
2. Central vomiting center.

SOMATOMOTOR EVENTS OF VOMITING

1. Diaphragm descends.
2. Inspiratory muscles contract versus closed glottis.
3. Esophagus dilates in response to negative intrathoracic pressure.
4. Stomach remains atonic, filled with refluxate from small intestine.
5. Abdominal muscle contractions compress the stomach, forcing gastric contents into the fundus and lower esophagus.

VOMITING SYNDROMES

REGURGITATION

Effortless regurgitation: secondary to spontaneous relaxation of lower esophageal sphincter.

CYCLIC VOMITING SYNDROME

1. Symptoms: Recurrent episodes of nausea and vomiting without identifiable organic cause. Rapid onset, usually during sleep or early morning. Children may vomit many times per hour, rarely persist > 72 h. Episodes are separated by symptom-free intervals. Family history of migraine in 47% first-degree relatives, irritable bowel syndrome in 62%.
2. Differential diagnosis: urea cycle defects, organic acid metabolism disorders, motility disorders, central nervous system lesions, familial dysautonomia, obstructive uropathy, obstructive cholangiopathy, familial pancreatitis, intestinal malrotation or duplication, intestinal strictures, adrenal insufficiency, diabetes, sinusitis, and porphyria.
3. Workup:
   a. Tests with highest yield are endoscopy (43%), sinus films (38%), and small bowel radiography (28%).
   b. Blood glucose, electrolytes, liver and pancreatic enzymes, NH$_3$, lactic acid, urinary organic acids, carnitine, δ-aminolevulinic acid, and porphobilinogen. Best performed during episodes to maximize chance of detecting intermittent (eg, disorder of fatty acid oxidation) or heterozygous (eg, partial ornithine transcarbamoylase deficiency) disorder.
   c. Surgical disorders best detected by small bowel radiography (6%), abdominal imaging (16%), and cranial imaging (17%).
   d. Evaluation for stress or psychiatric disease.
4. Treatment: propranolol, dilantin, and antihistamines (cyproheptadine) used prophylactically. Migraine drugs effective in treating attacks. Nasogastric (NG) suction and intravenous fluids (IVF) helpful in some patients. Stress management is important.

RUMINATION

1. Symptoms: frequent regurgitation of previously ingested food into the mouth; no accompanying nausea, retching, or forceful expulsion.
2. Most often presents in mentally retarded children.
3. Felt to be a form of self-stimulation with results of increased personal attention. Setting of neglect should raise suspicion of rumination.
4. Treatment: If untreated, may result in life-threatening inanition. Except in infants with reflux and in bulimia, the symptom often responds to increased personal attention and mild negative reinforcement.

BULIMIA

1. Symptoms: eating disorder characterized by recurrent episodes of bingeing and purging. Commonly affects adolescent females and adult females (10%). Patients have persistent anxiety over body shape and weight. Patients are often from dysfunctional families with enmeshment with over-controlling parents. Depression is common.
2. Complications: malnutrition, electrolyte imbalance, esophageal erosion or bleeding, dental erosion, dehydration; hyperamylasemia secondary to salivary gland stimulation.
3. Treatment: psychotherapy and antidepressants.

SUPERIOR MESENTERIC ARTERY SYNDROME

1. Point of obstruction: third part of duodenum, where duodenum sweeps anteriorly over spine at L2 posterior to superior mesenteric artery.
2. Usually occurs in older children.
3. Predisposing factors: rapid linear growth without weight, scoliosis, spinal surgery, weight loss, supine position, body cast, bed confinement, and high ligament of Treitz.
4. Symptoms: mild abdominal pain, anorexia, nausea, voluminous, and infrequent bilious vomiting.
5. Abdominal exam may reveal succession splash.
6. Radiograph: may be normal especially after emesis, but may show distended stomach with air or fluid. Upper gastrointestinal (GI) diagnostic.
7. Treatment: NG decompression, and IVF. Remain upright or lie prone or semiprone with left side down. Metoclopramide hydrochloride may help. Nutrition via nasojejunal placement and liquid diet. Rare to require surgery.

OTHER CAUSES

CHEMOTHERAPY

1. CTZ has the most important receptor for intravenous chemotherapy, particularly the dopamine-2 receptor.
2. Antihistamine and anticholinergic agents ineffective. High-dose metoclopramide blocks not only D2 but also 5-HT3 receptors.
3. 5-hydroxytryptamine (5-HT3) receptor antagonists are effective and block receptors in the peripheral ends of vagal afferents in the intestine, reducing the perception of emetic stimuli; fewer extrapyramidal side effects than metoclopramide.

DIAGNOSTIC APPROACH

1. Laboratory tests: complete blood count, electrolytes, blood urea nitrogen, urinalysis, urine culture, stool for occult blood, leukocytes, and parasites. Consider liver function tests, amylase, toxicity screen, pregnancy test, NH$_3$, urine organic acids, urine catecholamines, urinary porphyrins, and electroencephalography.
2. Imaging: consider upper GI series, abdominal ultrasound, and computed tomography or magnetic resonance imaging of head.
3. GI studies: endoscopy (upper) helpful if peptic disease or anatomic abnormality suspected. Manometry may be considered to diagnose motor abnormalities.

TABLE 1   DRUGS

CHEMICAL NAME	EXAMPLE OF AGENT	MECHANISM
Antihistamines		Labyrinthine suppression, possibly via anticholinergic and antihistamine H_2
Anticholinergics	Scopolamine (hyoscine)	Antimuscarinic effect, probably at labyrinth or central pattern generator
Substituted benzamides	Reglan, Tigan, Propulsid	D2 receptor blockade at CTZ and enteric nervous system
5-HT3 receptor antagonists	Zofran, Kytril	Most important at enteric level, possibly at CTZ
Cannabinoids	Marinol	Unknown
Benzodiazepines		Central GABA inhibition
Phenothiazines	Compazine, Phenergan	D2 receptor antagonist at CTZ
Butyrophenones	Haldol, domperidone	D2 receptor blockade at CTZ; D2 receptor blockade at enteric nervous system
Steroids		Unknown

CTZ = chemoreceptor trigger zone; GABA = γ-aminobutyric acid.

QUESTIONS

CHOOSE THE BEST ANSWER:

1. Which central nervous system center is involved in controlling vomiting?
   a. Chemoreceptor trigger zone.
   b. Central vomiting center.
   c. Substantia nigra.
   d. Both a and b.
   e. All of the above.

2. Which of the following are true regarding cyclic vomiting syndrome?
   a. Usually episodes are of gradual onset.
   b. Often episodes persist over 72 hours.
   c. Symptoms are persistent.
   d. Affected persons often have a family history of irritable bowel syndrome.
   e. Episodes usually occur in the evening.

3. Which of the following are false regarding rumination?
   a. It is not accompanied by nausea or retching.
   b. It is characterized by frequent regurgitation of previously ingested food into the mouth.
   c. It is often found in mentally retarded children.
   d. It is thought to have an organic cause.
   e. It is associated with inanition if not treated.

4. Which of the following are false regarding superior mesenteric artery syndrome?
   a. The point of obstruction is at the third portion of the duodenum.
   b. It can be diagnosed on upper gastrointestinal contrast study.
   c. It is seen in the setting of spinal surgery, weight loss, supine positioning, and bed confinement.
   d. It often requires surgical management.
   e. Abdominal examination may reveal succession splash.

5. Where do 5HT-3 receptor antagonists work?
   a. At the central nervous system.
   b. At motility receptors in the intestine.
   c. At vagal afferent receptors in the intestine.
   d. All of the above.
   e. None of the above.

COLIC AND GAS

SYNOPSIS

BEHAVIORAL CHARACTERISTICS

1. Age-dependent: starts at 2 weeks of age. Total daily crying increases for 2 months, declines in third and fourth months. 30% of cases persist into fourth and fifth months.
2. Diurnal: crying clusters in late afternoon and evening.
3. Behavioral: common: crying in prolonged bouts, some resistance to soothing; variable: clenched fists, legs flexed, back arched, flushed face or skin, grimacing, hard and distended abdomen, regurgitation, and passing gas. Paroxysmal: sudden, begin and end without warning.
4. Rule of three: colic if crying > 3 hr/d for > 3 d/wk for > 3 weeks.

ORGANIC DISEASES PRESENTING WITH "COLIC"

1. Strong evidence: cow's milk protein–intolerance, isolated fructose intolerance, maternal drug effects (especially fluoxetine hydrochloride), and anomalous left coronary artery from the pulmonary artery.
2. Moderate evidence: infantile migraine, reflux esophagitis, and "shaken baby."
3. Weak but suggestive evidence: congenital glaucoma, central nervous system abnormalities (Chiari malformation type I), urinary tract infection (weak, not suggestive).
4. Very weak evidence: lactose intolerance.

CONCEPTS

1. Crying and fussing is no different between breastfed and formula-fed infants.
2. Wet diapers not a cause of crying.
3. No evidence for medication effectiveness, except for dicyclomine hydrochloride (antispasmodic anticholinergic with hazardous side effects).
4. Strategy of not responding is ineffective. No negative side effects from responding.
5. Not much evidence for or against role of maternal anxiety. Increased crying not more common in firstborns.

6. Massage therapy or chiropractic therapy is not effective for the treatment of colic.

TREATMENT

1. No safe medication with proven efficacy.
2. Being responsive does not "spoil infant." Physically shaking the infant is *never* appropriate.
3. Diurnal crying patterns and weight gain are common findings of healthiness. Reassure, but let parents know that crying increases in second month.
4. Determine sources of pressure or stress. Watch for caregiver pressures, and need for help.

QUESTIONS

CHOOSE THE BEST ANSWER:

1. Organic diseases that are strongly related to colic like symptoms include all except:
   a. Cow's milk protein intolerance.
   b. Maternal Prozac use.
   c. Central nervous system abnormalities.
   d. Isolated fructose intolerance.
   e. Anomalous pulmonary return.

2. All are true about colic except:
   a. Crying tends to cluster in late afternoon and evening.
   b. Can be associated with weight loss.
   c. Daily crying increases in first 2 months then decreases.
   d. Crying bouts can be resistant to soothing.
   e. Crying can be prolonged.

TRUE OR FALSE:

3. Dicyclomine hydrochloride can be helpful in reducing colic symptoms.
4. It is effective to ignore colic and crying infants to reduce reinforcement of crying episodes.
5. Increased crying is more common in first-born infants.
6. Wet diapers cause colic-type crying.
7. Being too responsive to infants' crying in the first 3 months can lead to increased crying.

ABDOMINAL MASSES

Abdominal masses are outlined in Table 1.

SYNOPSIS

MULTICYSTIC DYSPLASTIC KIDNEY

1. Characteristics: most common form of cystic renal disease in infants; 20% of all urinary tract malformations; usually sporadic, present as asymptomatic flank mass; 15% bilateral. Associated with esophageal atresia, imperforate anus, and tracheoesophageal fistula.
2. Ultrasonography of kidney reveals "grape cluster pattern."

3. Treatment: removal of affected kidney to avoid hypertension, infection, mass effect, and abdominal pain.

AUTOSOMAL RECESSIVE POLYCYSTIC KIDNEY DISEASE

1. Characteristics: bilateral renal enlargement associated with congenital hepatic fibrosis.
2. Four types: mutation in *PKHD1* gene on chromosome 6.
   a. Perinatal (most severe): stillborn, Potter facies, renal agenesis, massive cystic kidneys, and pulmonary hypoplasia.
   b. Neonatal: renal failure in months to years. Hepatic involvement minimal.
   c. Infantile: renal failure later in life. More predisposed to hepatic disease.
   d. Juvenile: renal failure later in life. More predisposed to hepatic disease.

AUTOSOMAL DOMINANT POLYCYSTIC KIDNEY DISEASE

1. Clinical course: variable; 80% with mutations in *PKD1* gene.
2. Extrarenal associated anomalies: endocardial fibroelastosis, intracerebral vascular anomalies, pyloric stenosis, and hepatic fibrosis.

MESOBLASTIC NEPHROMA

1. Characteristics: most common renal tumor in neonatal period; generally benign.
2. Symptoms: massive flank mass with hematuria, hypertension, and vomiting.
3. Treatment: nephrectomy.
4. Prognosis: good.

RENAL VEIN THROMBOSIS

1. Results in infarction of renal parenchyma.
2. Infant or child risk factors: hemoconcentration or dehydration, polycythemia, and low perfusion states. Maternal risk factors: diabetes, toxemia, steroids, thiazide diuretics.
3. Symptoms: palpable flank mass, hematuria, thrombocytopenia, consumptive coagulopathy.
4. Treatment: hydration. Consider anticoagulation. Thrombectomy, if bilateral.

NEONATAL ADRENAL ABSCESS

1. Probably starts with hemorrhage into the adrenal gland.
2. Symptoms: adrenal hemorrhage, shock, abdominal mass, anemia, prolonged jaundice. Can be asymptomatic.
3. Differential diagnosis: lymphatic cyst, neuroblastoma, Wilm tumor, renal duplication, and hydronephrosis.
4. Treatment: percutaneous or surgical drainage.

FETUS IN FETU

1. Characteristics: occurs in 1/500,000 deliveries. Entrapped fetus, usually at upper abdominal retroperitoneal space. Painless mass.
2. Diagnosis: plain X-ray.

TABLE 1   ABDOMINAL MASSES IN INFANTS AND CHILDREN

NEONATES
Retroperitoneal—kidney
  Hydronephrosis
  Multicystic dysplastic kidney
  Autosomal recessive polycystic kidney disease
  Autosomal dominant polycystic kidney disease
  Mesoblastic nephroma
  Renal vein thrombosis
Retroperitoneal—other
  Adrenal abscess
  Fetus in fetu
Pelvic
  Hydrometrocolpos
  Ovarian cyst
Gastrointestinal
  Intestinal duplication, malrotation, obstruction
  Sacrococcygeal teratoma

INFANTS AND CHILDREN
Retroperitoneal
  Wilms tumor
  Neuroblastoma
  Pancreatoblastoma
  Rhabdomyosarcoma
  Lymphoma
  Ewing sarcoma
  Germ cell neoplasm
Liver—benign solid tumors
  Adenoma
  Mesenchymal hamartoma
  Focal nodular hyperplasia
Liver—malignant tumors
  Hepatoblastoma
  Hepatocellular carcinoma
  Germ cell neoplasm
  Angiosarcoma
  Intrahepatic mesenchymal tumor
  Embryonal rhabdomyosarcoma
Liver—vascular lesions
  Capillary hemangioendothelioma
  Solitary cavernous hemangioma

Liver—cystic hepatobiliary disease
  Choledochal cyst
  Caroli disease
  Caroli syndrome
  Congenital cysts
Alimentary tract
  Stomach
    Carcinoma
    Leiomyosarcoma
    Rhabdomyosarcoma
    Myosarcoma
    Fibrosarcoma
  Small bowel
    Anomalies: duplication, Meckel, malrotation
    Lymphoma
  Colon
    Fecal mass
    Adenocarcinoma
Omentum and mesentery
  Cysts
  Mesenteric fibromatosis
  Inflammatory pseudotumor
  Liposarcoma
  Leiomyosarcoma
  Fibrosarcoma
  Mesothelioma
  Metastatic tumor

ADOLESCENTS
Retroperitoneal
  Renal cell carcinoma
Pelvic
  Hematocolpos
  Ovarian cyst
  Teratoma
  Germ cell tumor
  Choriocarcinoma
  Gonadoblastoma
  Embryonal carcinoma
Liver
  Hepatocellular carcinoma

HYDROMETROCOLPOS

1. Symptoms: mass in lower midline of abdomen.
2. Associations: Bardet-Biedl syndrome, Kaufman-McKusick syndrome, and oral–facial–digital syndromes.
3. Cause: imperforate hymen is most common, then vaginal or cervical stenosis.
4. Treatment: surgical.

INTESTINAL DUPLICATION

1. Most common site: terminal ileum. Located on mesenteric border of adjoining bowel. Lined with intestinal or gastric mucosa.
2. Symptoms: intestinal obstruction or volvulus, perforation, and hemorrhage; intussusception rare.
3. Diagnostic: ultrasound is the best initial exam. Contrast radiology and Meckel scan can be used.

SACROCOCCYGEAL TERATOMA

1. Characteristics: most common neoplastic abdominal mass in neonate. Obvious at birth.
2. Majority benign, but delay in diagnosis associated with malignant transformation.
3. Treatment: surgical resection.

WILM TUMOR

1. Embryonal renal neoplasm. Most common childhood abdominal cancer.
2. Typical patient: 4 years old with asymptomatic abdominal mass.
3. Associations: aniridia, hemihypertrophy, genitourinary anomalies, neurofibromatosis, Beckwith-Wiedemann syndrome, hypospadias, cryptorchidism, gonadal dysgenesis, and duplication of renal collecting system.
4. Microscopic hematuria after minimal abdominal trauma should raise suspicion of Wilm tumor.
5. Treatment: surgery, chemotherapy, and radiation therapy.

NEUROBLASTOMA

1. Neural crest cell malignancy arising within adrenal medulla or sympathetic ganglia. Many with deletions at chromosome 1.
2. Characteristics: most common solid tumor of infancy; 60–75% arise in abdomen; ratio of boys to girls 2:1; 50–75% with advanced disease at presentation.
3. Symptoms: variable; immobile abdominal mass, fever, weight loss, failure to thrive, abdominal pain,

anemia, opsoclonus-myoclonus syndrome, and Horner syndrome.
4. Associations: Beckwith-Wiedemann syndrome, Hirschsprung disease, fetal alcohol syndrome, Waardenburg syndrome.
5. Tumor may secrete vasoactive intestinal peptide; catecholamine (vanilyllmandelic acid) in urine.
6. Treatment: based on stage. Local disease treated with tumor excision.
7. Prognosis: if < 1 yr old with no remote disease, best survival. Thoracic lesion and mature histology associated with good survival. Elevated lactate dehydrogenase, ferritin, or neuron-specific enolase: poor survival.

PANCREATOBLASTOMA
1. Rare pancreatic tumor that generally affects infants and young children.
2. Symptoms: palpable abdominal mass with abdominal pain, anorexia, vomiting, and weight loss; jaundice rare. 50% of cases occur in Asians.
3. Treatment: complete surgical resection.

HEPATIC ADENOMA
1. Benign encapsulated tumors of hepatic epithelium. Seen in women during reproductive years.
2. Symptoms: asymptomatic mass usually, but spontaneous rupture or hemorrhage in 25%.
3. Risk factors: glycogen storage disease (GSD) I and III, familial diabetes, oral contraceptive pills (OCP), androgenic steroids, hereditary tyrosinemia, and adenomatous polyp syndromes.
4. Laboratory tests: liver function tests and α-fetoprotein (AFP) are normal.
5. Ultrasonography: hypo- or hyperechoic lesions can appear like hepatocellular carcinoma. Diagnosis should not be based on imaging alone.
6. Potential malignant transformation if > 5 cm, OCP use, or GSD.
7. Treatment: surgical excision if lesions grow in size, if predilection for spontaneous hemorrhage exists, or if premalignant risk factors present.

MESENCHYMAL HAMARTOMA
1. Developmental anomaly of periportal mesenchyme, with bile ducts, liver cells, and angiomatous components. Benign hepatic tumor.
2. Occurs exclusively in children aged < 2 yr.
3. Symptoms: abdominal distention, respiratory distress secondary to mass effect, or congestive heart failure (CHF) from arteriovenous (AV) shunting; some children asymptomatic.
4. Ultrasonography: cystic mass usually in right lobe.
5. No malignant potential.
6. Treatment: conservative approach.

FOCAL NODULAR HYPERPLASIA
1. Rare, always benign.
2. Usually asymptomatic; acute abdominal pain if torsion. Most common in young women.

3. Computed tomography (CT): Large, homogenous, hypodense mass. Biopsy indicated since overlap with fibrolamellar cancer. Image enhanced with gadolinium.
4. Pathology: medium to large thick-walled muscular vessels contained within fibrous bands. Associated with micronodular cirrhosis.

HEPATOBLASTOMA
1. Arises in otherwise normal liver.
2. Symptoms: median age 16 months. Painless mass in right upper quadrant with weight loss, anorexia, and anemia. Usually not jaundiced.
3. Increased risk: Beckwith-Wiedemann syndrome, Meckel syndrome, diaphragmatic or umbilical hernias, Wilm tumor, fetal alcohol syndrome, familial adenomatous polyposis, and very low birth weight.
4. Laboratory aminotransferase levels normal in two-thirds of cases. Elevated AFP; amount of elevation not related to prognosis.
5. Prognosis: good if tumor confined to one lobe, resectable; poor if vascular invasion or distant metastases.
6. Treatment: surgical resection. Cisplatin and doxorubicin used to reduce tumor size. Orthotopic liver transplantation (OLT) is an option for patients with unresectable tumor despite chemotherapy.

HEPATOCELLULAR CARCINOMA
1. Epithelial neoplasm in older children and adolescents.
2. Symptoms: abdominal pain, fever, anorexia, malaise, and hepatomegaly.
3. Increased risk: chronic hepatitis B, hepatitis C, hemochromatosis, α-1 antitrypsin deficiency, hereditary tyrosinemia, porphyria, GSD, and hypercitrullinemia.
4. In adults, vast majority with cirrhosis. In children with hepatitis B virus (HBV), cirrhosis generally not present.
5. Most children present with advanced disease with metastases.
6. CT: hypodense mass; with intravenous contrast, ring enhancement. Vascular invasion characteristic.
7. Treatment: chemotherapy for unresectable lesions. OLT can be used.
8. Prognosis: unfavorable if large tumor size, HBV positive, nonfibrolamellar histology, local or metastatic spread.

GERM CELL TUMORS
Resection curative.

INTRAHEPATIC MESENCHYMAL TUMORS
Treatment: complete resection. Chemotherapy for extensive tumors.

ANGIOSARCOMA
1. Rare. Usually in girls aged 3–5 yr.
2. Rapidly expanding mass.
3. Treatment: surgery.

EMBRYONAL RHABDOMYOSARCOMA
1. Arise in extrahepatic biliary tree.
2. Prognosis: dismal.

3. Resection seldom possible, chemotherapy is ineffective, and radiation therapy is palliative.

CAPILLARY HEMANGIOENDOTHELIOMA

1. Massive AV connection.
2. Symptoms: high-output CHF and hepatomegaly in infants < 6 mo. Bruit over epigastrium. Can result in Kasabach-Merritt syndrome.
3. Associations: bilateral Wilm tumor, hemihypertrophy, Beckwith-Wiedemann syndrome, and meningomyelocele.
4. Imaging: best characterized using helical CT or magnetic resonance imaging.
5. Natural history: spontaneous resolution.
6. Treatment: medical support with digitalis and diuretics. May require thyroid hormone therapy with increased catabolism of thyroid hormone by hemangioendothelioma. Steroids helpful. Severe cases: antineoplastic drugs, steroids, and interferon. Surgical resection and hepatic artery embolization can be used.

SOLITARY CAVERNOUS HEMANGIONA

1. Localized usually to one lobe (right > left).
2. Risk: rupture with hemoperitoneum.
3. Treatment: surgical excision if localized, steroids, or hepatic artery embolization or ligation.

CHOLEDOCHAL CYST

1. Symptoms: hepatomegaly and palpable mass in 60% of patients. Consider in patients with cholestasis.
2. Risk of malignant transformation: increases with age, 12.5% risk overall.
3. Treatment: surgical excision not fully protective against future development of cancer.
4. Liver transplantation for extensive intrahepatic cysts.

CAROLI DISEASE

1. Characteristics: rare malformation consisting of multifocal nonobstructive dilations of the intrahepatic bile ducts (cystic or saccular); isolated finding (type 1, Caroli disease), or associated with congenital hepatic fibrosis (type 2 Caroli syndrome).
2. Symptoms: fever, abdominal pain, jaundice, and hepatosplenomegaly.
3. Median age onset of symptoms: 5.5 mo. Median age of diagnosis: 12 mo.
4. Congenital renal malformations in 80%, including autosomal recessive polycystic kidney disease (ARPKD) and renal tubular ectasia. In ARPKD, liver disease is diffuse or localized to left lobe.
5. Prognosis: dependent on frequency and severity of cholangitis.

CONGENITAL HEPATIC CYSTS

1. Large and detectable on physical exam.
2. Ultrasonography: diagnostic.
3. Symptoms: usually none, but torsion, hemorrhage, and perforation can bring to acute medical attention.
4. Treatment: depends on size and location; resection or drainage.

OMENTAL AND MESENTERIC CYSTS

1. Soft, thin-walled, freely mobile mass at mesentery near terminal ileum. Consequence of obstructed or ectopic lymphatics.
2. Symptoms: 90% no or minimal symptoms. Vague "pulling" sensation with mild discomfort and fullness. Can also present with crisis: ruptured cyst, obstruction, or volvulus.
3. Diagnosis: ultrasonography and CT.
4. Treatment: resection.
5. Prognosis: recurrences reported.

MESENTERIC FIBROMATOSIS

1. Rare benign intraabdominal tumor; aggressive.
2. Associations: Gardner syndrome, prior trauma, and prolonged estrogen.
3. Symptoms: variable. Abdominal pain, nontender abdominal mass, weight loss, and intestinal obstruction or perforation.
4. Prognosis: spontaneous regression < 20%, greater in congenital cases.
5. Treatment: surgical resection.
6. Prognosis: recurrence not uncommon. Likely to recur if age > 5 yr, incomplete excision, dermoid present on extremity, microscopic evidence of tumor at resection margins, mitotic index $\geq$ 5 per 10 high-power fields, areas of necrosis, or inflammation in tumor.

INFLAMMATORY PSEUDOTUMORS

1. Characteristics: firm, painless, well-circumscribed, and nonencapsulated masses; usually infiltrates surrounding viscera.
2. Associations: Hodgkin disease, Castleman disease, and peptic ulcer disease.
3. No report of malignant change.

OVARIAN CYSTS

1. 85% of cystic ovarian lesions benign. Teratoma is most common cystic lesion. Physiologic follicular cysts occur in 12–14 year olds.
2. If surgery needed: enucleation will preserve ovarian tissue.
3. If solid lesion present on pelvic ultrasound: warning sign of cancer.

RENAL CELL CARCINOMA

1. Mean age 14 yr.
2. Symptoms: flank pain and gross hematuria.
3. Prognosis: 60% survival in patients with complete resection. Resistant to chemotherapy. Poor prognosis with metastatic disease.

QUESTIONS

CHOOSE THE BEST ANSWER:

1. What is the most common renal tumor in the neonatal period?
   a. Renal vein thrombosis.
   b. Multicystic dysplastic kidney.

    c. Mesoblastic nephroma.
    d. Autosomal recessive polycystic kidney disease.
    e. Autosomal dominant polycystic kidney disease.

2. Where is the most common site of intestinal duplication?
    a. Stomach.
    b. Duodenum.
    c. Jejunum.
    d. Ileum.
    e. Colon.

3. Hepatocellular carcinoma is associated with all of the following except:
    a. Hepatitis B chronic infection.
    b. Hemochromatosis.
    c. Porphyria.
    d. α-1 antitrypsin deficiency.
    e. Hepatitis D infection.

4. Mesenteric fibromatosis is associated with all of the following except:
    a. Prior trauma.
    b. Prolonged estrogen exposure.
    c. Prolonged androgen exposure.
    d. Gardner syndrome.

TRUE OR FALSE:

5. Resection of choledochal cysts removes the risk of cholangiocarcinoma.
6. Pancreatoblastomas tend to occur in Asians.
7. Hepatoblastoma prognosis is related to tumor size and histology.

UPPER GASTROINTESTINAL BLEEDING

SYNOPSIS

UPPER GASTROINTESTINAL BLEEDING

1. Uncommon in children: 5% of patients for whom esophagogastroduodenoscopy (EGD) indicated.
2. More common in intensive care unit: 6–25% incidence.

DEFINITIONS

1. Bleeding: above the ligament of Treitz.
2. Hematemesis: frank red blood usually indicates more rapid bleeding than coffee ground emesis.
3. Melena: black, tarry stools (production requires minimum 50–100 cc of blood in stomach); may persist for 3–5 d (cannot be used as indication of ongoing bleeding).

DETERMINATION OF BLOOD

1. Gastroccult: determination of blood in gastric contents; detects hemoglobin.
2. Guaiac testing: guaiac leuko-dye not specific for blood; detects peroxidases.

3. Hemoccult false-positive: red meat, cantaloupes, radishes, turnips, cauliflower, broccoli, and grapes have peroxidase; false-negative: heme nonreactive because of heme degradation to porphyrin by stool bacteria.
4. HemoQuant: false-positive: affected by red meat but not dietary peroxidases or iron. No false negative since the test does report a positive in the presence of porphyrin.

DETERMINATION OF LOCATION

1. Evaluation for other sources: respiratory tract, nose, and oropharynx.
2. Initial laboratory evaluation: complete blood count, prothrombin time and partial thromboplastin time, blood type, and crossmatch. Also liver function tests and blood urea nitrogen (BUN) and creatinine levels. Elevated BUN–creatinine ratio may indicate upper gastrointestinal (GI) bleeding; azotemia may result from intestinal absorption of blood and hypovolemia.
3. Gastric aspiration: bloody aspirate indicates active upper GI bleeding; clear aspirate does not eliminate a duodenal bleeding source.
4. Dermatologic findings: for example, hemangioma and telangiectasias indicates upper GI lesions; caput medusa, spider angiomata, and jaundice indicate liver disease. Cutaneous purpura suggests Schönlein-Henoch purpura.
5. Ulcer: Causes: acid, *Helicobacter pylori*, nasogastric tube, medications, or Schönlein-Henoch purpura. Clean-based ulcer may rebleed < 3%. Flat spots on clean ulcer crater may rebleed < 7%.
6. Mallory-Weiss tear: after vomiting, hiccupping, and cough. In absence of coagulopathy, bleeding is self-limited.
7. Dieulafoy lesion: erosion into unusually large, submucosal artery. Usually present with massive hematemesis or hematochezia. Most cases have lesions at proximal stomach. Treat with epinephrine then thermal modality.
8. Duplication cysts: If cysts contain gastric mucosa, ulcerate and bleed. Antral duplications cause hypergastrinemia.

DIAGNOSTIC MODALITIES

1. Technetium 99m red blood cells scan: sample patient's own blood; label then reinject. Bleeding > 0.1 cc/min is detectable.
2. Angiography: require bleeding rate of > 0.5 cc/min to detect. Good urine output and renal function required.
3. Endoscopy: EGD is preferred method to evaluate the upper GI tract for bleeding. Most bleeding in children stops spontaneously; emergency EGD indicated only when findings will influence clinical decision (Figure 1). EGD contraindicated if patient unstable.
4. Newborn Apt-Downey test: adult hemoglobin denatures to alkaline globin with yellow-brown color when exposed to 1% NaOH; fetal hemoglobin remains pink.

TREATMENT

1. Resuscitation: restoration of hemodynamic stability.
2. Endoscopic therapy: electrocoagulation, laser photocoagulation, argon plasma coagulation, injection of

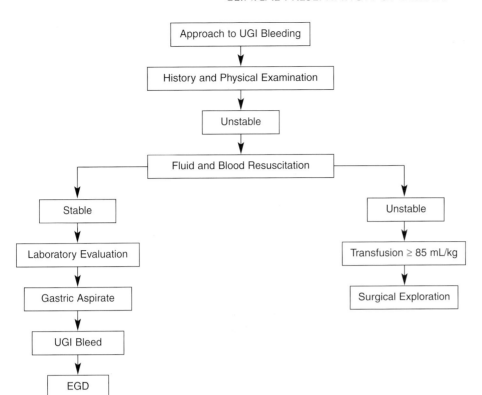

FIGURE 1 If > 50–70 cc/kg blood required over 4–6 h, invasive monitoring should be begun. EGD = esophagogastroduodenoscopy; UGI = upper gastrointestinal.

epinephrine, sclerosants, band ligation, and mechanical clipping. Little published data in children.

3. Endoscopic treatment: For active bleeding, visible vessels, and adherent clots: thermal modality or combined epinephrine and thermal modality; fair outcome. In infants aged < 2 yr: only injection therapy since heater probe will not fit small scope; inject 1–3 mm away from vessel (1/10,000 epinephrine); 4-quadrant injection (0.5–1 cc aliquots). Thermocoagulation: use heater probe or bipolar coagulator; apply tamponade force to bleeding vessel, then energy source to coagulate. For shallow tissue injury, use Bipolar Circumactive Probe.

4. Endoscopic varices: complications of sclerosing are ulceration, perforation, strictures, mediastinitis, and esophageal dysmotility. Banding more effective than sclerosants in eradicating varices and preventing rebleeding; esophagus must accommodate 1 cm scope for band ligation (usually > 1 yr old). Superficial ulceration usually within 1 wk of banding; ulcers may occa-

sionally bleed. First few sessions 2–4 wks apart. Once control established, therapy every 3–6 months until obliterated.

5. Sengstaken-Blakemore tube: serious complications in 20% of cases. Most complications from malpositioning and migration of tube. Excessive pressures carry risk of esophageal ulcer and perforation. Esophageal balloon should be decompressed in 12–24 hr. If fresh bleed again, reinflate and check in 6 hr. Sedate patient for comfort. Suppress cough to prevent sudden increase in abdominal pressure. If bleed stops, deflate esophageal balloon, then deflate gastric balloon in 12–24 hr.

6. Surgery: most common with posterior duodenal ulcer with arterial bleeding, bowel perforation with bleeding, and gastroesophageal varices. Exploratory laparotomy: reserved for uncontrollable bleeding. Portosystemic shunting: for varices. Esophageal transection and devascularization (Sugiura procedure): rare but potentially life-saving for uncontrollable bleeding of esophageal varices.

TABLE 1   ETIOLOGY OF UPPER GI BLEEDING IN CHILDREN BY AGE GROUP IN RELATIVE ORDER OF FREQUENCY

NEWBORN	INFANT	CHILD–ADOLESCENT
Swallowed maternal blood	Stress gastritis or ulcer	Mallory-Weiss tear
Vitamin K deficiency	Acid peptic disease	Acid peptic disease
Stress gastritis or ulcer	Mallory-Weiss tear	Varices
Acid peptic disease	Vascular anomaly	Caustic ingestion
Vascular anomaly	GI duplications	Vasculitis
Coagulopathy	Gastric or esophageal varices	Crohn disease
Milk-protein sensitivity	Duodenal or gastric webs	Bowel obstruction
	Bowel obstruction	Dieulafoy lesion, hemobilia

GI = gastrointestinal.

TABLE 2   MEDICATIONS FOR TREATMENT OF UPPER
GASTROINTESTINAL BLEEDING IN CHILDREN

ACID SUPPRESSION
Antacids
H₂ receptor antagonists
Proton pump inhibitors

VASOCONSTRICTION
Octreotide
Vasopressin

CYTOPROTECTION
Sucralfate
Misoprostol

QUESTIONS

CHOOSE THE BEST ANSWER:

1. A 5-year-old girl presents with a history of bright red
    hematemesis and hypotension following a history of
    recent *Mycoplasma* pneumonia. Total packed red cells
    volume infused is now > 90 cc/kg; patient is stabilized,
    but bright red blood is still coming out of the nasogas-
    tric (NG) tube. What should you do now?
    a. Plan for urgent endoscopy.
    b. Start octreotide.
    c. Consult surgery.
    d. Cold water lavage via NG tube.
    e. Start vasopressors

2. What is the minimum volume of blood loss required
    for angiography detection of gastrointestinal bleed?
    a. 0.1 cc/min.
    b. 0.3 cc/min.
    c. 0.5 cc/min.
    d. 0.7 cc/min.
    e. 1 cc/min.

3. If a newborn has swallowed maternal blood, what is
    the expected result of the Apt-Downey test?
    a. Yellow-brown color of solution after NaOH mixing.
    b. Pink color of solution after NaOH mixing.
    c. Blue color of solution after NaOH mixing.
    d. No change in color of solution after NaOH mixing.
    e. None of the above.

4. Which of the following is NOT associated with a false-
    positive Hemoccult test?
    a. Recent ingestion of red meat.
    b. Cantaloupes.
    c. Grapes.
    d. Iron.
    e. Radishes.

5. Where are most Dieulafoy lesions located?
    a. Esophagus.
    b. Stomach.
    c. Duodenal bulb.
    d. Small intestine.
    e. Oropharynx.

LOWER GASTROINTESTINAL BLEEDING

SYNOPSIS

LOWER GASTROINTESTINAL BLEEDING
Definition: bleeding with an origin distal to the ligament
of Treitz.

PRESENTATIONS
1. Hematochezia: bright red blood per rectum.
2. Melena: passage per rectum of black, tarry, foul-
    smelling stools (source of bleed usually proximal to
    ileocecal valve).
3. Occult gastrointestinal (GI) bleeding: with discovery
    of iron deficiency or anemia or by testing for presence
    of fecal blood
4. Symptoms of severe blood loss without objective
    bleeding.

ESSENTIAL ASSESSMENTS
1. Is it blood? Determine by fecal occult blood testing.
    False positive: ingestion of red meat or peroxidase
    containing fruits or vegetables (tomato, cherry, turnip,
    broccoli, radish, cantaloupe, and cauliflower). False
    negative: large doses of vitamin C, dry stool sample,
    outdated reagents, or prior conversion of hemoglobin
    to porphyrin by intestinal microbiota.
2. Is it blood from the child? Rule out maternal origin in
    an otherwise healthy baby (Apt-Downey test).
3. Is it blood from the GI tract? Possible epistaxis,
    nasopharyngeal lesions, menarche, or hematuria.
4. Is it blood from the lower GI tract? Nasogastric tube
    placement and aspiration can be used to differentiate
    upper from lower GI tract bleeding.
5. Assess hemodynamic status: vital signs, capillary refill.
6. Laboratory tests: complete blood count (cbc), clotting
    studies, routine chemistry, blood typing, and cross-
    matching.
7. Age: important for determining etiology of bleeding;
    different causes in different age groups.

CHARACTERISTICS AND SYMPTOMS
1. Hematochezia limited to outside of stools suggests an
    anal or rectal origin.
2. Hematochezia mixed through the stool suggests
    colonic source. If hematochezia mixed with mucus,
    loose stools suggests colitis.
3. Maroon-colored stools suggest vigorous hemorrhage
    from distal small bowel.
4. Currant jelly stools may indicate ischemic bowel lesions.
5. In general, the more proximal the hemorrhage is
    located in the GI tract, the darker the stool.

DIAGNOSTIC INVESTIGATIONS
1. Laboatory tests: cbc, clotting studies, routine
    chemistries. Hypereosinophilia suggests allergy. Iron
    deficiency anemia suggests history of chronic blood

TABLE 1   PRINCIPAL CAUSES OF LOWER GASTROINTESTINAL BLEEDING IN RELATION TO AGE

NEWBORN (BIRTH–1 MO)	INFANT (1 MO–2 YR)	PRESCHOOL AGE (2–5 YR)	SCHOOL AGE (> 5 YR)
Necrotizing enterocolitis	Anal fissure	Anal fissure	Anal fissure
Malrotation with volvulus	Infectious colitis	Infectious colitis	Infectious colitis
Allergic proctocolitis	Allergic proctocolitis	Polyp	Polyp
Hirschsprung disease enterocolitis	Intussusception	Meckel diverticulum	Henoch-Schönlein purpura
Hemorrhagic disease of the newborn	Meckel diverticulum	Henoch-Schönlein purpura	Inflammatory bowel disease
	Lymphonodular hyperplasia	Hemolytic uremic syndrome	
	Malrotation with volvulus	Lymphonodular hyperplasia	
	Hirschsprung disease enterocolitis		
	Intestinal duplication.		

loss. Inflammatory disorder or infectious colitis: erythrocyte sedimentation rates or C-reactive protein may be useful. Ratio of blood urea nitrogen to creatinine can help localize bleed, with a high ratio indicating an upper GI bleed. Bloody diarrhea: stool culture and viral, ova, parasite, and *Clostridium difficile* examination should be performed.

2. Radiology: abdominal radiograph can rule out obstruction or pneumoperitoneum. Ultrasonography can rule out intussusception.

3. Endoscopy: to find cause of lower GI bleed (colonoscopy). Rule out infection prior to endoscopy. Contraindicated in children with suspected intestinal obstruction or ischemia, fulminant colitis, toxic megacolon, suspected perforation or peritonitis, pneumatosis intestinalis, or suspected intussusception. Enteroscopy can be used to evaluate the small bowel. Capsule endoscopy allows for evaluation of obscure GI bleeding origin in the small bowel.

4. Radionuclide scanning: Meckel scan allows diagnosis of heterotopic gastric mucosa. Tagged red blood cell (RBC) scan can also localize bleeding if bleeding rate is 0.1 cc/min or more.

5. Angiography: identifies bleeding source with ongoing bleeding rate of 0.5 cc/min or more. Arterial embolization can control the bleed. Complications: arterial spasm, thrombosis, contrast reactions, and acute renal failure.

6. Laparoscopy: definitive diagnosis and treatment of GI bleeding of obscure origin in children with negative gastroscopy, colonoscopy, and RBC scan.

SPECIFIC CAUSES AND EVALUATIONS

1. Malrotation with volvulus: most commonly seen in the neonatal period; surgical emergency. Symptoms suggest bowel obstruction: bilious vomiting, pain, and abdominal distention. Melena can result from ischemia of volvulated bowel. Diagnose via ultrasonography (clockwise rotation of the superior mesenteric vein around the superior mesenteric artery) and upper GI series (duodenum does not cross the midline, small intestine lies to right of the midline).

2. Hemorrhagic disease of the newborn: hematochezia or melena may be a manifestation of vitamin K deficiency. Symptoms occur at 2–7 days of life.

3. Anal fissure: most common cause of lower GI bleeding in infants and young children. Passage of hard, large stools results in superficial tear of the squamous lining of the anal canal, usually at 6 and 12 o'clock position. Painful. When painless, suggests Crohn disease.

4. Intussusception: idiopathic or associated with lymphoid hyperplasia of the terminal ileum. In older children, lead point (polyp, Meckel diverticulum, intestinal duplication, or neoplasm) more likely to be found. May be a complication of Schönlein-Henoch purpura, cystic fibrosis, or Peutz-Jeghers syndrome. Typical scenario: episodes of colicky abdominal pain, vomiting, and passage of currant jelly stool. Exam may reveal palpable sausage-shaped abdominal mass. Diagnose by abdominal ultrasound. Hydrostatic or pneumatic enema allows reduction in 80%.

5. Meckel diverticulum: anomalous remnant of vitelline duct at the terminal 100 cm of the ileum. Most com-

TABLE 2   PRINCIPAL ASSOCIATED GASTROINTESTINAL SYMPTOMS IN RELATION TO THE UNDERLYING CAUSE(S) OF LOWER GASTROINTESTINAL BLEEDING

AMOUNT OF BLOOD LOSS	APPEARANCE OF BLEEDING	CHARACTERISTICS OF STOOLS	PAIN	UNDERLYING DISEASE
Small	Red	Hard	Yes (anorectal)	Anal fissure
Small to moderate	Red	Loose	Variable (abdominal)	Allergic proctocolitis, infectious colitis, hemolytic uremic syndrome, IBD
Small to moderate	Red	Normal, coated with blood	No	Polyp
Moderate	Red to tarry	Normal	Yes (abdominal)	Henoch-Schönlein purpura
Moderate	Red to tarry, currant jelly	Normal	Yes (abdominal)	Intussusception
Moderate	Red to tarry	Loose	Yes (abdominal)	Hirschsprung disease enterocolitis
Large	Red to tarry	Normal	No	Meckel diverticulum, angiodysplasia

IBD = inflammatory bowel disease.

TABLE 3   DIAGNOSTIC INVESTIGATIONS TO BE PERFORMED FOR IDENTIFYING THE MAIN CAUSES OF LOWER GASTROINTESTINAL BLEEDING IN CHILDREN

DISEASE	DIAGNOSTIC INVESTIGATION(S)
Newborn period: birth to 1 mo	
Necrotizing enterocolitis	Physical examination, plain radiographs of the abdomen
Malrotation with midgut volvulus	Plain radiographs of the abdomen, ultrasonography, upper gastrointestinal series, barium enema
Allergic proctocolitis	Diet history taking, exclusion of the allergen(s) from the diet, skin prick tests, total IgE and RAST, proctosigmoidoscopy
Hirschsprung disease enterocolitis	Barium enema, rectal manometry, rectal biopsies
Hemorrhagic disease of the newborn	Clotting studies
Infancy: 1 mo to 2 yr	
Anal fissure	Physical examination, anoscopy
Infectious colitis	Stool culture, stool examination for virus, ova, and parasites
Intussusception	Ultrasonography
Meckel diverticulum	Radionuclide scanning, exploratory laparoscopy or laparotomy
Lymphonodular hyperplasia	Proctosigmoidoscopy, biopsy, barium enema
Intestinal duplication	Ultrasonography, CT, upper gastrointestinal series, barium enema
Preschool age (2–5 yr)	
Polyps	Proctosigmoidoscopy, colonoscopy
Henoch-Schönlein syndrome	Physical examination
Hemolytic uremic syndrome	Complete blood count (anemia, thrombopenia, schizocytes), renal function (renal insufficiency)
School age (> 5 yr)	
Inflammatory bowel disease	Ultrasonography, small bowel follow-through or CT, esogastroduodenoscopy, colonoscopy, biopsy
Vascular causes	
Hemorrhoids	Physical examination, anoscopy
Angiodysplasia	Colonoscopy, angiography
Dieulafoy lesion	Colonoscopy, angiography
Telangiectasias	Colonoscopy
Miscellaneous	
Diversion colitis	Proctosigmoidoscopy, biopsy
Jejuno- or ileocolic perianastomotic ulceration	Barium enema, proctosigmoidoscopy, biopsy
Neoplasia	Colonoscopy, biopsy
Solitary rectal ulcer syndrome	Proctosigmoidoscopy, biopsy

CT = computed tomography; Ig = immunoglobulin; RAST = radioallergosorbent test.

mon congenital abnormality of the GI tract: incidence 1–4%. Ratio of boys to girls: 2:1. Typical presentation: lower GI bleeding resulting from ulceration of adjacent ileal mucosa by acid-secreting heterotopic gastric mucosa contained in the diverticulum. Bleeding is often brisk and painless. Diagnosis: Meckel scan (scintigraphy): sensitivity 85–90%; possible false-positive (intussusception, hydronephrosis, arteriovenous malformation, or inflammatory bowel disease). Treatment: surgical excision.

6. Lymphonodular hyperplasia: multiple yellowish nodules (enlarged lymphoid follicles). Diagnosed on upper GI series, barium enema, endoscopy, and histology. Common intestinal phenomenon in children aged < 10 yr. Etiology unknown but allergy should be excluded. Associated with abdominal pain and hematochezia. Unlikely source of GI bleeding in children > 7 yr.

RARE CAUSES

1. Angiodysplasia: identified by endoscopy or angiography. Endoscopic appearance is flat or slightly raised lesion 2–10 mm in diameter that is raised in color. Most bleeding episodes stop spontaneously. Surgical resection is first-line therapeutic modality.

2. Dieulafoy lesion: usually in stomach (80%) or duodenum (20%), but reported in distal small bowel and

colon. Characterized by congenitally abnormal enlarged arteriole running in submucosa. Symptom: massive recurrent bleeding. Therapy: injection, coagulative therapy, banding, and embolization.

3. Telangiectasia: frequently associated with the autosomal dominant condition of hereditary hemorrhagic telangiectasia (Osler-Weber-Rendu disease). GI hemorrhage unusual before typical skin and mucous lesions; usually presents with recurrent epistaxis.

4. Blue rubber bleb nevus syndrome or Bean syndrome: rare systemic disorder characterized by cutaneous, GI vascular malformations that cause occult blood loss as well as overt life-threatening GI bleeding. Can be inherited as autosomal dominant disease. Present with typical skin lesions: bluish, soft, compressible skin nodules especially at the soles of the feet and palms of the hands. Conservative therapy using endoscopic laser coagulation or bipolar electrocoagulation can be performed in the absence of massive bleeding. Resections are otherwise necessary.

5. Klippel-Trénaunay syndrome: capillary lymphaticovenous malformation resulting in limb hypertrophy. Can extend into the pelvis and colon.

6. Diversion colitis: surgical isolation of colonic mucosa from the normal fecal stream may provoke inflammation and ulceration. Symptoms include rectal bleeding,

mucoid discharge, tenesmus, and abdominal pain. Endoscopic, histologic findings may be indistinguishable from inflammatory bowel disease. Restoration of normal fecal flow results in complete resolution.

7. Jejuno- or ileocolic perianastomotic ulceration: may occur following ileocolic or jejunocolic anastomosis after intestinal resection in infancy or early childhood, many years after surgery. Cause unknown. Treatment: surgical resection.

8. Neoplasia: GI tumors revealed by lower GI bleeding are very uncommon in children.

9. Graft-versus-host disease: enteric graft-versus-host disease can present with hemodynamically significant lower GI hemorrhage.

10. Solitary rectal ulcer syndrome: benign chronic ulcerative disease; unusual in childhood. Symptoms: dyschezia, tenesmus, mucous discharge, pain in perineal area, rectal prolapse, and rectal bleeding. A relationship between solitary rectal ulcer syndrome and chronic constipation has been reported. Histopathologic diagnosis is based on the fibromuscular obliteration of the lamina propria with misorientation of smooth muscle cells.

QUESTIONS

CHOOSE THE BEST ANSWER:

1. What is the minimum bleeding rate required to be able to detect site of bleed by red blood cell scan?
   a. 0.1 cc/min.
   b. 0.2 cc/min.
   c. 0.4 cc/min.
   d. 0.5 cc/min.
   e. 1 cc/min.

2. What is the treatment for diversion colitis?
   a. Sulfasalazine.
   b. Steroids.
   c. Rectal decompression.
   d. Restoration of normal fecal flow.
   e. All of the above.

3. A 10-year-old boy presents with colicky abdominal pain and currant jelly stools. Sonogram verifies intussusception. Evaluation includes which of the following?
   a. Hydrostatic or pneumatic enema.
   b. Colonoscopy.
   c. Meckel scan.
   d. a and b.
   e. All of the above.

4. False-negative fecal occult blood testing results are associated with all of the following except:
   a. Large vitamin C intake.
   b. Dry, hard stools.
   c. Prior conversion of hemoglobin to porphyrin by intestinal bacteria.
   d. Old reagents.
   e. Peroxidase-containing foods.

TRUE OR FALSE:

5. Painless anal fissures are associated with Crohn disease.
6. Dieulafoy lesions are commonly found in the colon.
7. Lymphonodular hyperplasia is a common source of lower gastrointestinal bleeding in children older than 10 years old.
8. Meckel diverticula are more common in males.

GROWTH FAILURE

SYNOPSIS

ASSESSMENT OF GROWTH AND NUTRITION

1. Anthropometry (dimension measurements).
2. Clinical exam.
3. Biochemistry (tissue levels of nutrients).
4. Body composition (fat, fat-free mass, bone density).
5. Dietary assessment (food intake).
6. Functional test (muscle strength, nerve function).

PONDERAL ASSESSMENT

1. Assessment of mass.
2. Growth assessed by measuring change in weight, skinfold thickness, and mid upper arm circumference.
3. Generally more accurate than linear assessments of growth.

LINEAR ASSESSMENT

1. In children ≤ 2 years old: measure supine length.
2. In children > 2 years old: measure standing height with a stadiometer.

STUNTING

1. Deficit in height relative to age.
2. Reflects a chronic process.
3. Low height relative to age usually starts at 6–24 months of age; low height for age at 1 yr reflects current status, whereas low height for age at 6 yr reflects prior status.
4. Associated with a delay in the onset of the childhood phase of growth.
5. Nutritional interventions in first 2 years of life can reverse stunting, but if interventions occur later a degree of stunting will remain up to adulthood.

INDEX OF ACUTE RISK

1. Weight relative to height is a better index of acute risk than weight relative to age (Figure 1).
2. Indicator in developing countries for admission to hospital to treat severe malnutrition: < 70% reference of weight–height median.

LINEAR GROWTH PHASES

1. Infancy.
2. Childhood.
3. Puberty.

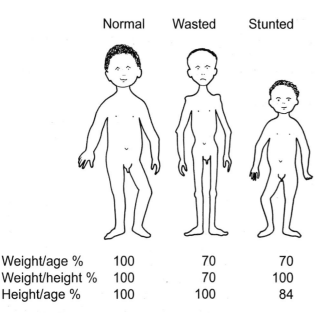

Normal   Wasted   Stunted

	Normal	Wasted	Stunted
Weight/age %	100	70	70
Weight/height %	100	70	100
Height/age %	100	100	84

FIGURE 1 Comparison of a normal, a wasted, and a stunted child, all aged 1 year. Reproduced with permission from Waterlow JC. Nutrition and growth. In: Protein energy malnutrition. London: Edward Arnold; 1992. p. 187–211.

INFANCY PHASE

1. Infant birth size linked to mother.
2. Continuation of the high fetal growth rate (maximum rate) with rapid decline to 3 years of age.
3. Size is a function of intrauterine environment and postnatal nutrition.
4. If birth length is less affected than weight: better prognosis; reflects a short-term insult in late pregnancy (placental insufficiency).
5. Baby with length and weight equally affected: chronic illness and malnutrition.
6. Requirements for dietary energy highest in first year of life.
7. Two-thirds of normal infants cross % in first 18 months of life. By 2 years of age, genetic potential predominates as principal determinant.
8. Breast-fed babies: gain less weight in the second half of the first year of life than formula-fed infants, but no deficits.
9. Truncal growth accounts for majority of linear growth.
10. Growth hormone (GH) secretion high but does not affect linear growth of the fetus.

CHILDHOOD PHASE

1. Onset occurs at 6–12 months; GH starts to affect linear growth. Trigger of onset unclear.
2. Abrupt increase in linear growth rate, then decelerating velocity.
3. GH action (long bone growth is GH-dependent) accounts for majority of linear growth in childhood phase.
4. Age of onset influences attained height: late onset common in populations with growth failure, resulting from malnourishment and chronic disease.
5. This phase is critical for catch-up growth.

PUBERTY

1. Onset marked by increased frequency of pulsatile gonadotropin-releasing hormone: luteinizing hormone and follicle-stimulating hormone.
2. Second increase in growth velocity: short-lived.
3. In girls: first sign of breast bud; menarche at end of growth spurt.
4. In boys: first sign of testicular enlargement, onset < 1 yr later than girls; growth spurt later with growth potential left after secondary sex organ development complete.
5. Adolescent growth spurt: consequence of both growth hormone and sex steroids; occurs 2 years earlier in girls than boys (thus 2 more yrs of growth).
6. Leg length increases first but increased growth due more to truncal growth, so trunk-to-leg ratio increases during puberty.

THRIFTY PHENOTYPE (BARKER) HYPOTHESIS

Impaired fetal and early infantile growth affects susceptibility to chronic adult degenerative disease.

CATCH-UP GROWTH

Ponderal catch-up growth easy to achieve with dietary rehabilitation: up to 10–20 g/k/d.
Linear catch-up growth more difficult: growth potential limited by severity and length of nutritional insult and age of occurrence and age at catch-up growth.

QUESTIONS

TRUE OR FALSE:

1. Growth hormone–deficient children present at birth with a deficit in birth length.
2. Ponderal catch-up growth is more difficult to achieve than linear catch-up growth.
3. Increased height in the pubertal years is mainly due to long bone growth.

CHOOSE THE BEST ANSWER:

4. Of the following, which is the best assessment of acute risk of malnutrition?
    a. Weight relative to age.
    b. Height relative to age.
    c. Weight relative to height.
    d. All of the above.
    e. None of the above.

5. Which of the following children has the best chance of not having any residual stunting as an adult?
    a. A stunted child at age 10 years with delayed puberty.
    b. A stunted child at age 12 months who is beginning aggressive nutritional interventions.
    c. A stunted child at age 24 months who is beginning aggressive nutritional interventions.
    d. Both b and c.

GASTROINTESTINAL SYSTEM IN MALNUTRITION

SYNOPSIS

MALNUTRITION

1. Major public health problem worldwide (Figure 1).
2. Most common among children < 5 yr.
3. Underweight children are at increased risk of dying from common infectious illnesses, and wasting has been specifically identified as a risk factor for mortality.

PRIOR CLASSIFICATIONS OF NUTRITIONAL DEFICIENCY

1. Marasmus: severe wasting without edema.
2. Kwashiorkor: underweight children with nutritional edema with or without dermatosis, hair changes, apathy, and irritability.
3. Marasmic kwashiorkor: children with edema who are severely underweight.

MALABSORPTION

Markedly reduced absorption of various nutrients has been demonstrated in malnourished children.

CARBOHYDRATES

1. Lactose intolerance is most consistent problem. Carbohydrate-free diet reduces stool weight and stool lactate in most children.
2. Malabsorption of other sugars variable.
3. Absorption of all sugars improved with clinical recovery.

NITROGEN

Increased nitrogen losses from gut related to malnutrition and gut infection.

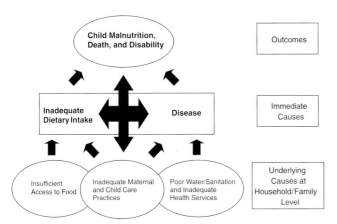

FIGURE 1 The vicious cycle of malnutrition, inadequate dietary intake, and disease (mostly infection) is related to underlying causes at the household and family level. Adapted from Bellamy C. The state of the world's children 1998: focus on nutrition. New York: Oxford University Press for UNICEF; 1997. p. 24.

FAT

1. Variable decreases in dietary fat absorption shown in malnutrition.
2. Absorption improves slowly during nutritional recovery.

VITAMIN B$_{12}$

Markedly reduced absorption in malnutrition that is slow to improve with clinical recovery. Absorption is not improved by giving intrinsic factor.

LIVER

1. Fatty infiltration in the liver in kwashiorkor: well documented. Begins at the periphery of the lobules and progresses to centrolobular areas. Moderate periportal and peripheral pericellular fibrosis and cellular infiltration at the portal areas have also been described. The degree of hepatic steatosis is not necessarily associated with the severity of malnutrition or transaminitis; in most cases, hepatic steatosis improves with weight gain.
2. Impaired hepatic synthesis: may be a risk factor for mortality.

PANCREAS AND BILE ACIDS

1. Marked atrophy of the acinar cells and a resulting small pancreas has been seen in kwashiorkor patients.
2. Pancreatic fibrosis: mild in kwashiorkor; uncommon in marasmus.
3. Histology correlates with decreased levels of pancreatic enzymes. Production of enzymes improves promptly with clinical recovery.
4. Deficiency of conjugated bile acids: can be main cause of fat maldigestion; may be secondary to small bowel bacterial overgrowth.

STOMACH

1. Histology in kwashiorkor: variable degrees of abnormality.
2. Basal acid output: generally low; may not return until complete recovery. *Helicobacter pylori* infection may play a role.

SMALL INTESTINE

1. Typically, intestinal wall is thin with a smooth, atrophic mucous membrane in malnutrition. Villous atrophy can occur and be marked. Brush border is often irregular. Intraepithelial lymphocytes are increased, as is the cellular infiltrate.
2. Mucosal lesions can persist even with clinical recovery—especially in marasmus.

IMMUNOHISTOCHEMISTRY

1. Immunohistochemistry studies show increased number of B cells in the intestinal lamina propria of malnourished children.
2. Density of mucosal cytokine immunoreactive cells: more proinflammatory cytokine-producing cells than regulatory cells.

INTESTINAL PERMEABILITY

1. Decreased surface area and increased leakiness are associated with worsening nutritional status.
2. Association between increased permeability and death suggests that sepsis caused by translocated bacteria from the gut may play a role.

LARGE INTESTINE

1. Sigmoidoscopy in kwashiorkor shows increased vascularity of the rectal mucosa.
2. Colitis appears to be a feature of protein-energy malnutrition even in the absence of gut infection and may contribute to diarrhea.

GASTROINTESTINAL FLORA

1. Increased bacteria and *Candida* demonstrated in gastric juice of the malnourished.
2. Increased bacterial colonization of the small bowel has been reported in malnutrition; unclear whether this reflects the environment rather than nutritional status.

MICRONUTRIENTS

1. Vitamin A: supplementation may reduce child mortality in some situations, but its effect on diarrhea and malnutrition effects in the gut is less clear.
2. Zinc: supplementation prevents episodes of diarrhea and reduces the duration and severity of acute and persistent diarrhea with some evidence of greater benefit in malnourished children.
3. Supplementation of both zinc and vitamin A have beneficial effects on the integrity of the intestinal mucosa in children, but the clinical importance of this remains to be studied.

QUESTIONS

TRUE OR FALSE:

1. The severity of steatohepatitis correlates to the degree of malnutrition in underweight children.
2. Small intestinal mucosal lesions do not heal promptly after nutritional recovery in malnourished children.

CHOOSE THE BEST ANSWER:

3. The following are malnutrition-associated changes in the gastrointestinal system except:
   a. Pancreatic atrophy.
   b. Steatohepatitis.
   c. Small bowel bacterial overgrowth.
   d. Lactose intolerance.
   e. Vitamin B_{12} malabsorption secondary to intrinsic factor deficiency.

OBESITY

SYNOPSIS

OBESITY

1. Definition:
   a. Weight/height ratio > 90%.
   b. Weight > 120% of median for weight given child's age and gender.
   c. At risk for obesity: body mass index (BMI) > 85%; obese: BMI > 95%.
2. Currently, 14% of children and adolescents in the United States are obese.

OBESITY AND RELATED COMPLICATIONS

1. Obesity is an important risk factor for both heart disease and type 2 diabetes.
2. Metabolic syndrome: hyperinsulinemia, dyslipidemia, obesity, and hypertension. Associated with nonalcoholic fatty liver disease (NAFLD). Increased ratio of visceral to subcutaneous adipose tissue predicts insulin resistance.
3. NAFLD: spectrum of liver disease associated with obesity in children and adults.
   a. Steatosis: accumulation of fat alone.
   b. Steatohepatitis: fat accompanied by inflammation and fibrosis.
   c. Obesity and diabetes: strongest predictors of fibrosis on biopsy.
   d. Nonalcoholic steatohepatitis (NASH): causes cirrhosis and liver failure; third leading indication for liver transplant in adults.
   e. NAFLD associated with 2–3-fold elevation in aminotransferases, particularly alanine aminotransferase (ALT); liver imaging is more sensitive for fatty liver.
   f. Elevated ALT is independently associated with measures of insulin resistance and not obesity.
   g. Inflammatory cytokines may also be involved and mediate insulin resistance.
4. A child's risk for obesity in adulthood also depends on the weight status of his parents; age < 3 yr, parental obesity status is the primary predictor of obesity in adulthood; age > 7 yr, child's own obesity status becomes the more important risk of obesity predictor.
5. Evidence of genetic influences: the more severe the obesity, the greater the heritability factor.
6. Newborns at both ends of the weight spectrum (high and low) are at increased risk for obesity-associated disease. Intrauterine nutritional environment may also predict obesity risk.

REGULATION OF BODY WEIGHT

1. Insulin: important regulator of nutrient partitioning in peripheral tissues and of centers regulating appetite in the brain.

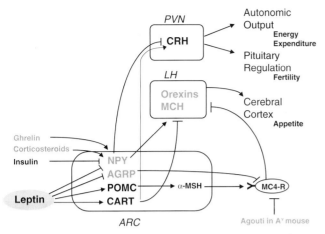

FIGURE 1 Central nervous system pathways regulating appetite and energy metabolism. Leptin positively regulates pro-opiomelanocortin (POMC) while negatively regulating agouti-related protein (AGRP)-releasing neurons in the arcuate nucleus (ARC) of the hypothalamus. POMC is a precursor of α-melanocyte-stimulating hormone (α-MSH), which is an antagonist at the MC4 receptor (MC4-R). AGRP and agouti protein are antagonists at MC4-R. The MC4-R pathway negatively regulates appetite, perhaps acting through appetite-stimulating neuropeptides in the lateral hypothalamus (LH), including melanin-concentrating hormone (MCH) and the orexins. Meanwhile, leptin has some actions that are independent of the POMC pathway, including negatively regulating neuropeptide Y (NPY), which is itself a potent appetite stimulant. Ghrelin also appears to act to stimulate appetite through the NPY pathway. NPY also influences autonomic and pituitary output through the paraventricular nucleus (PVN), acting in part through corticotropin-releasing hormone (CRH).

2. Gastrointestinal tract peptides (eg, cholecystokinin, ghrelin): affect short-term appetite and satiety; secreted in response to intraluminal nutrients and provides signals to the central nervous system. Ghrelin mediates short-term appetite via stimulation of receptors at the ventromedial hypothalamus; released from stomach during fasting, and suppressed by nutrient administration.
3. Leptin: produced in adipose tissue; provides negative feedback to the ventromedial hypothalamus, decreasing appetite and increasing energy expenditure (Figure 1).
4. Melanocortin pathway: leptin increases expression of various elements in the melanocortin pathway. Important regulator of body weight homeostasis; interruption in the melanocortin pathway can produce severe obesity.
5. Melanocortin-independent pathways: leptin inhibits the expression of the orexigenic agent neuropeptide Y, while increasing expression of cocaine- and amphetamine-related transcript, which affects energy expenditure via the autonomic nervous system.

GENETICS

1. Strong effects on obesity development: mutations in leptin and melanocortin pathways.

2. Other candidate gene associations: ghrelin, *PPAR*, uncoupling proteins, and adrenoreceptor genes.
3. Genetic syndromes associated with obesity: see Table 1.

EVALUATION

MEDICAL ASSESSMENT

1. Laboratory tests: thyroid-stimulating hormone, hemoglobin A1c, lipid panel (fasting), and fasting glucose and insulin (detection of insulin resistance).
2. Sleep studies: if strong clinical symptoms of sleep apnea.
3. Radiologic assessment: when slipped capital femoral epiphysis or Blount disease is suspected.
4. Indirect calorimetry: can predict the energy deficit necessary for weight loss.
5. Bone age: may help diagnose endocrinopathy.
6. Drug history: especially for drugs used to treat psychiatric illness, epilepsy, migraines, and diabetes, which are associated with weight gain.
7. Family history: to help establish genetic factors.

NUTRITIONAL, BEHAVIORAL, AND PSYCHOSOCIAL EVALUATION

1. Minimum evaluation: anthropometric measurements, history of onset of obesity, and history of weight loss attempts.
2. Dietary intake assessment: can determine diet composition, but not often a good estimate of energy intake owing to underreporting. Diet recall can detect micronutrient and mineral deficiencies. Assess frequency of types of food (dairy, fruits, vegetables, juices, soda, and fast food meals), meal patterns and social context of meals.
3. Exercise and sedentary behaviors should be evaluated with particular attention to frequency of TV and computer use (the American Academy of Pediatrics recommends limiting TV watching to 1–2 h/d).
4. Psychosocial health should be evaluated.

TREATMENT

NUTRITIONAL THERAPY

1. Traffic-light diet: color-coding scheme categorizes foods for consumption based on caloric density. Prescribed caloric content: 900 to 1,300 kcal/d.
2. Protein-sparing modified fast (PSMF) diet: high-quality lean protein while strictly limiting total calories. Effective for short-term weight loss, but not long term. Potential complications: protein losses, hypokalemia, inadequate calcium intake, cholelithiasis, and intravascular volume depletion with orthostatic hypotension.
3. Carbohydrate-restricting diets (eg, Atkins): short term: greater loss of body water than body fat; long term: loss of body fat. Nutritionally inadequate; supplementation of calcium and water-soluble vitamins required.

TABLE 1   CHARACTERISTICS OF THE MAJOR SYNDROMES ASSOCIATED WITH OBESITY

SYNDROME	COGNITIVE DEFICIT	OBESITY	FEATURES
Albright	Mild	Variable (general) Early onset	Neuroendocrine anomalies Normal or short stature Skin hyperpigmentation/vitiligo Polydactyly Bone fibrous dysplasia Precocious puberty
Alström	None	Moderate (central) Onset age 2–5 yr	Retinitis pigmentosa Deafness Neuroendocrine anomalies Normal or short stature Normal or hypogonadism
Bardet-Biedl	Moderate	Moderate (central) Onset age 1–2 yr	Normal or short stature Hypotonia Compulsive behavior Retinitis Heart anomalies Polydactyly Renal dysfunction Hypogonadism
Carpenter	Mild	Central	Acrocephaly Polydactyly Syndactyly Short stature Flat nasal bridge High arched palate Heart anomalies Hypogonadism
Cohen	Mild	Variable (central) Midchildhood	Short or tall stature Hypotonia Microcephaly Retinochoroidal dystrophy Short philtrum Low hairline Heart anomalies Normal or hypogonadism
POMC mutation (autosomal dominant)	None	Early onset	Red hair ACTH deficiency Hyperphagia
Prader-Willi	Mild to moderate	Moderate to severe (generalized) Onset 1–3 yr	Short stature Hypotonia Almond-shaped eyes V-shaped mouth Neuroendocrine anomalies Compulsive behavior High arched palate Hypogonadism

ACTH = adrenocorticotropic hormone; POMC = pro-opiomelanocortin.

BEHAVIOR THERAPY

1. Family-based treatments are better than patient-focused treatment.
2. Gradual behavioral treatment is better than rapid.
3. Positive reinforcement is better than restrictive or critical approaches, with frequent over less frequent positive reinforcement also having improved success.
4. The value of problem-solving techniques has not been consistently shown.

WEIGHT-LOSS DRUGS

In general, drugs demonstrate only modest efficacy. Weight regain typically occurs on discontinuation of the medication. The safety and efficacy of weight-loss drugs in children have not been established.

1. Sibutramine: appetite suppressant. Inhibits norepinephrine, serotonin, and dopamine reuptake. Side effects: modest increases in blood pressure (2 mm Hg average) and heart rate, dry mouth, constipation, and insomnia. United States Food and Drug Administration approved in adults for treatment of obesity.
2. Orlistat: inhibits gastrointestinal lipases, reducing fat digestion and absorption by about 30%. Side effects: steatorrhea and decreases in serum levels of fat-soluble vitamins. Daily multivitamin recommended. FDA approved in adults for obesity therapy.

TABLE 2   DIETARY SUPPLEMENTS FOR WEIGHT LOSS

DIETARY SUPPLEMENT	OTHER NAMES	MECHANISM	EFFECTIVENESS	SAFETY
Ephedra alkaloids	*Ma huang* Norepinephrine	Thermogenic	Yes, only in combination with caffeine	Unsafe (hypertension, palpitation, tachycardia, stroke, seizures, death)
Caffeine	Guarana (*Paullinia cupana*) Yerba maté (*Ilex paraguayansis*)	Thermogenic	No, when used alone	High doses or combinations may be unsafe (hypertenstion, tachycardia, nausea, dizziness)
Chromium	Chromium picolinate	↑ Insulin sensitivity	Uncertain	Uncertain
Ginseng	Korean ginseng (*Panax ginseng*)	↑ Insulin sensitivity	Uncertain	Uncertain
	American ginseng (*Panax quinquefolux*) Siberian ginseng (*Eleutherococcus senticosus*)	Thermogenic ↑ Lipolysis		May interfere with anticoagulant effect of warfarin
Fiber	Guar gum Psyllium Flaxseed Glucomannan	Malabsorption ↑ Insulin sensitivity	Unlikely	Generally safe, but some forms may have risk of gastrointestinal obstruction
Hydroxycitric acid	Malabar tamarind (*Garcinia cambogia*)	↓ De novo fatty acid synthesis	Unlikely	Uncertain
Dehydroepiandrosterone	Adrenal steroid hormone	↓ Fat synthesis	Uncertain	Uncertain Metabolites may stimulate breast and prostate tissue
Chitosan	Chitin (crustacean shells)	Blocks dietary fat absorption	Uncertain	Uncertain
Horsetail	*Equisetum* sp	Diuretic	Uncertain	Unsafe (may be K⁺-wasting)
Senna Cascara	*Cassia* sp *Rhamnus pushiana*	Laxatives	Uncertain	Unsafe for treatment of obesity
St. John's wort	"Herbal phen-fen" *Hypericum perforatum*	Antidepressant	Unlikely	Uncertain Phototoxicity; drug interactions with many psychoactive drugs

3. Metformin: improves insulin sensitivity; promotes modest weight loss in adults; may be useful in ameliorating psychotropic drug–induced weight gain in children.

4. Dietary "supplements" or herbal medicines (Table 2): popular but unregulated. Questionable substances: *Ephedra* (or *ma huang*), horsetail, herbal laxatives, and some forms of caffeine and fiber.

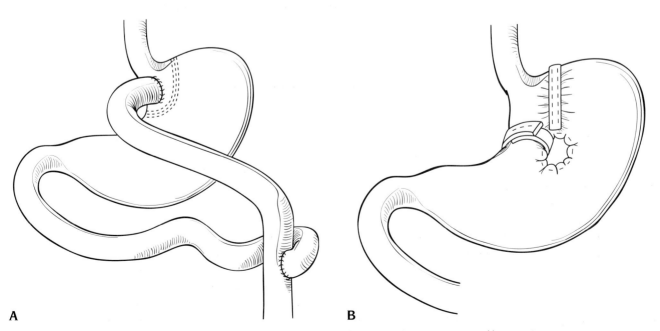

A   **B**

FIGURE 2   Gastric restrictive surgery for weight loss. *A,* Vertical banded gastroplasty; *B,* Roux-en-Y gastric bypass.

WEIGHT-LOSS SURGERY

1. Durable and substantial weight loss: > 80% of patients lose > 50% their excess body weight during the first year; stabilizes 12–24 months after surgery; 10–20% of patients regain significant weight.
2. Improves or resolves many medical complications: diabetes mellitus, hypercholesterolemia, and obstructive sleep apnea.
3. Limited data on adolescent patients.
4. Types:
   a. Jejunoileal bypass: frequent and unacceptable side effects, including intractable diarrhea, nutrient deficiencies, kidney stones, and hepatic failure. No longer used.
   b. Roux-en-Y gastric bypass and vertical banded gastroplasty (Figure 2): reduce gastric capacity to restrict caloric intake. Complications (10% of patients): anastomotic strictures, incisional hernias, gallstone formation requiring cholecystectomy, and dumping syndrome (1–2%). Malabsorption common; requires postoperative monitoring and treatment.

QUESTIONS

TRUE OR FALSE:

1. In a 9-year-old child, parental obesity status is the primary predictor of the child having obesity in adulthood.
2. Aspartate transaminase is more than alanine transaminase in nonalcoholic fatty liver disease.
3. Patients on the Atkins' diet require water-soluble vitamin supplementation.
4. Following gastric bypass surgery, 30% of patients regain a significant portion of the lost weight.

CHOOSE THE BEST ANSWER:

5. Which of the following is not an anthropometric determined definition of obesity?
   a. Weight/height ratio > 90%.
   b. Weight > 120% of median for weight given child's age, height, and gender.
   c. Body mass index (BMI) > 95%.
   d. BMI > 85%.
   e. All are defined as overweight status.

6. Complications of the protein-sparing modified fast include:
   a. Hypokalemia.
   b. Inadequate calcium intake.
   c. Cholelithiasis.
   d. Intravascular volume depletion.
   e. All of the above.

7. The following are complications of gastric bypass surgery except:
   a. Cholelithiasis.
   b. Hypotension.
   c. Anastomotic strictures.
   d. Dumping syndrome.
   e. All of the above.

8. Which of the following deficiencies are common after gastric bypass surgery?
   a. Iron.
   b. Niacin.
   c. Biotin.
   d. Folate.
   e. All of the above.

MUNCHAUSEN SYNDROME BY PROXY

SYNOPSIS

1. Asher described Munchausen syndrome in 1951. Meadow reported first cases of Munchausen syndrome by proxy in 1977.
2. Most cases involve gastrointestinal, genitourinary, and central nervous system symptoms.
3. Perpetrators usually familiar with medical environment and have some level of health training.
4. Children often present with symptoms incongruent with their general health.
5. Specific Axis II conditions most frequently associated with Munchausen syndrome by proxy: borderline and narcissistic personality disorders.

DIAGNOSIS

1. Phenolphthalein can be detected in stool when alkalinized to > 8.5 (turns pink). Check stool levels of magnesium and sulfate to detect laxatives.
2. Covert videotaping requires legal advice.
3. Do not confront prematurely: threat of legal action and discharge against medical advice often result.

TABLE 1   GASTROINTESINTAL DIAGNOSES FREQUENTLY CONFOUNDED BY FACTITIOUS DISORDER BY PROXY

PRESENTING DIAGNOSIS	METHOD OF FABRICATION
Colitis	Laxatives
Cystic fibrosis	Altered, contaminated sweat tests and fecal fat analysis
Diarrhea (intractable)	Laxatives
	Phenophtalein poisoning; salt poisoning
Failure to thrive	Withholding of food, fluids
Gastrointestinal hemorrhages (otherwise unexplained)	Patient's blood withdrawn from Broviac catheter; exogenous sources of blood (usually the perpetrators); warfarin poisoning
Rectovesical fistula	Altered urine specimens
Seizures/apnea secondary to gastroesophageal reflux	Asphyxiation (manual)
	Phenothiazine poisoning
	Salt poisoning
	Imipramine poisoning
	Perpetrator's fabricated report
Vomiting (with or without altered sensorium)	Emetic poisoning
	Salt poisoning, injecting air into a gastrostomy tube

TABLE 2   MANAGEMENT RECOMMENDATIONS
FOLLOWING THE ASSESSMENT OF
FACTITIOUS DISORDER BY PROXY (FDP)

Removal of the child from the care of the perpetrator and placement in a situation in which his/her safety is ensured. Placement with relatives is not necessarily a sufficient assurance of safety. Therapeutic foster care is indicated.

Separation of the child from the perpetrator should continue at least until the perpetrator has received a full psychiatric evaluation and a comprehensive social history has been obtained.

Primary pediatric medical care for the child should be coordinated by a practitioner specifically knowledgeable about FDP, who is also familiar with the case.

Comprehensive medical and psychosocial evaluations of siblings.

Long-term psychotherapy for both the perpetrator and the child provided by clinicians familiar with FDP. The perpetrator's partner should be included in therapy, as should siblings.

Ongoing monitoring of the child's medical, developmental, and psychosocial progress should be coordinated between providers of medical and psychosocial care, as well as coordinators of foster care arrangements.

If family reunification is eventually indicated, supervision should continue, with arrangements made through the courts for monitoring to continue regardless of relocation.

QUESTIONS

CHOOSE THE BEST ANSWER:

1. The following are warning signs of Munchausen syndrome by proxy except:
    a. Extraordinarily rare signs or symptoms.
    b. Repeated hospitalizations or evaluations have failed to provide a conclusive diagnosis or etiology.
    c. Noteworthy signs and symptoms do not recur when perpetrator is absent.
    d. Perpetrator is hypervigilant but comfortable in medical environment.
    e. Perpetrator freely gives access to prior medical records.
    f. All of the above are warning signs.

2. The following are useful evaluations with the complaint of chronic diarrhea if one is suspecting Munchausen syndrome by proxy except:
    a. Toxicology screen of feces and urine.
    b. Fecal magnesium and electrolytes.
    c. Stool osmolality.
    d. Acidification of the stool.
    e. Stool electrolytes.

3. Which are the most common specific Axis II conditions most frequently associated with Munchausen syndrome by proxy (can be more than one)?
    a. Borderline personality.
    b. Violent personality.
    c. Aggressive personality.
    d. Narcissistic personality.
    e. All of the above.

TRUE OR FALSE:

4. Covert videotaping is the best way to establish Munchausen syndrome by proxy.

5. If one is suspecting Munchausen syndrome by proxy, it is best to confront early rather than later.

ANSWERS

ACUTE DIARRHEA
1. b.
2. b.
3. False. At the crypt.
4. False.
5. False. At the small intestine.
6. False. Usually both coexist.
7. False.
8. False.
9. b.
10. a.
11. b.
12. a.
13. b.

PERSISTENT DIARRHEA
1. b.
2. d.
3. e.
4. False.
5. True.

PROTEIN-LOSING ENTEROPATHY
1. b.
2. d. Globulin infusions often not necessary.
3. e. A1AT degraded at pH < 3; does not account for gastric losses well.

VOMITING
1. d.
2. d.
3. d.
4. d.
5. c.

COLIC AND GAS
1. c.
2. b.
3. True.
4. False.
5. False.
6. False.
7. False.

ABDOMINAL MASSES

1. c.
2. d. Terminal ileum.
3. e.
4. c.
5. False.
6. True.
7. False.

UPPER GASTROINTESTINAL BLEEDING

1. c.
2. c.
3. a.
4. d.
5. b.

LOWER GASTROINTESTINAL BLEEDING

1. a.
2. d.
3. e. Intussusception is often associated with a lead point in older children. Workup should be performed to rule out polyp, neoplasia, and Meckel diverticulum.
4. e.
5. True.
6. False. 80% in stomach.
7. False. Source of lower GI bleeding in younger children.
8. True

GROWTH FAILURE

1. False. Fetal growth is not growth hormone-dependent.
2. False. Linear growth is more difficult to achieve.
3. False. Although long bone growth contributes initially, truncal growth is more significant.
4. c.
5. b. Interventions started within the first 2 years have the best chance of reversing stunting.

MALNUTRITION

1. False.
2. True.
3. e. Vitamin B_{12} malabsorption in malnutrition is not responsive to intrinsic factor supplementation.

OBESITY

1. False. After 7 years of age, the child's obesity status is the primary predictor of obesity in adulthood.
2. False. ALT elevations are more characteristic of NAFLD.
3. True.
4. False. 10-20%.
5. d. BMI > 85% indicates risk for overweight status.
6. e.
7. b.
8. a.

MUNCHAUSEN SYNDROME BY PROXY: FACTITIOUS DISORDER BY PROXY

1. e.
2. d.
3. a and d.
4. False. Covert videotaping requires legal advice.
5. False. Confrontation prematurely often leads to discharge against medical advice and threat of legal action.

CLINICAL MANIFESTATIONS AND MANAGEMENT:
The Mouth and Esophagus

DISORDERS OF THE ORAL CAVITY

SYNOPSIS

TOOTH ABNORMALITIES

1. Amelogenesis imperfecta: characterized by defects of enamel. Requires evaluation by pediatric dentistry.
   a. Hypocalcified: most common form; normal thickness at eruption but soft and rapidly lost.
   b. Hypomaturation: normal thickness, but mottled, brown-yellow, or white appearance.
   c. Hypoplastic: reduced thickness.
2. Dentine dysplasia: crowns of the teeth are of normal shape but have an amber or opalescent appearance owing to abnormal dentinal structure.
3. Dentinogenesis imperfecta: early loss of overlying enamel.
   a. Dentinogenesis imperfecta Shields type II: blue-gray or translucent amber appearance of teeth and tendency for enamel to shear off.
   b. Dentinogenesis imperfecta Shields type III: abnormally large pulp chamber.
   c. Dentinogenesis imperfecta is associated with osteogenesis imperfecta, Ehlers-Danlos syndrome, Goldblatt syndrome, Schimke immuno-osseous dysplasia and skeletal dysplasia, and rootless teeth.
4. Ectodermal dysplasia: large group of genetically determined disorders clinically characterized by alteration of 2 or more ectodermally derived structures. Characterized by congenitally missing primary teeth and hypodontia; anhidrosis, predisposition to heat intolerance, and hyperthermia; and sparse blonde hair.

GINGIVAL DISEASE IN CHILDHOOD

1. Acute necrotizing ulcerative gingivitis (Vincent gingivitis): common in adulthood but can arise in children, especially in the malnourished or immunocompromised; poor oral hygiene most common cause.

   Characteristics: notable, painful, necrotic gingival ulceration, and edema with bleeding and malodor; associated with *Borrelia vincentii*, fusiform bacteria, *Treponema denticola*.

   Treatment: improved oral hygiene; systemic metronidazole or penicillin for severe disease.
2. Long-term cyclosporin therapy: gingival enlargement (not correlated with plasma levels)

PERIODONTAL DISEASE IN CHILDHOOD

1. Aggressive periodontitis: uncommon in childhood; usually reflects underlying primary defect of phagocyte number of function, deficiency of cathepsin C, or structural defect of cementum or connective tissue of the periodontium.
2. Management: reducing the infection with *Actinobacillus* by thorough subgingival mechanical cleaning, antimicrobial agents, or periodontal surgery.

RECURRENT ORAL ULCERATION

1. Recurrent aphthous stomatitis (RAS): characteristics: one or more oral ulcers; heal then reappear at regular intervals. Prevalence 20–30%: 30% of affected persons have first attack by age 14 yr, 10% before age 10 yr.
2. Three distinct types: no distinguishing histopathologic features. Subepithelial connective tissue infiltrated with inflammatory cells.
   a. Minor aphthous ulceration.
   b. Major aphthous ulceration.
   c. Herpetiform ulceration.
3. Minor aphthous ulcers: 80% of RAS cases. Most common in people age 10–40 yr. Ulcers affect nonkeratinised oral mucosa lips, cheeks, vestibule, and margins of tongue. Hard palate, gingivae, and dorsum of tongue typically unaffected. Painful ulcer preceded by prodrome 1–3 d. Ulcers last 10–14 d. Healing complete but ulceration occurs at 1–4 mo intervals. Individual ulcers shallow surrounded by reddened mucosa.
4. Major aphthous ulcers: much larger than minor aphthous ulcers; appear singly or up to 3–4 at a time. Very painful: extensive tissue destruction. Both keratinized and nonkeratinized oral mucosa may be affected. Heal over weeks, can leave scarring. Cervical lymph nodes may be enlarged.
5. Herpetiform ulcers: affect keratinized and nonkeratinized oral mucosa, usually mouth floor and lateral and ventral surface of tongue. Heal within 10 d without mucosal scarring. Discrete ulcers may coalesce to form a large painful lesion with serpiginous outline.
6. Etiology: unknown.
7. Therapy: oral hygiene (mouthwash with 0.2% chlorhexidine); topical antibacterial agents; thalidomide is the most effective agent.

BEHÇET DISEASE

1. Almost all patients exhibit recurrent RAS-like ulceration, all 3 types.
2. Histologically and clinically RAS-like ulcers. Local management similar to that for RAS.

ORAL CANDIDIASIS

1. Acute pseudomembranous candidiasis: most common fungal infections in oral cavity in children; caused by *Candida albicans* (commensal in the mouths of 70% of the general population). Also seen in patients with human immunodeficiency virus (HIV), poorly controlled diabetes, immunosuppression, and in neonates.
2. Chronic mucocutaneous candidiasis (CMC): can be widespread and recurrent in children. Four types: diffuse CMC, sporadic CMC, candidiasis endocrinopathy syndrome (can include hypoparathyroidism and enamel hypoplasia), and late-onset CMC. Long-standing iron deficiency in CMC may give rise to glossitis and postcricoid webbing.
3. Acute atrophic candidiais: very occasionally seen in children; result of candidal overgrowth after broad-spectrum

antibiotics or immunosuppressants. Mucosa sore, inflamed, and sensitive to hot and spicy foods. Treat with nystatin or amphotericin lozenges sucked qid after food. Continue treatment for 48 h after lesions resolved.

4. Chronic atrophic candidiasis ("denture sore mouth"): red, inflamed mucosa, precisely limited to area covered by well-fitting denture (usually upper). Local therapy: antifungal agents; nystatin or amphotericin lozenges; suspension on fitting surface of denture; appliance should be immersed overnight in weak hypochlorite solution to eliminate organisms.

5. Angular cheilitis: red, ulcerated areas at corners of mouth. Lesions often colonized by *C. albicans* or *Staphylococcus aureus*. May reflect iron deficiency, neutropenia, or cell-mediated immunodeficiency. Treatment: miconazole cream applied tid.

6. Median rhomboid glossitis (a candidal infection manifesting as painless erythematous atrophic area in center of dorsum of tongue).

POTENTIALLY MALIGNANT AND MALIGNANT DISEASE

1. Oral squamous cell carcinoma: rare in children; may manifest as solitary white patch, speckled area, or ulcer.

2. Human *Papillomavirus* (HPV): manifests as warts, usually on lips, palate, or gums.

3. Lichen planus: common (1–2% of population), mid to late life, in women more than men. White patches typically arise bilaterally on buccal mucosa, dorsum of tongue, or labial and buccal aspects of gingivae. Usually asymptomatic. Erosions within white patches can be painful. Can be caused by drugs but in children usually idiopathic. Warrants therapy when erosive, ulcerative, or bullous; topical corticosteroids. Rarely resolve.

4. Oral mucosal pigmentation: usually racial in origin. Malignant melanoma rare. Kaposi sarcoma is the most common oral malignancy of HIV in childhood; manifests as blue, red, or purple macule, papule, nodule, or ulcer of the hard palate or gingivae; associated with human herpesvirus 8. Addisonian pigmentation can manifest as diffuse hypermelanosis of the buccal mucosa.

SALIVARY GLAND DISEASE IN CHILDHOOD

1. Mumps: acute generalized paramyxovirus infection of children and young adults. Affects major salivary glands; usually bilaterally enlarged; salivary swelling diminishes after 4–5 d. Diagnosis based on clinical picture; may be confirmed by detection of viral-specific immunoglobulin G and A.

2. HIV salivary gland disease: 4–8% of acquired immunodeficiency syndrome patients (arises late). Recurrent or persistent swelling or xerostomia; reflects underlying bacterial sialadenitis, intraparotid lymphadenopathy, primary or metastatic non-Hodgkin lymphoma, or Kaposi sarcoma. Clinical picture can mimic Sjögren syndrome, but anti-Ro or anti-La antibodies are absent. Fine-needle aspiration biopsy may be useful to rule out malignancy. Course is nonprogressive, thus

therapy only necessary with cosmetic deformity or xerostomia. Resolution with highly active antiretroviral therapy.

3. Suppurative sialadenitis: painful swelling, purulent discharge from the duct and cervical lymphadenopathy. Highest incidence in children age 3–6 yr. Causative organism often not identified. Therapy includes effective hydration and antibiotics. If no improvement in 3–5 d, surgical drainage.

4. Recurrent parotitis: usual age of onset 3–6 yr. Tends to be unilateral. Frequency of recurrence peaks between 5–7 yr, 90% resolve disease by puberty. Etiology unknown. Analgesia is mainstay of therapy; antibiotics do not shorten attacks.

5. Xerostomia: radiotherapy can cause profound and irreversible xerostomia. Symptoms: oral dryness, dysarthria, dysphagia, and loss of taste; dry oral mucosa, lack of saliva; depapillation, redness, and crenation of dorsal tongue. Increased caries, gingivitis, and risk of sialadenitis.

6. Sjögren syndrome: characterized by xerostomia and xerophthalmia owing to lymphocytic infiltrate into the salivary and lacrimal glands. Secondary disease associated with rheumatoid arthritis and lupus. Uncommon in childhood. Etiology unknown. Investigation requires histopathology of labial gland tissue and detection of serum anti-Ro or anti-La antibodies. For treatment of oral complications see Table 1.

DIETARY DISEASE

1. Dental caries: most common diet-related disease of mouth. Principal etiologic factor: diet high in sugars, carbonated drinks (low pH of these drinks causes ero-

TABLE 1   MANAGEMENT OF LONG-STANDING XEROSTOMIA

THERAPY	COMMENTS
SALIVARY SUBSTITUTES	
Nonsynthetic agents	Sips of water; convenient but of limited benefit. Soft drinks should be avoided in view of the risk of caries or dental erosion.
Synthetic agents	A variety of sprays, mouthrinses, and gels are available; no one agent is better than another; benefit can be transient.
SALIVARY STIMULANTS (SIALOGOGUES)	
Nonspecific	Nonsucrose confectionary can be of benefit, but there may still be a risk of dental erosion. Sorbitol-containing pastilles may be helpful.
Specific	Pilocarpine (and possibly cevimeline) may be helpful, but there are no detailed studies of their application in children with long-standing xerostomia.
Oral hygiene care and dietary advice	Minimized risk of caries and gingivitis
Fluoride supplements	Reduces risk of caries

sion of all dental surfaces, but as with reflux-associated erosion, palatal surfaces of upper teeth particularly vulnerable).

2. Malnutrition: gives rise to gingival and oral mucosal disease. Profound malnutrition gives rise to severe acute necrotizing ulcerative gingivitis and later necrotic ulceration and loss of orofacial skin and muscles.
3. Anorexia and bulimia: oral mucosal ulceration is a consequence of resulting anemia. In bulimia, trauma of finger over palate can cause traumatic ulceration, palatal petechiae, and rarely necrotizing sialometaplasia. Acid reflux causes erosion of deciduous and permanent dentition. Erosion affects posterior teeth and palatal aspects of upper anterior teeth. Painless bilateral enlargement of parotids can occur without xerostomia owing to reflux of acidic gastric contents.

DEFICIENCIES
1. Vitamin C: gingival enlargement; friable gingivae.
2. Hematinic deficiencies: anemia secondary to hematinic deficiency may give rise to superficial ulceration of nonkeratinized (mobile) oral mucosa. Deficiencies of iron, B_{12}, and folate predispose to angular stomatitis (cheilitis) and glossitis (sore, erythematous, smooth tongue). B_{12} deficiency rarely gives rise to linear erythematous patches of dorsum tongue (Moeller glossitis).
3. Zinc deficiency: generally does not cause oral disease. Acrodermatitis enteropathica: oral mucosal ulceration, angular stomatitis.
4. Hypocalcemia: with celiac disease: hypocalcification of dentition (areas of whiteness and brown staining of enamel). With severe hypocalcemia: enamel pitting; secondary to autoimmune hypoparathyroid hormone in candidiasis endocrinopathy syndrome: enamel hypoplasia, especially of the permanent teeth.
5. Fluorosis: excess fluoride intake will cause some staining of enamel of developing teeth. Most commonly affects permanent dentition. Mild: chalky white patches of enamel. More severe: intrinsic brown staining. Severe: brown pitting, mottling, and brittleness of enamel. Enamel associated with fluorosis is resistant to caries.
6. Other causes of intrinsic dental staining: hyperbilirubinemia (yellow), tetracycline therapy, congenital erythropoietic porphyria (orange or red). Topical chlorhexidine, iron, and minocycline may cause more long-standing discoloration. Teeth can be stained orange, black, or green as consequence of chromogenic bacteria.

ORAL MANIFESTATIONS OF GASTROINTESTINAL DISEASE
1. Gluten-sensitive enteropathy (GSE): 3% with undiagnosed or poorly controlled GSE can develop superficial oral ulceration, usually of nonkeratinized oral mucosa. RAS unrelated. Additional oral features include glossitis, angular stomatitis secondary to hematinic deficiencies, enamel hypoplasia as consequence of longstanding hypocalcemia. Defects in children similar to those in dermatitis herpetiformis.

2. Cystic fibrosis: tetracycline staining of teeth most likely oral feature. Degree of staining depends upon age at which given, duration of therapy, and type of tetracycline provided. Vary in color from yellow to gray. Tetracycline does not influence risk of caries. Minocycline causes profound melanotic hyperpigmentation of oral mucosa that can mimic Addison disease. Vitamin K deficiency may predispose to spontaneous gingival bleeding.
3. Peutz-Jeghers syndrome: oral features rare, but notable circumoral melanosis (discrete brown-to-bluish black macules). Lower lip more affected than upper lip.
4. Ulcerative colitis: oral pyostomatitis vegetans more likely than in Crohn disease; course may follow bowel disease. Multiple small ragged superficial pustules, ulcers, and fissures of reflected mucosa of lips (usually upper), soft palate, and buccal mucosa; superficial ulceration related to hematinic deficiency.
5. Gardner syndrome: commonly affects mouth; up to 69% have clinical or radiologic evidence of oral lesions by adolescence. Multiple odontomas and supernumerary teeth common; delayed or failed eruption of permanent teeth (malocclusion); osteomas at mandible and maxilla.
6. Crohn disease: may give rise to persistent or recurrent lip swelling of one (typically the lower) or both lips. Enlargement can result in angular stomatitis and median fissuring, exacerbated by accompanying iron and vitamin B_{12} deficiency. Swollen buccal mucosa (cobblestoned appearance); ragged deep ulcers; superficial oral mucosal ulceration secondary to hematinic deficiencies. Melkersson-Rosenthal syndrome: combination of orofacial swelling, facial nerve palsy, fissured tongue, and mucosal swelling. Orofacial granulomatosis may represent intolerance to food additives; patch-testing and elimination diets may be helpful.

HEPATIC DISEASE AND VIRAL HEPATITIS
1. Kernicterus can cause intrinsic yellow staining of teeth.
2. Penicillamine therapy in primary biliary cirrhosis may cause lichenoid drug reaction in mouth clinically identical to idiopathic lichen planus.
3. Hepatitis C virus infection gives rise to destructive sialadenitis identical to Sjögren syndrome; not seen in children.

QUESTIONS

MATCH THE CONDITIONS WITH THE SYMPTOM OR SYNDROME:
a. Peutz-Jeghers syndrome.
b. Crohn disease.
c. Gardner syndrome.
d. Minocycline.
e. Celiac disease.

f.   Cyclosporine therapy.
g.   Chronic atrophic candidiasis.
h.   Malnutrition.
i.   Bulimia.

1.   Supernumerary teeth.
2.   Melkersson-Rosenthal syndrome.
3.   Palatal petechiae.
4.   Circumoral melanosis.
5.   Profound melanotic hyperpigmentation of oral mucosa.
6.   Gingival hyperplasia.
7.   Glossitis, angular stomatitis, and enamel hypoplasia.
8.   Acute necrotizing ulcerative gingivitis.
9.   Dental sore mouth.

MATCH THE CONDITIONS WITH THE CHARACTERISTICS:

a.   Minor aphthous ulceration.
b.   Major aphthous ulceration.
c.   Herpetiform ulceration.
d.   All of the above.
e.   None of the above.

10.   No scarring
11.   More females than males.
12.   Dorsum of tongue unaffected.
13.   Behçet disease.

CHOOSE THE BEST ANSWER:

14.   Causes of intrinsic dental staining include all except:
   a.   Hyperbilirubinemia.
   b.   Tetracycline therapy.
   c.   Iron therapy.
   d.   Chlorhexidine therapy.
   e.   Chromogenic bacteria.
   f.   Zinc deficiency.

CONGENITAL ANOMALIES

SYNOPSIS

PALATOGENESIS AND ANOMALIES

1.   Fetal facial development: starts at 5 weeks gestation. Frontonasal processes grow downwards to meet the maxillary processes, which grow laterally. Failure of fusion and incomplete penetration of mesoderm between ecto- and endoderm results in clefting anomalies.
2.   Palatogenesis: 7–12 weeks' gestation.
3.   Clefts: incidence of isolated cleft palate 1/2,000 live births. More females than males. More lip clefts than palate clefts. Multifactorial. Children with cleft lip or palate at risk for dental caries.
4.   Diagnosis: start at 15 weeks gestation via ultrasonography. Sensitivity 20–40%.

5.   Therapy: special nipples; evaluation by orthodontist, audiologist or otologist, surgeon, and feeding team. Cleft repair usually at 3 mo of age. Palate closure timing controversial, but most repaired in child aged 12–24 mo.

PIERRE ROBIN SYNDROME

1.   Essential features: micrognathia, posterior displacement of tongue into pharynx (glossoptosis), and respiratory obstruction secondary to anatomic and neuromuscular components. 20–40% nonsyndromic. Most associated with syndromes: Stickler syndrome (34%), velocardiofacial (11%), fetal alcohol syndrome (10%), and Treacher Collins syndrome (5%). Feeding problems common; can lead to failure to thrive. Full catch-up growth typically occurs during early childhood.
2.   Receding chin, high arched palate with or without cleft, and flattened nasal bridge. Cleft palate may also be feature. Associated cardiac anomalies not unusual.
3.   Therapy: nurse in prone position. Use of oral or nasopharyngeal airways may avoid need for tracheostomy. Nasogastric (NG) and gastrostomy tube feeds.

TONGUE ABNORMALITIES

1.   Osseous christmas: lesions composed of normal bone within soft tissue. When at tongue, usually posterior near foramen cecum. Increased frequency in those aged 20–40 yr, predominantly in females. Treatment: surgical excision. No recurrences or malignant transformation reported.
2.   Hamartomas: benign tumor-like proliferation of tissue at usual anatomic location. Lingual hamartomas occur in > 50% orofaciodigital syndrome. Airway obstruction is a problem with large lesions. Treatment: resection.
3.   Lingual teratomas: at foramen cecum. Typically encapsulated masses that may contain hair, skin, cartilage, or mucous membrane.
4.   Aglossia: extremely rare. Typically occurs in association with aglossia-adactylia syndrome and Goldenhar syndrome.
5.   Microglossia: often associated with other syndromes including Pierre Robin syndrome; patients may have difficulty with articulation. Tongue hemihypertrophy or hemiatrophy: associated with auricular, mandibular, and maxillary hypoplasia. Found in Parry-Romberg syndrome: congenital hemifacial hyperplasia.
6.   Macroglossia: enlarged tongue that protrudes beyond teeth or alveolar ridge.
   a.   Primary macroglossia: Beckwith-Wiedemann syndrome, mucopolysaccharidoses (Hurler and Hunter syndromes), neurofibromatosis (neurofibromas at tongue usually unilateral, slow growing), congenital hypothyroidism (secondary to myocyte hypertrophy and myxedematous tissue deposition).
   b.   Pseudomacroglossia: in Down syndrome and Pierre Robin syndrome where there is a small mandible.
   c.   Secondary macroglossia: lymphangioma (cystic hygroma), hemangiomas, and cystic lesions.

d. Initial management: ensuring patent airway. Nursing prone. NG tube as needed for feeding. Surgical debulking or partial glossectomy may be required.

7. Long tongue: seen in Ehlers-Danlos syndrome. No clinical symptomatology.

8. Accessory tongue: rare, usually attached to tonsil or from one side of base of the tongue.

9. Lingual thyroid: occurs when thyroid gland elements persist in area of foramen cecum. Usually along midline, color varies from red to purple. Usually grows with child. Thyroid scan required to determine amount of active thyroid tissue as this may be patient's only functional thyroid tissue. Surgical resection may be warranted. Increased risk of thyroid carcinoma in lingual thyroid tissue.

10. Ankyloglossia (tongue-tie): minor but common abnormality caused by an excessively short frenulum between floor of mouth and undersurface of tongue.
    a. Sequelae debated: unable to predict based on exam who will have problems. Mobility of tip of tongue may be impaired.
    b. Therapy: frenotomy or frenoplasty. Repair in child older than 1 yr often requires general surgery; younger children tolerate procedure in clinic setting.

11. Other abnormalities: Melkersson-Rosenthal syndrome (folded tongue), Coffin-Lowry syndrome (deep central lingual groove, thickened lips), Riley-Day syndrome (decreased numbers of fungiform and circumvallate papillae), and Klippel-Trénaunay-Weber syndrome (angiomatosis of tongue).

CYSTIC HYGROMA

1. Benign lymphangiomatous lesion affecting head and neck, usually at posterior neck. Typically develops between late first and early second trimester of pregnancy. Tendency to infiltrate tissue planes, including tongue and floor of the mouth. Can lead to life-threatening airway compromise.

2. Histology: fluid-filled (serous lymphatic fluid) spaces lined by endothelium.

3. Associations: numerous syndromes, including Turner and other karyotypic abnormalities. Also, exposure to alcohol, trimethadone, and aminopterin.

4. Antenatal diagnosis common. Large lesions (associated with fetal hydrops) have very poor outcome.

5. Therapy: complete surgical excision. Injection of lesion with substance OK 432 (mixture of group A *Streptococcus pyogenes*) or bleomycin shrinks lesions.

6. Recurrence following resection common if initial excision not complete.

EPIGNATHUS

1. Uncommon mature teratoma tumor that protrudes from mouth and arises from craniopharyngeal canal. Female-to-male ratio 3:1. More frequent in children with young mothers.

2. Obvious at birth; can be detected antenatally by ultrasonography. Associated with polyhydramnios.

3. Tumor benign. Well-recognized tissue, including formed limb and other body elements. Malignant degeneration never described.

4. Large lesions have high mortality due to airway obstruction. Initial treatment includes urgent establishment of airway.

5. Therapy: resection. Recurrence not reported.

EPULIS

1. Benign soft-tissue tumor arising from alveolar margin of upper or lower jaw, usually close to midline. Female-to-male ratio 8:1. Occurs 3 times more often at maxilla than at mandible.

2. Therapy: local excision. Metastases do not occur. Small amounts of residual tumor can regress spontaneously.

HAMARTOMA

1. Airway obstruction with large lesions: anywhere in body, including mouth and tongue.

2. Therapy: local resection.

NATAL AND NEONATAL TEETH

1. Natal teeth: observed in oral cavity at birth. Neonatal teeth: those that erupt during first month of life. Etiology unknown.

2. Teeth may be conical or normal in shape, normal in size, and opaque yellow-brown in color. Often absent root formation, irregular dentin formation, and hypoplastic enamel. Most are primary teeth and not supernumerary. Usually at region of lower incisors (85%).

3. Treatment depends on tooth's implantation, degree of mobility, and interruption of suckling. Removal only if difficulty in feeding or highly mobile.

RANULA

1. Retention cyst of a mucous gland in floor of the mouth. Bluish in color and displaces tongue upwards. Soft and slow to enlarge.

2. Rare in neonatal period. In newborn period, rarely reaches a size that causes significant symptoms.

3. Therapy: deroofing of cyst and marsupialization. May recur.

LARYNGOTRACHEOESOPHAGEAL CLEFT

1. Symptoms: respiratory difficulties, aspiration, choking, cyanosis, recurrent chest infections, and poor cry.

2. Diagnosis: direct endoscopic visualization most reliable method of diagnosis. See Figure 1. Presence of an intact arytenoid fold excludes the diagnosis of a cleft.

3. Management: minor cleft may not require therapy. Longer clefts: protect airway. Gastrostomy may be needed for nutrition. Esophageal dysmotility present after repair may still place patient at risk for aspiration.

ESOPHAGEAL ATRESIA AND TRACHEOESOPHAGEAL FISTULA

1. Incidence 1/3,000 to 1/4,000 live births. Highest rate among whites (Figure 2).

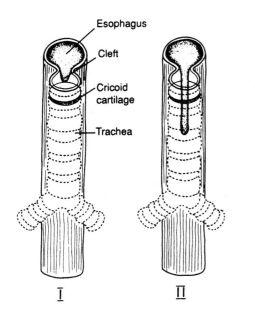
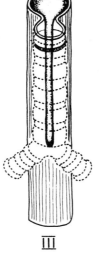
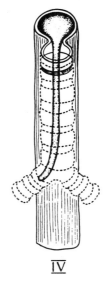

FIGURE 1   Types of defect. Type I, laryngeal cleft only. Type II, partial cleft involving the larynx, trachea, and esophagus. Type III, cleft extends distally to the carina. Type IV, cleft extends into the main bronchus.

2. Prolonged maternal use of oral contraceptives and exposure to progesterone and estrogen during pregnancy implicated as teratogens.
3. Clinical presentation: maternal polyhydramnios in one-half of cases. No fetal stomach after 20 weeks' gestation suggests of esophageal atresia (EA) but nondiagnostic. Neonate with EA: frothing saliva at mouth and nose and respiratory distress, worsening with feeds and aspiration. In isolated tracheoesophageal fistula (TEF): chronic respiratory symptoms and infections; bronchospasm.
4. Associated congenital anomalies common, 50–70%. VACTERL association.
5. Trachea often has more muscle than cartilage resulting

in tracheomalacia (in 75%). Lower esophageal sphincter (LES) typically incompetent; vagus nerve defective resulting in dysmotility.
6. Diagnosis: attempt NG tube. Plain chest and abdominal radiograph: gas in hollow viscera in abdomen indicates presence of coexisting TEF in the setting of EA. Can see associated skeletal abnormalities. Prenatal ultrasonography: positive predictive value 56% in setting of polyhydramnios and smaller than usual gastric bubble. For isolated TEF: pullback esophagogram in prone position necessary to detect isolated fistula. Bronchoscopy may identify isolated TEF.
7. Management: maintaining airway and preventing aspiration. Nursing in prone position with sump suction

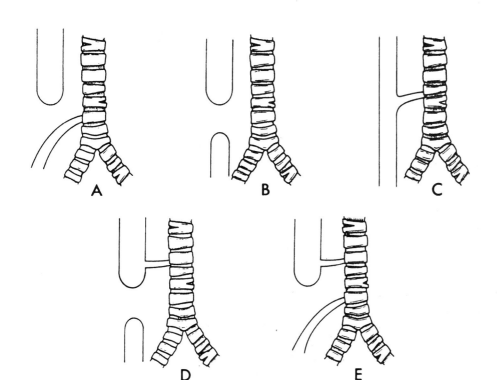

FIGURE 2   Types of esophageal atresia (EA) with or without tracheoesophageal fistula (TEF). A, EA with distal TEF (85%). B, EA without TEF (8%). C, Isolated TEF (4%). D, EA with proximal TEF (2%). E, EA with distal and proximal TEF (<1%).

in upper pouch on continuous aspiration. Endotracheal intubation should be avoided (places gas in bowel without ability to release).

8. Therapy: surgical TEF ligation and end-to-end anastomosis of esophagus. Long gap: gastrostomy with suction at upper pouch; colonic interposition required.

9. Postoperatively: risk of anastomotic leak (10–17%) and strictures. Gastroesophageal reflux (GER) common (70% via pH probe). Poor outcome if low birth weight or major cardiac anomalies.

CONGENITAL ESOPHAGEAL STENOSIS

1. Incidence 1/25,000 to 1/50,000 live births. Segmental stenosis attributable to tracheobronchial rests and segmental hypertrophy of the muscularis; submucosal fibrosis associated with esophageal atresia and tracheoesophageal fistula; membranous diaphragm type is least common.

2. Most at mid and distal third of esophagus with cartilaginous remnants.

3. Clinical presentation: may be asymptomatic. Respiratory symptoms if stenosis high. Regurgitation of feeds, failure to thrive, and solid food dysphagia.

4. Diagnosis: upper gastrointestinal (UGI) series: constant stenotic area. Esophagogastroduodenoscopy (EGD) may allow identification. Deep biopsy may reveal cartilaginous tissue.

5. Therapy: dilatations usually unsuccessful; requires surgery. Consider fundoplication at time of resection.

ESOPHAGEAL WEB AND RINGS

1. Rare abnormalities composed of mucosal membrane, which occludes lumen. Associated with TEF. Esophageal web tends to occur proximally. More common in females than males.

2. Plummer-Vinson syndrome: esophageal web associated with glossitis, iron deficiency anemia, and koilonychias (concave or spoon-shaped nails).

3. Associated diseases with webs: epidermolysis bullosa, cicatricial pemphigoid, Stevens-Johnson syndrome, psoriasis, idiopathic eosinophilic gastroenteritis, and graft-versus-host disease.

4. Esophageal rings:
   a. A-ring: asymptomatic, involves hypertrophied muscle; usually 1.5–2 cm above squamocolumnar junction.
   b. B-ring: synonymous with Schatzki's ring (occurs at squamocolumnar junction), only mucosa.
   c. C-ring: indentation of esophagus caused by diaphragmatic crura.
      Muscular ring varies caliber on barium swallow and may disappear with full distention (A-ring) but Schatski ring does not vary in appearance (B-ring).

5. Clinical presentation: identical to EA if complete membrane or web. When membrane perforates (Schatzki ring), symptoms may be absent. Steakhouse syndrome (acute dysphagia due to food impaction) commonly associated with Schatzki ring.

6. Diagnosis: EGD or UGI series; passing an orogastric tube can be diagnostic and demonstrate patency of the esophagus.

7. Therapy: surgical resection. In incomplete membranes: dilatation and EGD incision of membrane by cautery or laser. GER may require antireflux procedure

ESOPHAGEAL DUPLICATIONS, DORSAL ENTERIC CYSTS, AND BRONCHOGENIC CYSTS

1. Duplications: lined by gastrointestinal (GI) epithelium, have well-developed smooth muscle wall, and are attached to normal GI tract at some point through their length. Esophageal duplications are the most frequently encountered foregut duplication cysts, but rare. 80%: cysts are without luminal connection. Location: distal third of esophagus (80%), then proximal third (23%). Associated vertebral malformation (50%).

2. Bronchogenic cysts: mainly benign; most found within parenchyma of lung, but one-third present as mediastinal masses. Occasionally found in wall of esophagus; more often, compress esophagus from outside. Clinically difficult to distinguish from esophageal duplication cysts.

3. Clinical presentation: respiratory distress in neonatal period caused by enlarging cyst pressing on adjacent lung or airway. Dysphagia common in older children. In older children: erosion of duplication wall by acid secreted by gastric mucosa can cause massive GI or bronchial hemorrhage or spinal meningitis.

4. Diagnosis: barium swallow examination may reveal a communicating duplication or indentation of the esophagus. Chest computed tomography most useful.

5. Treatment: excision if possible. Excise bulk of duplication with mucosectomy.

ESOPHAGEAL DIVERTICULUM

1. True diverticula comprising all layers are rare. False or pulsion diverticula: herniations of mucosa through muscular layers are more common.

2. Zenker diverticulum: most common false diverticulum at esophagus at posterior midline between inferior constrictor and cricopharyngeal muscle. Usually present in patients aged 60–80 yr.

3. Causes of mid-esophageal and epiphrenic diverticula: motility disorders, including achalasia, diffuse esophageal spasm, nutcracker esophagus (high pressure waves at distal esophagus), and hypertensive LES.

4. Presentation: depends on size and position. Dysphagia from compression on esophageal wall. Halitosis from retained matter can occur.

5. Diagnosis: EGD and barium study.

6. Therapy: surgery when associated with aspiration. No treatment if asymptomatic. Treat underlying disorder.

ESOPHAGEAL INTRAMURAL PSEUDODIVERTICULOSIS

1. Multiple, small (1–3 mm) flask-shaped outpouchings of the esophagus. These are cystic dilations of esophageal gland ducts.

2. Associations: esophageal candidiasis (33%), strictures (almost always with stricture at upper or mid-esophagus with pseudodiverticula distal to stricture), and GER.

ESOPHAGEAL BRONCHUS

1. Most common congenital bronchopulmonary foregut malformation with the origin of a bronchus arising from the esophagus. May be associated with EA/TEF.
2. Clinical presentation: asymptomatic or respiratory symptoms; recurrent sepsis from consolidated or collapsed lung.
3. Diagnosis: initial chest radiograph may reveal lung opacity. Barium swallow study may show barium in lung. EGD may reveal fistula at middle or lower third of esophagus. Bronchoscopy shows absence of major bronchus. Angiography to determine blood supply to lung.
4. Therapy: surgical excision of bronchus and associated lung tissue.

FELINE ESOPHAGUS

1. Transient transverse fold of esophagus seen on upper EGD and double contrast esophagogram.
2. Seen as normal variant in GER.

VASCULAR RINGS

1. Usually presents during infancy or early childhood.
2. Variants include double aortic arches, right aortic arch with patent ductus arteriosus and ligamentum arteriosum.

QUESTIONS

MATCH THE CONDITION TO THE TIME PERIOD:

a. 12 mo of life.
b. 3–6 mo of life.
c. 5 wk of gestation.
d. 7–12 wk of gestation.

1. Palatogenesis.
2. Facial development starts.
3. Repair of cleft lip.
4. Repair of hard palate.

MATCH THE TERM TO ITS DESCRIPTION OR SYNONYM:

a. Ranula.
b. Epulis.
c. Tongue-tie
d. Cystic hygroma.

5. Ankyloglossia.
6. Retention cyst of a mucous gland in floor of the mouth.

7. Benign lymphangiomatous lesion affecting head and neck
8. Benign soft-tissue tumor arising from alveolar margin of upper or lower jaw.

CHOOSE THE BEST ANSWER:

9. The following represent correct associations except:
   a. Riley-Day syndrome and decreased numbers of fungiform papillae.
   b. Coffin-Lowry syndrome and thickened lips.
   c. Klippel-Trénaunay-Weber syndrome and angiomatosis of tongue.
   d. Melkersson-Rosenthal syndrome and folded tongue.
   e. Ehlers-Danlos syndrome and aglossia.

10. True macroglossia is seen in all except:
    a. Down syndrome.
    b. Hurler syndrome.
    c. Congenital hypothyroidism.
    d. Beckwith-Wiedemann syndrome.
    e. It is seen in all of the above.

11. Esophageal atresia occurs in:
    a. 1/500 live births
    b. 1/3,000 live births
    c. 1/10,000 live births
    d. 1/100,000 live births

12. Which is the most common type of esophageal atresia (EA)/tracheoesophageal fistula (TEF)?
    a. EA, distal TEF.
    b. H-type TEF, no esophageal atresia.
    c. EA, proximal TEF.
    d. EA with both proximal and distal TEF.
    e. EA without TEF.

13. The following are associated with esophageal webs except:
    a. Plummer-Vinson syndrome.
    b. Epidermolysis bullosa.
    c. Lupus.
    d. Psoriasis.
    e. Stevens-Johnson syndrome.

TRUE OR FALSE:

14. The presence of an intact arytenoid fold excludes the diagnosis of a laryngotracheoesophageal cleft.
15. Congenital esophageal stenosis is often successfully treated with dilatation therapy.
16. The majority of patients with Pierre Robin syndrome have an associated syndrome.

DISORDERS OF DEGLUTITION

SYNOPSIS

PHASES OF SWALLOWING
1. Oral: voluntary.
2. Pharyngeal: reflexive, lasts 1 second.
3. Esophageal: bolus transported via primary peristalsis.

ANATOMY OF SWALLOWING
1. Upper esophageal sphincter (UES): manometrically high-pressure zone distal to hypopharynx, composed of striated muscle. Cricopharyngeal (CP) muscle is main contributor to UES. Tonically closed at rest, opens during swallowing, belching. Major motor nerve of CP muscle is pharyngoesophageal nerve. Sensation via glossopharyngeal nerve and sympathetic nervous system.
2. Swallowing center: activated by cerebral cortex (voluntary) and peripheral receptors in mouth and pharynx (reflex); includes glossopharyngeal (IX), superior laryngeal (X), and recurrent laryngeal (X) nerves (reflex).
3. Tongue: infant: tongue lies entirely in oral cavity; at age 2–4 yr: tongue moves posteriorly; at age 9 yr: posterior third of tongue in neck.
4. Larynx: infant: third or fourth cervical vertebrae; child: sixth cervical vertebrae; adult: seventh cervical vertebrae.

DEGLUTITION
1. In utero: occurs at 16–17 weeks gestation. Important in amniotic fluid resorption, recirculation of urine, lung fluids, and maintaining amniotic fluid volume.
2. Nutritive sucking: Characterized by series of short bursts and pauses; one suck per second.
3. Nonnutritive sucking: rhythmic movements on a non-feeding nipple. Short bursts and pauses occur at a faster frequency.
4. Complications of impaired deglutition: apnea, bradycardia, choking, chronic noisy breathing, reactive airway disease, chronic or recurrent pneumonia, bronchitis, atelectasis, and aspiration; sialorrhea (excessive drooling) in patients with neurologic disease.
5. Preterm infant: suckle-feeds at 34 weeks gestation; coordination of swallowing and breathing may not be mature.
6. Critical period of learning: inadequate oral stimulation during a critical period may result in oral aversion.

DISORDERS
1. Isolated CP dysfunction and CP achalasia: rare in children and infants.
2. Most patients with CP achalasia present at birth with feeding difficulties.
3. Diagnosis difficult (Table 1). On upper GI, horizontal bar in proximal esophagus seen in CP dysfunction; is also seen in up to 5% of adults and may be normal in infants.

TABLE 1   DIFFERENTIAL DIAGNOSES OF DYSPHAGIA IN PEDIATRIC PATIENTS

PREMATURITY

UPPER AIRWAY-FOODWAY ANOMALIES
Nasal and nasopharyngeal
    Choanal atresia and stenosis
    Nasal and sinus infections
    Septal deflections
    Tumors
Oral cavity and oropharynx
    Defects of lips and alveolar processes
    Cleft lip and/or cleft palate
    Hypopharyngeal stenosis and webs
    Craniofacial syndromes (eg, Pierre Robin, Crouzon, Treacher Collins, Goldenhar)
Laryngeal
    Laryngeal stenosis and webs
    Laryngeal clefts
    Laryngeal paralysis
    Laryngomalacia

CONGENITAL DEFECTS OF THE LARYNX, TRACHEA, AND ESOPHAGUS
Laryngotracheoesophageal cleft
Tracheoesophageal fistula/esophageal atresia
Esophageal strictures and webs
Vascular anomalies
    Aberrant right subclavian artery (dysphagia lusorum)
    Double aortic arch
    Right aortic arch with left ligamentum

ACQUIRED ANATOMIC DEFECTS
Trauma
    External trauma
    Intubation and endoscopy

NEUROLOGIC DEFECTS
Central nervous system disease
    Head trauma
    Hypoxic brain damage
    Cortical atrophy, microcephaly, anencephaly
    Infections (eg, meningitis, brain abscess)
    Myelomeningocele
    Chiari malformation
Peripheral nervous system disease
    Traumatic
    Congenital
Neuromuscular disease
    Myotonic muscular dystrophy
    Myasthenia gravis
    Guillain-Barré syndrome
    Poliomyelitis (bulbar paralysis)
Miscellaneous
    Achalasia
    Cricopharyngeal achalasia
    Esophageal spasm
    Esophagitis
    Dysautonomia
    Paralysis of esophagus (atony)
    Tracheoesophageal fistula/esophageal atresia–associated nerve defects
    Aberrant cervical thymus
    Conversion dysphagia

Adapted from Weiss MH. Dysphagia in infants and children. Otolaryngol Clin North Am 1988;21:727–735; and Cohen SR. Difficulty with swallowing. In: Bluestone CD, Stool SF, editors. Pediatric otolaryngology. Philadelphia: W.B. Saunders; 1983.

4. CP achalasia may resolve spontaneously or after dilatation. Myotomy may be required but is contraindicated in patients with gastroesophageal reflux or poor pharyngeal peristalsis.

CLINICAL ASSESSMENT

1. Feeding history.
2. Nutritional assessment.
3. Physical exam: facial, oral cavity, oropharynx structure, and gag reflex.
4. Observational feeding trial.

DIAGNOSTIC TESTS

1. Videofluoroscopy: modified barium swallow, with liquids, pastes, and pureed foods.
2. Pharyngeal manometry.
3. Ultrasonography: poor visualization of oropharynx and lack of standardization.
4. Nuclear scintigraphy: poor resolution of image.
5. Cervical auscultation: lack of standards.
6. Fiberoptic endoscopic evaluation of swallowing: observes pharyngeal phase.
7. Fiberoptic endoscopic evaluation of swallowing with sensory testing: determination of laryngopharyngeal sensation.

TREATMENT

TABLE 2   IMPAIRED SWALLOWING: MANAGEMENT TECHNIQUES

Alteration of the oral bolus—modify volume, physical properties (eg, consistency, temperature)

Proper intraoral bolus placement

Adjust position of the head, neck, and body during deglutition

Provide jaw control and stabilization during deglutition

Decrease oral hypersensitivity/increase oral hyposensitivity—thermal sensitization/stimulation

Extinguish abnormal feeding behaviors

Swallowing exercises
    Tongue resistance/range of motion
    Laryngeal adduction

Protection maneuvers—supraglottic swallow procedure

Cricopharyngeal myotomy

Suckle-feeding—valved feeding bottle

Provide alternate means of enteral nutrition
    Nasogastric feeding
    Gastrostomy tube (surgical or endoscopic)

Adapted from Tuchman DN. Dysfunctional swallowing in the pediatric patient: clinical considerations. Dysphagia 1988;2:203–8.

QUESTIONS

TRUE OR FALSE:

1. The oral phase of swallowing is voluntary.
2. The tongue lies entirely in the oral cavity in infants.
3. The larynx is at its final position at birth.
4. Cricopharyngeal achalasia can resolve spontaneously.

MATCH THE FOLLOWING:

a. Cerebral cortex.
b. Cranial nerve IX.
c. Vagus nerve.
d. All of the above.

5. Activates swallowing center.
6. Recurrent laryngeal nerve.
7. Glossopharyngeal nerve.

CHOOSE THE BEST ANSWER:

8. When is a fetus able to suckle-feed?
    a. 28 weeks.
    b. 30 weeks.
    c. 32 weeks.
    d. 34 weeks.
    e. 36 weeks.

9. When during gestation does deglutition begin?
    a. 10 weeks.
    b. 12 weeks.
    c. 14 weeks.
    d. 16 weeks.
    e. 18 weeks.

GASTROESOPHAGEAL REFLUX

SYNOPSIS

PRESENTATION AND SYMPTOMS

1. Manifests differently in infants and in older children.
2. Infants: regurgitation, crying, malnutrition, and apnea.
3. Children: pain and asthma.

NATURAL HISTORY

1. Regurgitation resolves in most symptomatic infants by 12–24 mo.
2. By 9 years of age, if still present reflux symptoms tend to persist.

PATHOPHYSIOLOGY

1. Predominant mode of gastroesophageal reflux (GER) in infants and older children: transient lower esophageal sphincter relaxation (TLESR) unassociated with normal peristalsis allow gastric contents to reflux.
2. Tonic lower esophageal sphincter (LES) pressure is usually maintained above 4 mm Hg (adequate to prevent reflux). Relaxation of LES via vagal pathways occurs via the brainstem.
3. Esophageal peristalsis:
    a. Gravity: crude clearance in upright persons.
    b. Primary peristalsis: initiated by swallowing.
    c. Secondary peristalsis: stimulated by esophageal distention.
    d. Esophagitis impairs peristaltic function.
    e. Saliva washes down the esophagus and neutralizes residual acid.
4. Nocturnal reflux uncommon in normal children, but occurs in children with gastroesophageal reflux disease (GERD) (Figure 1).
5. Components of the refluxate determine pathogenicity to esophageal mucosa. Pepsin when acidified produces an irreversible lesion at esophageal squamous epithelium.

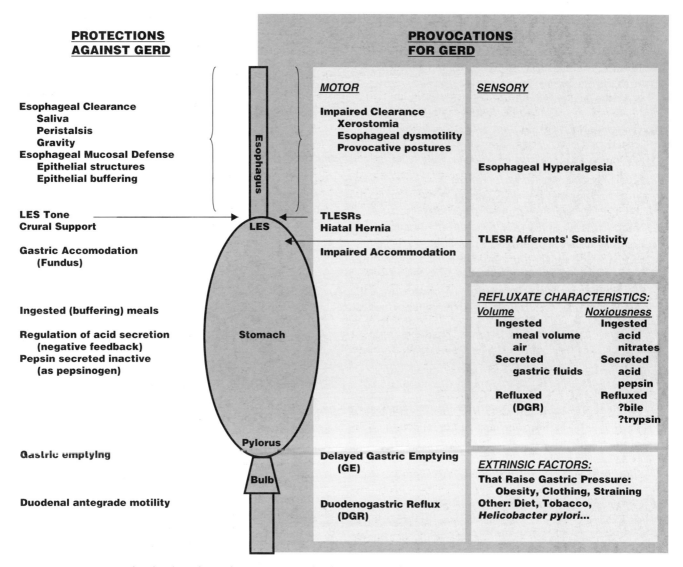

FIGURE 1   Cartoon of pathophysiology of GERD. DGR = duodenogastric reflux; GE = gastric emptying; GERD = gastroesophageal reflux disease; LES = lower esophageal sphincter; TLESRs = transient LES relaxations.

Acid and pepsin increased in patients with esophagitis, strictures, and Barrett syndrome.

6. *Helicobacter pylori* gastritis with its decreased acidity and volume of refluxate may protect against GERD.

DIAGNOSIS

1. Upper gastrointestinal series: to rule out anatomic abnormality.
2. 24h pH probe monitoring of physiologic conditions has notable variability, postprandial detection difficult with food buffering. Most useful for determining effectiveness of therapy and temporal correlation with symptoms.
3. Endoscopy: most accurate method of demonstrating esophageal damage by reflux. Histologic criteria of GERD: in adults, basal zone hyperplasia and increased stromal papillae. In infants, normal thickening of basal zone at distal esophagus. Presence of intraepithelial eosinophils correlates with presence of GERD in infancy but can indicate eosinophilic esophagitis if > 20 per high power field. Pain: correlation with endoscopic or histologic esophagitis is incomplete.

4. Impedance: demonstrates bolus reflux without regard for acidity; may complement pH monitoring. Cumbersome to perform and analyze.
5. Scintigraphy: noninvasive, low radiation. Assesses postprandial GER and severity. Detects stomach emptying rate. Milk scan detects pulmonary aspiration.
6. Manometry: demonstrates volumetric reflux and TLESR and defective peristalsis.
7. Bilirubin monitoring: developed owing to potential pathogenicity of duodenogastric reflux, which does not cause esophagitis unless with acid.
8. Bronchial lavage: detects intratracheal lipid-laden macrophages; useful to detect aspiration but not whether secondary to swallowing or reflux.
9. Empiric treatment trial: brief trials to spare more invasive, costly diagnostic testing; nonresponding or relapsing symptoms require more testing.

THERAPY

1. Prone positioning: helpful, but limited in ages where sudden infant death syndrome is an issue. Reduced

volume, frequent feeds: effective in many infants. Thickened feeds: reduce emesis, crying, and wakenings, but not number of reflux episodes, per pH probe.
2. Medications:
    a. Antacids.

es gastric emptying.
yramidal neck pain
gyric crisis).
efit.
e United States.
gonist resulting in
. Major side effect:
ythmias.

ommon procedure:
st 3.5 cm of esoph-
ostsurgical compli-
wrap, vagal injury,
ne.
usly surgeons used
t patients; current
as fundoplication
tying.

NS

esult in esophageal
cid ± pepsin. Gen-
ird of esophagus,
hagus. Treatment:
therapy; for resis-
of steroids at time
ion.
aplasia of distal
with neurologic
isease, repaired
d hiatal hernia.
a size, length of
cid reflux are all

ease in sinusitis,
bronchiectasis;
laryngomalacia.
n or sinusitis can
apy.
way response to
airway response

ns makes GERD
studies, scintig-
py, laryngobronchoscopy, and endoscopy.
4. Therapy: aggressive in potency and duration to affect

respiratory symptoms with bid proton pump inhibitor therapy for at least 3 months. Fundoplication surgery provides better results.

NEUROLOGIC IMPAIRMENT
Neurologically impaired children have more GERD and more complicated GERD than neurologically normal counterparts.

QUESTIONS

CHOOSE THE BEST ANSWER:
1. A barium swallow or upper gastrointestinal (UGI) series is helpful to determine all except:
    a. Atypical pyloric stenosis.
    b. Duodenal web.
    c. Malrotation.
    d. Hiatal hernia.
    e. Gastric emptying.
    f. All of the above can be determined by a UGI series.

2. The following have proved useful in the assessment of gastroesophageal reflux (GER) except:
    a. pH probe.
    b. Endoscopic evaluation and biopsy.
    c. Manometry.
    d. Scintigraphy.
    e. Bronchial lavage.
    f. All of the above are helpful in GER assessment.

3. The following are true of cisapride except:
    a. Enhances acetylcholine release.
    b. Is a 5-HT4 receptor antagonist.
    c. Prolongs QTc interval.
    d. Carries an increased risk for side effects in young infants owing to decreased hepatic metabolism.
    e. Has no significant central nervous system effects.
    f. All of the above.

TRUE OR FALSE:
4. Placement of a gastrostomy tube can initiate or worsen GER.
5. Bethanechol has been shown to be effective in reducing GER by pH probe.
6. Thickened feeds have been shown to reduce the number of reflux episodes.
7. The presence of subglottic stenosis should prompt an evaluation for GERD even in the absence of other GER symptoms.
8. Patients with familial dysautonomia and GERD often can be managed with aggressive medical therapy.
9. Histologic severity of esophagitis correlates with pH-measured reflux.

ESOPHAGITIS

SYNOPSIS

ETIOLOGIES

1. Chemical: owing to reflux or swallowed substances.
2. Immunologic: owing to specific responses to specific antigens.
3. Infective.
4. Traumatic.
5. Systemic: Crohn disease and chronic granulomatous disease.
6. Miscellaneous: Munchausen syndrome by proxy.
7. Idiopathic: for example, idiopathic eosinophilic esophagitis.

GASTROESOPHAGEAL REFLUX

1. Natural history: improves with age.
2. Cause of infantile gastroesophageal reflux: combination of anatomic relationship of the lower esophageal sphincter (LES) preventing effective pressure generation and inappropriate LES relaxation. Acid with pepsin causes severe esophagitis. Role of duodenogastroesophageal reflux remains controversial.

CHEMICAL ESOPHAGITIS OWING TO SWALLOWED SUBSTANCES

1. Alkaline substance ingestion can result in acute perforation at the esophagus and mediastinitis and subsequent stricture.
2. Medications associated with esophageal damage and esophagitis: tetracyclines, acne medications, and non-steroidal antiinflammatory drugs.

IMMUNOLOGIC

Multiple food antigens may induce esophagitis; most common precipitant is cow's milk protein. Eosinophilia at esophageal mucosa < 10–15 eosinophils per high power field. Dietary exclusion of cow's milk and oral steroids can induce remission with decreased mucosal eosinophilia. Eotaxin (eosinophil-specific chemokine) found to have increased expression in cow's milk protein–associated esophagitis along with activated T lymphocytes

INFECTIVE

Most infective esophagitis occurs in immunocompromised child: due to herpes simplex virus (HSV), cytomegalovirus (CMV), and *Candida*.

1. HSV esophagitis: can occur in normal immune function but more common in immunocompromised. Characteristic nuclear inclusions and multinucleate giant cells may not be seen on histology. Volcano ulcers seen on endoscopy. Acyclovir or foscarnet (if acyclovir-resistant) recommended in immunocompromised.
2. CMV esophagitis: basophilic nuclear inclusions on biopsy of ulcer edge. Predominantly found in immunocompromised. Treat with ganciclovir or foscarnet.

3. *Candida* is the most common infectious cause of esophagitis; white mucosal plaques. Oral *Candida* is not predictive of esophageal involvement except in the immunocompromised host (even then esophageal candidiasis can be seen without oral involvement). Diagnosis confirmed by presence of hyphae in biopsies. Complications: fistulae, perforation, stricture formation, dysmotility, transient achalasia, and systemic candidiasis. Treatment: 2–6 weeks of oral nystatin or fluconazole or liposomal amphotericin.

TRAUMATIC

1. Nasogastric tube can be associated with abrasive esophagitis.
2. Radiation-induced esophageal strictures are described in children receiving mediastinal irradiation (usually > 4000 cGy) and doxorubicin.

SYSTEMIC DISEASE MANIFESTATIONS

1. Crohn disease lesions at the esophagus are usually distinct rounded ulcers. Diffuse disease may also occur.
2. Glycogen storage disease type 1B may present with a similar phenotype to Crohn disease.
3. Inflammation, stricturing of the esophagus can occur in chronic granulomatous disease.
4. Scleroderma and vasculitic conditions have significant esophageal pathology in adults; rare in children.

MISCELLANEOUS

1. Passive smoking has strong association with esophagitis.
2. Munchausen syndrome by proxy can lead to esophagitis via the deliberate introduction into the esophagus of caustic substances.

IDIOPATHIC EOSINOPHILIC ESOPHAGITIS

1. Characteristics: dense eosinophilic infiltrate > 20–40 eosinophils/high power field in the absence of reflux or parasite infection. Interleukin (IL)-5 and eotaxin play a role.
2. Symptoms: dysphagia, odynophagia, and chest pain. Result in narrowing or stricturing of proximal or mid esophagus.
3. Endoscopy shows concentric indentations for most of the length of the esophagus. Distal esophagus may be spared. Allergy testing usually does not identify a responsible allergen.
4. Treatment with topical steroid, systemic steroids, or azathioprine may be effective. Elimination diet usually not therapeutic.

SYMPTOMS

1. Infants: irritability, Sandifer syndrome with paroxysmal head posturing described, refractory wheezing, and hematemesis.
2. Children age 1–5 yr: feeding disorders, food refusal, and sleeping disorders. No clear relationship between symptoms and severity of esophagitis.
3. Older children: symptoms similar to adults. Rarely, hypertrophic osteoarthropathy has been reported with esophagitis in childhood.

DIAGNOSIS

1. Ambulant esophageal pH analysis: indication of the nature and severity of acid or alkali reflux.
2. Endoscopy with biopsy: reveals nature and severity of esophagitis. In general, esophageal endoscopic appearances do not reliably differentiate between reflux and other causative pathologies.
3. Upper gastrointestinal series (barium): provides an anatomic evaluation.
4. Intraluminal impedance: determination of reflux episodes independent of pH; can describe patterns of antegrade and retrograde bolus movement.
5. Manometry: limited usefulness.

HISTOLOGY

1. Elongation of stromal papillae and basal zone hyperplasia is a useful indicator of reflux.
2. Esophageal mucosal eosinophilia has been described in cow's milk–associated, eosinophilic esophagitis and in primary reflux esophagitis.
3. Immunohistochemical markers have been used. An increase in Ki-67 has been shown in the longer papillae seen in reflux. Eotaxin has an increased expression colocalized with activated T lymphocytes to the basal and papillary epithelium in cow's milk protein–associated esophagitis.
4. Electron microscopy demonstrates ultrastructural changes associated with esophagitis. Eosinophil activation can help distinguish between reflux and cow's milk protein esophagitis.

MANAGEMENT

1. Dictated by etiology: spontaneous resolution may occur. 60% will be symptom-free by 18 months of age, greatest improvement at 8–10 months when the child sits upright. Normal or mildly erythematous mucosa or only histologic esophagitis: simple measures (positioning), thickening agents, increasing frequency and decreasing the volumes of feeds. Erosive esophagitis or refractory to conservative measures: medications (Zantac, proton pump inhibitor [PPI], metoclopramide, domperidone). Cases refractory to maximal medical therapy: surgery (Nissen fundoplication: full wraparound of gastric fundus at distal esophagus; Thal procedure: 80% circumferential wrap) to prevent full LES relaxation and reduce transient LES relaxations.
2. Cow's milk protein–associated esophagitis: removal of cow's milk protein from diet. 30–40% cross reaction with soy protein. Casein hydrolysate products often used. May be necessary to put the infant on elemental (amino acids) formulas. Some infants may be helped by oral sodium cromoglycate.
3. Idiopathic eosinophilic esophagitis: oral or inhaled steroids.
4. Infective esophagitis: specific therapies (as described above).
5. Caustic esophagitis: initially conservative treatment with barium swallow 4–6 weeks post-ingestion, endo-

scopic evaluation, and stricture dilation as needed. To prevent restenosis: antifibrotic (mitomycin C) applied topically to the mucosa poststricture dilation.
6. Barrett esophagus (gastric metaplasia that develops after long-term acid exposure): antireflux surgery or long-term PPI. Requires frequent monitoring for associated adenocarcinoma.

QUESTIONS

CHOOSE THE BEST ANSWER:

1. The following are true of childhood gastroesophageal reflux except:
   a. In children, tends to improve spontaneously with age.
   b. Is associated with transient lower esophageal sphincter relaxation.
   c. Esophagitis results from exposure to acid and pepsin.
   d. Is associated with elongation of stromal papillae and basal zone hyperplasia.
   e. All of the above are true.

2. The most common food antigen causing esophagitis is:
   a. Soy protein.
   b. Cow's milk protein.
   c. Peanuts.
   d. Environmental allergies.
   e. Wheat.

3. The following are true of idiopathic eosinophilic esophagitis except:
   a. Associated with well-identified food allergies.
   b. Characterized by eosinophilic infiltrate > 20–40 eosinophils/high power field.
   c. May result in stricturing at the proximal or mid esophagus.
   d. Can spare the distal esophagus.
   e. Responds to topical or systemic steroids.

4. Symptoms associated with esophagitis in children include:
   a. Irritability.
   b. Paroxysmal head posturing.
   c. Hematemesis.
   d. Food refusal.
   e. Hypertrophic osteoarthropathy.
   f. All of the above.

TRUE OR FALSE:

5. *Candida* is the most common infectious cause of esophagitis.
6. Herpes simplex virus esophagitis is easily diagnosed on endoscopy.
7. Ambulant pH evaluation can evaluate all episodes of reflux.
8. Children with cow's milk protein allergy–induced esophagitis should have intact cow's milk protein and soy protein eliminated from their diet.

OTHER MOTOR DISORDERS

SYNOPSIS

CRICOPHARYNGEAL DISORDERS

1. Cricopharyngeal muscle:
   a. Disorders usually appear shortly after birth or during first 2 months of life.
   b. Symptoms: repeated aspirations, choking, and pooling of saliva at pharynx.
   c. Upper gastrointestinal (UGI) series: holding up of barium at upper esophageal sphincter (UES).
   d. Major 2 defects: abnormalities of sphincter resting pressure and abnormalities in UES relaxation.
2. Cricopharyngeal hypertension: horizontal esophageal bar on UGI series, although normal finding in 5% of adults and in infants; manometry may be helpful.
3. Cricopharyngeal hypotension: seen in myoneural disorders including amyotrophic lateral sclerosis, myasthenia gravis, and polymyositis.
4. Abnormalities of relaxation: may see on UGI series or manometric studies.
5. Treatment:
   a. Achalasia: in adults: treatments range from bougienage (effects short-lived) to surgery; Botox available for those at high risk for surgery. In children: possible spontaneous improvement, good response after dilatation. Conservative approach is best.
   b. Premature cricopharyngeal closure: may spontaneously resolve.
   c. Delayed relaxation (found in Riley-Day syndrome): nitrazepam administration.

STRIATED MUSCLE OF ESOPHAGUS

MYOPATHIC DISEASES

1. Muscular dystrophies: dysphagia rare except for 2 types.
   a. Myotonic muscular dystrophy: symptoms: myotonic facies, muscle wasting, frontal baldness, testicular atrophy, and cataracts. Myotonia presents 2–15 yr before dysphagia. Involves both striated and smooth muscle. UGI series shows barium stasis, and hypomotility owing to pharyngeal weakness.
   b. Oculopharyngeal dystrophy.
2. Inflammatory myopathies: inflammation of skeletal muscle affects striated muscles of pharynx and esophagus; dysphagia related to pharyngeal muscle weakness; may respond to steroids.
3. Arnold-Chiari malformation: associated with dysphagia and UES dysfunction. Outcome after surgical correction depends on severity of preoperative symptoms. Patients with unexpected cricopharyngeal dysfunction should be evaluated for Chiari malformation.
4. Motor neuron disease: degeneration of upper or lower motor neurons. In children, bulbar palsy: leads to sucking, swallowing, and drooling. Jaw jerk exaggerated (diagnostic clue). In lower motor neuron form: poor suck and nasal regurgitation. If facial bulbar paralysis and facial diplegia = Möbius syndrome.

OTHER

1. Myasthenia gravis: affects the motor end plate of striated muscle. Dysphagia, choking, and aspiration of food. Difficulties as meal progresses. Recovery of abnormalities with Tensilon (edrophonium chloride).
2. Multiple sclerosis: swallowing difficulties common.
3. Polio: bulbar poliomyelitis may cause dysphagia.
4. Botulism: binding of toxin to peripheral cholinergic terminals preventing release of acetylcholine at the neuromuscular junction. Symptoms: peripheral muscle weakness, hypotonia, respiratory depression, and diminished suck and swallow. Disruption of UES function and peristalsis in proximal esophagus. No significant effect on lower esophageal sphincter (LES) and distal esophagus.
5. Drugs: delayed cricopharyngeal relaxation associated with nitrazepam, also neuroleptics.

SMOOTH MUSCLES OF ESOPHAGUS

PRIMARY DISORDERS

Achalasia

1. Characteristics: increased LES pressure, partial or incomplete LES relaxation, loss of esophageal peristalsis. Incidence 1/10,000; usual presentation age 20–40 yr, but can present as neonate; < 5% manifest before age 15 yr. Involves Auerbach plexus with progressive ganglion loss. Possible nitric oxide and vasoactive intestinal polypeptide deficiency and lack of inhibitory innervation.
2. Associations:
   a. Allgrove (triple-A) syndrome: adrenocorticotropic hormone deficiency, alacrima, and achalasia.
   b. Rozychi syndrome: autosomal recessive. Deafness, vitiligo, short stature, muscle weakness, familial dysautonomia, and hypophosphatemic rickets.
   c. Suggested to be associated with: Down syndrome, pyloric stenosis, Hodgkin disease, and Hirschsprung disease.
   d. Symptoms in children: vomiting (80%), dysphagia (76%), weight loss, respiratory symptoms, odynophagia, failure to thrive, and nocturnal regurgitation (21%).
3. Diagnosis:
   a. Radiology: chest radiograph: widened mediastinum and air-fluid level; UGI series: beaking and sigmoid esophagus.
   b. Endoscopy: used for exclusion of other inflammatory processes.
   c. Manometry: test of choice. Demonstrates increased LES pressure (if normal does not exclude diagnosis) and absence of peristalsis (pathognomic). Amplitude of tertiary contractions: if > 50–

60 mmHg, vigorous achalasia. Incomplete or abnormal relaxation of LES. Intraesophageal pressure greater than gastric pressure.

   d. Radionucleotide tests: ingestion of labeled solid meal with retention in esophagus even in upright position.

   e. Provocative tests: mecholyl test: increase in esophageal baseline pressure and high amplitude contractions; positive for achalasia if rise in pressure > 25 mm Hg, lasting for at least 30 s; contraindicated in patients with asthma or heart disease. cholecystokinin octapeptide: causes paradoxical contraction in achalasia (nonspecific result for impaired innervation to LES)

4. Treatment:

   a. Anticholinergic drugs: no value.

   b. Nitrates: isosorbide dinitrate; acts on LES; allows patient to eat meal. High incidence of side effects with long-term use.

   c. Ca-channel blockers: nifedipine, good temporizing option.

   d. Botox: intrasphincteric injection; short-term efficacy; may lead to inflammation and fibrosis at LES making future surgery more difficult. Suboptimal to pneumatic dilatation (PD) or myotomy; considered in poor candidates for invasive surgery or other procedures.

   e. Bougienage: disappointing.

   f. PD: complications: perforation, gastroesophageal reflux (GER), bleeding. Perform after failed myotomy.

   g. Heller myotomy: suggested as primary therapy. Antireflux procedure if pathologic GER documented preoperatively.

5. Possible relationship between achalasia and esophageal cancer: no information about incidence of cancer complication in patients who developed achalasia as children.

Chagas Disease

1. Destruction by *Trypanosoma cruzi* of Auerbach plexus (widely seen in South America).

Diffuse Esophageal Spasm

1. Primary disorder of motor activity in the smooth muscle portion of the esophagus. Only case reports in children.

2. Symptoms: chest pain may be initiated by cold or hot meals; not associated with weight loss. In infants: apnea and sudden infant death syndrome; in children: aspiration pneumonia.

3. Diagnosis: established by manometry with repetitive nonperistaltic contractions at least 10% wet swallows, normal peristaltic sequence periods, alterations in contractions (increased duration and amplitude), and normal LES.

4. Barium swallow shows frequent nonpropulsive contractions usually at lower third.

5. Treatment: symptom reduction: calcium channel blockers, nitrates, peppermint oil, antidepressants, PD, surgery, and botulinum toxin injection.

SECONDARY DISORDERS

1. Esophageal atresia and tracheoesophageal fistula: esophageal peristalsis dysfunction probably reflects both congenital abnormalities and injury following surgical repair.

2. Idiopathic intestinal pseudo-obstruction: ≥ 85% have abnormal esophageal motility.

3. Hirschsprung disease: abnormal esophageal motility more associated with total colonic aganglionosis than short segment.

4. Caustic ingestion: strictures and dysphagia common; motility abnormalities present.

5. Esophageal sclerotherapy and band ligation: both affect esophageal motility. Possibly reversible.

6. Collagen vascular disease, especially scleroderma: incompetent LES and low amplitude esophageal contractions at smooth muscle portion of esophagus; later, alterations in striated muscle section. Treatment mainly directed at GER symptom relief.

7. Graft-versus-host-disease: esophagogastroduodenoscopy: desquamative esophagitis at upper and middle third and frequent webs. Distal esophagus: usually normal. Manometry: frequently abnormal. Pathology: no nerve or muscle abnormalities; motor alterations may be related to mucosal abnormalities or immunologic phenomena.

QUESTIONS

MATCH THE CHARACTERISTICS TO THE CONDITIONS:

a. Cricopharyngeal disorders.
b. Myotonic muscular dystrophy.
c. Möbius syndrome.
d. Myasthenia gravis.
e. Pyloric stenosis.
f. Loss of esophageal peristalsis.
g. Increased lower esophageal sphincter pressure.
h. Allgrove syndrome.
i. Rozychi syndrome.
j. Down syndrome.
k. Hirschsprung disease.
l. Chagas disease.
m. Sudden infant death syndrome.
n. Supranuclear bulbar palsy.

1. Diffuse esophageal spasm.
2. Proven association with achalasia.
3. Progressive dysphagia with meal intake.
4. Presents in first 2 months of life.
5. Associated with frontal baldness and hypogonadism.
6. Jaw jerk.
7. Facial diplegia and facial bulbar dysfunction.
8. Hallmark finding of achalasia.
9. Hypophosphatemic rickets, vitiligo, and deafness.
10. Achalasia, alacrima, and Addison disease.

TRUE OR FALSE:

11. Muscle and nerve histopathology is present in persons with esophageal graft-versus-host disease with dysphagia.

CHOOSE THE BEST ANSWER:

12. Of the following muscular dystrophies, which is associated with dysphagia in children?
    a. Becker muscular dystrophy.
    b. Duchenne muscular dystrophy.
    c. Myotonic dystrophy.
    d. None of the above are associated.

INJURIES OF THE ESOPHAGUS

SYNOPSIS

FOREIGN BODY AND COIN INGESTIONS

1. Pharyngeal and cricopharyngeal foreign bodies: best approached with laryngoscope.

2. Esophageal foreign body: most pass spontaneously especially if diameter < 2 cm. Transit retarded at cricopharyngeal ring (in 60–65% of cases), aortic arch (10–15%), lower esophageal sphincter (20–25%), pylorus, duodenal curve, ligament of Treitz, Meckel diverticulum, ileocecal valve, appendix, and rectosigmoid junction. Once in stomach, generally passes through remainder of gastrointestinal (GI) tract without difficulty. Sharp or pointed objects may perforate or become impacted at ileocolic valve. High incidence of complications reported with objects > 5 cm in length, > 2.5 cm in diameter, and batteries.

3. Symptoms: choking, hoarseness, refusal to eat, vomiting, drooling, blood-stained saliva, and respiratory distress. Long-standing foreign bodies can present as neck mass, chronic cough or stridor, or dysphagia. Crepitus, erythema, tenderness, and swelling may be present with pharyngeal or esophageal perforation.

4. Diagnosis: plain films for opaque items: posteroanterior and lateral. Handheld metal detector for swallowed metallic objects. Thin barium for contrast study or computed tomography (CT). Avoid Gastrografin: can cause pulmonary edema.

5. Therapy: back blows and chest thrusts in young children and infants. Remove obstruction in upper third of the esophagus endoscopically; monitor asymptomatic child (12–24 h) if in middle or lower two-thirds. If still in esophagus after 24 h, remove. If below diaphragm, examine stools for passage. If still in stomach at 4–6 wk, remove; Foley balloon extraction under fluoroscopy may be considered for removal of esophageal foreign bodies.

     Objects longer than 5 cm or wider than 2 cm unlikely to pass through pylorus. Long narrow objects (> 6 cm in children, > 13 cm in adults) may fail to pass through duodenal loops.
    a. Safety pins: if opened proximally, push into stomach and removed with overtube; if open distally, pull out through overtube.
    b. Razor blades: with rigid esophagoscope, pull blade into instrument or by using rubber hood.
    c. Straight pin: if > 5 cm may fail to pass; remove endoscopically with protector hood.
    d. Crack vials or "body bags" of heroin or marijuana: appear as double condom on radiograph; remove with basket as forceps extraction carries danger of perforation.

6. Complications: increase with time foreign body remains in esophagus; perforations after 24 h. Also aspiration pneumonia, abscess, mediastinitis, pseudodiverticula, fistulae, and aortic pseudoaneurysm. Nickel, copper, and zinc toxicity reported after coin ingestion.

FOOD AND MEAT OBSTRUCTION

1. Impaction of food in esophagus occurs with congenital anomalies, stricture, achalasia, esophageal spasm, and motor disorders.

2. Bolus should not remain > 24 h because risk of perforation; remove endoscopically. Intravenous glucagons (decrease lower esophageal sphincter [LES] and smooth muscle spasm) or nifedipine helpful. Glucagon contraindications include pheochromocytoma, insulinoma, and allergy. Gas-forming agents associated with perforations. Enzymatic digestion with papain has risk of perforation (absolute contraindications: meat impaction > 36 h, suspected perforation, and bone within bolus).

CAUSTIC INJURY

1. Lye ingestion: causes liquefaction necrosis of mucosa; chemical reactions in stomach between gastric acid and lye generate heat; stomach should be suctioned prior to cold water lavage; caustic burns at oropharynx and upper esophagus.

2. High-density liquid drain cleaners: causes lesions at lower esophagus and stomach; lesions in upper esophagus usually occur where aorta and left main stem bronchus cross.

3. Ammonia: caustic esophageal injury, chemical pneumonitis, and pulmonary edema.

4. Grades of caustic injury at esophagus (Table 1):
    a. First degree: superficial involvement of mucosa.
    b. Second degree: transmural involvement with or without muscularis damage. No extension into periesophageal or perigastric tissues.
    c. Third degree: full-thickness extending into periesophageal and perigastric tissue; may extend into peritoneum and mediastinum. Perforation: several hours to days later. Fibrosis: second week. Ulcerations: for several months. Esophagus weakest at 10–12 d when connective tissue appears. Strictures: develop at 3–4 wk. Total obliteration of lumen from edema, charring, eschar, and full-thickness necrosis often with perforation.

5. Symptoms: often no complaints. Respiratory distress and stridor more frequent in children < 2 yr. Edema and ulceration or white, fragile, bleeding membranes of oropharynx; fever; slight leukocytosis (30%). Serious esophageal burns or perforation can occur in absence of oropharyngeal burns or abdominal complaints. Burns to the mouth do not predict esophageal burns.

6. Diagnosis: esophagogastroduodenoscopy (EGD) within 12–36 h to grade lesions. Radiology studies usually not done until later, owing to false-negative.

7. Treatment: severe symptoms: resuscitation and airway control. Emergency esophagectomy only if massive quantities of strong caustic agent ingested with esophageal necrosis. Gastric resection must be sparse and limited to antrum if possible. See Table 2.

8. Prognosis: 1000-fold increased incidence of squamous cell esophageal carcinoma in patients with history of caustic lesion. Time interval between ingestion and carcinoma 13–71 yr with latent time correlating with age at time of ingestion. Risk of cancer has led authors to advocate early surgery.

ACID INGESTION

1. Acid burns cause coagulation necrosis; damage limited to mucosa. Strong acids usually pass rapidly through esophagus, cause most significant damage in stomach and duodenum.

2. Prolonged drooling and dysphagia for 12–24 h associated with esophageal scar formation. Steroids not effective for acid burns. Strictures develop in 25% of patients. Esophageal cancer has occurred in an adult with acid ingestion as a child.

BLEACH INGESTION

1. Mean age 24 mo.
2. Esophageal irritant: low concentration (5%) does not cause tissue necrosis.
3. Problems with drooling and dysphagia: associated with airway edema; laryngoscopy.

DISC BATTERY INGESTION

1. Esophageal lodging requires urgent removal. Esophageal injury secondary to electrolyte leakage from battery, alkali produced from current, mercury toxicity, pressure necrosis, and direct current. More damage with lithium battery (within 15 min) than button alkali battery.

TABLE 1   ENDOSCOPY LESION GRADING*

GRADE	CHARACTERISTICS
0	Normal
1	Erythema, edema
2A	Noncircumferential superficial mucosal ulcerations with necrotic tissue, white plaques extending over less than one-third of esophagus
2B	Superficial noncircumferential ulcerations extending over > one-third of esophagus.
3A	Deep mucosal ulcerations, area of necrosis in circumferential pattern extending < one-third of esophageal length.
3B	Extensive necrosis, deep ulcerations over > one-third of esophagus.
4	Signs of transmural necrosis: shock, coagulopathy, and metabolic acidosis.

*Grade 2 and 3 not clearly distinguished as no standard method to determine depth of injury.

TABLE 2   TREATMENT OF CAUSTIC INJURY TO THE ESOPHAGUS

GRADE	TREATMENT
0–1	No treatment indicated; patient discharged.
2A	Observation for 1–3 d in hospital. In some patients, oral broad-spectrum antibiotics and antacids.
2B and greater	Prevention of stricture formation. Optimal nutrition imperative—with liquids by mouth—introducing dairy products as tolerated. Antacids for GER and esophageal dysmotility. If unable to eat, gastrostomy and TPN. High-dose dexamethasone may be helpful in prevention of secondary stricture. Use of antibiotics controversial. Stenting used with variable degrees of success (disadvantages: GER, inflammatory reaction, and perforation when placed blindly). EGD evaluation after 2–3 wk establishes healing or development of stricture. If stricture, dilatation after 1–2 months after ingestion, repeated q2–3 wk as needed. Topical mitomycin C has been used after dilatation to prevent restenosis. Esophageal replacement with colon may be necessary if fail.

EGD = esophagogastroduodenoscopy; GER = gastroesophageal reflux; TPN = total parenteral nutrition.

2. Symptoms: children usually asymptomatic after button battery ingestion.

3. Diagnosis: double density on chest radiograph, anterior projection. On lateral films, the edges are round and show a step-off at the junction of anode and cathode.

4. Therapy: no ipecac, no neutralizing solutions. Chest radiograph: if lodged in esophagus, immediate EGD removal with anesthesia. Foley catheter, balloon, or magnetized catheter removal has been described. If damage, barium study in 10–14 d to rule out stricture or fistula formation. Battery in stomach will pass if < 20 mm, but some advocate removal. If still in stomach at 1 wk, remove endoscopically. Administer prokinetic agent. If in intestines at 5 d, remove surgically.

5. Complications: tracheoesophageal fistula, perforation, stricture, and death. Mercury toxicity rare but reported. Rashes owing to presumed nickel hypersensitivity in 2% children.

RADIATION-INDUCED DAMAGE

1. Risk greater in children receiving 4000 cGy to chest. In general, esophagus considered relatively radiotherapy resistant.

2. Acute effects: dysphagia, odynophagia, and mucositis; usually starting by 10–12 days after beginning radiation therapy.

3. Most frequent complications: altered motility, ulcerations, and pseudodiverticula and strictures owing to fibrosis at lamina propria and submucosa. Squamous cell carcinoma can be a late complication.

4. Treatment: with sucralfate throughout therapy and fluconazole starting at 4 wk after therapy. Acute esophagitis: viscous lidocaine, antacid, or Benadryl or antacid with Reglan, bethanechol, or nifedipine. Strictures: stenting, bougienage, and balloon dilatation.

INTRAMURAL HEMATOMA OF THE ESOPHAGUS

1. Characteristics: rare, usually idiopathic; represents intramural perforation; associated with minor trauma in bike accidents.
2. Symptoms: dysphagia, acute epigastric or substernal pain, and hematemesis. Not usually preceded by vomiting.
3. Can be infrequent complication of sclerotherapy (can obstruct lumen); symptoms within few hours of procedure. Responds within 1 week to conservative therapy.

FOOD-RELATED ESOPHAGEAL TRAUMA

1. Esophageal burns: from hot chili peppers (requiring handling with gloves).
2. Chips and other pointed foods can cause hematoma or laceration.

PILL-INDUCED ESOPHAGEAL INJURY

1. Pills and gelatin capsules tend to adhere to esophageal mucosa. In adults: at level of aortic arch. Risks increased in patients who take pills with little or no fluid, have decreased salivation or swallowing, or take pill at night or supine.
2. Continuous retrosternal pain and dysphagia shortly after pill ingestion.
3. EGD shows circumferential lesions, ulcers, and longitudinal exudates over linear ulcerations with histologic changes showing inflammation, erosion, or necrosis.
4. Treatment: prevention: upright positioning during pill taking, with plenty of water and not at bedtime. Discontinue offending drug or reformulate. In severe cases, intravenous nutrition may be required. Strictures require dilatation.

BAROTRAUMA

1. Pressurized soft drinks and aerosols with explosion of pressurized gas or liquid in mouth.
2. Symptoms: immediate; respiratory distress, blood-tinged sputum, hematemesis, hemoptysis, and neck pain.
3. Diagnosis: pneumothorax, air at mediastinum, or perforation by Hypaque swallow.
4. Treatment: conservative; broad-spectrum antibiotics and chest tube or surgical procedure.

MALLORY-WEISS SYNDROME

1. Most common form of esophageal trauma: spontaneous laceration of esophagus after forceful and prolonged vomiting; one-half of adults have hiatal hernia, especially with gastric tears. Generally, laceration at gastroesophageal junction; can extend into cardia. Bleeding more severe with tear extending into more vascularized cardia.
2. EGD: longitudinal cracks at mucosa with little inflammation; after 24 h, white, raised streak with erythema and granulation tissue.
3. Treatment: spontaneous resolution. Rarely patient requires transfusion. If hemostasis does not occur, aggressive therapy with octreotide, balloon tamponade, sclerotherapy ligation, epinephrine injection, and cautery.

NEONATAL TRAUMATIC ESOPHAGITIS

Can result from too vigorous suctioning or passage of nasogastric tube.

BOERHAAVE SYNDROME

1. True, spontaneous tear through all layers of left lateral wall of esophagus (left posterolateral wall where smooth muscle the weakest). Adults: usually preceded by forceful retching or vomiting. Neonates: spontaneous rupture consistently on right side at lower esophagus just above hiatus without prior history of emesis.
2. Symptoms: pain, tenderness, swallowing, tachycardia, and fever if related to trauma. With iatrogenic causes, can present an hour or more later. Crepitus usually not appear for hours after fever. Cold-water polydipsia frequent.
3. Diagnosis: cervical and chest film: shows mediastinal widening or air in paracervical region or near esophagus. Esophagogram with water-soluble contrast: identifies site of perforation. CT helpful. EGD: procedure of choice to localize site precisely.
4. Treatment: pharyngoesophageal perforations: antibiotics, total parenteral nutrition (TPN), and nothing by mouth. Penetrating injury below arytenoids: neck exploration and drainage. Small esophageal tear: treat conservatively. Large perforations: cervical esophagostomy with TPN.
5. Complications: fulminant mediastinitis is major threat. Delayed complications: fistula. Mortality rates for penetrating perforation of cervical esophagus 9–15% with immediate therapy or 25% if treatment delayed. Perforation after sclerotherapy for varices at high risk with mortality up to 80% owing to liver disease. In children, most cases can be closed primarily. Little difference in mortality between iatrogenic and Boerhaave perforation.

TRAUMATIC RUPTURE AND PERFORATION OF ESOPHAGUS

1. Symptoms related to trauma immediate. Iatrogenic: may not be obvious for > 1h. Pharyngoesophageal perforations common in newborns: usually iatrogenic. Perforation usually at posterior wall of esophagus. Pain and tenderness at and under neck, difficulty swallowing, tachycardia, fever, crepitus, and cold water polydipsia.
2. Diagnosis: plain films: mediastinal widening or air in paracervical region. Hypaque esophagogram: identify site of perforation. EGD: procedure of choice.
3. Treatment: broad-spectrum antibiotics, TPN, and nothing by mouth. Majority treated surgically. Treat medically if clinically stable and detected before mediastinal contamination or esophageal disruptions. Esophagectomy may be better option in those with stricture or diffuse esophageal disease.
4. Complications: fulminant mediastinitis (major threat); continued swallowing difficulty requiring dilatation and reconstruction in one-third of patients surviving primary repair (4% mortality in children).

ESOPHAGEAL TRAUMA IN EPIDERMOLYSIS BULLOSA

1. Oral, pharyngeal, and esophageal blistering common. Recurrent blistering leads to progressive contraction of mouth and fixation of tongue. Associated pain and dysphagia lead to reduction of nutritional intake. Gastroesophageal reflux common; esophageal scarring leads to dysmotility and stricturing. Poor dentition and dental caries owing to oral infection compounded by poor dental hygiene owing to pain of teeth brushing.

2. Autosomal dominant form: moderate bullous skin lesions and oral, esophageal, or anal lesions without stricture formation; autosomal recessive form; associated with extensive lesions of skin, mouth, esophagus, and anus.

3. Mucosa bullae develop between birth and age 30 yr. Bullae can cause esophageal obstruction. Strictures frequent with one-half at proximal esophagus, one-quarter at lower, one-quarter random. Also, esophageal webs (largely proximal). Major symptom: dysphagia.

4. Diagnosis: radiology.

5. Therapy: nutritional support. Steroids 2 mg/kg/d, taper over 6–8 wk. Antacids and oral antibiotic suspensions prevent superinfection. Balloon dilation of strictures recommended. Webs can fracture spontaneously with a pop. Dilantin (collagenase inhibitor) used successfully at onset of symptoms to prevent bullae (less successful when used at time of dilation); plasma level 10 mg/mL. If performing surgical bypass, monitor with CT for development of carcinoma in bypassed esophagus.

QUESTIONS

1. The following are true of Boerhaave syndrome except:
   a. Occurs on the left in adults.
   b. Occurs on the left in neonates.
   c. In children, usually primary surgical repair is possible.
   d. Presents as a catastrophic event.
   e. Stricturing may occur as a late complication.

2. The following are false about intramural hematoma of the esophagus except:
   a. This is a common condition.
   b. Is usually preceded by vomiting.
   c. Is associated with bike accidents.
   d. Is not associated with esophageal obstruction.
   e. All of the above.

3. The following are true of foreign bodies in the esophagus except:
   a. Majority pass spontaneously, especially once in the stomach.
   b. Need to be removed if still present in esophagus after 24 h.
   c. Should remove objects > 6 cm in length.
   d. Distally opened safety pins should be directly removed with overtube.
   e. Crack vials and drug bags should be removed with a basket.

TRUE OR FALSE:

4. Mallory-Weiss syndrome tears usually start at the gastroesophageal junction.
5. Disc batteries lodged at the esophagus should be managed first with an observation period for possible self-passage, followed by endoscopic removal.
6. The most common site of injury for drug-induced injury is at the distal esophagus at the gastroesophageal junction in adults.
7. Radiation injury at the esophagus is more likely to occur in children receiving 4000 cGy.
8. Most strictures in epidermolysis bullosa occur at the lower esophagus.
9. Most webs in epidermolysis bullosa occur proximally.
10. Dilantin is a therapy for epidermolysis bullosa esophageal complications.
11. Bleach ingestion is associated with severe esophageal injury.

CHOOSE THE BEST ANSWER:

12. Which of the following is false regarding food impaction at the esophagus?
    a. Many impacted foods will pass.
    b. Food boluses lasting longer than 24 h should be removed endoscopically.
    c. Glucagon is especially useful for meat impaction.
    d. Papain digestion is useful for meat impactions longer than 36 h.

13. Children with a history of lye ingestion are at increased risk for which of the following?
    a. Squamous cell carcinoma of the esophagus.
    b. Adenocarcinoma of the esophagus.
    c. Gastrinoma.
    d. Gastric adenocarcinoma.
    e. Lymphoma.

ANSWERS

DISORDERS OF THE ORAL CAVITY

1. c.
2. b. Melkersson-Rosenthal syndrome: orofacial swelling, facial nerve palsy, fissured tongue, and mucosal swelling.
3. i.
4. a.
5. d. Similar to Addison disease.
6. f.
7. e.
8. h.
9. g.
10. a.
11. e.
12. a.
13. d.
14. f.

CONGENITAL ANOMALIES

1. d.
2. c.
3. b.
4. a.
5. c.
6. a.
7. d.
8. b.
9. e.
10. a. Down syndrome has pseudomacroglossia.
11. b.
12. a.
13. c.
14. True.
15. False.
16. True.

DISORDERS OF DEGLUTITION

1. True.
2. True.
3. False. In adulthood.
4. True.
5. d.
6. c.
7. b.
8. d.
9. d.

GASTROESOPHAGEAL REFLUX

1. e.
2. c. Too burdensome-used mainly in research.
3. b. Cisapride is a 5-HT4 receptor agonist.
4. True.
5. False.
6. False. But clinical improvement demonstrated.
7. True.
8. False.
9. False.

ESOPHAGITIS

1. e.
2. b.
3. a.
4. f.
5. True.
6. False. Difficult diagnosis.
7. False. Only those episodes where the refluxate has an acidic pH.
8. True.

OTHER MOTOR DISORDERS

1. m.
2. h, i.
3. d.
4. a.
5. b.
6. n.
7. c.
8. f.
9. i.
10. h.
11. False.
12. c.

INJURIES OF THE ESOPHAGUS

1. b.
2. c.
3. d. If open proximally then push into stomach.
4. True.
5. False. Need immediate removal.
6. False. Where aorta crosses.
7. True.
8. False. 50% proximal.
9. True.
10. True. It is a collagenase inhibitor at 10 mg/mL plasma levels.
11. False.
12. d. This is a contraindication to the use of glucagon.
13. a.

CLINICAL MANIFESTATIONS AND MANAGEMENT:

AND MANAGEMENT:

The Stomach and Duodenum

CONGENITAL ANOMALIES

SYNOPSIS

STOMACH

MICROGASTRIA

1. Very rare: only 45 cases described.
2. Occurs sporadically. Slight female predominance. Genetic cause unknown, but bone morphogenetic protein (BMP) signaling may play a role.
3. Associated anomalies common: malrotation, asplenia, transverse liver, tracheoesophageal anomalies, atrioventricular septal defects, upper limb and spinal deformities, micrognathia, renal dysplasia or aplasia, corpus callosum agenesis, and anophthalmia.
4. Symptoms: postprandial vomiting and reflux; recurrent chest infections common; rapid gastric emptying causing diarrhea.
5. Diagnosis: upper gastrointestinal (UGI) series: stomach small, tubular, midline. May be associated with

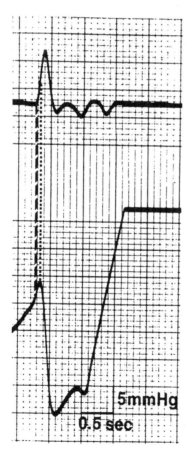

FIGURE 1 Delayed cricopharyngeal relaxation in a patient taking nitrazepam. The upper tracing represents hypopharyngeal contraction (onset at broken line); the lower tracing represents cricopharyngeal relaxation (onset at dotted line). Note that the hypopharyngeal contraction preceded the cricopharyngeal relaxation by 0.3 seconds. Reproduced with permission from Wyllie E et al.[6]

megaesophagus or gastroesophageal reflux (GER).
6. Treatment: adequate nutrition, prevention of aspiration, creation of adequate gastric reservoir.

GASTRIC ATRESIA OR STENOSIS

1. Most commonly affects the pylorus or antrum. Occurs either as a true atresia or secondary to complete or partial occlusion of the lumen by a membrane or diaphragm.
2. Rare: 1% of intestinal atresias.
3. Defects: isolated or in association with other genetic defects or syndromes (junctional epidermolysis bullosa, intestinal atresias, Down syndrome, or aplasia cutis congenital).
4. Symptoms: Complete atresia: within few hours of birth, persistent nonbilious emesis and hypochloremic hypokalemic acidosis; gastric rupture reported.
5. Diagnosis: abdominal radiograph shows no intestinal air. Diagnosis of incomplete atresia endoscopy or UGI can show gastric membrane.
6. Management: surgery. Gastroduodenostomy if atretic or pyloroplasty if stenotic. Endoscopic transection of webs with balloon dilatation or laser ablation.

GASTRIC DIVERTICULUM

1. Very uncommon. Usually occurs at posterior wall, antrum, or pylorus; comprises all layers of stomach wall.
2. Presentation: usually found in adults; children may present with recurrent abdominal pain or vomiting.
3. Diagnosis: UGI endoscopy or contrast studies.
4. Treatment: surgical excision.

GASTRIC DUPLICATION CYSTS

1. Characteristics: presents in infancy. Females more affected than males. 4–8% of foregut duplications, usually at greater curvature, do not communicate with gastric lumen. Common blood supply and outer smooth muscle coat. Mucosal lining usually gastric or intestinal. Associated anomalies common: 50%.
2. Symptoms: depend on size and location of cyst; nonbilious vomiting, weight loss, failure to thrive, abdominal pain, and distention. Ulceration, bleeding, or inflammation of enclosed mucosa can cause gastrointestinal (GI) hemorrhage, perforation, or fistula. If ectopic pancreatic tissue, associated with hyperamylasemia or pancreatitis. May feel mass on examination.
3. Diagnosis: radiology (ultrasonography, computed tomography, and magnetic resonance imaging). UGI to determine if communication with the GI tract exists.
4. Treatment: surgical excision, or leave cyst intact but strip mucosa of cyst. Excellent outcome.

GASTRIC TERATOMA

1. Very rare: < 1% of all teratomas. Almost exclusively in males. Contains all three embryonic germ layers. Usually extragastric, near greater curvature of stomach.
2. Presentation: abdominal mass with or without emesis, possibly GI bleed.

3. Usually not associated with other congenital abnormalities.
4. Treatment: surgical excision.

CONGENITAL MUSCULAR DEFECT OF THE STOMACH
1. Muscular defect total or in part. Body of stomach most commonly affected. Predisposition to gastric perforation usually shortly after birth.
2. BMP signaling abnormalities may be a cause.
3. Management of perforation: emergency decompression of free air in abdomen, intravenous antibiotics, fluid resuscitation, and surgery.

GASTRIC VOLVULUS
1. Abnormal rotation of one part of the stomach around another resulting in obstruction, possible ischemia. Recognition essential, surgical emergency.
2. Normally, stomach is resistant to abnormal rotation, as it is fixed at the gastroesophageal junction and pylorus, in addition to four ligaments.
3. Two types: majority secondary to gastric malfixation.
   a. Organoaxial: rotation along longitudinal axis; most common but rare in children. Associated with diaphragm defects. Strangulation and necrosis common.
   b. Mesentericoxial: rotation along transverse axis through greater and lesser curves. Rotation incomplete, occurs intermittently.
4. Symptoms: Borchardt triad: pain, violent retching with little emesis, and inability to pass NG tube past distal esophagus; not usually seen in children. In children, tends to present in first few months of life with reflux, recurrent emesis, and failure to thrive.
5. Diagnosis: UGI. Chest radiograph and kidney, ureter, bladder (KUB) exam: large, gas-filled viscus in chest or abdomen.
6. Management: surgical emergency. Gastropexy if viable, with fixation to abdominal wall.

DUODENUM

DUODENAL ATRESIA
1. Most common site: GI tract; at level of the ampulla of Vater. Presents within first few days of life. Bilious emesis.
2. Associations: malrotation (50%), Down syndrome (one-third), anorectal malformations, esophageal atresia, vertebral, cardiac, genitourinary, prematurity, and polyhydramnios.
3. Diagnosis: double bubble on KUB exam with no distal gas. Contrast study usually not necessary.
4. Treatment: surgical. Side-to-side or end-to-side duodenoduodenostomy or duodenojejunostomy.

DUODENAL STENOSIS
1. Incomplete duodenal atresia owing to hole in membrane, often eccentrically placed; accounts for 70% of intestinal stenoses (the most common GI stenosis).
2. Presentation later in life: emesis and failure to thrive. Association with Down syndrome.

3. Diagnosis: esophagogastroduodenoscopy; radiology not helpful.
4. Treatment: surgical (see Duodenal Atresia).

DUODENAL DUPLICATIONS
1. Rare. Tend to occur on mesenteric border of first two parts of duodenum.
2. Presenting symptoms: usually related to duodenal obstruction. Also, ulceration, hemorrhage within the cyst, pancreatitis, and biliary obstruction.
3. Treatment: surgical.

QUESTIONS

CHOOSE THE BEST ANSWER:
1. Which of the following is true of microgastria?
   a. Is demonstrated by a small, tubular sac in the midline on contrast studies.
   b. Is associated with asplenia.
   c. May be associated with megaesophagus.
   d. All of the above.
   e. None of the above.

2. Which of the following is true of gastric diverticulum?
   a. Is a false diverticulum.
   b. Arises most commonly at the cardia.
   c. Is usually found in children.
   d. Is treated conservatively.
   e. None of the above.

3. Which of the following is true of congenital muscular defect of the stomach?
   a. Predisposes infants to visceral perforation shortly after birth.
   b. Occurs at the body of the stomach.
   c. Requires surgery.
   d. All of the above.
   e. None of the above.

4. Which of the following is the most common type of intestinal atresia?
   a. Gastric.
   b. Duodenal.
   c. Jejunal.
   d. Ileal.
   e. Colonic.

5. Which is not true of gastric teratomas?
   a. Occur almost exclusively in males.
   b. Contain all three germ cell layers.
   c. Usually found extragastrically.
   d. Usually located at lesser curvature of the stomach.
   e. All of the above are true.

TRUE OR FALSE:
6. Duodenal atresias usually occur proximal to the ampulla of Vater.
7. Duodenal duplications tend to occur at the mesenteric border of the first and second part of the duodenum.

GASTRITIS AND PEPTIC ULCER DISEASE

SYNOPSIS

PRIMARY GASTRITIS

Helicobacter pylori INFECTION

1. Gram-negative spiral flagellated bacterium. Colonizes only gastric tissue.
2. Onset: usually acquired by age 5 yr.
3. Prevalence: developing countries: up to 80% in children under age 10 yr; developed countries < 10% of young children, up to 50% in children with low socioeconomic status. In developed countries the prevalence is 10% by 10 yr, 60% by 60 yr.
4. Risk factors: poor socioeconomic status, bed sharing, large sibships.
5. Transmission mode: unknown.

Virulence Factors

1. Urease: protect bacteria against gastric acid.
2. Flagella: enables motility.
3. Cytotoxin-associated gene (cag) A–positive: possibly more virulent strain. In Western countries, cagA+ strains commonly found in adults with peptic ulcer disease. Not true in children.
4. Vacuolating cytotoxin (VacA): more commonly associated with ulcer disease.
5. CagE+ strains associated with ulcer disease in children and associated with interleukin-8 production and inflammation.
6. Acute infection associated with transient hypochlorhydria, which may facilitate transmission.
7. *H. pylori* gastritis causes increase in gastrin release and depletion of somatostatin D cells, but basal acid output does not differ between infected and noninfected.
8. Pepsinogen 1 elevated in children infected with *H. pylori*
9. Reinfection rate: < 1%/yr in adults; 2% total in children over age 5 yr.

Disease Associations

1. Chronic gastritis: all children. Majority asymptomatic; 15% peptic ulcer disease (PUD), 1% gastric cancer.
2. Duodenal ulcer disease: 90% of children have *H. pylori* on antral mucosa. Symptoms: episodic epigastric pain, vomiting, nocturnal awakening, and meal-associated pain in 50–75%. Eradication of *H. pylori* leads to healing of duodenal ulcer disease.
3. Gastric ulcer disease associated with *H. pylori* antral gastritis in adults. In children, gastric ulcers rare, usually secondary.
4. Gastric cancer: 2–6-fold increased risk for gastric cancer among infected. Highest risk among those with corpus-predominant gastritis, gastric atrophy, and intestinal metaplasia. Those with duodenal ulcers and antral-predominant gastritis do not develop gastric cancer. Increased risk with family history.
5. Mucosa-associated lymphoid tissue lymphomas: *H. pylori* implicated as an etiology. Tumors often multifocal, located at antrum or distal body. 75% completely responsive to treatment of *H. pylori*. If translocation t(11;18)(q21;q21) present in tumor, will not respond to *H. pylori* therapy.
6. No association with recurrent abdominal pain. Possible association with sideropenic or iron deficiency anemia.

Diagnosis

1. Esophagogastroduodenoscopy (EGD): investigation of choice; *H. pylori* at antrum in 90% with duodenal ulcer, especially if gastric metaplasia in duodenum (need to biopsy as gross EGD appearance correlates poorly with presence of gastritis); antral nodularity and cobblestoning described in children. Biopsy: lymphoid follicles with germinal centers suggestive. Warthin-Starry silver stain: *H. pylori* seen.
2. Culture: difficult. Requires 5–7 days; Skirrow medium.
3. Urease test: color change within 30 min, but can take up to 24 h; with full biopsy, test sensitivity is about 100%.
4. Urea breath test (UBT): fast for 2 h, collect baseline sample of expired air, then ingest ^{13}C urea. Second breath sample 30 min later. Ratio of ^{13}C to ^{12}C measured and subtracted from baseline is delta over baseline (DOB). If DOB > 5, *H. pylori*. 100% sensitivity; 92% specificity in older children. In children age < 2 yr, reduced specificity of UBT. Specimens taken at 15–20 min can be false-positive (possible oral urease organisms). Following therapy, 100% sensitivity in following status.
5. Serology: children's mean antibody levels are lower than adults. Commercial tests not sensitive or specific enough to detect *H. pylori* if younger than age 12 yr.
6. Salivary immunoglobulin G (IgG) antibodies: in children, sensitivity 93% and specificity 82%.
7. Stool antigen enzyme immunoassay: monoclonal antibody test positive predictive value 98% and negative predictive value 99% in children.

Treatment

1. Children with peptic ulcer disease secondary to *H. pylori* as well as those who are asymptomatic should receive therapy.
2. Failure of treatment: failed eradication in 5–30% of children. Treatment is less effective if < 75% of medications ingested. Flagyl resistance more common than clarithromycin resistance. Amoxicillin resistance not reported in children. Tetracycline resistance reported.

Helicobacter heilmannii GASTRITIS

1. Gastritis mainly at antrum; mild mononuclear inflammatory response without neutrophil activity. Importance as a gastric pathogen in children not yet clear.
2. Prevalence: 0.08–1% adults, 0.3% in children.

SECONDARY PEPTIC DISEASE: EROSIVE GASTRITIS

STRESS: ACUTE EROSIVE GASTRITIS

1. Stressors: burns, head injury, major surgery, sepsis, multiple trauma, respiratory failure, and coagulopathy; generally occurs within 24 h of onset of critical illness.
2. Etiology: impaired blood flow and ischemia. Risk factors for hemorrhage: gastric hypersecretion, mechanical ventilation, and use of steroids.
3. Symptoms: 75% asymptomatic; hematemesis and melena. Newborns and infants prone to perforations.
4. EGD. Early lesions predominate at fundus, and proximal body, later spreading to antrum to produce diffuse erosive appearance. Antral involvement alone uncommon.
5. Treatment: proton pump inhibitor (PPI). Prophylaxis with H_2 receptor antagonists.

NEONATAL GASTROPATHIES

1. Most due to physiologic stress. Hemorrhagic gastropathy has also been reported in otherwise healthy full-term infants presenting with severe upper gastrointestinal (UGI) hemorrhage.
2. Prolonged infusions of prostaglandin E associated with antral mucosal thickening and gastric outlet obstruction.

TRAUMATIC GASTROPATHY

1. Forceful retching or vomiting produces typical hemorrhages at fundus and proximal body of the stomach secondary to prolapse of the proximal stomach into distal esophagus.
2. Nasogastric suctioning causes severe subepithelial hemorrhage.
3. Trauma by foreign bodies cause hemorrhages and erosions.

DRUGS AND INGESTIONS

1. Nonsteroidal antiinflammatory drugs (NSAIDs) and aspirin: cause mucosal damage primarily at stomach but also duodenum. Exert effects via inhibition of cyclooxygenase (COX) conversion of arachidonic acid to prostaglandins. Aspirin also inhibits thromboxane production by platelets enhancing gastrointestinal (GI) bleeding. Characteristic histologic NSAID lesion is reactive gastropathy. Risk for gastroduodenal injury in children 5 times that in those not taking NSAIDs. Consider selective COX-2 inhibitors instead or prophylax with PPI in those requiring long-term NSAID use. Eradication of *H. pylori* is also recommended.
2. Corrosives: prepyloric area vulnerable to injury. Presence of food may limit injury. Endoscopic findings range from mild friability and erythema to hemorrhage and perforation. Can develop gastric outlet obstruction within 4–8 wk of corrosive exposure. Treat with steroids, antibiotics, and antacids. Do not induce vomiting or perform gastric lavage.
3. Oral ferrous sulfate may cause mild endoscopic abnormalities in stomach of uncertain clinical significance.

4. Erosive or hemorrhagic gastropathies described with valproate, dexamethasone, chemotherapy, alcohol, KCl, and cysteamine.
5. Cystinosis: inherited lysosomal storage disorder with cystine deposited within macrophages. Therapeutic cysteamine is ulcerogenic and a potent secretagogue causing hypergastrinemia and gastric acid hypersecretion 1–2 h after drug ingestion. In addition, delayed gastric emptying and inhibition of gastric bicarbonate and mucus production contributes to formation of ulcers. EGD: fine nodularity throughout stomach in children.
6. Radiation gastropathy: abdominal radiation causes erosions and ulcers at antrum and prepyloric region and severe diffuse hemorrhagic gastritis. Subsequent fibrosis and strictures can occur and cause gastric outlet obstruction. Risk factors: high total radiation dose and high daily fraction. Treatment difficult; may require surgery.

UREMIC GASTROPATHY

1. In acute renal failure, gastropathy may be due to physiologic stress. Associated with erosions and ulcers in 71% cases with increased mortality.
2. Chronic renal failure associated with increased parietal, chief, and gastrin-producing cells. Gastric pH higher than expected, perhaps secondary to ammonia neutralization. Little data in children. In adults, hemorrhagic gastropathy prevalent in patients on hemodialysis; often present with bleeding rather than pain and with multiple *H. pylori*-negative ulcers.

CHRONIC VARIOLIFORM GASTRITIS

1. Reported in middle-aged and elderly men; few children.
2. Symptoms: insidious (UGI symptoms, anemia, protein losing enteropathy [PLE], elevated immunoglobulin E [IgE], and eosinophilia).
3. Endoscopy: prominent nodules (similar to chicken pox) at fundus and proximal body with thickened gastric rugae.

BILE GASTROPATHY

1. Alkaline gastropathy: most reports in adults. Well-documented in postoperative stomach.
2. Endoscopy: bile in the stomach usually of little clinical significance; however, duodenogastroesophageal reflux can be accompanied by beefy erythema and erosions on endoscopy. Biopsies: little or no increase of cellular infiltrate in lamina propria, lamina propria edema, venous congestion, and foveolar hyperplasia.

SCHÖNLEIN-HENOCH GASTRITIS

1. Multisystem disorder: nonthrombocytopenic skin purpura, arthralgias, renal disease, and colicky abdominal pain. GI symptoms: pain, nausea, vomiting, and bleeding.
2. Endoscopic findings at stomach include erythematous or hemorrhagic swollen mucosa with erosions or ulcers. Findings can be patchy or diffuse with similar

lesions at small intestine. Biopsies may show leuko-clastic vasculitis similar to that seen in skin.

EXERCISE-INDUCED GASTROPATHY

1. Recognized in long distance runners. Usually presents with blood loss anemia with symptoms after exercise (abdominal cramps or pain, nausea, and vomiting).
2. Erosive and nonerosive gastritis described. Gastritis usually acute with hemorrhagic inflammation on biopsy.
3. Proposed mechanisms: ischemia, with reports of 80% reduction in visceral blood flow during exercise.

NONEROSIVE GASTRITIS

INFLAMMATORY BOWEL DISEASE

Gastroduodenal involvement common. Macroscopic or histologic abnormalities seen in up to 80% of children with Crohn disease.

PPI GASTROPATHY

1. Hyperplasia of parietal cells with cystic changes in the glands, caused by long-term or high-dose PPI therapy. Benign fundic gland polyps may be present. Reversible with cessation of PPI therapy. No reported association with dysplasia.
2. Gastric polyps unrelated to PPI therapy are rare in children.

ALLERGIC GASTRITIS

1. Allergic gastritis always mucosal (erosion in eosinophilic gastritis is deeper).
2. Usually associated with a specific allergen (in infants, mainly cow or soy milk protein, egg, or wheat). Reintroduction of antigen almost always possible by age 2 yr. Disease benign and self-limited.
3. Biopsy reveals eosinophilic infiltration at lamina propria and surface epithelium. On endoscopy, normal mucosa or changes similar to eosinophilic gastritis (endoscopic changes are milder in allergic versus eosinophilic gastritis).

EOSINOPHILIC GASTRITIS

1. Chronic severe disease of unknown etiology.
2. Symptoms: upper GI symptoms, poor growth, GI bleeding, diarrhea; iron deficiency and PLE common; elevated serum IgE and peripheral eosinophilia.
3. Diagnosis: EGD: findings nonspecific; friability, erythema, erosions, edema, and nodularity.
4. Biopsy: striking eosinophilic infiltrate. All layers of gastric wall may be involved with eosinophilic infiltrate being patchy, thus, surgical full-thickness biopsy may be needed.
5. Treatment: oral steroids; dietary manipulations and cromolyn usually of no benefit.

CELIAC GASTRITIS

Lymphocytic gastritis usually in presence of normal EGD. Lymphocytic infiltrate usually at intraepithelial location.

COLLAGENOUS GASTRITIS

1. Rare. Characterized by subepithelial collagen deposition and associated gastritis. Described in collagenous sprue and colitis, lymphocytic colitis, and celiac disease.
2. Presentation in children: upper abdominal pain, GI bleeding, and anemia.
3. Treatment: gluten-free diet, steroids, and acetylsalicylic acid preparations to improve symptoms.

GRAFT-VERSUS-HOST DISEASE

1. Acute graft-versus-host disease (GVHD) occurs 3–4 weeks after transplant with varying degrees of involvement of the gut, liver and skin. Upper GI symptoms commonly seen.
2. Stomach important in acute GVHD for histologic diagnosis even when diarrhea is main symptom. Chronic GVHD rarely involves the stomach.
3. Biopsy findings range from normal to extensive mucosal sloughing. Early biopsy findings unique to GVHD with crypt epithelial cell apoptosis.

CHRONIC GRANULOMATOUS DISEASE

1. Rare immunodeficiency. Gastric wall involvement common. Delayed gastric emptying.
2. Diagnosis: UGI series: narrowed antrum; EGD: nonspecific.
3. Histology: focal, chronic active inflammation at antrum with granulomas and multinuclear giant cells. Typical yellow pigment in histiocytes may not be present.

CYTOMEGALOVIRUS GASTRITIS

1. Common in immunosuppressed patients. Cytomegalovirus (CMV) infection in immunocompetent children manifests as Ménétrier disease.
2. Tends to occur in gastric fundus and body; causes wall thickening, ulceration, bleeding, and perforation.
3. Histology: active inflammation with edema, necrosis, and CMV inclusion bodies. Usually involves deeper mucosa.
4. Diagnosis: viral culture and CMV antigen detection.
5. Treatment: spontaneous recovery in 1–2 mo; ganciclovir may be beneficial.

MÉNÉTRIER DISEASE

1. Rare in children. Generally clinically benign, self-resolving in children with mean age of onset 4–5 years.
2. Characteristics: large mucosal folds at stomach, associated with excess mucus secretion, hypochlorhydria, and PLE at stomach. Associated with CMV.
3. Symptoms: vomiting. Associated with abdominal pain, anorexia, and edema.
4. Diagnosis: barium radiograph and EGD: large, irregular mucosal folds especially at upper stomach. Biopsy: hypertrophy, hyperplasia gastric glands, cyst formation, and edema at lamina propria. Inflammatory cell infiltrate. CMV testing should be performed.
5. Therapy: supportive care; disease self-limited 4–6 wk. If chronic: acid suppression, octreotide, H. pylori elimination, or potential partial gastrectomy.

PERNICIOUS ANEMIA

1. Autoimmune process; parietal cell components attacked, resulting in absolute achlorhydria and megaloblastic anemia secondary to intrinsic factor absence and resulting in vitamin B_{12} deficiency. Associated conditions: autoimmune thyroid disease, diabetes, vitiligo, immunoglobulin A deficiency, chronic candidiasis, abnormal cell immunity, and collagen vascular disease.
2. EGD: thin rugae of gastric body. Biopsy: severe atrophic fundic gland gastritis with absence of parietal cells. Adenocarcinoma can occur as a complication; rare in children. Endoscopic surveillance is indicated.
3. Childhood or juvenile pernicious anemia is a separate entity; consists of a heterogeneous group of conditions with megaloblastic anemia and hypo- or achlorhydria, but no gastric atrophy. Etiology: secretion of abnormal intrinsic factor (IF) or abnormalities in the secretion of IF.
4. Cobalamin C disease: congenital anomaly of vitamin B_{12} metabolism, rare, cystic dysplastic changes at stomach, and total absence of parietal and chief cells.

VARIOLIFORM GASTRITIS

1. Only 2 cases in pediatric patients.
2. Radiograph or EGD show radiolucent halos and volcano-like elevations.
3. Biopsy at central erosion shows lamina propria with inflammatory cells, lymphocytes, and plasma cells.

GASTRITIS ASSOCIATED WITH AUTOIMMUNE DISEASES

1. Gastritis with and without atrophy seen in children with autoimmune thyroiditis, some with achlorhydria and gastric parietal cell antibodies.
2. In subjects with connective tissue disease, mast cell gastritis with or without an eosinophilic gastritis has been described.
3. In children with insulin-dependent diabetes mellitus, 48% had erosions and ulcers and 25 of 27 had histologic gastritis negative for *H. pylori*.

GRANULOMATOUS GASTRITIS

1. Except when attributable to Crohn disease, rare. Condition limited to stomach; diagnosis of exclusion. Only one report in a teenager.
2. Differential diagnosis: foreign body reaction, tuberculosis, histoplasmosis, Wegener syndrome, Langerhans cell histiocytosis, sarcoidosis.

PHLEGMONOUS GASTRITIS AND EMPHYSEMATOUS GASTRITIS

1. Phlegmonous gastritis: rare and life threatening. Rapidly progressive bacterial inflammation of gastric submucosa resulting in necrosis or gangrene. Most due to α-hemolytic *Streptococcus*, *Staphylococcus aureus*, *Escherichia coli*, and *Clostridium welchii*.
2. Acute emphysematous gastritis is a complication; where gastric wall infection occurs with gas-forming bacteria. Usually fatal. Risk factors: caustic ingestion, abdominal surgery, and immunosuppression. Treatment: gastrectomy, drainage of intramural collections, and antibiotics. Need to distinguish from gastric emphysema and cystic pneumatosis, which follow instrumentation or gastric outlet obstruction.

OTHER INFECTIOUS GASTRITIDES

1. *Giardia*: may be pathogen in the stomach in some patients.
2. Herpes simplex virus and varicella-zoster virus: rare cause of gastritis in immunosuppressed patients. Biopsies demonstrate typical intranuclear inclusion bodies.
3. Influenza A: rare cause of bleeding in children, occasionally fatal.
4. Fungal infections of stomach may occur especially in sick neonates, burn victims, and children with malnutrition or immunodeficiencies.
5. Gastric anisakiasis simplex infections occur commonly in Japan, where there is high consumption of raw fish. Gastric symptoms occur within 3 h and systemic allergic symptoms within 5 h of ingestion in sensitized patients. Peripheral leukocytosis and eosinophilia. EGD: worms protruding into the lumen with a surrounding erythematous ring, mucosal swelling, and occasional erosions. Favor greater curvature. Treatment: endoscopic removal of worm.

ZOLLINGER-ELLISON SYNDROME

1. Triad: severe PUD, gastric acid hypersecretion, and gastrinoma (usually in pancreas but can be at stomach or duodenum).
2. Symptoms: multiple gastric, duodenal, and jejunal ulcers. Diarrhea secondary to stimulation effect of gastrin on motility and pancreatic secretion. More males than females; age 7–90 yr; peak age 30–50 yr; one-third with multiple endocrine neoplasia, type I (MEN I) (parathyroid, pancreatic, and pituitary tumors) but association is rare in children.
3. Conditions suggesting testing for gastrinoma in children: ulcers distal to first portion of duodenum, multiple UGI ulcers, PUD unresponsive to standard medical therapy, PUD and diarrhea, strong family history of PUD, personal or family history of MEN I, PUD and urinary tract calculi, recurrent PUD negative for *H. pylori* and without prior NSAID use, and gastric acid hypersecretion or hypergastrinemia.
4. Gastrinomas very small and multiple tumors common; 60% malignant. Typically found in gastrinoma triangle, between cystic duct, third portion duodenum, neck of pancreas and head of pancreas, duodenum, and porta hepatic. Metastasize to local lymph nodes and liver.
5. Diagnosis:
   a. Fasting serum gastrin $\geq$ 125 pg/mL (after 8 h fast).
   b. Secretin stimulation test: 2 U/kg secretin injected over 30 s. Blood samples taken for gastrin 5 min before injection, just before injection, and at 5 min intervals for 30 min after injection. Secretin has no effect on gastrin in normal patients or on benign G-cell hyperplasia but doubles gastrin in gastrinoma.
   c. Gastric acid secretion stimulated by pentagastrin.
   d. Somatostatin receptor scintigraphy.
   e. Biopsy.

f. Endoscopic ultrasonography.
g. Angiography.

6. Treatment: resection (normal fasting serum gastrin and secretin stimulation test postoperatively = long-term cure). In unresectable cases and MEN I: vagotomy makes medical therapy easier. Metastases: streptozotocin ± 5-fluorouracil. Medication: PPI bid, intravenous H_2 blockade. Goal: reduce acid secretion to < 10 meq/h.

7. Prognosis: 30% cure. If no cure, 15 yr survival is 83%. MEN I cure rare, but long-term survival usual.

QUESTIONS

MATCH THE CONDITION TO THE GASTRITIS TYPE:
a. Primary gastritis
b. Secondary gastritis

1. Pernicious anemia.
2. *Helicobacter pylori* infection.
3. Chemical ingestion.
4. Crohn disease.

MATCH THE CONDITION TO THE OUTCOME:
a. Requires immediate intervention, life-threatening.
b. Benign.

5. Phlegmonous gastritis.
6. Gastric emphysema.
7. Emphysematous gastritis.
8. Cystic pneumatosis.

TRUE OR FALSE:
9. *Helicobacter pylori* colonizes gastric and nongastric tissue.
10. All children infected with *Helicobacter pylori* have chronic gastritis.
11. The reinfection rate of *Helicobacter pylori* is 2% in children less than 5 years old.
12. *Helicobacter pylori* infection results in peptic ulcer disease in 15% of cases.
13. *Helicobacter pylori* infection advances to gastric cancer in 1% of cases.
14. D cells make gastrin.
15. G cells make somatostatin.
16. Ménétrier disease in children often requires prolonged intervention.

MATCH THE CHARACTERISTICS TO THE CONDITIONS:
a. Stress gastritis.
b. Nonsteroidal anti-inflammatory drug use.
c. Cobalamin C deficiency.
d. Crohn disease.
e. Pernicious anemia.
f. Eosinophilic gastritis.
g. Ménétrier disease.

17. Total absence of parietal and chief cells.
18. Local mucosal ischemia.
19. Inhibition of prostaglandins.
20. Granulomatous associated changes.
21. Cytomegalovirus infection in immunocompetent children.
22. Protein-losing enteropathy and peripheral eosinophilia.

ESOPHAGEAL AND GASTRIC NEOPLASMS

SYNOPSIS

ESOPHAGEAL TUMORS
1. Rare in childhood.
2. Most benign tumors are small, > 50% asymptomatic, discovered incidentally during upper endoscopy.
3. Symptoms: Larger tumors: dysphagia and feeding and respiratory problems. Larger, malignant tumors: bleeding, weight loss, and vomiting.
4. Evaluation: upper endoscopy, upper gastrointestinal (UGI) series, computed tomography (CT), magnetic resonance imaging (MRI), and endoscopic ultrasonography.
5. Biopsy diagnosis usually possible. Endoscopic procedures may be curative. Surgical resection treatment choice for the remainder. Data on adjuvant chemotherapy and radiation therapy not available in children given rarity of malignant tumors.

BENIGN EPITHELIAL ESOPHAGEAL TUMORS
1. Esophageal squamous papilloma: benign polypoid tumor usually at lower esophagus. Incidence rates 0.1–0.4%. Usually asymptomatic. Etiologic factors: physical trauma (acid reflux, radiation, irritation from chemicals, and foreign bodies) and human papillomavirus infection. At endoscopy, usually solitary mucosal protrusions with a stalk. Overlying mucosa normal or roughened, white with keratinization. Pathology: central fibrovascular core covered by benign mature squamous epithelium. Papillomatosis rare, occurs predominantly in children. Most are reactive, do not recur or progress. No malignant esophageal squamous papilloma found in children
2. Esophageal cysts and reduplications: esophageal cysts; duplications usually seen in lower third of the esophagus and toward right side. Communication with gastric reduplication common, but only 10% communicate with esophageal lumen. Usually single. Most present in the first year of life with respiratory difficulty, dysphagia, and feeding problems. Mucosal lining of cyst may be ciliated columnar, gastric, or esophageal squamous. Wall contains smooth muscle, nerves, blood vessels. Treatment is surgical resection. Small risk of malignant transformation of the epithelial lining of untreated cysts.
3. Pseudodiverticulosis: duct orifices of submucosal glands become dilated and form multiple intramural

cysts. Esophageal dysmotility presumptive cause; achalasia may be present. Usually at upper esophagus but can be diffuse. Endoscopy: small pit-like openings. Biopsy: squamous lining, with candidal superinfection.

4. Glycogen acanthosis: appears as white patch of esophageal mucosa. Biopsy: esophageal squamous mucosa with enlarged superficial keratinocytes. Sporadic. Multiple glycogen acanthoses may indicate hamartomatous polyposis related to germline mutation *PTEN* associated with thyroid and breast cancers.

BENIGN NONEPITHELIAL ESOPHAGEAL TUMORS

1. Esophageal leiomyoma: most common benign neoplasm of the esophagus. Derived from the muscularis mucosa. Most cases reported in teenage years. More females than males. Diffuse, multiple forms more common. May occur in multiple, often confluent form (leiomyomatosis) as part of Alport syndrome (nephropathy, sensorineural hearing loss) or in association with reflux. Appear as submucosal bumps or sessile polyps at endoscopy with intact overlying mucosa. Most intramural; common site is distal esophagus and gastroesophageal junction. Treatment: enucleation for single tumors and surgical resection for multiple esophageal leiomyomas.

2. Granular cell tumor: mesenchymal tumor composed of epithelioid or plump-spindled cells with granular eosinophilic periodic acid–Schiff stain positive cytoplasm. Most are small, found incidentally on upper endoscopy as a sessile, yellow-white firm nodule with intact overlying mucosa (overlying squamous mucosa is markedly hyperplastic on histology). Occurs on lower esophagus more so than on proximal esophagus, in males more than females, in blacks more than whites.

3. Vascular tumors: hemangioma and lymphangioma reported at the esophagus of children. Lesions apparent at endoscopy.

MALIGNANT EPITHELIAL TUMORS

1. Barrett esophagus: acquired defect resulting from acid reflux resulting in intestinal metaplasia. Preneoplastic state (progression from Barrett esophagus to adenocarcinoma takes about 20 yr). Endoscopy: velvety red tongues extending up the esophagus from the gastroesophageal junction with areas of residual white squamous mucosa, ulceration, and friability. Requires presence of goblet cells for diagnosis. Short segment (3 cm or less) has less risk of adenocarcinoma compared with classic or long-segment Barrett esophagus.

2. Adenocarcinoma: if arising in Barrett esophagus usually occurs at distal esophagus. Long-term survival possible with mucosal carcinoma, but submucosal invasion and lymph node metastases associated with poor survival.

3. Squamous cell carcinoma: rare tumor in children; more blacks than whites; male-to-female ratio 3.7:1. In United States, predisposing factors: alcohol and tobacco. Outside United States: associated with ingestion of hot foods, vitamin-deficient diets, mineral deficiencies, nitrosamines, diets low in fresh foods, high benzopyrenes from coal smoke. Inherited or sporadic disorders affecting keratin synthesis (palmoplantar keratosis and tylosis) associated with high rates of squamous cell carcinoma. Celiac disease associated with increased risk of esophageal squamous cell carcinoma, as is caustic ingestion, presence of esophageal stricture, achalasia, and dysmotility. Endoscopy: white plaques, nodules, and occasional polyps. Granular surface and ulceration associated with higher grades of dysplasia. Mid and lower esophagus most often affected. Biopsy: thickened squamous mucosa with layers of keratin. Inflammation is common. Prognosis grim for advanced tumors. Death usually related to local disease with fistulization into the tracheobronchial tree and hemorrhage. Surgical resection after chemoirradiation.

4. Malignant melanoma: presents with dysphagia, usually forms a sessile polyp at lower esophagus. Surrounding esophageal squamous mucosa heavily pigmented. Often diagnose at late stage; curative therapy is rare.

NONEPITHELIAL ESOPHAGEAL MALIGNANT TUMORS

1. Esophageal sarcoma: very rare. Rhabdomyosarcoma, malignant schwannoma, leiomyosarcoma (not reported in children), carcinosarcoma reported. Most present with dysphagia and a large submucosal mass usually with ulceration or necrosis on endoscopy.

2. Gastrointestinal stromal tumor: arises from the interstitial cells of Cajal, which uniformly express the receptor tyrosine kinase KIT. Not reported in children.

GASTRIC TUMORS

BENIGN TUMORS OF THE STOMACH

1. Gastric polyps: sporadic or more common manifestations of a polyposis syndrome, polyps in the stomach are less frequent than in the lower gastrointestinal (GI) tract. Can be adenomatous, fundic gland type, juvenile, or hamartomatous. Fundic gland polyps are neoplastic in nature, but development of carcinoma rare and not usual in childhood. Gastric adenomas should be completely excised. Endoscopic follow-up necessary owing to high risk of new adenomas.

2. Peutz-Jeghers syndrome: 40% present with gastric polyps usually at the antrum. May present with antral obstruction but usually asymptomatic. Histologically, polyps with arborizing framework of smooth muscle covered by hyperplastic fundic or antral type mucosa. Risk of malignancy low.

3. Juvenile polyposis: stomach involved in generalized juvenile polyposis and juvenile polyposis of infancy. Most sessile hamartomatous polyps measure 5–40 mm. Characterized by large cystic spaces lined by foveolar epithelium with mixed inflammatory infiltrate at the lamina propria. Risk of malignant transformation in stomach lower than in the colon. Reasonable to require periodic upper endoscopy.

4. Gastric teratoma: Rare tumor composed of mesodermal, endodermal, and ectodermal elements. Occurs exclusively in the pediatric population. Nearly all patients are male, usually age < 2 yr. Present with large intra-abdominal masses that can lead to obstruction and upper GI bleeding owing to ulceration of the overlying mucosa. Imaging studies may demonstrate calcifications. Excision curative.

MALIGNANT TUMORS OF THE STOMACH

1. Adenocarcinoma: 2–10% of gastric carcinomas in patients ages < 40 yr. Cases in children extremely rare.
2. Risk factors: in childhood, not well established. 10–25% affected children have positive family history; cases associated with familial diffuse gastric carcinoma syndrome are associated with mutations in the E-cadherin/CDH2 gene. Helicobacter pylori infection not associated with gastric cancer in children.
3. Associated conditions: immunoglobulin A deficiency, common variable immunodeficiency, ataxia telangiectasia, and Rothmund-Thomson syndrome (short stature, cataracts, skin pigmentation, baldness, and abnormalities of bone, nails, and teeth). Polyposis syndromes (familial polyposis coli and Peutz-Jeghers syndrome) also associated, but later in life.
4. Symptoms: pain, vomiting, anorexia, and weight loss. Abdominal mass can be palpated in 70%.
5. Treatment: surgery; various chemotherapy protocols and radiation therapy. Lymphatic, vascular, and direct extension and seeding of peritoneum reported.

HEMATOPOIETIC NEOPLASMS

1. Gastric lymphoma: 2.5–17% of GI non-Hodgkin lymphomas in children. Predisposing condition: primary immunodeficiency. B-cell lymphomas (most frequent neoplasia in human immunodeficiency virus) frequently involve the stomach. Clinical presentation: abdominal pain, abdominal mass, and GI bleeding. Gastric outlet obstruction has been reported. Most are cytologically high-grade cancers. Treatment: resection; postoperative chemotherapy and radiation therapy.
2. Langherhans cell histiocytosis: rarely involves stomach. Diffuse antral and fundic polyposis and granulomatous pattern of histiocytosis is noticeable.

MESENCHYMAL NEOPLASMS

Gastrointestinal stromal tumor (GIST): rare. Spindle or epithelioid mesenchymal neoplasms expressing KIT. Firm, tan, well-circumscribed masses. Described as a component of Carney triad (gastric epithelioid stromal sarcoma, functioning extra-adrenal paraganglioma, and pulmonary chondroma). GIST have oncogenic mutations of the KIT gene. Most in stomach, intraluminal or subserosal masses. Commonly present with GI bleeding and intestinal obstruction.

MISCELLANEOUS

1. Gastric hemangiomas: frequently associated with vascular lesions of skin and intestine. Hematemesis frequent initial symptom. Benign; require surgery.

2. Gastric lipomas: slow-growing tumors. Frequently originate from submucosa. Usually located at antrum as sessile and polypoid lesions that may intussuscept into the pylorus or duodenum. Mucosal ulceration with chronic blood loss reported. MRI T1 images show fat enhancement. On endoscopy, the mass will sink if poked with forceps. If small, can remove via polypectomy; larger lesions may require laparotomy.
3. Inflammatory myofibroblastic tumor: rare cases in stomach. Histologically, spindle-shaped myofibroblasts (smooth muscle markers) embedded in collagenized stoma with chronic inflammatory cells. May be aggressive and invade, requiring surgical resection.
4. Gastric hamartoma: benign lesions composed of abnormal admixture of components of the gastric wall.
5. Gastric leiomyosarcoma: Leiomyomas and leiomyosarcomas reported with Alport syndrome, acquired immunodeficiency syndrome, pulmonary osteoarthropathy, and Carney triad.

QUESTIONS

MATCH THE CONDITIONS WITH THE ASSOCIATED TUMOR TYPE:

a. Barrett esophagus.
b. Caustic ingestion.
c. Achalasia.
d. Alport syndrome.
e. KIT gene.

1. Squamous cell carcinoma of esophagus.
2. Adenocarcinoma of the esophagus.
3. Gastrointestinal stromal tumor.
4. Leiomyomatosis.
5. Pseudodiverticulosis.

6. The following is true about gastric carcinoma in children except:
   a. Extremely rare in children.
   b. There is a positive family history in 10–25% of affected children.
   c. Associated with Helicobacter pylori infection in children.
   d. Associated with primary immunodeficiencies.
   e. Associated with polyposis syndromes.

7. Esophageal squamous cell carcinoma is associated with all the following except:
   a. Tylosis.
   b. Celiac disease.
   c. Nitrosamines.
   d. Achalasia.
   e. Gastroesophageal reflux.

8. The following is false about gastric teratoma except:
   a. Has no age predilection in children.
   b. Tends to occur in adults.
   c. Is more common among females.

d. Requires chemotherapy for cure.

e. Imaging may demonstrate calcifications.

9. Which of the following are false regarding gastric polyps in Peutz-Jeghers syndrome?

    a. Usually located at the antrum.

    b. Usually asymptomatic.

    c. High risk of malignancy.

    d. Can present with gastric outlet obstruction.

    e. All of the above are true.

10. The following are true of esophageal cysts except:

    a. Usually seen in upper third of esophagus.

    b. Communicate with esophageal lumen in 10% of cases.

    c. Small risk of malignant transformation.

    d. Treatment is surgical resection.

    e. Usually single.

MOTOR DISORDERS, INCLUDING PYLORIC STENOSIS

SYNOPSIS

NORMAL MOTOR ACTIVITY OF STOMACH AND DUODENUM

1. Motor activity requires integrity of smooth muscle, interstitial cells of Cajal, innervation, and humoral secretion.

2. Proximal half of stomach is a reservoir, allowing for large changes in volume. Receptive relaxation of proximal muscles occurs to accommodate ingested food and is mediated by a vagal reflex. Recent evidence favors nitric oxide (NO) as inhibitory transmitter. Weak tonic contractions move intragastric contents to antrum and pylorus (under vagal, intrinsic cholinergic stimulation).

3. Distal stomach half includes antrum and pylorus. Contraction is phasic, organized to break up food and move contents to duodenum in an aboral direction. Antral waves occur at 3 cycles/min.

4. When digestible food emptied from stomach, digestive phase ends and fasting phase begins. (Liquids empty faster than solids. In infants, increased caloric density delays gastric emptying.) Remaining gastric contents are swept into duodenum by forceful rhythmic contractions (phase 3 of fasting state). Antral waves occur at 3 cycles/min, determined by a pacemaker region at the greater curvature (interstitial cells of Cajal).

5. In duodenum, when receiving chyme from stomach, continuous segmenting activity ensures maximal mixing and mucosal exposure. Duodenal waves occur at 11 cycles/min.

6. In fasting state, a band of forceful contractions propagates contents in aboral direction down the gut. This is the migrating myoelectric complex (MMC), occurring at intervals of 100 minutes.

DISORDERED GASTRODUODENAL ACTIVITY

1. Emesis: activation of the emetic reflex results in preejection and ejection phase. Initiated by inputs (dorsal vagal nuclei and chemoreceptor trigger zone):

    a. Preejection phase: autonomic responses (eg, nausea or skin pallor).

    b. Ejection phase: forcible contraction of the abdominal, diaphragmatic, and intercostal muscles.

2. Rapid gastric emptying: most frequently occurs after surgery (especially gastric resection) and in some patients with peptic ulcer.

3. Delayed gastric emptying: many causes (anatomic, metabolic or electrolyte disorder, drugs, neuronal or muscle dysfunction, infection, idiopathic).

4. Duodenogastric reflux: bile-stained vomiting.

DISEASES OF STOMACH AND DUODENUM

1. Hypertrophic pyloric stenosis: grossly thickened circular muscle at pylorus developing in first few weeks of life. More common in firstborn; 2.5 times more common in whites; male-to-female ratio 5:1. Inheritance polygenic. Risk highest in firstborn male of an affected mother. Etiology unknown; appears related to defective NO innervation. Presentation: nonbilious projectile emesis, hypochloremic alkalosis, and jaundice. Ultrasonography: muscle thickness > 4 mm and pyloric length > 16 mm. Treatment: pyloromyotomy following rehydration and correction of metabolic alkalosis. Postoperative complications: incomplete myotomy (usually resolves with conservative management) and wound dehiscence.

2. Idiopathic gastroparesis: may develop in healthy children, preceded by flu-like illness or gastroenteritis.

3. Gastric antral dysrhythmias: dysfunction and alteration of the usual slow wave frequency of 3 cycles/min.

4. Migraine and nonulcer dyspepsia: nausea and vomiting are common symptoms. Conditions not rigorously defined in children.

5. Lesions of extrinsic innervation:

    a. Local lesions of vagal, vestibular nuclei, labyrinth, and increased intracranial pressure may result in disordered gastroduodenal motility and emesis.

    b. Infectious, metabolic, or degenerative disorders: infections (eg, varicella-zoster virus and Epstein-Barr virus) reported to cause pseudo-obstruction. Guillain-Barré syndrome causes autonomic dysfunction, may affect motility. Common metabolic causes of gastroparesis in adults (diabetes and amyloidosis) occur only rarely in children. Riley-Day syndrome (pandysautonomia) can lead to vomiting, constipation, internal ophthalmoplegia, lack of tears or sweating, and orthostatic hypotension; degeneration of sensory and autonomic nerves occurs secondary to mutations of IKBKAP kinase gene.

    c. Vagotomy: after vagotomy, impaired relaxation of proximal stomach leads to early satiety or epigastric fullness. Rapid initial emptying of liquids (dumping). Truncal or total vagotomy: entire stomach loses vagal innervation with defective relaxation of the proximal stomach, defective antral motility, and delayed emptying of solids. Also, MMCs contribute less frequently to stasis of solids.

6. Enteric nervous system disorders: may be familial, limited entirely to the gut as in congenital absence of

argyrophil nerves (X-linked or autosomal recessive) and familial megaduodenum as part of a familial visceral neuropathy.

7. Disorders affecting gastroduodenal smooth muscle: smooth muscle disease as part of a systemic disease very rare in children. Most suffer from 2 syndromes: hollow visceral myopathy and megacystis-microcolon–intestinal hypoperistalsis syndrome. Pathogenesis of both not understood.

8. Drugs: cholinergic agents, adrenergic, dopaminergic, chemotherapeutic compounds, opioids, and calcium channel blockers.

9. Postfundoplication: some may develop gas-bloat syndrome with early satiety, bloating, nausea, retching, and vomiting, especially children with severe neurologic impairment.

10. Small intestinal malrotation: common feature of pseudo-obstructive disorders. Aberrant antroduodenal dysmotility shown in surgically corrected children with prolonged feeding difficulties.

DIAGNOSTIC TECHNIQUES

1. Contrast studies to delineate anatomic abnormalities.
2. Manometry: in patients with suspected pseudo-obstruction, study at least three areas: esophagus, small intestine, and rectosigmoid colon. Need to observe in fasting and fed states. In myopathic processes, low-amplitude, poorly propagated contractions. In neuropathies, normal-amplitude contractions with abnormalities in waveform and propagation. Disturbances in neuroendocrine environment can manifest as increased slow wave frequency (catecholamine excess diseases: hyperthyroidism, pheochromocytoma, ganglioneuroma) or decreased slow wave frequency (preterm infants and hypothyroidism).
3. Gastric emptying studies and scintiscan.
4. Electrogastrography: recording of myoelectric activity of the smooth muscle of the stomach by electrodes.
5. Histology: full-thickness biopsies to demonstrate disease of smooth muscle or enteric nerves; sampling error is problematic.

TREATMENT

1. Patients without anatomic abnormalities: not possible to treat surgically. Patients with isolated tachygastria: antrectomy successful after pseudo-obstruction ruled out. Children with duodenal pseudo-obstruction or superior mesenteric artery syndrome: gastroenterostomy sometimes beneficial. In patients with general-ized pseudo-obstruction, adhesional obstruction often occurs after laparotomy.

2. Prokinetic agents are usually unsuccessful. Treatment of malnutrition and primary disease is helpful and necessary.

PROGNOSIS

1. Excellent in uncomplicated pyloric stenosis and malrotation.
2. Pseudo-obstruction: uncertain.
3. In conditions affecting extrinsic innervation: prognosis affected by underlying condition.
4. In patients with intrinsic neuromuscular disease: mortality may be as high as 25%, especially in early years of life.

QUESTIONS

MATCH THE PROCESS TO ITS FREQUENCY:

a. 3 cycles/min.
b. Every 100 min.
c. 11 cycles/min.

1. Migrating motor complex.
2. Antral contraction waves.
3. Duodenal contraction waves.

CHOOSE THE BEST ANSWER:

4. Which of the following is false of hypertrophic pyloric stenosis?
   a. It is a congenital disorder.
   b. It occurs more commonly in males.
   c. It appears to be a defect in nitric oxide innervation.
   d. It can often be corrected by pyloromyotomy.

5. Mutations in which gene leads to autonomic nerve degeneration in Riley-Day syndrome?
   a. RET tyrosine kinase gene.
   b. *IKBKAP* kinase gene.
   c. *BCL2* gene.
   d. Endothelin 3 gene.

6. Which of the following are associated with a decreased slow wave frequency?
   a. Pheochromocytoma.
   b. Hyperthyroidism.
   c. Ganglioneuromas.
   d. Prematurity.

ANSWERS

CONGENITAL ANOMALIES
1. d.
2. e.
3. d.
4. b.
5. d. Located at greater curvature.
6. False. Occur at level of ampulla of Vater.
7. True.

GASTRITIS
1. b.
2. a.
3. b.
4. b.
5. a.
6. b.
7. a.
8. b.
9. False. Only gastric tissue.
10. True.
11. False. 2% in children older than 5 years old.
12. True.
13. True.
14. False. D cells make somatostatin.
15. False. G cells make gastrin.
16. False. Usually self-limited.

17. c.
18. a.
19. b.
20. d.
21. g.
22. f.

ESOPHAGEAL AND GASTRIC NEOPLASMS
1. b.
2. a.
3. e.
4. d.
5. c.
6. c. *Helicobacter pylori* association is in adults.
7. e.
8. e.
9. c. Low risk.
10. a. Usually seen in lower third.

MOTOR DISORDERS INCLUDING PYLORIC STENOSIS
1. b.
2. a.
3. c.
4. a. Not congenital.
5. b.
6. d.

CLINICAL MANIFESTATIONS AND MANAGEMENT:
The Intestine

ANATOMIC ANOMALIES

SYNOPSIS

DEFINITIONS

1. Foregut: from pharynx to proximal duodenum down to level of bile duct, liver, pancreas, and biliary system. Arterial supply: celiac artery.
2. Midgut: gives rise to small intestine beyond the opening of the bile duct up to the proximal transverse colon. Arterial supply: superior mesenteric artery.
3. Hindgut: distal transverse colon to superior portion of anal canal. Caudal hindgut: cloaca. Arterial supply: inferior mesenteric artery. Epithelium of anal canal derived from endoderm of hindgut rostrally and ectoderm caudally as marked by pectinate line.

OMPHALOCELE (SEE ALSO HERNIA SECTION)

1. Congenital defects in abdominal wall. Eviscerated abdominal organs contained in membranous sac. When coexists with defects of diaphragm, sternum, pericardium, and heart: pentalogy of Cantrell.
2. Associations: other congenital abnormalities, especially trisomies 13, 18, and 21.

GASTROSCHISIS (SEE ALSO HERNIA SECTION)

1. Abdominal wall defect to right of umbilicus.
2. No overlying membrane.
3. Abnormalities of intestine (especially atresia) occur in 10%.
4. Extra abdominal anomalies and chromosome abnormalities rare.

OMPHALOCELE AND GASTROSCHISIS

Develop at 5–10 weeks of gestation. High alpha fetoprotein.

OMPHALOMESENTERIC DUCT

1. Can be completely patent or completely closed, leaving a diverticulum (most commonly Meckel) or cords (which can cause obstruction or volvulus). If patent, fistula presents with persistent umbilical discharge.
2. Diagnosis: patent omphalomesenteric duct: pass nasogastric (NG) tube through fistula and inject contrast or aspirate small bowel contents. Meckel diverticulum: use Meckel scan with H2 antagonists, glucagon, and pentagastrin to increase sensitivity.
3. Treatment: resection.

CONGENITAL HERNIA AND HYDROCELE

1. Common abnormalities of childhood; peak incidence in neonatal period. Hernias/hydroceles result from persistent patency of the processus vaginalis.
2. Congenital inguinal hernia: presence of abdominal viscus in processus vaginalis. Spontaneous resolution does not occur; surgical revision is advised.
3. Congenital hydrocele: associated with a narrow patent processus vaginalis that becomes distended by peritoneal fluid. Most hydroceles spontaneously resolve in the first 6 months of life. Treatment is conservative; if hydrocele not closed by 2 yr, operative closure recommended.

INTESTINAL DIVERTICULA

Lesions on mesenteric border; may be multiple; rare. Involves jejunum more than ileum.

BOWEL ATRESIAS

1. Affected areas in order of frequency: duodenum, jejunum, ileum, and colon; 5 types (Figure 1); 1/5,000 to 1/3,000 live births. Polyhydramnios seen in gastrointestinal atresias of proximal gut.
2. Duodenal atresia: occurs at 4–8 wk of gestation with a recanalization defect of the intestinal lumen. Obstruction at level of ampulla of Vater. Incidence: 1/10,000 to 1/6,000. Associated anomalies: trisomy 21, congenital heart disease, esophageal atresia, anorectal anomalies, and malrotation. Annular pancreas may encircle duodenum at point of atresia. Abdominal radiograph demonstrates double-bubble sign. Preferred surgery: duodenoduodenal anastomosis.
3. Jejunoileal atresia: develops as a result of ischemic infarction of a segment of fetal intestine. Distal ileal atresia must be distinguished from meconium ileus and long-segment Hirschsprung disease.
4. Colonic atresia: rare. Presents with abdominal distention, failure to pass stool, and vomiting. Contrast enema will distinguish from distal ileal atresia and Hirschsprung disease. Treat with local excision.

MIDGUT MALROTATION

1. Most common: third part of the duodenum lies to the right of the vertebral column and the cecum lies in the upper abdomen to the left of the duodenum. Mesentery of the midgut is narrow, twists at any time with torsion leading to midgut ischemia. Risk of volvulus highest during the neonatal period.

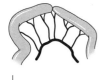 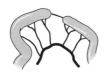 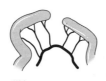 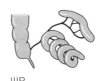 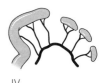

| I | II | IIIA | IIIB | IV |

FIGURE 1 *Type I,* Complete membrane and mucosal diaphragm obstructing lumen. *Type II,* Proximal and distal blind segments joined by fibrous cord. *Type IIIA,* Complete disruption without connection. *Type IIIB,* Proximal jejunal atresia and absence of distal superior mesenteric artery (apple peel atresia). *Type IV,* Multiple string of sausages from duodenum to colon.

2. Presentation: bilious emesis, abdominal pain, distention, and tenderness; hematochezia suggests ischemia. With ischemia, hypovolemia and metabolic acidosis will result.

3. Treatment: urgent laparotomy required after fluid and electrolyte resuscitation and NG decompression. At surgery, the volvulus derotated in the anticlockwise direction. If viability of the bowel uncertain, bowel reexamined after 24–36 h.

DUPLICATIONS

1. Congenital tubular or spherical cysts attached to gut, most commonly at ileocecal region. Blood supply with adjacent normal structure is shared. Intestinal duplications lie on the mesenteric side of the small intestine and antimesenteric side of large bowel.

2. Presentation: abdominal mass or obstruction. Ulceration secondary to acid secretion may lead to gastrointestinal bleeding or perforation. Ultrasonography and radiography may help to distinguish duplication from ovarian cyst.

3. Treatment: excision or extraction of just mucosa if too much gut needs to be resected.

MECONIUM PLUG SYNDROME

1. Whitish plug of epithelial cells causing obstruction to passage of meconium.

2. Common in premature infants.

3. Cystic fibrosis and Hirschsprung disease need to be excluded.

MECONIUM ILEUS

1. Almost unique to cystic fibrosis. Definitive diagnosis: sweat Cl > 60 meq/L. Two forms:
   a. Simple: distal small bowel obstructed by meconium. Accompanied by microcolon.
   b. Complicated: includes other features such as atresias or volvulus, necrosis, perforation or peritonitis, and meconium pseudocyst.

2. Differential diagnosis: ileal atresia, Hirschsprung disease, colonic atresia, meconium plug, or small left colon syndrome (infants of diabetic mothers). Difficult to distinguish from ileal atresia on radiograph; may see ground glass at right lower quadrant and lack of air fluid levels on upright.

3. Treatment: Gastrografin enema. Success rate 60%, perforation 3%. Children who recover from meconium ileus have same prognosis as those without.

ANORECTAL ANOMALIES

1. Most often detected during routine postnatal examination; 1/2,500 live births. Lesion usually associated with fistulous communication between rectum and either the genitourinary (GU) tract or perineum. Spectrum is anterior malposition of the anus to anal agenesis. Up to 60% of infants will have malformations affecting other organ systems (vertebral, anal, cardiac, tracheal, esophageal, renal, and limb).

2. Surgical options are to form a colostomy or perform definitive reconstruction (only low lesions). Long-term outcome variable and dependent on initial anatomy; high malformations have poorer outcome and higher rates of fecal incontinence.

CLOACAL EXSTROPHY (SEE ALSO HERNIA SECTION)

1. Rare and complicated birth defect; 1/250,000 births. Cause unknown.

2. Genitalia usually ambiguous. Often need to send for chromosomal analyses to determine gender. Small bowel may be shorter than normal. Normal intelligence.

3. Can be part of OEIS complex which includes: omphalocele, exstrophy of the cloaca, imperforate anus, spinal defects; varying degrees of spina bifida.

4. Treatment: surgery to repair omphalocele. Major urinary reconstructive surgery, in which a neobladder is created; vagina may also be created at this time.

5. Prognosis: very good chance of survival. Quality of life will depend on severity of anomalies.

HIRSCHSPRUNG DISEASE

1. Absence of ganglion cells in a variable length of distal bowel; 1/5,000 newborns. In 80% aganglionosis confined to rectum and sigmoid. Most common associated mutation: involves RET gene. Common in Down syndrome. Suspect in infants who have not passed meconium in 48 h of birth and with signs of bowel obstruction. Diagnosis by rectal suction biopsy at 2–4 cm above anal verge. Histopathology: absence of ganglion cells, thickened nerve trunks, and increased acetylcholinesterase. Anorectal manometry diagnostic: in older children, absent rectoanal inhibitory reflex.

2. Surgical reconstruction principles: excision of aganglionic colon and pull through of ganglionic colon with coloanal anastomosis.

3. Hirschsprung enterocolitis: potentially life-threatening complication that can occur before or after surgery. Characterized by pyrexia, abdominal distention, malaise, and constipation or diarrhea. Treatment is empiric, consisting of rectal washouts, antibiotics, probiotics, and sodium cromoglycate. Chemical (botulinum toxin) or surgical internal sphincterotomy may be of benefit.

PANCREATIC CONGENITAL ANOMALIES

Abnormalities of rotation and fusion account for most; 60–70% have normal ductal anatomy.

PANCREAS DIVISUM

1. Most common variant of human pancreas (10%).

2. Results from incomplete fusion of dorsal and ventral pancreatic ductal systems (at second month of gestation), thus no formation of main pancreatic duct of Wirsung.

3. Most pancreatic exocrine secretions enter duodenum via minor duct (accessory duct of Santorini) and papilla.

4. Affects males and females equally.

5. Most cases asymptomatic.

6. If symptomatic, present with acute pancreatitis usually at 20–40 yr of age.

7. Diagnosis: endoscopic retrograde cholangiopancreatography (ERCP). Treatment: sphincterotomy.

HETEROTOPIC PANCREAS

1. Ectopic or aberrant pancreas: presence of pancreatic tissue that lacks anatomic and vascular continuity with main body of pancreas; 70% located at upper GI tract. Most asymptomatic.
2. Endoscopy: well-defined dome-shaped defect with central umbilication. Histology: usually normal gastric mucosa since pancreatic tissue is submucosal or subserosal. Incidental lesions: leave alone.

ANNULAR PANCREAS

1. Flat band of pancreatic tissue completely encircling second portion of duodenum.
2. Symptoms: in newborn: polyhydramnios, poor feeding tolerance. In adults: postprandial obstructive symptoms.
3. Associations: Down syndrome and duodenal atresia.
4. Diagnosis: double-bubble sign on abdominal radiograph needed in adults to diagnose ERCP.
5. Treatment: surgical bypass.

CONGENITAL CYSTS OF PANCREAS

1. Associations: polycystic disease, cystic fibrosis, and von Hippel-Lindau disease.
2. If symptomatic and only one solitary cyst: surgical resection and drainage. Surgery not usually advisable for multiple cysts.

QUESTIONS

MATCH THE LOCATION:

a. Foregut.
b. Midgut.
c. Hindgut.

1. Pharynx to proximal duodenum.
2. Superior mesenteric artery.
3. Celiac artery.
4. Cloacal exstrophy.

TRUE OR FALSE:

5. Intestinal duplications are located on the antimesenteric side of the colon.
6. Duodenal atresia is the most common type of intestinal atresia.
7. In a male newborn with imperforate anus, meconium at the perineum is a sign of a low lesion.
8. In a female newborn with imperforate anus, meconium at the perineum is a sign of a low lesion.
9. Most persons with pancreas divisum will present with signs and symptoms consistent with acute pancreatitis.
10. Usual or typical pancreatic duct anatomy occurs in 95% of cases.
11. Midgut volvulus is reduced in a clockwise fashion.

MATCH THE FIGURE TO THE CONDITION:

a. IV   b. I   c. IIIB   d. II

12. Type II intestinal atresia.
13. Type I intestinal atresia.
14. Type IV intestinal atresia.

CHOOSE THE BEST ANSWER:

15. Which is not true?
    a. Meckel diverticulum is a true diverticulum.
    b. Meckel diverticulum is a form of intestinal duplication.
    c. Meckel diverticulum is associated with malignancy.
    d. Meckel diverticulum arises from the mesenteric border.
    e. Meckel diverticulum is a variant of the omphalomesenteric duct.
    f. None of the above.

16. Annular pancreas:
    a. Encircles the third portion of the duodenum.
    b. Presents with gastrointestinal bleeding in the newborn.
    c. Is associated with Down syndrome.
    d. Is not associated with duodenal atresia.
    e. Is medically managed.

HERNIAS

SYNOPSIS

OMPHALOCELE

1. Prevalence: 1/20,000 to 1/5,000 live births. More males than females. No racial differences in incidence.
2. Associations: trisomy 18 (10–40%) and Beckwith-Wiedemann syndrome. If no associated chromosomal anomalies, survival and quality of life is good.
3. Diagnosis: prenatal ultrasonography. Hernia of abdominal contents into umbilical stalk with viscera covered by gelatinous, translucent sac.
4. Repair soon after birth; may require a silo with progressive squeezing of contents into the abdomen in the ensuing postoperative days. Intestinal necrosis may occur owing to increased abdominal pressure and ischemia and lead to short gut.
5. Associated malrotation usually does not cause problems but may lead to volvulus. Surgical correction may be required.

TABLE 1   TYPES OF HERNIAS IN CHILDREN

Omphalocele (exomphalos)
Cloacal exstrophy
Gastroschisis (laparoschisis)
Congenital diaphragmatic hernia
Hernia of Morgagni
Inguinal hernia
Femoral hernia
Umbilical hernia
Epigastric hernia

6. Gastroesophageal reflux detected in one-half of cases; may require fundoplication.

CLOACAL EXSTROPHY

1. Very rare. Prevalence 1/400,000 to 1/200,000. Slightly more males than females.
2. Major defect of abdominal wall: omphalocele, bladder exstrophy, ileal prolapse, absent anus, vertebral bodies malformed, and other malformations. Short bowel may exist at onset, aggravated by use of intestine for reconstruction of genitourinary tract or stomas. Fecal incontinence or permanent stomas often unavoidable.
3. Gender assignment difficult at birth on visual inspection alone. Often requires sex chromosomal analyses.
4. Surgical corrections multiple and require coordination with multiple specialty services.

GASTROSCHISIS

1. Abdominal wall defect on right side of umbilical cord insertion allowing evisceration of part of abdominal contents without an overlying membrane.
2. Etiology unknown. Lack of association with chromosomal diseases. Prenatal diagnosis possible on ultrasound.
3. Prevalence: 1/20,000 to 1/3,000 gestations; affects males and females equally.
4. Prenatally, patients usually small for gestational age because of fetal malnutrition; at birth, normal except for gastroschisis.
5. After birth, repositioning of bowel into abdomen urgently required to reduce fluid depletion and bacterial contamination. Silo may be required.
6. May have associated intestinal atresias. Malrotation almost constant.
7. Invariably intestinal dysmotility and delays in start of enteral feeding. Gastroesophageal reflux (GER) common. Need to provide adequate nutrition via parenteral nutrition.

CONGENITAL DIAPHRAGMATIC HERNIA

1. Intra-abdominal organs displaced into thorax through posterolateral diaphragmatic orifice (usually on left side). Lung hypoplasia seen as well as associated malformations. Intestines not normally rotated.
2. Prevalence 1/4,000 live births. No gender or racial differences.
3. Diaphragmatic orifice due to incomplete growth of posthepatic mesenchymal plate prior to pleuroperitoneal canal closure. Lung hypoplasia is primary.
4. Prenatal diagnosis: ultrasound.
5. Presentation: at birth, hollow abdomen with displacement of heart sounds and severe respiratory distress. Radiographs show displacement of abdominal viscera into chest.
6. Perinatal treatment: endoscopic fetal surgery followed by ventilatory support and extracorporeal membrane oxygenation at birth increases survival.
7. With survival, chronic respiratory insufficiency, pectus excavatum, sensorineural sequelae, GER abnormal

motility, and malrotation. Complication: necrotizing enterocolitis.

MORGAGNI HERNIA

1. Herniation of abdominal viscera through anterior, retrosternal orifice of diaphragm. Prenatal diagnosis possible on ultrasound.
2. Rare; associated with trisomy 21.
3. Often asymptomatic, but may induce repeated respiratory infections, abdominal pain, and vomiting because of gastric malposition or malrotation.
4. Surgical repair advised.

UMBILICAL HERNIA

1. Caused by failed closure of fascial orifice of umbilicus shortly after birth. Can contain bowel; rarely, can strangulate, incarcerate, or rupture bowel.
2. Common in otherwise healthy newborns and especially in premature infants. No gender difference; 5–10 times more common in black than white infants.
3. Fascial orifice reduces spontaneously and closes itself. If persists > 4 yr (rare), requires surgical correction.
4. More common in Beckwith-Wiedemann syndrome, Hurler syndrome, Ehlers-Danlos syndrome, congenital hypothyroidism, and trisomy 13 or 18 with reduced spontaneous closure.

EPIGASTRIC HERNIA

1. Defects of linea alba where fascial layers of anterior abdominal wall fuse; may allow protrusion of intra-abdominal contents.
2. Frequent. Asymptomatic in most cases. Slim persons more affected.
3. On physical exam, defect can be palpated.
4. Surgical reinforcement of defect is corrective.

INGUINAL HERNIA

1. Fetal communication (processus vaginalis testis) between peritoneum and vaginal celomic compartments persists (usually obliterated at eighth month of gestation) partially or entirely allowing intestinal loops to pass into the inguinal canal. Involved viscus: bowel or omentum in boys, ovary or fallopian tube in girls. Prevalence: 1/50 boys, 1/500 girls. In boys, two-thirds appear on right; no side predilection in girls. Bilateral hernias more common in girls (50%).
2. Associations: diseases with increased intra-abdominal pressure (chronic respiratory disease), connective tissue disorders, or abundant peritoneal fluid (ventriculoperitoneal shunting or peritoneal dialysis).
3. Main symptom: bulge in groin or scrotum that reduces spontaneously usually. Bowel incarceration: painful swelling. Strangulation often presents with bowel obstruction.
4. Littre hernia: strangulation of Meckel diverticulum into an inguinal hernia.
5. Treatment: surgical. Controversial whether contralateral inguinal exploration should be performed. Recurrence rare.

FEMORAL HERNIA

Occurs through femoral canal medial to femoral vein, posterior to inguinal ligament, and lateral to lacunar ligament. Swelling occurs below inguinal ligament.

HIATAL HERNIA

1. Sliding:
   a. Symptoms: GER, vomiting, failure to thrive, recurrent chest infections, dysphagia, and stricture or hemorrhage.
   b. Diagnosis: upper gastrointestinal series. Esophagogastroduodenoscopy: bell sign.
   c. Treatment: may not be necessary. Surgery involves tightening of right crus of diaphragm posteriorly and partial or complete esophageal wrap.
2. Paraesophageal:
   a. Coincidental finding. Dysphagia can be prominent symptom; pain often a feature. Normal gastroesophageal junction position.
   b. Treatment: surgery always indicated because risk of incarceration stomach, gastric volvulus, and gastric perforation.

QUESTIONS

CHOOSE THE BEST ANSWER:

1. Umbilical hernias:
   a. Are more common in white infants.
   b. Can close spontaneously up to 5 years of age.
   c. Are more common in fullterm than premature infants.
   d. Are less likely to close spontaneously when associated with chromosomal anomalies.
   e. All of the above.

2. Inguinal hernias:
   a. Are more common on the right in boys.
   b. Occur more commonly in boys.
   c. Are often bilateral in girls.
   d. Are more likely to occur in patients with chronic lung disease.
   e. All of the above.

3. Congenital diaphragmatic hernias:
   a. Occur more commonly on the right.
   b. Are more common in males.
   c. Are associated with lung hypoplasia.
   d. Are not associated with malrotation.
   e. All of the above.

4. Umbilical hernias are associated with all of the following except:
   a. Beckwith-Wiedemann syndrome.
   b. Hurler syndrome.
   c. Ehlers-Danlos syndrome.
   d. Down syndrome.
   e. Trisomy 18.

5. Malrotation is found in all of the following except:
   a. Omphalocele.
   b. Gastroschisis.
   c. Congenital diaphragmatic hernia.
   d. Umbilical hernia.
   e. Cloacal exstrophy.

6. The following are associated with chromosomal abnormalities except:
   a. Omphalocele.
   b. Morgagni hernia.
   c. Umbilical hernia.
   d. Gastroschisis.
   e. All of the above are associated with chromosomal anomalies.

TRUE OR FALSE:

7. Not all hiatal hernias require surgical management.
8. Epigastric hernias occur more frequently in obese persons.
9. Paraesophageal hernias are often coincidentally found.

PERITONITIS

SYNOPSIS

PERITONEUM

1. Functional membrane lining the intra-abdominal wall and viscera. Normally, peritoneal cavity is a sterile environment with serous fluid. Normal peritoneal cells are 50% macrophages, 44% lymphocytes, 2% dendritic cells, and a few eosinophils and mast cells.
2. Peritonitis: local or systemic response is initiated to eradicate pathogens; characterized by hyperemia, exudation of protein-rich fluid, and influx of neutrophils. Mesothelial cells play an active role through secretion of cytokines and adhesion receptor upregulation for leukocyte recruitment.

ETIOLOGY OF PERITONITIS ACCORDING TO AGE

ANTENATAL

1. Meconium peritonitis after intestinal perforation (most common cause is meconium ileus associated with cystic fibrosis followed by intestinal atresia, Hirschsprung disease, antenatal appendicitis, and intrauterine parvovirus B19 infection).
2. Diagnosis: prenatal ultrasound shows ascites or calcifications in bowel wall.
3. Management: depends on clinical or radiologic presentation. If asymptomatic, surveillance. If obstruction or pneumoperitoneum, laparotomy indicated.

NEWBORN

1. Clinical presentation: bilious emesis with fever. Can have septic shock picture with multiorgan failure.

Abdomen is tender and edematous. Radiographs can show ileus or pneumoperitoneum.

2. Treatment: fluid resuscitation, nasogastric (NG) decompression, and surgery for etiology with antibiotics intra- and postoperatively.

3. Etiology: necrotizing enterocolitis (NEC), intestinal perforation, spontaneous biliary perforation, omphalitis, and perforation of the urachal cyst.

CHILD

Etiologies: appendicular peritonitis, gastric ulcer perforation, Meckel diverticulum perforation, traumatic intestinal perforation, neutropenic colitis, tuberculosis peritonitis, salpingitis, and primary peritonitis.

SPECIFIC ENTITIES

MECONIUM PERITONITIS

Chemical inflammation from digestive enzymes in meconium.

NEC

1. Most common surgical emergency in newborns, especially premature infants.

2. Etiology: unclear; factors include ischemia or hypoxia, luminal factors, enteral feeding, and infection. Inflammatory factors lead to coagulation necrosis of digestive mucosa, followed by inflammatory invasion.

3. Lesions can be located anywhere in the gastrointestinal (GI) tract, but generally localized to the terminal ileum, right colon, and left colonic angle.

4. Clinical presentation: usually within 3 wk of birth, with septic appearance (abnormal gastric residues, abdominal distention with tenderness, and bloody stools). Radiographs important in looking for pneumatosis intestinalis and portal venous gas.

5. Treatment: initially medical: nothing by mouth, gastric aspiration, total parenteral nutrition (TPN), and intravenous (IV) antibiotics. Surgery limited to perforation and pneumoperitoneum.

IDIOPATHIC GASTROINTESTINAL PERFORATION

1. Occurs in premature infants with low birth weight; perforation located in terminal ileum or jejunum in antimesenteric position. Spontaneous neonatal gastric perforation rare but 4 times more frequent in boys; 85–95% occur at anterior part of greater curvature of the stomach usually within first week of life.

2. Risk factors: twin pregnancy, neonatal ventilation, umbilical artery catheter, nonsteroidal antiinflammatory drug (NSAID) use, steroid use, *Staphylococcus epidermidis* infection, and candidiasis.

3. Etiology: Histologically, discontinuous absence of internal layer of muscularis mucosae.

4. Clinical presentation: neonates with extensive abdominal distention; bluish discoloration of abdomen. Abdominal radiograph reveals pneumoperitoneum.

5. Therapy: needle puncture to relieve pneumoperitoneum. If pneumoperitoneum recurs after 2–3 needle punctures, laparotomy indicated. In the case of gastric perforation, stomach must be explored completely, as perforations often multiple.

INTESTINAL PERFORATION IN HIRSCHSPRUNG DISEASE

Usually involves the appendix in long segment disease.

SPONTANEOUS BILIARY PERFORATION

1. Occurs between 1 wk and 3 mo of age. Etiology unclear. In majority, perforation occurs at junction of cystic and common hepatic ducts.

2. Clinical presentation: abdominal distention; can be accompanied by vomiting and fever. Classic subacute presentation: 80% of infants; fluctuating mild jaundice, normal to acholic stools, slowly progressive ascites, and abdominal distention. Abdominal ultrasonography: fluid located around the gallbladder and porta hepatic without dilatation of bile duct. Hepatobiliary scan is diagnostic. Laboratory tests without elevation of transaminases. Bilirubin in ascitic fluid is higher than serum.

3. Preoperative fluid resuscitation mandatory. Surgical drainage is main recommendation. Biliary intestinal anastomosis is needed if obstruction or stenosis on cholangiogram.

OMPHALITIS

1. Common problem in neonates from developing countries owing to poor cord care.

2. Peritonitis results from direct spread of infection of umbilical cord to peritoneal cavity.

3. If intraperitoneal abscess, laparotomy and drainage must be performed.

PERFORATION OF THE URACHAL CYST

1. The urachus is the fibrous cord extending from bladder dome to the umbilicus. Disorders are due to incomplete regression.

2. Urachal cysts can become infected (usually with *Staphylococcus aureus*) and lead to peritonitis when the infected cyst perforates into the peritoneum.

3. Presentation: inflammatory mass with peritoneal irritation.

4. Diagnosis: abdominal ultrasonography and computed tomography (CT).

5. Treatment: surgical drainage and resection with part of bladder dome to reduce risk of subsequent carcinoma.

APPENDICULAR PERITONITIS

1. Most frequent form of peritonitis in children; appendix has perforated or bacteria diffused through the appendiceal wall.

2. Most common organisms: *Escherichia coli*, *Enterococcus*, *Bacteroides*, and *Pseudomonas aeruginosa*.

3. Mortality 1%.

4. Symptoms: abdominal pain with vomiting, fever, and deterioration; possible intestinal obstruction. Clinical exam: swollen, rigid abdomen. Laboratory tests: elevated white blood cell count and C-reactive protein level. Kidney, ureter, and bladder (KUB) exam: appendicolith or ileus. Ultrasonography: can demonstrate thickening of appendiceal wall.

5. Treatment: appendectomy and rinsing of peritoneal cavity. Fluid resuscitation and antibiotics important.

PERFORATION OF MECKEL DIVERTICULUM

1. Occurs in 14.5% of cases; due to ectopic gastric mucosa or ileoileal intussusception.
2. *Helicobacter pylori* infection of gastric mucosa plays minor role.
3. In newborns, NSAIDs can contribute to perforation when neonatal ischemia present.
4. Treatment: surgical resection.

GASTRIC ULCER PERFORATION

1. Rare in children. Occurs in settings of stress.
2. Symptoms: intense abdominal pain, hemorrhage, and emesis. KUB exam: pneumoperitoneum.
3. Therapy: NG tube insertion, laparoscopy, and suture of perforation. May require laparotomy or drainage in cases of abdominal distention, intestinal obstruction, or septic shock.
4. Treatment with proton pump inhibitor indicated for 1 month after surgery.

TRAUMATIC PERFORATION OF INTESTINE

1. Associated in 30–60% of cases with additional intra- or extra-abdominal lesions. Can be associated with lumbar fracture (seat belt syndrome). Usually localized at junction of fixed and mobile bowel segment (Treitz angle and ileocecal junction). Diagnosis difficult; be vigilant to avoid increased morbidity and for early surgical intervention.
2. Clinical signs: abdominal tenderness, fever, and tachycardia. KUB exam: rarely shows pneumoperitoneum. CT: shows localized pneumoperitoneum and thickened bowel wall with intraperitoneal effusion; if questionable, repeat CT in a few hours.
3. Treatment: surgical repair. If severe, surgical resection with anastomosis or colostomy.

NEUTROPENIC COLITIS

1. Inflammatory process involving colon, especially cecum in immunocompromised patients. Secondary to immunocompromise, neoplastic infiltration, ischemia, and bacterial overgrowth. Preferential location at cecum owing to distensibility, high bacterial load, and predisposition to ischemia or stasis.
2. Most common in children with acute leukemia or lymphoma or who are postrenal transplant.
3. Symptoms: diarrhea, abdominal pain, GI hemorrhage with emesis, fever, or with acute abdomen if perforation has already occurred.
4. Diagnosis: KUB: pneumatosis; CT: bowel wall thickening and dilated loops.
5. Therapy: IV antibiotics, antifungals, bowel rest, and TPN. Surgery if perforation, abscess, or GI hemorrhage. Prognosis poor with mortality rate 50–100%.

TUBERCULOSIS PERITONITIS

1. Diagnosis difficult; must be distinguished from lymphoma.
2. Two essential historical elements: contact with adult tuberculosis (TB) and documented weight loss.

3. Normal chest radiograph does not eliminate diagnosis.
4. Abdominal ultrasonography and CT: lymphadenopathy, ascites, thickened bowel wall, and omental masses. Paracentesis: may reveal presence of TB but culture can take up to 4–6 wk; can be measured for elevated adenosine deaminase activity where adenosine is converted to inosine in activated T cells (activated by mycobacterial antigens).

SALPINGITIS

1. Mode of contamination: ascending and hematogenous. Can be similar in presentation to appendicular peritonitis.
2. Diagnose and treat by laparoscopy—allows fluid sample for bacterial analysis and rinsing of peritoneum. In addition, deliver IV antibiotics.

PRIMARY PERITONITIS (SPONTANEOUS BACTERIAL PERITONITIS)

1. Infection of peritoneum without perforation of intestine. Pathogens may reach peritoneum via blood or lymphatics, vagina (ascension), translocation through bowel wall, or inserted foreign bodies.
2. Primary peritonitis characteristically develops in patients with impaired ability to clear intraperitoneal bacteria, especially in those with nephrotic syndrome (usually *Streptococcus pneumoniae*) or albumin < 1.5 g/L.
3. Presentation: fever, diffuse abdominal pain, peritoneal irritation, and vomiting.
4. Diagnosis: paracentesis and laparoscopy with fluid sampling.
5. Treatment: parenteral antibiotics.

RESULT OF PERITONITIS: ADHESIONS

1. Adhesion formation secondary to peritoneal injury.
2. Bowel obstruction secondary to adhesions occurs in 7% of patients after laparotomy.
3. Prevention of contact between peritoneal surfaces by using methylcellulose has been successful.

INTRA-ABDOMINAL ABSCESS

1. Most cases secondary to intestinal or appendiceal perforation. Tend to form in most dependent parts of abdominal cavity: at pelvis, paracolic gutters, and subphrenic spaces. Small intestinal perforation can result in interloop abscesses. Duodenal and posterior gastric perforation can result in abscess in lesser sac.
2. Most common organisms include gram negative bacilli and intestinal anaerobes.
3. Diagnose: ultrasonography or CT.
4. Treatment: percutaneous drainage and IV antibiotics.

QUESTIONS

CHOOSE THE BEST ANSWER:

1. The following are true regarding spontaneous perforation of the common bile duct except:
    a. It spontaneously occurs at all ages.
    b. It has no gender or racial predilection.

c. Bile in ascites is greater than serum bilirubin.

d. It occurs commonly where cystic and common hepatic ducts join to form the common duct.

e. All of the above are true.

2. The following are true regarding primary peritonitis except:
   a. It is associated with chronic liver and renal disease.
   b. *Streptococcus pneumoniae* is commonly cultured in patients with nephrotic syndrome.
   c. It requires ascites fluid sampling for diagnosis.
   d. It is associated with intestinal perforation.
   e. All of the above are true.

TRUE OR FALSE:

3. Intra-abdominal abscesses are most commonly caused by intestinal perforation.

4. Free air in the abdomen is not an absolute indication for laparotomy.

5. Perforation of Meckel diverticulum occurs mainly in the setting of *Helicobacter pylori* infection of gastric mucosa.

6. Traumatic perforation of the intestine occurs throughout the intestine without preferential locations.

WHAT IS THE DIAGNOSIS:

7. A full-term 10-week-old boy was examined for marked abdominal distention, irritability, and anorexia over the past week. Stools were reported to be intermittently acholic during the past month. There was no history of hyperbilirubinemia, anemia, blood transfusions, or total parenteral nutrition during the neonatal period. Medical history and family history were unremarkable. There was no history of suspected physical abuse or trauma. He had received no medications.

    On physical examination, he was irritable but well nourished and anicteric. He was afebrile with normal vital signs. His weight was 75% and length was 50% for age. Results of chest and cardiovascular examinations were normal. The abdomen was very distended, firm but not discolored. Normal bowel sounds were present. The liver was palpable just below the right costal margin but was not nodular or hard. There was no splenomegaly. There were marked ascites but no peripheral edema.

    Laboratory evaluations included mildly elevated transaminases (60s) and normal bilirubin (direct and indirect) and albumin levels. Hemoglobin and hematocrit were normal. Serum electrolytes, glucose, amylase and lipase, thyroid stimulating hormone, and T4 were normal. Abdominal findings on ultrasonography examination confirmed the presence of ascites. Technetium-99m hepatobiliary scan demonstrates extravasation of the radiopharmaceutical into the peritoneum on delayed images

BENIGN PERIANAL LESIONS

SYNOPSIS

ANATOMY

1. The rectum has 2–3 lateral curves that form mucosal folds known as valves of Houston, which terminate in the anal canal, opening on to the anal verge (Figure 1).

2. The posterior rectum is free of peritoneum, with the most distal third of the rectum devoid of peritoneum circumferentially.

3. Dentate line: marks transition from columnar epithelium of rectum to squamous epithelium of anal canal. Longitudinal folds of mucosa at dentate line: columns of Morgagni.

4. Internal and external hemorrhoid plexuses drain veins of anus and rectum.

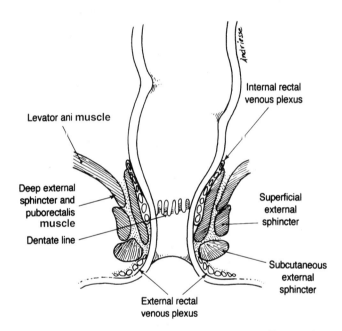

FIGURE 1   The anatomy of the rectum and anus is illustrated in coronal section.

ANAL FISSURE

1. Tear in epithelium and superficial tissues of anal canal (Figure 2). Most frequent cause of rectal bleeding in first 2 years of life.

2. Majority located at posterior midline (90%). Chronic (longer than 6 wk, with fibrosis) fissures associated with hypertrophy of anal papilla, fibrosis, and skin tag. Large fissure with bruising may indicate child abuse.

3. Pathogenesis: predisposing factors: trauma to anoderm, sphincter hypertonicity, and poor perfusion of anoderm at posterior midline.

4. By the time patient develops symptomatic fissure, sphincter hypertonicity is present.

5. Symptoms: pain at defecation; may last for hours afterwards.

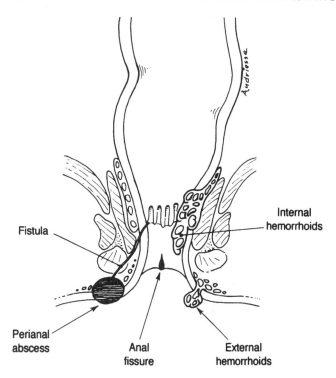

FIGURE 2 A diagrammatic representation of perianal lesions and their anatomic relationships is depicted in coronal section.

6. Treatment: stool softeners, lubricants, and fiber supplementation. Warm baths: reduce anal tone and promote good anal hygiene. Topical steroids or anesthetic do not improve healing rates. If fissure persists after therapy, consider inflammatory bowel disease, group A streptococci infection, or leukemic infiltration.

7. Chronic fissure therapy: unlikely to heal with high fiber diet and warm baths. Reduce pressure: topical 0.2% glyceryl trinitrate ointment tid. With botox injection: 95% of cases heal. In infants: gentle anal dilatation is helpful. Very infrequently, surgery required. In older children, lateral internal sphincterotomy is procedure of choice.

PERIRECTAL ABSCESS AND FISTULA IN ANO

1. Localized abscess in perirectal tissues classified by location relative to levator and sphincteric muscles; in order of most common location: perianal, ischioanal, intersphincteric, and supralevator.

2. Fistula in ano: spontaneous drainage of perirectal abscess forms a chronic infected tract from dentate line to skin. Usually occurs during first year of life. Communicates directly with rectum at crypts Morgagni. Low fistula: internal opening usually located radially opposite to external opening.

3. Often encountered in infants in diapers. Group A β-hemolytic streptococcus infection of perianal tissue sometimes associated.

4. Clinical presentation: persistent rectal pain. Onset can be acute. Sign: indurated tender area of perianal skin with or without erythema. External perianal and digital rectal exam identifies abscess in 95%.

5. Treatment: incision and drainage. Persistence of anal fistula is indication for surgery.

6. Consider Crohn disease and immune deficiency in older children.

HEMORRHOIDS

1. Hemorrhoid: varicose vein from either internal or external rectal venous plexuses.

2. Internal: painless. Lined with columnar epithelium, not innervated by sensory nerves. 3 positions: left lateral, right posterior or posterolateral, and right anterior or anterolateral.
   a. First degree: present on anal exam.
   b. Second degree: may prolapse below dentate line and reduce spontaneously.
   c. Third degree: must be manually reduced.
   d. Fourth degree: irreducible.

3. External: involve skin of anoderm external to dentate line with cutaneous innervation. Lined with squamous epithelium. Newly thrombosed external hemorrhoids associated with pain.

4. Constipation, straining, and diarrhea often associated with hemorrhoid development. Internal hemorrhoids can also be associated with chronic liver disease and portal hypertension.

5. Symptoms: external hemorrhoids rare to cause symptoms unless thrombosed; will drain spontaneously. In children, primary internal hemorrhoids virtually unknown; presence should raise questions of portal vein obstruction. Internal hemorrhoids are painless.

6. Therapy: external: do not require surgery; may be surgically removed during acute thrombosis. Internal: range from diet alterations (1st degree: stool softeners and bulk agents) to surgical removal (4th degree).

RECTAL PROLAPSE

1. Mucosal or full thickness herniation of rectum through anus. Can be confused with chronic prolapsed internal hemorrhoids; concentric rings of mucosa seen with rectal prolapse whereas usually seen in only one sector (lateral) with hemorrhoids.

2. Pathogenesis: increased intra-abdominal pressure, diarrhea, neoplasia, malnutrition, and pelvic floor weakness (surgery).

3. Most common causes: chronic constipation, diarrhea, and cystic fibrosis.

4. Clinical presentation: affects more males than females. Self-limited; tends to appear during toilet training. If recurrent, consider cystic fibrosis.

5. If recurrent: sweat test.

6. Treatment: manual reduction; treat constipation with bulk laxatives. If persistent, surgical intervention (injected sclerosant). May require more complex surgery if prior surgery (pelvic weakness present).

PILONIDAL DISEASE

1. Pilonidal abscess: inflammatory cavity overlying sacrococcygeal region at midline, often accompanied by multiple draining sinus tracts (Figure 3).

2. Pathogenesis: starts at site of ingrown hair follicle, usually 1–2 inches above anus, and leads to cavity

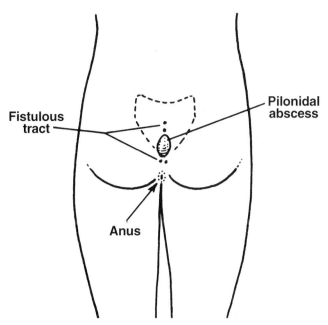

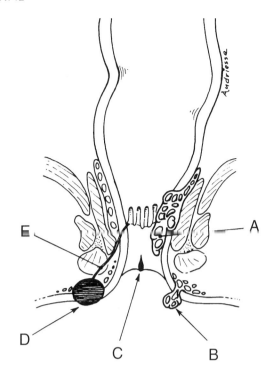

FIGURE 3 A pilonidal abscess and its associated tracts are shown in relation to the sacrum.

underlying skin. Pilonidal cyst may then drain spontaneously. If opening of tract is occluded, an abscess forms. Spontaneous drainage of a pilonidal abscess often results in chronic pilonidal sinuses.
3. Clinical presentation: persistent pain at sacrum with boil at midline just above anus
4. Diagnosis: physical examination including digital rectal exam.
5. Therapy: incision and drainage.

PRURITIS ANI
1. Persistent anal itching.
2. Primary: diagnosis of exclusion.
3. Secondary: chronic moisture, *Enterobius vermicularis*, and excessive soap use. Caffeine intake (reduces anal pressure) most common cause in older subjects. Aggressive use of soaps changes cutaneous pH and continues the irritation.
4. To diagnose: pinworm: apply transparent adhesive tape to skin around anus before bathing or using toilet in morning for pinworm egg evaluation.
5. Treatment for pinworm: pyrantel pamoate or mebendazole for 2–3 wk, plus handwashing, laundering of bedsheets twice weekly, and cleaning toilet seats. Nonpinworm therapy: discontinue excessive anal hygiene, use of ointments, steroids, or anesthetics, and scratching. Psyllium (promotes complete bowel evacuation) and loperamide (increases anal pressure) may be helpful.

QUESTIONS

MATCH THE LOCATION:
1. Internal hemorrhoids.
2. Fistula.
3. Anal fissure.

4. External hemorrhoids.
5. Perianal abscess.

CHOOSE THE BEST ANSWER:
6. All of the following are true of rectal prolapse except:
   a. It can be confused with prolapsed internal hemorrhoids.
   b. It is often associated with chronic constipation.
   c. It can be treated with laxative therapy.
   d. It occurs in more girls than boys.
   e. If it is a chronic condition, sweat test should be considered.

7. All of the following are true of hemorrhoids except:
   a. External hemorrhoids generally not associated with pain.
   b. Internal hemorrhoids in children deserve further workup.
   c. Dietary and laxative therapy is primary mode of therapy for all hemorrhoids.
   d. External hemorrhoid thrombosis often resolves spontaneously.
   e. None of the above.

8. All of the following are true of anal fissures except:
   a. They are usually linear and extend from dentate line distally.
   b. They are the most frequent etiology of rectal bleeding in first 2 years of life.
   c. If associated with bruising, child abuse must be ruled out.
   d. They are associated with sphincter hypotonicity and poor perfusion of anoderm.
   e. If condition is chronic, it will not respond to high fiber diet and warm baths.

SURGICAL ABDOMEN

SYNOPSIS

INTESTINAL OBSTRUCTION

1. Clinical symptoms: bile-stained emesis, abdominal distention, failure to pass stool, and colicky abdominal. Depends on level of obstruction and presence of complications (strangulation).
2. Radiographs most commonly used to confirm diagnosis and identify level of obstruction. Erect films will show air-fluid levels. Contrast studies may be helpful.
3. Management: nasogastric (NG) drainage, intravenous (IV) fluids for pain control. Surgical repair: only after fluid resuscitation and correction of electrolyte and acid-base abnormalities; urgency dependent on whether intestinal viability being compromised. Operation may be delayed if possibility that obstruction will resolve spontaneously; in uncomplicated intestinal obstruction, nonoperative therapy may be continued as long as evidence of progressive resolution. If no improvement by 12–24 h, operative intervention advisable.

INCARCERATED OR STRANGULATED INGUINAL HERNIA

1. Congenital inguinal hernia: presence of abdominal viscus in processus vaginalis. Spontaneous resolution does not occur. Prompt surgery advised because of high risk of incarceration during first 3 months of life (10–28%).
2. Incarcerated hernia: admit to hospital. Under sedation, reduction of hernia is performed with repair after 2 days to allow resolution of swelling. If reduction not possible then urgent surgery to reduce and repair.

MECKEL BAND OBSTRUCTION

1. Band arises from persistence of primitive omphalomesenteric duct between umbilicus and Meckel diverticulum.
2. Intestinal obstruction may result from entrapment of loop of intestine or volvulus around the band.
3. Urgent surgery required to prevent strangulation.

PERITONEAL ADHESIONS

1. Occur most commonly following surgical procedure; may occur as result of inflammatory or infectious conditions.
2. Adhesive obstruction is result of bowel entrapment and may lead to closed-loop obstruction or strangulation.
3. No reliable method for preventing adhesions.
4. Management: initially nonoperative; in most patients, obstruction will resolve in 24–48 h. However, because of risk of strangulation, operation advisable if no improvement in 6–12 h. Urgent operation if signs of compromise.

HYPERTROPHIC PYLORIC STENOSIS

1. Most common condition requiring surgery in first 2 mo of life.
2. 3/100,000 births; male-to-female ratio 4:1.
3. Underlying mechanism not understood. notable reduction in nitric oxide. Also, abnormalities shown in neural components.
4. Infants are well for the first 2–3 weeks of life; the lesion is acquired not congenital. Nonbilious emesis develops after feeds; progressive in frequency and volume. Severe dehydration and metabolic alkalosis may result.
5. Diagnosis: palpation of pylorus; confirm by ultrasonography or contrast study with elongation and narrowing of pyloric lumen.
6. Preoperative correction of fluid, electrolyte, and acid-base abnormalities essential. NG initially placed for decompression. Pyloromyotomy is treatment of choice. Postoperatively, oral feeds given on demand.

MECONIUM ILEUS EQUIVALENT (DISTAL INTESTINAL OBSTRUCTION SYNDROME)

1. Patients with cystic fibrosis may develop acute intraluminal obstruction mimicking neonatal meconium ileus.
2. Oral Gastrografin may clear the obstruction; surgical requirement rare.

MILK CURD INSPISSATION

1. Attributed to use of concentrated formula.
2. Therapy: If irrigation by radiology unsuccessful, surgery required.

FOREIGN BODY INGESTION

1. Diagnosis by plain films if radiopaque object. Commercially available metal detectors useful as radiographs for screening.
2. Asymptomatic patients allowed normal diet as outpatient (special diets and laxatives not necessary). If symptoms develop or impaction, foreign body should be removed endoscopically or surgically.

INTESTINAL STRICTURES

Pathologic narrowing of intestine by local injury, impaired blood flow, or inflammation may result in partial or complete obstruction.

SUPERIOR MESENTERIC ARTERY SYNDROME

1. Rare. Third part of duodenum obstructed between the superior mesenteric artery anteriorly and vertebral column posteriorly.
2. Predisposing factors: rapid linear growth without weight gain, weight loss, scoliosis, spinal surgery, bed confinement, or body cast. Absence of cushion of retroperitoneal fat may be a factor.
3. Clinical features: nonspecific; intermittent abdominal pain associated with anorexia, nausea, and vomiting. Exam may reveal succession splash.
4. Diagnosis: Upper gastrointestinal series demonstrating cutoff at the third to fourth portion of the duodenum where the superior mesenteric artery crosses over the duodenum.
5. Management: NG decompression and IV fluids. Symptoms may resolve with improved nutrition. Operative therapy occasionally required to mobilize ligament of

Treitz and realign duodenum. Duodenojejunostomy also has been used.

DISORDERED PERISTALSIS

PARALYTIC ILEUS

1. Form of functional intestinal obstruction owing to loss of intestinal peristalsis. Common after abdominal surgery.
2. Causes: local factors (peritonitis), intestinal ischemia, surgical manipulation, retroperitoneal bleeding, spinal surgery, sepsis, hypokalemia, diabetic ketoacidosis, and uremia.
3. Clinical picture resembles obstruction except for absence of bowel sounds.
4. Abdominal radiograph: gas throughout small and large intestine with no focal obstruction.
5. Management: NG drainage and IV fluids.

CHRONIC IDIOPATHIC INTESTINAL PSEUDO-OBSTRUCTION

1. Rare cause of functional obstruction in children with ganglionic bowel. Acute episodes may occur on background of chronic peristaltic dysfunction.
2. Treatment: symptomatic; avoid laparotomy if possible.

ACUTE ABDOMINAL PAIN

APPENDICITIS

1. Commonly, young children (under age 5 yr) present late, with perforation. Abdominal distention common.
2. Diagnosis: ultrasonograpy and computed tomography (CT).
3. Treatment: IV fluid resuscitation and IV antibiotics should be started when needed. Appendectomy is treatment of choice.

MESENTERIC ADENITIS

1. Self-limited inflammatory process that afffects the mesenteric lymph nodes in the right lower quadrant. May mimic appendicitis.
2. If no definitive cause can be identified, rule out appendicitis.

INTUSSUSCEPTION

1. Intestinal obstruction and impaired blood flow results from telescoping of a bowel segment into adjacent distal bowel. Most cases idiopathic; Peyer patches may play a role as lead point. In older children, a pathologic lead point such as Meckel diverticulum or small bowel lymphoma may be found.
2. Clinically, infants experience colicky abdominal pain associated with bilious emesis. Peak incidence at age 4–14 mo. Passage of blood and mucus per rectum is later sign of intussusception. Sausage shaped abdominal masses may be felt. In patients with gastroenteritis, sudden cessation of stools and increasing pain raises possibility of secondary intussusception.
3. Radiographs show intestinal obstruction with occasional outline of intussuscepted bowel. Confirm diagnosis by ultrasonography or contrast enema.

4. Treatment: pneumostatic or hydrostatic reduction by radiology. Resuscitation before procedure is necessary. Enema reduction is contraindicated in children in shock or with signs of peritonitis. In minority, open surgical reduction required. Necrotic bowel will need to be resected. Children over 2 yr treated nonoperatively must be investigated to exclude underlying pathology.

MIDGUT MALROTATION

1. Volvulus typically occurs in infancy but may occur in later years. Most episodes are self-correcting and not associated with intestinal ischemia. Patients present with intermittent abdominal pain with or without vomiting and history of chronic constipation.
2. Diagnosis: upper and lower intestinal contrast studies.

CONSTIPATION

1. Can be presenting feature of wide range of disorders. Examination should include evaluation for pelvic mass, anorectal pathology, and neurologic deficit and examination of lumbosacral spine.
2. Therapy should be centered on clear discussion of problem with advice on diet, toileting, and laxatives.

PARASITIC INFESTATION: ASCARIASIS

1. Infestation occurs as result of ingesting larvae. Intestinal ascariasis mimicks intussusception (with obstruction of intestine with worms), and is associated with small bowel volvulus, or appendicitis. Biliary colic and pancreatitis may result from ascaris entering the biliary tree.
2. Diagnosis: passing worms in stool and > 1 abdominal mass palpated. Kidney, ureter, bladder (KUB) examination may visualize worm bolus. Contrast enemas and ultrasound may be helpful.
3. Management: IV fluid replacement, NG drainage as needed for significant emesis, IV antispasmodic, and analgesics. Anthelmintic after acute symptoms subsided. If no resolution of biliary colic or pancreatitis with above measures, remove worm endoscopically or by surgery. Late complications include biliary and pancreatic duct strictures.

INTESTINAL POLYPS

1. Commonly present with abdominal pain; may be accompanied by hematochezia.
2. Initial investigation and therapy: endoscopic biopsy or excision.

PANCREATITIS

1. Uncommon in childhood. May present acutely, chronically, or in association with trauma. Acute pancreatitis may follow viral illnesses or in children with hyperlipidemia, cystic fibrosis, or polyarteritis nodosa. Gallstone pancreatitis rare in children. Pancreatitis may complicate intestinal ascariasis. Chronic pancreatitis may lead to irreversible changes in the pancreas. Severe fulminant pancreatitis rare.

2. Diagnosis via detection of raised serum or urinary amylase levels > 5 times normal.
3. Treatment: supportive therapy with IV fluids, bowel rest, analgesia, and antibiotics (as needed). Surgery rarely indicated.

CHOLECYSTITIS
1. Consider in child with right upper quadrant pain (Murphy sign) and pyrexia. Family history of gallstones and hemolysis are important diagnostic clues.
2. Diagnosis: confirm by ultrasonography.
3. Treatment: cholecystectomy.

GYNECOLOGIC CAUSES
1. Adolescent girls may present with acute lower abdominal pain owing to ruptured follicular cyst, hemorrhage into a cyst, ovarian torsion, or premenstrual pain. Pelvic inflammatory disease may present with acute or chronic abdominal pain.
2. Ultrasonography has important role in identifying ovarian and uterine abnormalities.
3. Urgent laparoscopy or laparotomy indicated when ovarian torsion or acute appendicitis cannot be excluded.

URINARY TRACT INFECTION
1. Common in children.
2. Typical symptoms: pain at lower abdomen, dysuria, pyrexia, and vomiting.
3. Diagnosis: bacteria on microscopy or culture of > 10^7/mL bacteria.
4. Urinary tract infection (UTI) associated with vesicoureteric reflux may lead to renal scarring and ultimately renal failure. All children with recurrent UTI should therefore be screened with renal tract ultrasonography to rule out genitourinary obstruction and calculus disease and with voiding cystourethrogram (diagnostic test for vesicoureteric reflux). Technetium 99m dimercaptosuccinate scans may also be used.
5. Treatment: antibiotics, fluids, and surgery when appropriate. Suppurative infection is a surgical emergency.

INFLAMMATORY CONDITIONS

NEONATAL NECROTIZING ENTEROCOLITIS
1. Multifocal progressive ischemic necrosis of intestine. Risk factors: low birth weight, coexistent disease such as congenital heart disease, umbilical vein catheterization, sepsis, and hypoglycemia.
2. Presentation: passage of blood per rectum, refusal to feed, bilious emesis, abdominal distention, and sepsis.
3. Radiographs: pneumatosis intestinalis and portal venous gas with pneumoperitoneum secondary to intestinal perforation in advanced cases.
4. Treatment: nothing by mouth, total parenteral nutrition, and IV antibiotics. Operation for perforation or intestinal necrosis with persistent sepsis.

HIRSCHSPRUNG ENTEROCOLITIS
1. Hirschsprung disease may be complicated by enterocolitis characterized by malaise, pyrexia, abdominal distention, constipation, or diarrhea. Pathologic basis poorly understood.
2. Therapy: empiric; rectal washouts, antibiotics, probiotics, and sodium cromoglycate. Botox, topical glyceryl trinitrate, or surgical internal sphincterotomy may be beneficial. If refractory to medical management, may be necessary to perform urgent colostomy.

INFLAMMATORY BOWEL DISEASE
Urgent operative intervention may be required for acute complications of ulcerative colitis or Crohn disease.

TRAUMA

BLUNT ABDOMINAL TRAUMA
1. Falls are most frequent cause (> 50%).
2. Patients with abdominal injury must be fully assessed.
3. Diagnosis: CT scan with IV enhancement for evaluating intra-abdominal organs, retroperitoneum, and head injury.
4. Management: appropriate IV fluids with NG and foley catheter insertion as needed. Urgent laparotomy indicated if hemodynamically unstable owing to ongoing intra-abdominal bleeding or if evidence of peritonitis or pneumoperitoneum.
5. Most injuries to solid abdominal organs will heal without surgery.

PENETRATING INJURY
1. If entry wound between level of nipples and symphysis pubis, possibility of intra-abdominal injury needs to be considered.
2. High risk of multiple intestinal injuries.
3. Safest approach is laparotomy to exclude organ injury.

NONACCIDENTAL INJURY
1. Especially in infants age < 1 yr.
2. Risk factors: delay in seeking medical attention and historical inconsistencies.
3. Thorough documentation of injuries essential.
4. If perineal injury, examination under anesthesia to minimize trauma; perform in presence of child protection clinician or expert.

QUESTIONS

MATCH THE THERAPY TO THE CONDITION:
a. Rectal irrigation and antibiotics.
b. Nothing by mouth, total parenteral nutrition, and intravenous antibiotics.
c. Intravenous fluids, analgesia, and bowel rest.
d. Antispasmodic, fluid resuscitation, and analgesic initially.

e. Immediate surgery.
f. Pneumostatic or hydrostatic enema.

1. Hirschsprung enterocolitis.
2. Ascariasis.
3. Necrotizing enterocolitis.
4. Pancreatitis.
5. Intussusception.
6. Meckel band obstruction.

TRUE OR FALSE:

7. Congenital inguinal hernias tend to resolve spontaneously.
8. Most injuries to solid abdominal organs heal without surgical intervention.

APPENDICITIS

SYNOPSIS

DEVELOPMENT

1. Cecum: visible by 5th week of gestation.
2. Appendix: a diverticulum arising from the cecum; appears by 8th week.
3. Lymphoid nodules: appear at 7 months of gestation.

PATHOPHYSIOLOGY

1. Obstruction of lumen by fecalith or lymphoid tissue.
2. Obstruction and multiplication of bacteria leads to infection of wall of appendix and swelling with activation of stretch receptors perceived at the 10th dermatome (periumbilical region).
3. Inflammatory fluid exudes from organ and causes peritoneal pain.
4. If inflammation unchecked for 36 h, then perforation occurs.

SYMPTOMS

1. Incidence: one-third of acute appendicitis cases occur in children; male-to-female ratio 1.4:1; one-quarter of cases perforated at time of presentation.
2. Peak ages 10–14 yr in boys and 15–19 yr in girls.

3. Earliest: periumbical pain. Vomiting usually follows; pain relocates to right lower quadrant.
4. McBurney's point: point of maximal tenderness located ⅔ laterally between anterior iliac spine and umbilicus.

DIAGNOSIS

Most reliable sign of acute appendicitis: localized tenderness at right lower quadrant.

LABORATORY AND RADIOLOGY EXAMINATIONS

1. Urinalysis: important to rule out genitourinary pathology, especially urinary tract infection.
2. White blood cell (WBC) count: only test correlated with appendicitis (elevated WBC count). Generally, WBC < 20 K in patient with nonperforated appendicitis.
3. C-reactive protein: elevated in 85% if tested > 12 h after infection onset.
4. Radiograph: most common finding is curvature of spine to the right. Dilated cecum with air-fluid levels may be seen. Perforated appendicitis in ½ of children presenting with abdominal pain and a fecalith.
5. Chest radiograph: to rule out right lower lobe pneumonia.
6. Ultrasonography useful in experienced hands (Table 1).
7. Rectal contrast computed tomography (CT): best results; highest sensitivity, accuracy, and specificity (all 94%).

DIFFERENTIAL DIAGNOSIS

1. Gastroenteritis: can be confused with retrocecal appendicitis (Table 2).
2. Constipation with right lower quadrant pain: pain rarely progresses.
3. Urinary tract infections: often characterized by fever and leukocytosis rather than abdominal signs. With pyelonephritis, pain usually localized to the flank area.
4. Crohn disease: usually presents with a much longer history. Occasionally, initial presentation can be similar; Crohn disease discovered on pathology review or at surgery with creeping mesenteric fat at the bowel wall.
5. Pelvic inflammatory disease (PID): often preceded by menstrual period with pain localized to the lower

TABLE 1   FINDINGS SUGGESTIVE OF APPENDICITIS

ULTRASONOGRAPHY	COMPUTED TOMOGRAPHY
Fluid-filled, noncompressible, distended tubular structure (≥ 6 mm)	Fluid-filled tubular structure measuring > 6 mm in maximum diameter
No peristalsis in appendix	Fat stranding, abscess or phlegmon in adjacent tissue
± Appendicolith	± Appendicolith
Location: anterior to psoas or retrocecal	Focal cecal apical thickening
Pericecal inflammatory changes	

TABLE 2   DIFFERENTIATING APPENDICITIS FROM ACUTE GASTROENTERITIS

ACUTE GASTROENTERITIS	APPENDICITIS
Pain improves with time	Pain worsens with time
Vomiting with or after abdominal pain	Abdominal pain precedes emesis
High stool volume and frequency	Low volume stool (mucoid)
Peristalsis present	Absent peristalsis
No peritoneal or rectal pain signs	Peritoneal signs and rectal pain

TABLE 3   PROTOCOL FOR MANAGEMENT OF PERFORATED APPENDICITIS

1. Fluid resuscitation; control fever and administration of intravenous antibiotics (ampicillin 100 mg/kg/24 h, gentamicin 5 mg/kg/24 h, and clindamycin 30 mg/kg/24 h on admission, or piperacillin/tazobactam 240 mg/kg/24 h of piperacillin component, up to 18 g/24 h).
2. Explore peritoneal cavity via right lower quadrant incision.
3. Perform appendectomy in all cases.
4. Perform limited peritoneal débridement.
5. Irrigate peritoneal cavity with cephalothin solution (4 g/L).
6. Place Penrose drains in pelvis and right pericolic space, which exit through the lateral margin of the wound.
7. Close the muscle layers, Scarpa fascia, and skin around the drains with absorbable sutures.
8. Encourage postoperative activity and position at will.
9. Continue parenteral antibiotics for 9 days, adjusting gentamicin dosage based on serum levels.
10. Remove drains slowly from the seventh to the ninth postoperative days. If the patient has been discharged for home antibiotics, he is usually seen sometime during this period in the clinic.
11. Discharge patient generally on the tenth postoperative day.

quadrants rather than the periumbilical area. Cervical motion tenderness is the hallmark of PID. Erythrocyte sedimentation rate is often > 15 (normal in appendicitis).

6. Ovarian pathology: most common cause is rupture of an ovarian cyst. Ultrasonography may be helpful.
7. Pneumonia: right lower lobe pneumonia may refer pain to the abdomen; often fever and cough. Chest radiograph for diagnosis.
8. Mesenteric adenitis: lymph node inflammation clustered at mesentery of terminal ileum usually due to viral infection. Laparotomy or laparoscopy for diagnosis.
9. Typhlitis: severe leukopenia with right lower quadrant pain. Related to invasive infection of bowel wall at cecum. Responds to bowel rest and intravenous antibiotics. CT: thickened, irregular cecum and occasional pneumatosis coli. Surgery is associated with high morbidity and mortality.

TREATMENT

1. Treatment of choice: appendectomy on day of diagnosis. Exception: perforated appendicitis with drainable, well-defined abscess (Table 3).
2. In periappendiceal abscess: CT- or ultrasonography-guided drainage of the abscess, broad-spectrum antibiotics, and delayed removal of the appendix (~8 wk).
3. Laparoscopic appendectomy is widely gaining favor.
4. Most institutions report a 10–20% false-positive surgical rate.

COMPLICATIONS

1. Incidence of wound infectious complications: primary closure without drains: > 10%; with drains < 1%.
2. Abdominal and pelvic abscesses after perforated appendicitis: most frequent complication. Many pelvic or abdominal abscesses subside with intravenous antibiotics; if abscess does not subside, drain.
3. Fecal fistula at wound site after severe perforated appendicitis: virtually all will resolve with intravenous antibiotics, bowel rest, and total parenteral nutrition. Rule out distal obstruction.

4. Intestinal obstruction: paralytic ileus may persist for 3–5 d after removal of a perforated appendix. Most managed conservatively with nasogastric drainage until inflammatory adhesions resolve. Obstructions occurring more than 1 mo postoperatively usually require surgery.
5. Antibiotic-associated colitis: check stool for *Clostridium difficile* and treat appropriately.

QUESTIONS

TRUE OR FALSE:

1. The incidence of acute appendicitis is equal in boys and girls.
2. Perforation occurs in 25% of pediatric appendicitis cases.
3. Ultrasonography is the most sensitive radiologic test for appendicitis.

MATCH THE TIMING OF GESTATIONAL DEVELOPMENT TO THE CONDITION:

a. 5th week.
b. 8th week.
c. 7th month.

4. Appendix.
5. Lymph nodes in cecum.
6. Cecum.

MATCH THE TREATMENT TO THE SITUATION:

a. Surgery.
b. Percutaneous drainage.
c. Nasogastric drainage.
d. Antibiotics.

7. Nonperforated acute appendicitis.
8. Well-defined abscess cavity with perforated appendicitis.
9. Fecal fistula.
10. Early intestinal obstruction after appendicitis.
11. Intestinal obstruction more than 1 mo after appendicitis.

INTESTINAL BACTERIAL INFECTIONS

SYNOPSIS

Cholera

1. Most rapidly fatal diarrheal disease in humans.
   a. *Vibrio cholerae*: single short curved gram-negative rod with single flagellum.
   b. Agglutinating *Vibrio* is pathogenic (O1); nonagglutinating also causes disease (non-O1).
2. Transmission: O1; fecal-oral and through contaminated food and water. Non-O1: associated with eating raw or undercooked shellfish. Infectious dose 106 organisms.
3. Incubation: a few hours to 5 days.
4. Most forms are asymptomatic: mild disease with few watery stools; nausea and vomiting are rare; no significant dehydration.
5. Cholera gravis: most severe form. Profuse rice water diarrhea with mucus and vomiting; fluid or water loss 1 L/hr. Most severe during first 48 hr. Resolves in 4–6 d.
6. For *Vibrio vulnificus*: associated with eating raw oysters. Alcoholics or those with hemochromatosis especially susceptible. Most common cause of serious Vibrio-related disease in United States. Symptoms: bacteremia, bullous skin lesions, and hypotension. Mortality: bacteremia 50%; hypotension 90%. Diagnosis: culture of blood or bullous fluid. Treatment: early antibiotics; susceptible to tetracycline, ciprofloxacin, Bactrim, chloramphenicol, and ampicillin
7. Diagnosis: stool culture.
8. Cornerstone of therapy: oral rehydration solutions.
9. Antibiotics reduce volume and duration by half and reduce excretion by 1 day. Tetracycline resistance reported. Furazolidone, Bactrim, and erythromycin prescribed for children.

Salmonella

1. Genus of family of Enterobacteriaceae.
2. Gram-negative, nonlactose-fermenting, motile bacilli.
3. Human pathogens usually belong to *S. enterica*. Most common reported human pathogen in United States is *S. enteritidis*. Acid is first line of defense.
4. *S. typhi* and *S. paratyphi*: colonize only humans.
   a. Acquisition only through close contact with person with typhoid fever or carrier. Fecal-oral transmission.
   b. Incidence decreasing.
5. Nontyphoidal salmonella: incidence increasing.
   a. Risk factors for infection: immunodeficiency, age < 3 mo, achlorhydria, antacid therapy, and rapid gastric emptying.
   b. *S. enteriditis*: leading cause of foodborne disease outbreaks in United States; intact eggs and egg-containing foods incriminated > 80%.
   c. Incidence: greatest among children aged < 5 yr; peak in children aged < 1 yr.
6. Clinical manifestations: incubation range 6 hr to 10 d.
   a. Nontyphoidal: acute, self-limited enterocolitis occasionally accompanied by bacteremia (highest incidence in first year of life, peak in first 3 mo). Watery diarrhea occurs but may contain blood, mucus, and fecal leukocytes. Headache, abdominal pain, and emesis may occur. Fever in at least 70%. Most patients recover in 1 wk, but some have persistent diarrhea. *Salmonella* detected in stool for 5 wk; will be excreted for 1 yr in 5%.
   b. Extraintestinal manifestations: mainly in young infants or in patients with impaired immunity. Life-threatening sepsis or focal infections at any body site. *Salmonella* is the most common cause of osteomyelitis in sickle cell disease patients. Meningitis carries a high mortality and morbidity and high relapse rate in neonates. Prolonged diarrhea, weight loss, persistent bacteremia, and disseminated infection in patients positive for human immunodeficiency virus (HIV).
   c. Enteric fever: Typhoid or paratyphoid fever in humans. Severe systemic illnesses with fever and gastrointestinal (GI) symptoms. Incubation 5–21 d, followed by enterocolitis for several days; symptoms resolve before onset of fever. Constipation (10–38%). Nonspecific symptoms: chills, headaches, and muscle pain. Neuropsychiatric manifestations (5–10%). Truncal rose spots (30%). Resolves by 4th week of infection without antibiotics in 90%.
7. Diagnosis: culture.
8. Therapy:
   a. Nontyphoidal: No antibiotics for asymptomatic carriage or uncomplicated infections (antibiotics may prolong excretion or induce relapse). Antibiotics for infants < 3 mo, patients with hemolytic anemia, cancer, immunodeficiency, or chronic colitis, and patients who are ill or with bacteremia and extraintestinal infection. Increasing antibiotic resistance. Treat bacteremia for 2 wk, osteomyelitis 4–6 wk, and meningitis 4 wk. Prevention: hygiene. Avoid raw or undercooked eggs and meat. Thaw food in fridge or microwave or under cold water, not room temperature. Hand washing a must. Infected children should be excluded from day care centers if symptomatic. No vaccine currently.
   b. Typhoid or enteric fever: Treatment of choice: chloramphenicol; high availability after oral administration. Effective attenuated vaccine Ty21a available.

Shigella

1. Gram-negative, nonlactose-fermenting, nonmotile bacilli. Enterobacteriaceae.
2. Four species: *S. dysenteriae*, *S. flexneri*, *S. boydii*, and *S. sonnei* (*S. sonnei* account for 60–80% of disease in United States). *S. sonnei* is the main type in industrialized countries. *S. flexneri* and *S. dysenteriae* predominate in less-developed countries. Developing countries, *S. flexneri* endemic. *S. dysenteriae* type 1 capable of pandemic transmission.

3. Humans are the only natural hosts for *Shigella*. Fecal-oral transmission.

4. Low infectious inoculum (as few as 10 organisms); highly contagious.

5. Symptomatic persons are the main reason for transmission.

6. Elevated risk: day care facility. Incidence highest in children aged 1–4 yr (worldwide). However, uncommon cause (< 5%) of diarrhea disease in United States in children aged < 5yr.

7. Clinical presentation: incubation 1–4 d. Watery diarrhea: sole clinical manifestation in mild infection. Progression to frank dysentery can occur in hours to days with frequent small bloody stools with mucus. Microangiopathic hemolytic anemia can complicate infection with organisms producing Shiga toxin: hemolytic-uremic syndrome (HUS) in children and thrombotic thrombocytopenic purpura in adults. Most shigellosis self-limited; resolves within 5–7 d. Life-threatening complications in malnourished infants and children in developing countries. Bacteremia reported in HIV-positive cases.

8. Fastidious to culture. Obtain stool (not swab), rapidly inoculate specimens onto selective culture plates, and incubate at 37°C.

9. Antibiotics decrease duration of symptoms. In United States, in cases where susceptibility is unknown, treatment is with Bactrim for 5 d.

Campylobacter

1. Most common bacterial cause of acute gastroenteritis in developed countries. Transmission via mainly raw meats (especially poultry).

2. Small, nonsporing, spiral gram-negative bacteria, single flagellum. Microaerophilic.

3. Reservoir in animals is extensive; virtually all surface waters contaminated. Does not multiply in food like *Salmonella*.

4. Occurs in industrialized countries with temperate climates, with a peak incidence in summer; common in rural communities. *C. jejuni* causes 90% of cases; *C. coli* causes the remainder.

5. Age-specific incidence: climax 0–5 yr, 15–29 yr. In less-developed countries, hyperendemic.

6. Clinical presentation: incubation is 3–6 d. Begins abruptly with abdominal cramps and diarrhea. Watery diarrhea precedes bloody diarrhea. Abdominal pain can mimic appendicitis. Diarrhea lasts 4–5 days. Mean duration of fecal excretion: 1 mo; carriage prolonged in immunodeficient persons. Neonates have a milder illness with hematochezia without fever, diarrhea, but severe or systemic infection can occur. *C. fetus* causes most cases of neonatal *Campylobacter* meningitis.

7. Diagnosis: culture, PCR, enzyme immunoassays

8. Complications: cholecystitis, hepatitis, acute appendicitis, pancreatitis, and focal extraintestinal infections. Long-term complications: reactive arthritis, Reiter syndrome, uveitis, and Guillain-Barré syndrome (owing to molecular mimicry between core oligosaccharides of *Campylobacter* and neuronal glycosphingolipids; usually occurs 1–6 wk after infection).

9. Treat with erythromycin. Reserve antibiotics for patients with severe illness or risk factors (eg, pregnancy, systemic infection, immunosuppression).

Yersinia

1. Family Enterobacteriaceae. Two important enteropathogens: *Y. enterocolitica* and *Y. pseudotuberculosis*.

2. Nonlactose-fermenting gram-negative aerobic, facultatively anaerobic bacilli that grow better at 25°C than 37°C.

3. Distributed widely in environment. Foodborne transmission. High infectious inoculum. Prefer cool temperature; more common in northern latitudes.

4. Clinical presentation: incubation 3–7 d. Most often affects children aged < 5yr. Watery diarrhea, fever, and abdominal pain. Bloody diarrhea (25–30%). Pharyngitis (20%): can be exudative, associated with adenitis. Diarrhea lasts 14–22 d; fecal excretion persists for 6–7 wk longer. Abdominal complications: appendicitis, diffuse ulceration of intestine or colon, perforation, peritonitis, intussusception, toxic megacolon, cholangitis, and mesenteric venous thrombosis. Pseudoappendicitis symptoms: occur primarily in older children and adults; fever, abdominal pain, and tender right lower quadrant, with or without diarrhea. Computed tomography can help distinguish from appendicitis, case fatality can reach 50%. Bacteremic spread: abscess formation and lesions at liver, spleen, lungs, kidneys, and bone. Iron overload states predispose to *Y. enterocolitica* septicemia (hemochromatosis, cirrhosis, and hemolysis). *Y. enterocolitica* associated with immunosequelae: reactive arthritis, uveitis, Reiter's syndrome, and erythema nodosum.

5. Diagnosis: stool culture.

6. Most cases resolve without therapy. Therapy mainly for patients with severe infection or who are immunocompromised: includes third-generation cephalosporins, imipenem, and aztreonam (β-lactamases) for 2–6 wk. No vaccines.

Aeromonas, Plesiomonas, and Edwardsiella

1. *Aeromonas*: Gram-negative, facultative anaerobic motile bacilli. Associated with acute gastroenteritis. High attack rate in children aged < 3 yr. More frequent in the warm months. Symptoms: watery diarrhea, dysentery, and prolonged or chronic diarrhea; abdominal pain, fever, and nausea or vomiting are common. Usually self-limited. < 7 d; dehydration or persistent diarrhea in one-third of cases. *A. caviae* most common (present with failure to thrive, sepsis, HUS). Mainstay of therapy is rehydration. Chronic forms may benefit from antibiotic therapy: Bactrim.

2. *Plesiomonas*: Enterobacteriaceae. Gram-negative facultative anaerobic, motile, freshwater organism. Fish and shellfish frequently harbor plesiomonads; can also be isolated from feces of asymptomatic animals. Common in Bangladesh; less in United States. Increased infection prevalence in warm season. Symptoms:

secretory or colitis or proctitis diarrhea (frank bloody diarrhea in one-third), abdominal pain, nausea or vomiting and fever. Fatal outcomes from severe GI infection without dissemination reported. Quinolones or Bactrim shorten course; used for the therapy of uncomplicated infections.

3. *Edwardsiella*: gram-negative, facultative anaerobic rods. *E. tarda* is only species associated with intestinal and extraintestinal human illness. Isolated from persons with diarrhea, fish, freshwater, animals that inhabit these locales. Clinical entity: generally benign secretory diarrhea or dysentery or enterocolitis. Most common symptoms: low-grade fever, vomiting, and watery stools; can be severe with pseudomembranous colitis and enterocolitis. Can disseminate (septicemia, hepatic abscess) in subjects with liver dysfunction or iron overload. Treat with ampicillin, Bactrim, or ciprofloxacin.

Escherichia coli

1. Gram-negative lactose-fermenting bacilli Enterobacteriaceae.
2. Six categories: enteropathogenic (small intestine); enterotoxigenic (small intestine); enteroinvasive (colon); enterohemorrhagic (colon); diffusely adherent; and enteroaggregative.

ENTEROPATHOGENIC

1. Leading cause of persistent diarrhea in children in developing countries.
2. Produce attaching, effacing lesion at enterocyte.
3. Infective dose high (10^9); fecal-oral transmission.
4. Self-limited watery diarrhea. Short incubation period: 6–48 h.
5. Antibiotics diminish morbidity and mortality.

ENTEROTOXIGENIC

1. Important cause of diarrheal disease in humans and animals.
2. Elaborate heat-stable (ST) or heat-labile (LT) enterotoxins without invading or damaging enterocytes.
3. High inoculum, short incubation (14–30 h).
4. Watery diarrhea; severe form is cholera-like. Traveler's diarrhea. Self-limited < 5 d; few cases > 3 wk. Antibiotics shorten course by 1–2 d. Prevention: avoid contamination.

ENTEROINVASIVE

1. Genetically, biochemically, clinically similar to *Shigella*.
2. Endemic in developing countries. In industrialized countries, foodborne outbreaks.
3. Inoculum higher than *Shigella*. Produce dysentery as with *Shigella*, but watery diarrhea more common.
4. Treatment as for *Shigella*.

ENTEROHEMORRHAGIC

1. Produce one or both phage encoded cytotoxins Shiga-like toxin I or II. *E. coli* O157-H7 prototype is the predominant Shiga-like toxin producing *E. coli*.

2. Predominant mode of transmission is contaminated, undercooked ground beef. Also raw fruits (apple juice), vegetables, raw milk, processed meats, and contaminated water. Person-to-person at day care. Infection more frequent in northern United States; peaks June through September. Highest rates in 5–9 year olds and 50–59 year olds. Onset: 3–9 d after ingestion of as few as 100 organisms.
3. Symptoms: crampy abdominal pain and nonbloody diarrhea with occasional emesis. By day 2 or 3, diarrhea bloody in 90% of cases and abdominal pain worsens. Bloody diarrhea lasts 1–22 d (4 d average). Fever usually absent or low grade. Younger children excrete organism (3 wk) longer than older persons. In outbreaks 25% require hospitalization, 5–10% have HUS, and 1% die.
4. Complications: rectal prolapse, appendicitis, intussusception, and pseudomembranous colitis. HUS: diagnosed 2-14 days after onset diarrhea.
5. Risk factors: young or old age, bloody diarrhea, fever, elevated white blood cell count, and undergoing treatment with antimotility agents.
6. Diagnosis: special stool culture exploits inability of *E. coli* O157 to rapidly ferment sorbitol after 24 h incubation on sorbitol-MacConkey agar in contrast to 90% of *E. coli* species that can. Sorbitol-negative colonies can then be screened for O157 antigen. Of those who develp HUS, two-thirds are no longer excreting the organism in their stools.
7. Therapy: antibiotics not recommended; prevention is key.

DIFFUSELY ADHERENT

1. Causes diarrheal disease in children 2–6 years old. More frequently isolated from cases of prolonged diarrhea. Seasonal pattern: occurs more frequently in warmer season.
2. GI symptoms: indistinguishable from those of enterotoxigenic *E. coli*.
3. Diagnosis: deoxyribonucleic acid (DNA) probe and adherence pattern on HE-2 cells.

ENTEROAGGREGATIVE

1. Associated with cases of persistent diarrhea in developing world. Causes sporadic diarrhea.
2. Watery, mucoid, and secretory diarrhea. Grossly bloody stools in up to one-third of cases. Incubation 8–18 h. Link with growth retardation in infants. High prevalence of asymptomatic enteroaggregative *E. coli* excretion in many areas. Fecal-oral transmission.
3. Diagnosis: isolation from stools and aggregative pattern in HEp-2 assay; DNA probe highly specific in detection. Forms stacked pattern when adheres to epithelium.
4. Self-limited. More persistent cases may benefit from antibiotic therapy. High rate of antibiotic resistance.

Clostridium difficile

1. Single most common cause of bacterial diarrhea in hospitalized patients. Mild diarrhea to fatal

pseudomembranous colitis (PMC). Almost all cases of PMC are secondary to *C. difficile*; 25% of antibiotic-associated diarrhea associated with *C. difficile*.

2. Gram-positive anaerobe. Spore production not associated with toxin production.

3. Person-to-person transmission; persists in environment owing to spore formation. Can persist in curtains and floors of rooms of infected persons for 5 mo.

4. Symptoms: asymptomatic to severe diarrhea, PMC, toxic megacolon, and death. Onset of symptoms usually several days after starting antibiotics to up to 2 mo after cessation.

5. Stool culturing, latex agglutination, tissue culture assay, and enzyme-linked immunosorbent assay help diagnosis.

6. Usually self-limited; responds to withdrawal of antibiotics. Severe infection or PMC requires antibiotic therapy with oral vancomycin or Flagyl. Relapse rate 40–50%. Use of probiotics (*Lactobacillus GG* and *Saccharomyces boulardii*) significantly eradicates *C. difficile* and decreases recurrent infection.

PATHOGENESIS

1. Toxins (1) activate enterocyte signal pathways (cyclic adenosine monophosphate [cAMP], cyclic guanosine monophosphate [cGMP], and calcium-dependent pathways); (2) are pore-forming; (3) block protein synthesis; and (4) affect enterocyte skeleton.

2. Cholera toxin: made of 1 A subunit and 5 B subunits. B subunit binds holotoxin to cell receptor. A subunit has intracellular enzyme function (A1 enters cell, activates adenylate cyclase, and increases intracellular cAMP, which activates protein kinase A, which phosphorylates proteins, which increase chloride secretion). Cholera toxin receptor GM1 is ubiquitous (intestine, ovary, and neurons). Neuraminidase produced by *Vibrio cholera* can increase GM1 receptors. Maximal activity at duodenum, minimal at ileum. Heat-labile *E. coli* enterotoxin can also bind to GM2 and asialo GM1 receptors.

3. Heat-stable *E. coli* enterotoxin increases intracellular cGMP, which also stimulates chloride secretion and diarrhea.

4. Pore-forming toxins: *Clostridium perfringens*: hydrophobic protein released by bacterial lysis, binds to brush border receptor, and associates with another membrane protein to form pores. Maximal activity at ileum, minimal at duodenum.

5. Protein synthesis blockage: A1 subunit of Shiga toxin and Shiga-like toxins inactivates 60S subunit of host cell ribosome, interrupting protein synthesis.

6. Toxins affecting cytoskeleton: *Clostridium difficile*: toxins A (enterotoxin) and B (cytotoxin). Both cytotoxic. Both are glucosyltransferases and use uridine diphosphate glucose to inactive Rho proteins (guanosine triphosphatases), which regulate cytoskeleton functions such as cell adhesion, motility, cell transformation, and apoptosis. Dramatic effects include increased intestinal permeability, diarrhea, cell retraction or rounding, disruption cell adhesion, and apoptosis. *Clostridium botulinum*: toxins C2 and C3 similarly act by inactivating actin and Rho, respectively.

QUESTIONS

1. Which of the following is the most rapidly fatal diarrheal disease in humans?
   a. *Salmonella enteritis*.
   b. *Shigella enteritis*.
   c. Cholera.
   d. *Campylobacter enteritis*.
   e. *Yersinia enteritis*.

2. What is the most common bacterial form of acute gastroenteritis in developed countries?
   a. *Salmonella enteritis*.
   b. *Shigella enteritis*.
   c. Cholera.
   d. *Campylobacter enteritis*.
   e. *Yersinia enteritis*.

3. Which type of *Escherichia coli* causes hemorrhagic colitis and hemolytic-uremic syndrome and has a high fatality rate?
   a. Enteropathogenic.
   b. Enterotoxigenic.
   c. Enteroinvasive.
   d. Enterohemorrhagic.
   e. Diffusely adherent.
   f. Enteroaggregative.

4. The following conditions predispose to *Yersinia enterocolitica* septicemia except:
   a. Hemochromatosis.
   b. Cirrhosis.
   c. Renal failure.
   d. Hemolytic processes.
   e. None of the above.

TABLE 1   IDENTIFICATION OF BACTERIAL ENTERIC PATHOGENS IN SYMPTOMATIC PATIENTS FROM DEVELOPING AND INDUSTRIALIZED COUNTRIES

AGENT	INDUSTRIALIZED COUNTRIES (%)	DEVELOPING COUNTRIES (%)
Vibrio cholerae	< 1	0–3
Non-O1 *Vibrio* species	—	?
Salmonella	3–7	4–6
Shigella	1–3	5–9
Campylobacter	6–8	7–9
Yersinia	1–2	?
Escherichia coli	2–5	14–17
Clostridium difficile	?	?
Aeromonas, Plesiomonas, and *Edwardsiella*	0–2	4–5

5. Which infection can look like appendicitis?
   a. Shigellosis.
   b. *Salmonella enteritis.*
   c. Enteropathogenic *Escherichia coli.*
   d. *Yersinia.*
   e. *Edwardsiella.*

MATCH THE SEASON TO THE BACTERIA:

a. Summer.
b. Winter.
c. Fall.
d. Spring.

6. Enterohemorrhagic *Escherichia coli.*
7. *Campylobacter jejuni.*

MATCH THE LOCATION OF ACTION:

a. Duodenum.
b. Ileum.
c. Jejunum.
d. Colon.

8. *Clostridium perfringens* toxin.
9. *Vibrio cholera* toxin.
10. Enteroinvasive *Escherichia coli.*

TRUE OR FALSE:

11. Antibiotics should be used to treat *Escherichia coli* O157:H7 infection.
12. Blood cultures are usually negative in shigellosis.
13. Stools from enterotoxigenic *Escherichia coli*–infected patients are bloody.
14. Achlorhydria increases susceptibility to *Salmonella* infection.

MATCH THE MECHANISM TO THE AGENT:

a. Acts via cyclic adenosine monophosphate.
b. Acts via cyclic guanosine monophosphate.
c. Blocks protein synthesis.
d. Encourages protein synthesis.
e. Affects the cytoskeleton.
f. Pore-forming.

15. *Campylobacter jejuni* enterotoxin.
16. *Shigella* Shiga toxin.
17. *Vibrio cholera* toxin.
18. *Salmonella* enterotoxin.
19. *Yersinia enterolytica* Shiga toxin (ST) I and STII.
20. *Clostridium difficile* toxins A and B.
21. *Clostridium perfringens* enterotoxin.

FOODBORNE ILLNESS

SYNOPSIS

PREFORMED TOXINS

Clostridium botulinum

1. Gram-positive, spore-forming, toxin-producing obligate anaerobe.
2. Natural habitat: soil and spores on fruits and vegetables. Toxin A–G (A, B, E, F, and G associated with human disease), A accounts for 25% of cases, B for 8%.
3. Toxin heat-labile. Majority of outbreaks from home-produced foods.
4. Absorbed from proximal intestine; spreads via blood stream to peripheral cholinergic nerves, blocks acetylcholine release resulting in flaccid paralysis. Does not cross blood-brain barrier. Symptoms occur 18–36 h after ingestion. Cranial nerves affected first, then respiratory muscles, leading to death.
5. No major gastrointestinal (GI) symptoms.
6. Detect toxin or organism in patient or food for diagnosis. Patients affected by type A toxin have 25% mortality. Horse serum antitoxin available.

Staphylococcus aureus Toxin

1. Toxins A, B, C1–3, D, and E. Type A toxin with or without D most frequently associated with outbreaks. Ingestion of 100–200 ng is sufficient to cause disease.
2. Symptoms: within 6 h of ingestion; nausea, vomiting, abdominal cramps, and diarrhea. Fever rare.
3. Transmission: foods, especially dairy-based. Bacteria grow in room temperature food and produce toxin.
4. Heat-stable; also stable against pH, protease, and radiation. Once formed in food, impossible to remove.
5. Toxin not absorbed systemically, so protective immunity not induced.
6. Treatment: supportive. Symptoms usually abate within 8 h with good outcome.

Bacillus cereus Toxin

1. Gram-positive, spore-forming aerobe.
2. Two distinct clinical syndromes
   a. If short incubation: emetic symptoms
      - Incubation: 1–6 h.
      - Nausea and vomiting predominant; no fever. Usually recover well.
   b. If longer incubation: diarrhea predominant.
3. Present in soil, water, and most raw foods; Transmission often via starchy food contamination 10–40% of humans are colonized. Heat-stable. Reheating food does not ensure destruction.

NATURAL TOXINS

CIGUATERA

1. Neurotoxin from fish. Toxin produced in dinoflagellates (*Gambierdiscus toxicus*); accumulates in flesh of tropical

and subtropical marine fin fish (mackerel, grouper, snapper). Most common type of fish poisoning in the United States (Florida and Hawaii) and the Caribbean.
2. Incubation 5 min to 30 h (mean 5 h).
3. GI and neurologic symptoms: nausea, vomiting, watery diarrhea, ataxia, and blurred vision. Some develop cranial nerve (CN) palsies, respiratory paralysis. Symptoms last 1 wk, then resolve.
4. Diagnosis is clinical. Confirmation of toxin presence is difficult; use mouse bioassay.

SCOMBROID

1. Occurs after ingestion of spoiled fish, especially tuna and mackerel, especially if not frozen shortly after being caught. Probably caused by excess levels of histamine in fish, produced by bacteria. Associated also with other foods (eg, Swiss cheese).
2. Symptoms: 10 min to 3 h after ingestion; nausea, vomiting, diarrhea, flush, and headache. Respiratory distress rare. Resolve in few hours.
3. Clinical diagnosis; elevated levels of histamine in suspected food can be detected.

SHELLFISH POISONING

1. Four types: paralytic, neurotoxic, diarrheic, and toxic-encephalopathic. Toxins made by algae (dinoflagellates) that accumulate in shellfish.
   a. Paralytic: due to saxitoxin (Na channel toxin). Symptoms within 1 h: nausea, vomiting, and paralysis limited to CNs or respiratory muscles.
   b. Neurotoxic: due to brevitoxin; lipophilic and heat-stable. Toxin stimulates postganglionic cholinergic neurons within 3 h of exposure. Paresthesia but no paralysis.
   c. Diarrheic: nausea, vomiting, and diarrhea.
   d. Toxic-encephalopathic (amnesic): has caused outbreaks with mussel consumption. Symptoms may not occur for 24–48 h: nausea, vomiting, diarrhea, severe headache, and occasional memory loss.
2. Symptoms: usually occur within 2 h and resolve spontaneously (except toxic-encephalopathic).
3. Diagnosis is clinical. Toxins can also be detected with mouse bioassays.

TETRODOTOXIN

1. Puffer fish; if ingested, rapid paralysis and death.
2. Symptoms: can occur in as little as 20 min; GI disturbance, total paralysis, cardiac arrhythmias, and death within 4–6 h.
3. Diagnosis is clinical and by history.

MUSHROOM TOXINS AND AFLATOXINS

Mushroom

1. Four different toxins:
   a. Protoplasmic (amatoxins): cell damage and organ failure.
   b. Neurotoxins (muscarine and psilocybin): coma, convulsions, and hallucinations.

   c. GI irritants: nausea, vomiting, and diarrhea.
   d. Disulfiram-like toxins: problematic if person has had exposure to alcohol in prior 48–72 h.
2. Diagnosis usually clinical, by history.
3. Treatment: supportive; reduce toxin absorption via GI lavage, charcoal, or plasmapheresis.

Aflatoxins

1. Produced by certain fungi (*Aspergillus flavus* and *A. parasiticus*) growing on various foods (nuts and oil seeds).
2. Various types: B1 is most toxic; causes liver damage resulting in cirrhosis or cancer.
3. Acute condition: high-dose aflatoxicosis; fever, jaundice, abdominal pain, and emesis.
4. Diagnosis clinical.

OTHER

1. Grayanotoxin: found in honey from rhododendrons. Nausea, vomiting, and weakness. Self-limited to 24 h.
2. Hypoglycin A: in Akee fruit from Jamaica; causes hypoglycemia and emesis in 4–10 h.
3. Cucurbitacin E: from bitter cucumber; cramps and diarrhea within 1–2 h.
4. Hydrogen cyanide: lima beans or cassava root; death within minutes.
5. Hemagglutinin: castor beans; nausea and vomiting.
6. Phytohemagglutinin: associated with eating raw or undercooked red kidney beans. Symptoms within 1–3 hours: severe nausea, vomiting, and diarrhea. Heat-sensitive toxin, but needs high temperature to be inactivated.

MICROBES THAT PRODUCE TOXINS FOLLOWING INGESTION

Vibrio

1. *V. cholerae* O1: transmission: contaminated water and food. Toxin activates cyclic adenosine monophosphate; profound secretion of chloride and fluid in watery diarrhea.
2. *V. parahaemolyticus*: shellfish consumption. Thermostable direct hemolysin. Self-limited.
3. *V. vulnificus*: associated with eating raw oysters.

Clostridia

1. *Clostridium perfringens*: anaerobic, spore-forming gram-positive rod.
2. Type A: predominantly associated with foodborne diarrheal disease. Associated with ingestion of meat and poultry. Clostridial spores germinate in food, begin vegetative growth, then colonize bowel, where they produce toxin. *Clostridium perfringens* enterotoxin: heat-labile; inserts itself into host membrane and causes permeability changes. Diagnosis difficult: *Clostridium perfringens* found in normal bowel flora of many persons; use tests to detect toxins.
3. Type C: causes necrotizing enterocolitis in context of poor nutrition. Three toxins; enterotoxin, α toxin, and

b toxin. B toxin causes necrosis: inactivated by proteolysis in intestine; associated with disease in persons whose enzymes are inadequate (as in malnutrition) or in the presence of trypsin inhibitors (undercooked pork or sweet potatoes).

Escherichia coli

1. Enterotoxigenic *E. coli* (ETEC) and Shiga toxin-producing *E. coli* (STEC).
2. ETEC: colonizes bowel and produces toxins. Heat-stable toxins (ST) and heat-labile toxins (LT). ST: increase cyclic guanosine monophosphate. LT: similar to *V. cholerae*. Transmission: contaminated water and food.
3. STEC: *E. coli* O157:H7. Main virulence factor is Shiga toxin. Toxins cross intestinal epithelium and damage target sites (kidney, brain).

FOODBORNE INFECTIONS, CAUSING DISEASE BY OTHER MECHANISMS

Salmonella

1. *S. typhi* and *S. paratyphi* infect only humans. Causes typhoid fever. Infectious dose: < 100 to 10^6.
2. *S. enteritidis*: nontyphoidal; 1/10,000 eggs contaminated. Penetrates intact eggs lying in contaminated feces and transovarially during egg development before shell formed. Can invade epithelium and interact with lymphoid tissue.
3. See section entitled "Intestinal Bacterial Infections" for more information.

Campylobacter

1. Pathogenicity depends on motility. Nonmotile strains are not infective. Causes notable intestinal invasion, inflammation and direct spread to other organs.
2. Molecular mimicry between core oligosaccharides of *Campylobacter* and neuronal glycosphingolipids leads to Guillain-Barré syndrome.
3. See section entitled "Intestinal Bacterial infections" for more information.

Yersinia

1. *Y. enterocolitica* and *Y. pseudotuberculosis* are foodborne. *Y. pestis* is not foodborne.
2. Serotype O1 accounts for 80% cases.
3. Transmission: food, especially pork and milk.
4. Symptoms: can last weeks; usually self-limited. Complications: ulceration and perforation. Long-term complications: reactive arthritis (more likely in *HLA B27+*).
5. All pathogenic strains contain plasmal pYV, which encodes virulence proteins allowing intestinal invasions.
6. Treatment: uncomplicated cases resolve; antibiotics such as ceftriaxone and quinolones for serious infections.

Listeria

1. Only *L. monocytogenes* is a significant pathogen for humans; high mortality rate.
2. Occurs sporadically and in outbreaks. Commonly spread via milk, cheese, raw vegetables, undercooked meat, and hot dogs. Common in environment.
3. Nonspecific symptoms: fever, myalgia, and GI upset (diarrhea and nausea). Case fatality rate: 20%.
4. Groups at risk: pregnant women, elderly, immunocompromised. Can cause spontaneous abortion, prematurity, neonatal sepsis, and meningitis as complications of transplacental transmission.
5. Killed by heat and cooking but ubiquitous: risk of recontamination. Grows at standard refrigerator temperature.
6. Treatment: penicillin and aminoglycosides.

Shigella

1. Highly host-adapted. Infects only humans and some nonhuman primates.
2. Enteroinvasive.
3. Shiga toxin leads to hemolytic uremic syndrome (HUS).

ENTEROINVASIVE *Escherichia coli* (EIEC)

Causes disease similar to shigellosis. Invasive but no Shiga toxins.

Aeromonas

1. Gram-negative organism facultatively anaerobic, motile, oxidase-positive bacilli.
2. Present in soil and fresh water. Peaks in summer.
3. *A. hydrophila*, *A. caviea*, *A. veronii*, and *A. jandaei*: most frequently associated with gastroenteritis.
4. Watery persistent diarrhea. Fecal leukocytes; red cells absent. Abdominal pain. Nausea, vomiting, and fever in 50%. Asymptomatic carriage reported; finding in stool may not be enough to confirm diagnosis; immunologic tests to prove recent infection.
5. Treatment: usually self-limited; no antibiotics required unless persistent symptoms with no other etiology.

Plesiomonas shigelloides

1. Freshwater organism with increased disease prevalence in warm months.
2. Gram-negative, motile, facultative anaerobes.
3. Contamination of food products with water.
4. Symptoms: usually within 24–48 h; abdominal cramps and bloody stools reported.
5. Treatment: rehydration key. Antibiotics: quinolones or Bactrim if required.

ENTEROPATHOGENIC *Escherichia coli*

1. Fecal-oral.
2. No animal reservoir. Important cause of enteric disease in developing countries.
3. Watery diarrhea without blood. Low-grade fever and emesis. In developing countries: high mortality in infants.

PROTOZOAL FOODBORNE PATHOGENS

Cryptosporidium parvum

1. Can infect both normal hosts and patients with acquired immunodeficiency syndrome (AIDS). Domestic and wild animal reservoirs. Organism

ingested as cysts: sporozoites invade epithelium; do not penetrate beyond epithelium.
2. Symptoms: watery diarrhea (which can be profuse), abdominal cramps, nausea, and vomiting. No fever or GI bleeding.
3. Treatment: self-limited; recovery in 1–2 wk. In immunocompromised hosts: no clearance and malabsorption; life-threatening; no treatment available.

Giardia lamblia
1. Most frequent enteric protozoan worldwide.
2. Transmission: fecally contaminated water and food.
3. Only *G. lamblia* species infects humans. Infectious dose: 10–100 organisms. After ingestion, cysts excyst in proximal small intestine and release trophozoites that divide and attach to epithelium.
4. Clinically variable: asymptomatic to severe chronic diarrhea leading to malabsorption. In acute cases: usually watery diarrhea and abdominal discomfort.
5. Treatment: Flagyl.

Entamoeba histolytica
1. One of leading causes of parasitic death in the world.
2. Fecal-oral or food contamination.
3. Cyst infective: excysts at small bowel and forms trophozoites that infect large bowel. In colon, can invade lumen, causing ulceration and amebic dysentery. If gains access to portal system, destroys hepatic parenchyma, leading to amebic abscess in liver (1%).
4. Diagnosis: stool wet mount or serology.
5. Treatment: Flagyl, paromomycin, or iodoquinol.

Cyclospora cayetanensis
1. Transmission: undercooked meat and poultry and water. Infected by ingested sporulated oocysts.
2. Symptoms: self-limited diarrhea; nausea, vomiting, and abdominal pain in immunocompetent (persistent diarrhea in immunocompromised).
3. Diagnosis: stool microscopy.
4. Treatment: Bactrim.

Balantidium coli
Only ciliate known to parasitize humans. Most persons are not symptomatic but can present with dysentery.

Microsporidia
Watery diarrhea and malabsorption in immunocompromised patients (*Enterocytozoon bieneusi* and *Septata intestinalis* cause human disease).

Blastocystis hominis
Anaerobic protozoan causing diarrhea, abdominal pain, nausea and vomiting, anorexia, and malaise.

CESTODES AND WORMS

Taenia saginata
1. Beef tapeworm highly endemic to South America, Africa, South Asia, and Japan. Largest human parasite. Cattle are intermediate hosts.
2. Pass by blood or lymph to muscle, subcutaneous tissue, or viscera in cattle (larva), then ingested by humans.
3. Clinically asymptomatic: feeling of fullness may be only symptom; nausea, vomiting, and diarrhea may occur.
4. Diagnosis: stool.
5. Treatment: praziquantel or albendazole.

Taenia solium
1. Pork tapeworm.
2. Transmission: ingestion of infected pork. Larva invade humans and cause central nervous system infection. Adult worm in humans sheds proglottids, is eaten by pigs, and migrates to muscle. Humans eat larva and complete cycle.
3. Diagnosis: stool; discovery of proglottids.
4. Treatment: praziquantel or albendazole.

Diphyllobothrium latum
1. Fish tapeworm. Most common in Northern Europe (Scandinavia).
2. Greatest risk factor: eating raw fish. Eggs passed in human feces, are eaten by freshwater crustaceans, develop into larva, are eaten by fish, reside in muscle of fish, then are eaten by humans.
3. Clinically asymptomatic; diarrhea, fatigue, and paresthesia have been described. Pernicious anemia occurs; tapeworm absorbs free vitamin B_{12}.
4. Diagnosis: stool exam.
5. Treatment: praziquantel or niclosamide.

Ascaris
1. Most common intestinal helminth worldwide.
2. *Ascaris lumbricoides* specific for humans; infected by ingesting food with mature ova. Larva released in small intestine, enter circulation, reach pulmonary alveoli where develop. Pneumonitis and allergic manifestations. Soil necessary for development of eggs. Transmission: contaminated food or water.
3. Diagnosis: stool discovery of adult worms, larvae, or eggs.
4. Treatment: mebendazole or pyrantel pamoate.

Trichuris trichiura
1. Whipworm. Found in same parts of world as *Ascaris*.
2. Humans are the host with eggs passed in stool to soil. Transmission: ingestion of contaminated food.
3. Symptoms: asymptomatic or chronic diarrhea; dysentery and malnutrition with heavy work burden.
4. Diagnosis: discovery of adult worms or eggs in stool.
5. Treatment: mebendazole.

Trichinella spiralis
1. Nematode.
2. Ingested as larvae or nurse cell in striated muscle. Larvae released in stomach and pass to small intestine where infects epithelium. Larvae penetrate lymph or blood to muscle cells where nurse cell forms. Transmission: undercooked meat, especially pork.
3. Clinical features: cell destruction secondary to penetration of cardiac or nervous tissue; GI symptoms (nausea and vomiting) are common.

4. Diagnosis: histologic discovery of nurse cells within infected muscle; serology helpful.
5. Treatment: thiabendazole.

ANISAKIDAE
1. Anisakiasisis caused by ingestion of larval nematodes of the family Anisakidae. In North America, infection due to *Anisakis* simplex (herring worm) or *Pseudoterranova decipiens* (cod or seal worm).
2. Anisakis embeds itself in the gastric mucosa along the greater curvature. Acquired by eating contaminated sushi and raw fish.
3. Symptoms: severe abdominal pain, which subsides within a few days. Infection associated with gastric-fold swelling, erosions, and ulcers.
4. Treatment: none, but worms may need to be endoscopically removed. Prevention: avoid undercooked fish and flash freezing of fish at catch.

VIRAL FOODBORNE INFECTIONS

HEPATITIS A
1. Ribonucleic acid (RNA) Picornaviridae.
2. Transmission: fecal-oral; contaminated food or water.
3. Incubation: 30 d. Virus rapidly disappears after acute illness. Excrete 3 wk before symptoms, 1wk after.

HEPATITIS E
1. Small RNA virus from Caliciviridae.
2. Transmission: contaminated drinking water; also person-to-person.
3. Incubation 2–9 wks. Similar to disease seen with hepatitis A with constitutional symptoms followed by jaundice. Recovery is usual, but mortality as high as 3% in pregnant women.

NORWALK
1. Small, round structured virus; *Calicivirus*.
2. Transmission: fecally contaminated drinking water, swimming water, undercooked shellfish, and salads.
3. Incubation: 48 h. Symptoms: vomiting, watery diarrhea without blood or mucus. Resolves within 24 h. No therapy.

QUESTIONS

CHOOSE THE BEST ANSWER:
1. Which is true of *Clostridium botulinum*?
   a. Type A toxin is most associated with human disease.
   b. Crosses the blood-brain barrier.
   c. Is associated with notable gastrointestinal symptoms.
   d. Is a gram-negative organism
   e. Has a mortality rate of 50%.

TRUE OR FALSE:
2. Staphylococcal toxin is easy to eradicate.
3. Reheating food does not neutralize *Bacillus cereus* toxin.

MATCH THE AGENT TO THE INDUCED SYMPTOM:
a. Ciguatera.
b. Scombroid.
c. Tetrodotoxin.
d. Saxitoxin.
e. Brevitoxin.
f. Toxic-encephalopathic.
g. Aflatoxin.
h. Akee fruit.
i. Red kidney beans.
j. Lima beans.

4. Can cause death within minutes from hydrogen cyanide.
5. Histamine reaction.
6. Paresthesias without paralysis.
7. Amnesia.
8. Hypoglycemia.
9. Cirrhosis and liver cancer.
10. Most common fish poisoning in United States.
11. Cardiac arrhythmias, severe paralysis, and death.
12. Cranial nerve or respiratory paralysis.

CHOOSE THE BEST ANSWER:
13. Which is the only ciliate known to infect humans?
   a. *Giardia lamblia*.
   b. *Enterocytozoon bieneusi*.
   c. *Blastocystis hominis*.
   d. *Balantidium coli*.
   e. *Cyclospora cayetanensis*.

14. Which is false of *Vibrio* infections?
   a. *V. cholerae* toxin activates cyclic adenosine monophosphate and causes notable secretory diarrhea.
   b. *V. parahaemolyticus* is associated with shellfish consumption.
   c. *V. vulnificus* is associated with increased mortality in iron overload states.
   d. All of the above are true.
   e. All of the above are false.

15. Which is true of *Clostridium perfringens*–associated diseases?
   a. Type A causes necrotizing enterocolitis.
   b. Type C is the most common.
   c. Necrotizing enterocolitis occurs in well-nourished patients.
   d. *Clostridium perfringens* can be part of normal bowel flora.
   e. All of the above are true.

16. *Salmonella* infection:
   a. *Salmonella typhi* and *Salmonella paratyphi* infect only humans.
   b. Salmonella enteritidis can infect intact eggs through contaminated soil contact.
   c. Is increasingly resistant to various antibiotic therapies.
   d. Invades epithelium.
   e. All of the above are true.
   f. None of the above is true.

17. *Campylobacter* infection:
    a. Is the most common bacterial foodborne infection in the United States.
    b. Is linked with Guillain-Barré syndrome and probably occurs via molecular mimicry.
    c. Is associated with uveitis.
    d. Diarrhea by this organism is mainly caused by *Campylobacter jejuni*.
    e. All of the above are true.
    f. None of the above is true.

18. *Listeria monocytogenes* infection is associated with the following except:
    a. Spontaneous abortion.
    b. Case mortality rate of 20% in pregnant women.
    c. Meningitis in the newborn.
    d. Is not common in the environment.
    e. Causes infection in several risk groups including pregnant women, elderly, and immunocompromised individuals.

MATCH THE INDUCED SYMPTOM WITH THE ORGANISM/AGENTS:

a. *Taenia saginata*.
b. Anisakiasis.
c. *Diphyllobothrium latum*.
d. Norwalk virus
e. *Ascaris lumbricoides*.
f. *Taenia solium*.

19. Associated with pernicious anemia.
20. Associated with notable abdominal pain and embeds in the gastric mucosa at greater curvature of the stomach.
21. Largest human parasite.
22. Pneumonitis.
23. Rapid spread.

VIRAL INFECTIONS

SYNOPSIS

1. Viral infections account for up to 40% of cases of severe infectious diarrhea in children in developing countries (Table 1).
2. Transmission: person-to-person and fecal-oral.
3. Viruses causing diarrhea show strong tropism for epithelial cells in the small intestine. In contrast to invasive bacterial pathogens, host inflammatory response in viral enteritis is mild and not thought to contribute much to diarrhea.
4. Malnutrition may delay recovery from viral infections, particularly if vitamin A and zinc deficient. Viral infections are common in the immunodeficient.
5. Breastfeeding reduces incidence of diarrhea in infants and reduces mortality in children with diarrhea in developing countries.

QUESTIONS

MATCH THE VIRUS TO THE CHARACTERISTIC:

a. Cytomegalovirus.
b. Epstein-Barr virus.
c. *Rotavirus* A.
d. Norwalk virus.
e. Adenovirus.
f. Aichi virus.
g. *Rotavirus* B.

1. Only types 40 and 41 associated with diarrhea.
2. Associated with Ménétrier disease.
3. Major cause of infantile dehydrating diarrhea requiring hospitalization.
4. Immunoproliferative syndrome in transplant patients.
5. Rapid spread.
6. Infection associated with eating oysters.

CHOOSE THE BEST ANSWER:

The following have a peak incidence in winter in temperate climates except:
a. Norwalk virus
b. *Rotavirus* group A
c. Enteric adenovirus
d. Sapporo virus

TRUE OR FALSE:

8. The host inflammatory response in viral infections is mild.
9. Host immunity to caliciviral infections wanes over time.

PARASITIC AND FUNGAL INFECTIONS

SYNOPSIS

PARASITES OF THE STOMACH

Anisakis anisakis
1. Transmission: ingestion of uncooked fish. Most common in Japan, Holland, and Pacific coast of South America.
2. Symptoms: upper gastrointestinal (GI) illness, epigastric pain, and nausea or vomiting. Symptoms secondary to attachment of larvae to gastric mucosa where cause ulceration and ultimately perforation.
3. Treatment: may need to be endoscopically removed.
4. See "Foodborne Illness".

PARASITES OF THE SMALL INTESTINE

Giardia
1. Flagellate protozoan.
2. Transmission: food, water, and person-to-person.
3. Asymptomatic carriage recognized.

TABLE 1   VIRAL AGENTS OF GASTROENTERITIS

AGENT	VIROLOGY	CLINICAL EPIDEMIOLOGY	DIAGNOSIS AND THERAPY
Rotavirus group A	80 nm, segmented dsRNA. 4 major groups, A–D. Group A responsible for most *Rotavirus* infection in humans. Infects only mature villus enterocytes. Diarrhea by 2 mechanisms: undigested or unabsorbed carbohydrates leading to osmotic diarrhea; loss of active absorption of water in face of intact crypt secretion chloride, water with subsequent low-grade secretory diarrhea.	Most important cause of diarrhea requiring admission to hospital during first 6–24 mo of life. Neonatal rotavirus often asymptomatic in full term infant (possible passive immunity from breast milk). Peak incidence in winter in temperate climates. Incubation 2–7 d, then vomiting, fever, and profuse watery diarrhea.	EIA, EM, PAGE, RT-PCR. Treatment: correct dehydration, acidosis, and electrolyte imbalance. Early resumption of normal feeds encouraged. If lactose malabsorption: lactose-free diet. Drugs contraindicated. Breastfeeding may delay infection rather than prevent. Passive IgG: delays onset and decreases severity. Bovine antibody: hastens recovery and protects versus infection. Live attenuated vaccine possibly associated with intussusception.
Astrovirus	34 nm, ssRNA; 8 human serotypes, serotype 1 most common.	Diarrhea in infants; outbreaks in elderly and immunocompromised. Peak incidence in winter. Fecal-oral transmission. Asymptomatic infection common, especially in day care or hospital. Most children develop antibodies by age 5 yr. Important cause of diarrhea in AIDS and bone marrow transplant patients. Moderate gastroenteritis symptoms; less severe than *Rotavirus*. Incubation 1–4 d. Immunocompromised hosts: more prolonged symptoms.	EIA, EM, RT-PCR. Treatment: hydration and nutrition.
Calicivirus (Norwalk and Sapporo viruses); hepatitis E virus is another strain	28 nm, ssRNA. Nonenveloped.	Common cause of outbreaks among adults, children, and infants. Outbreaks usually at schools, camps, or cruise ships. Peak incidence in winter in temperate climates. Transmission: contaminated food. Incubation 12–24 h. Common nosocomial pathogens. Notably rapid onset of symptoms; rapidly spreads through groups. Predominant vomiting. Self-limited to 12–24 h.	EM, RT-PCR (most efficient). No specific treatment. Immunity to *Calicivirus* develops after infection but wanes rapidly.
Enteric adenoviruses	80 nm, dsDNA. Only serotypes 40 and 41 definitely associated with diarrhea. Ubiquitous: cause of range of symptoms from respiratory disease to hepatitis.	Prolonged diarrhea in infants and young children; year-round prevalence. No seasonal peak. Often asymptomatic infection, especially in day care.	EIA, EM. No specific therapy. Use of ribavirin in immunocompromised.
Picobirnavirus	Segmented dsRNA.	Possible diarrhea in immunocompromised	EM, PAGE.
CMV, EBV	Enveloped dsDNA	CMV: enterocolitis in immunocompromised; protein-losing gastropathy (Ménétrier disease), GI ulcerations, and enterocolitis similar to Crohn disease. EBV: immunoproliferative syndrome in transplant patients with fever and diarrhea.	Culture, serology, PCR. Histology: characteristic nuclear inclusions. Treatment: restoration of immune function and ganciclovir; CMV IgG for CMV infection.
Rotavirus groups B and C	Segmented dsRNA; do not grow in tissue culture.	Animal pathogens, with occasional human outbreaks.	EM, PCR, PAGE.
Torovirus	ssRNA, enveloped.	Livestock diarrhea. Possible infantile gastroenteritis.	EM, experimental EIA.
Measles		Developing world. Accompanied by severe diarrhea.	Prevention: vaccine.
HIV	Retrovirus	AIDS patients frequently develop diarrhea even in absence of pathogens.	Diarrhea often responds to multiagent antiviral therapy.
Aichi virus	ssRNA	Associated with gastroenteritis in persons eating oysters. Also found in Pakistani children, Southeast Asia travelers.	Cultured in cells.

AIDS = acquired immunodeficiency syndrome; CMV = cytomegalovirus; dsDNA = double-stranded deoxyribonucleic acid; dsRNA = double-stranded ribonucleic acid; EBV = Epstein-Barr virus; EIA = enzyme immunoassay; EM = electron microscopy; GI = gastrointestinal; HIV = human immunodeficiency virus; IgG = immunoglobulin G; PAGE = polyacrylamide gel electrophoresis; PCR = polymerase chain reaction; RT-PCR = real-time polymerase chain reaction; ssRNA = single-stranded ribonucleic acid.

4. Diagnosis: fecal specimens, duodenal fluid, and biopsy (gold standard). Multiple stool specimens will identify 80%.
5. Treatment: metronidazole (drug of choice) and furazolidone.
6. See "Foodborne Illness".

Cryptosporidium

1. Intracellular but extracytoplasmic location in host's intestinal epithelial cells. Usually found in immunocompromised individuals. Found in small and large intestine; reproduces sexually and asexually. Able to complete life cycle within human host.
2. Transmission: water and person-to-person. Two different strains of *C. parvum* (one infects only animals, other humans and animals). Acute infection: incubation 1–7 d, then fever, abdominal discomfort, nausea, vomiting, and high-volume watery diarrhea. Illness resolves in 2 d to 2–3 wk. Asymptomatic carriage well recognized.
3. Diagnosis: oocysts in stool and duodenal fluid.
4. Treatment: nitazoxanide may eradicate. In patients with human immunodeficiency virus (HIV): zidovudine may eradicate or reduce stool volume. Antidiarrheals and octreotide may help.

Microsporidia

1. *Enterocytozoon bieneusi* and *Encephalitozoon intestinalis* (also known as *Septata intestinalis*) known to infect humans. Obligate intracellular spore-forming organisms with wide range of hosts. Infection in humans confined to small intestine with atrophy.
2. Clinically, *Enterocytozoon bieneusi* resembles *Cryptosporidium*. Associated also with sclerosing cholangitis in HIV. *Encephalitozoon intestinalis* similar diarrheal disease with spread to kidneys, shedding in urine.
3. Diagnosis: detection of spores in stool, at small intestine biopsies.
4. Treatment: albendazole; usually results in suppression rather than eradication.

Isospora belli AND Sarcocystis

1. Rare in immunocompetent, but seen in HIV.
2. Ingested in undercooked food, especially pork and beef.
3. Various degrees of small intestine atrophy and inflammation. Carried without symptoms, but children can develop profuse diarrhea or steatorrhea and weight loss.
4. Diagnosis: oocysts in feces and duodenal fluid; biopsy.
5. Treatment: furazolidone and Bactrim effective, but recurrence is common. May need to treat for weeks.

Cyclospora cayetanensis

1. Infection is seasonal; peak prevalence in periods of high rainfall.
2. Symptoms: prolonged diarrhea.
3. Diagnosis: oocysts in feces.
4. Treatment: Bactrim.

NEMATODES

Strongyloides stercoralis

1. Adult worms live in the duodenum and jejunum. Found in tropics and subtropics. Adult worms invade intestinal mucosa, producing inflammatory response.
2. Penetration of skin produces a local reaction; 1 wk later, respiratory symptoms; 2 wk later, diarrhea, as small intestine invaded. Autoinfection at colon and perianal area can result in larva currens (hyperinfection), usually in immunocompromised individuals (often fatal).
3. Diagnosis: larvae can be detected in feces and sputum; jejunal biopsy. Negative stool exam can be misleading. Serology positive in 80%.
4. Treatment: albendazole (drug of choice). Thiabendazole will eliminate in 80% of patients. Side effects: nausea and vomiting, dizziness, and headache.

Capillaria philippinensis

1. Southeast Asia. Occurs after ingestion of raw fish.
2. Symptoms: after 1–2 months incubation: severe diarrhea and malabsorption.
3. Diagnosis: parasite found in stool and biopsies.
4. Treatment: eradicated by mebendazole or thiabendazole if used for 3–4 wk.

Trichinella spiralis

1. Occurs worldwide in communities that eat pork.
2. Requires 2 hosts to complete its life cycle. (Figure 1)
3. Initially, diarrhea and abdominal pain, usually several days after ingestion; 1–2 wk later, fever with periorbital edema, erythematous rash, and severe muscle pains lasting up to 6 wk. Associated complications: myocarditis, pneumonitis, and encephalitis.
4. Diagnosis: larvae in skeletal muscle biopsies. Eosinophilia; creatine kinase and serum glutamic-oxaloacetic transaminase elevation.
5. Treatment: prolonged mebendazole. If systemic infection, treat with steroids to reduce allergic reaction.
6. See "Foodborne Illness".

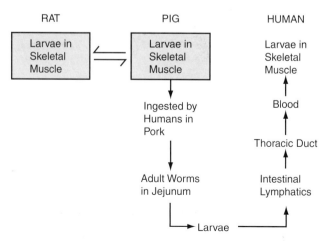

FIGURE 1 Life cycle of *Trichinella spiralis*.

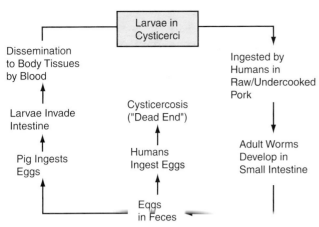

FIGURE 2   Life cycle of *Taenia solium* (pork tapeworm).

Trichostrongylus orientalis
1. Small roundworm.
2. Transmission: contaminated food and drink.
3. Diagnosis: ova in duodenal fluid and feces.
4. Treatment: one dose levamisole.

Ascaris lumbricoides
1. Largest intestinal nematode.
2. Symptoms: most are not symptomatic; pulmonary phase can have wheezing, eosinophilia, and fever. Heavy infections in children: abdominal pain and anorexia.
3. Diagnosis: ova and worms in feces; larvae in sputum or gastric washings.
4. Treatment: albendazole, mebendazole, and levamisole (one dose) drugs of choice. Intestinal obstruction may require surgery.
5. See "Foodborne Illness".

Ancylostoma duodenale AND Necator americanus
1. *Ancylostoma duodenale*: Africa, Asia, Australia, and southern Europe. *Necator americanus*: Central and South America.
2. Adult worms attach firmly to small intestinal mucosa. Larvae penetrate skin with local inflammation.

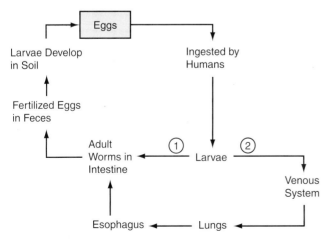

FIGURE 3   Life cycle of (1) *Trichuris trichiura* and *Enterobius vermicularis* and (2) *Ascaris lumbricoides*. The shaded area indicates the infective form of parasites.

3. Dominant response: iron-deficiency anemia. Occasionally, heavy infection can lead to protein-losing enteropathy.
4. Diagnosis: ova and larvae in stool and duodenal fluid.
5. Treatment: mebendazole, albendazole, and iron.

CESTODES
1. Four types: *Taenia solium*, *Diphyllobothrium latum*, *Taenia saginata*, and *Hymenolepis nana*. Adult worms reside in intestinal tract; larvae exist in tissues.
2. *Taenia saginata* (beef tapeworm): usually asymptomatic; mild abdominal discomfort and occasional diarrhea. Occasionally adult worms obstruct appendix or pancreatic duct. Praziquantel is drug of choice, niclosamide effective. Freeze at −10°C for 5 d, cooking at 57°C to kill.
3. *Taenia solium* (pork tapeworm): similar to *Taenia saginata*. Disseminates to eye, central nervous system, skeletal muscle, and myocardium: cysticercosis. Cysts remain alive for many years: inflammatory reaction and calcification (Figure 2). Treatment: praziquantel.
4. *Diphyllobothrium latum* (fish tapeworm): usually asymptomatic but can have abdominal discomfort, vomiting, and weight loss. Cleaves B₁₂-intrinsic factor complex and consumes 80–100% of dietary B₁₂; can lead to vitamin B₁₂ deficiency in host. Treatment: praziquantel or niclosamide.
5. *Hymenolepis nana*: usually no symptoms; heavy infection can lead to diarrhea and abdominal pain. Treatment: praziquantel or niclosamide.
6. See "Foodborne Illness".

TREMATODES

Fasciolopsis buski
1. Largest human fluke. Found in Far East; attaches to proximal small intestine.
2. Can cause ulceration, bleeding. Asymptomatic infections can occur but with large burden: diarrhea, abdominal pain, and protein losing enteropathy.
3. Treatment: praziquantel.

Heterophyes heterophyes and Metagonimus yokogawai
1. Small flukes in Far East.
2. Infection asymptomatic. Heavy infection: abdominal pain and intermittent diarrhea.
3. Diagnosis: ova in feces.
4. Treatment: praziquantel.

PARASITES OF COLON AND RECTUM

PROTOZOA
Entamoeba histolytica and *Balantidium coli* (ciliate) important ones. *Cryptosporidium* can affect colitis as well. *Giardia* can occasionally cause colitis.

Entamoeba histolytica
1. Amebiasis rare in infancy and childhood, but morbidity and mortality high in this age group.

2. Two forms: trophozoite and cyst. Cyst can exist outside human host for long periods.
3. Transmission: food, water, and person-to-person. *Entamoeba dispar* is not pathogenic.
4. Most cases are asymptomatic. Acute amebic dysentery can lead to toxic megacolon (most likely in pregnancy and malnourished infants and children). Chronic amebic colitis insidious; bowel function can return to normal or result in constipation. Complications of strictures or inflammatory masses (ameboma) can occur. Liver abscess can occur in 50% without colonic involvement. Distant spread to lung, brain, and kidney occurs when abscess bursts into hepatic vein.
5. Diagnosis: feces; fresh saline wet mount reveals trophozoites with ingested red cells. Also biopsy. Rare trophozoites seen in pus of liver abscess. Serology positive in 70–80% of colitis and 100% of liver abscess.
6. See "Foodborne Illness".

Balantidium coli
1. Only ciliate to cause disease in humans. Restricted to communities exposed to pigs (preferred host).
2. Cyst infects; trophozoite can survive outside human for 1 wk. Clinically similar to amebiasis.
3. Diagnosis: trophozoite in feces.
4. Treatment: tetracycline; also Flagyl and ampicillin.
5. See "Foodborne Illness".

Trypanosoma cruzi
1. Chagas disease. Does not directly affect GI tract. Infection occurs early in childhood. Transmitted via bite of insect family Reduviidae. Deposited in insect feces on skin and rubbed into mucous membranes or bite wound.
2. Vast majority of initial illness unnoticed; some cases with marked fever, hepatosplenomegaly, and lymphadenopathy. Severe infection can be accompanied by myocarditis. Megasyndromes (ie, megaesophagus) occur years later.
3. Treatment: nifurtimox or benznidazole.

NEMATODES
Most common to infect colon: *Trichuris trichiuria* (whipworm) and *Enterobius vermicularis* (threadworm). *Strongyloides stercoralis* also colonizes large intestine in

TABLE 1   TREATMENT OF AMEBIASIS IN CHILDREN

INTESTINAL AMEBIASIS
Metronidazole
50 mg/kg daily for 10 d, followed by diloxanide furoate, 20 mg/kg daily for 10 d
AMEBIC LIVER ABSCESS
Metronidazole
50 mg/kg daily for 10 d
ASYMPTOMATIC CYST PASSER
Diloxanide furoate
20 mg/kg daily for 10 d + metronidazole

hyperinfection (autoinfection), causing ulceration and inflammatory changes.

Trichuris trichiuria
1. Transmission: ingestion of ova (Figure 3).
2. Symptoms: light infections often asymptomatic. With more parasites: diarrhea, blood, and mucous; also abdominal pain, anorexia or weight loss, tenesmus, and rectal prolapse.
3. Diagnosis: eggs in feces or worms at mucosal biopsy, usually with ulceration and inflammation.
4. Treatment: mebendazole, drug of choice for people aged > 2 yr. Albendazole can also be given as one dose. May need multiple treatment courses.

Enterobius vermicularis
1. Direct transmission of ova person-to-person or indirect via house dust or clothing (see Figure 3).
2. Anal pruritis is usually the only symptom, occurring at night. Symptoms can mimic appendicitis when *Enterobius vermicularis* enters appendix.
3. Diagnosis: ova detected by applying tape to perianal skin. Also under fingernails.
4. Treatment: albendazole, drug of choice; also pyrantel pamoate and piperazine. Wise to treat entire family and consider retreatment in 2–4 wk.

Oesophagostomum
1. Occasional human infection.
2. Penetrates intestinal wall; resulting in multiple nodules along intestine.
3. May require intestinal drainage of abscesses.

Angiostrongylus costaricensis
1. Inflammatory mass involving cecum, appendix, and terminal ileum characteristic. Acute form can be confused with appendicitis. Inflammatory reaction is a result of intramural eggs discharged from adult worms living in terminal mesenteric arterials.
2. Treatment: surgery may be required.

TREMATODES
1. Five *Schistosoma* species: *Schistosoma mansoni*, *Schistosoma japonicum*, *Schistosoma haematobium*, *Schistosoma mekongi*, and *Schistosoma intercalatum*. Human infection totally dependent on freshwater snail (Figure 4).
2. Inflammatory reaction at skin: swimmer's itch. Within 1 wk: generalized allergic response with fever, urticaria, myalgia, malaise, and eosinophilia.
3. Acute phase (*Schistosoma japonicum*): Katayama fever. Clinical symptoms consist of skin rashes, asthma-like episodes, daily fever, malaise, diarrhea, swollen lymph nodes and aching joints, and a number of other nonspecific symptoms.
4. Gut involvement: Hepatosplenomegaly occurs in early stages. Extensive intestinal polyp formation and ulceration typical of *Schistosoma mansoni* infection. Stricture formation and obstruction are characteristic; localized granulomatous masses within gut wall (bil-

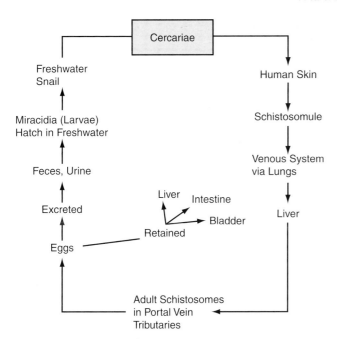

FIGURE 4 Life cycle of *Schistosoma* species.

harziomas). *Schistosoma japonicum* involves both small intestine and large intestine: has premalignant potential. Inflammation at intestine owing to T-cell mediated reaction to eggs.

5. *Schistosoma haematobium* produces rectal inflammation and bladder involvement.
6. Diagnosis: ova in stool; biopsy.
7. Treatment: praziquantel (1 dose), drug of choice. Oxamniquine also effective.

FUNGAL INFECTIONS

Candida

1. Isolated in 15% of gastric ulcers but not part of pathogenesis. Candida peritonitis: seen after bowel surgery and peritoneal dialysis.
2. Infection associated with watery diarrhea in infants. Can invade intestine in terminally ill patients. Esophagitis in immunocompromised. In disseminated candidiasis, the major risk factor is neutropenia.
3. Treatment: nystatin thrush, fluconazole, ketoconazole, and amphotericin.

Aspergillus

1. Disease form: hyphae. Most seen in severely immunocompromised patients.
2. 20% of cases involve intestine in addition to esophagus and stomach.
3. Treatment: amphotericin B, drug of choice.

Zygomycetes

1. Mucormycosis and phycomatosis.
2. In debilitated disease can cause acute fulminant invasive infection.
3. Can infect subcutaneous and submucosal tissues in immunocompetent host.

Coccidioidomycosis

1. Dimorphic fungus endemic to southwestern United States.
2. Usually pulmonary infection. Spores can escape chest.
3. In disseminated disease; terminal ileum and colon can rarely be involved.

QUESTIONS

MATCH THE SITE OF HUMAN INFECTION TO THE PARASITE OR FUNGI:

a. Stomach.
b. Small intestine.
c. Colon.
d. Bladder.
e. Lung.
f. Muscle.
g. None of the above.

1. *Giardia* .
2. Microsporidia.
3. *Isospora.*
4. *Cryptosporidium.*
5. *Cyclospora.*
6. *Strongyloides.*
7. *Capillaria.*
8. *Trichinella.*
9. *Balantidium coli.*
10. *Trichuris trichiuria.*
11. *Trichostrongylus.*
12. *Ascaris* .
13. *Metagonimus yokogawai.*
14. Ancylostoma.
15. *Enterobius vermicularis.*
16. *Taenia solium.*
17. *Entamoeba histolytica.*
18. *Taenia saginata.*
19. *Diphyllobothrium latum.*
20. *Hymenolepis nana.*
21. *Fasciolopsis buski.*
22. *Heterophyes heterophyes.*
23. *Oesophagostomum.*
24. *Angiostrongylus costaricensis.*
25. *Schistosoma mansoni.*
26. *Schistosoma haematobium.*
27. *Entamoeba dispar.*
28. Coccidioidomycosis.
29. *Anisakis anisakis.*

MATCH THE TREATMENT OF CHOICE TO THE PARASITE OR FUNGI:

a. Metronidazole.
b. Albendazole.
c. Bactrim.
d. Mebendazole.
e. Levamisole.
f. Praziquantel.
g. Niclosamide.

h. Nifurtimox.
i. Tetracycline.
j. Pyrantel pamoate.
k. Amphotericin.
l. Nitazoxanide.

30. *Schistosoma.*
31. *Cryptosporidium.*
32. *Enterobius vermicularis.*
33. *Trichuris trichiuria.*
34. Microsporidia.
35. *Trypanosoma cruzi.*
36. *Trichinella spiralis.*
37. *Giardia*
38. *Entamoeba histolytica.*
39. *Isospora.*
40. *Taenia solium.*
41. *Cyclospora cayetanensis.*
42. *Diphyllobothrium latum.*
43. *Hymenolepsis nana.*
44. *Fasciolopsis buski.*
45. *Metagonimus yokogawai.*
46. *Ascaris lumbricoides.*
47. *Trichostrongylus orientalis.*
48. *Balantidium coli.*
49. *Strongyloides stercoralis.*

SMALL BOWEL BACTERIAL OVERGROWTH

SYNOPSIS

CHARACTERISTICS
1. Abnormal colonization of upper small intestine by organisms that usually reside in colon (Table 1).
2. Steatorrhea.
3. Anemia.

NORMAL PROTECTIVE MEASURES
1. Gastric acidity (pH < 4 is bactericidal for most organisms).
2. Peristaltic propagation of luminal contents distally; migrating motor complex is particularly important in this role (Figure 1).

TABLE 1   COMMENSAL ENTERIC FLORA OF THE NORMAL INTESTINAL TRACT

PROXIMAL SMALL INTESTINE
< 10^6 organisms/mL
Aerobic, oral flora dominate
Streptococcus, Lactobacillus, Neisseria

DISTAL SMALL INTESTINE
> 10^9 organisms/mL
Greater numbers of anaerobic and facultative anaerobic bacteria
Bacteroides, Escherichia coli, Bifidobacterium

COLON
10^{9-10} organisms/mL
Anaerobic and facultative anaerobic bacteria
Bacteroides, Escherichia coli, Bifidobacterium, Clostridium

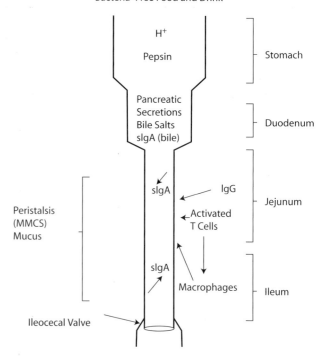

FIGURE 1   Prevention of small bowel bacterial overgrowth in health.

3. Enzymatic digestion (pancreatic juice has antibacterial activity).
4. Intestinal secretions dilute the bacterial mass and prevent access to preferential growth sites.
5. Mucus entraps bacteria intraluminally while moving them distally.
6. Ileocecal valve prevents retrograde bacterial colonization of distal small bowel.
7. Immunoglobulins: Secretory immunoglobulin A (sIgA) prevents bacterial attachment to intestinal membranes. Hypo- and agammaglobulinemic patients are at increased risk of small bowel bacterial overgrowth (SBBO), although some say achlorhydria must also be present (Table 2).

TABLE 2   FACTORS PREDISPOSING TO THE DEVELOPMENT OF SMALL BOWEL BACTERIAL OVERGROWTH

ANATOMIC ABNORMALITIES
Diverticula, duplication
Stricture, stenosis, web
Blind loop
MOTILITY DISORDERS
Pseudo-obstruction
Absence of migratory motor complexes
Autonomic neuropathy (eg, diabetes mellitus)
Collagen vascular diseases (eg, scleroderma)
EXCESSIVE BACTERIAL LOAD
Achlorhydria
Fistula
Loss of ileocecal valve
ABNORMAL HOST DEFENSES
Immunodeficiency
Malnutrition
Prematurity

TABLE 3   INTRALUMINAL BACTERIA: EFFECTS ON THE HOST

INTRALUMINAL EFFECTS	MUCOSAL EFFECTS	SYSTEMIC EFFECTS
Bile salt deconjugation	Disaccharidase loss	Absorption of bacterial toxins, antigens
11α-Hydroxylation	Enterocyte damage	Hepatic inflammation
Bile salt depletion		
Lipid malabsorption	Inflammation	Immune complex formation
Vitamin B_{12} malabsorption	Protein loss	Cutaneous vasculitis
Fermentation—short-chain fatty acids	Bleeding	Polyarthritis
Release of proteases, toxins		

PATHOPHYSIOLOGY

1. Intraluminal:
   a. Bacteria deconjugate bile salts, which reduces bile salt concentration below the critical micellar concentration, reducing the effectiveness of pancreatic enzymes. Result: steatorrhea (Table 3).
   b. Bacteria compete with host for vitamin B_{12}. Vitamin B_{12} malabsorption not correctable by exogenous intrinsic factor is most consistent feature of SBBO.
2. Mucosal effects:
   a. Enterocyte damage via enzyme and metabolic products.
   b. Mucosal disaccharidases reduced; monosaccharide transport may be impaired, as well as transport of Na and Cl.
   c. May cause protein loss and protein-losing enteropathy.
   d. Intestinal blood loss also documented.
3. Systemic effects:
   a. Bacterial products and antigens are absorbed through damaged mucosa causing immune responses and immune complex formation.
   b. Hepatobiliary injury in rat. Many studies show that liver disease is associated with SBBO in humans.

CLINICAL FEATURES

Overgrowth in proximal small intestine (SI) results in greater disability than SBBO in distal SI.

DIAGNOSIS

HISTORY

1. Previous abdominal surgery leading to alterations in motility or stasis (adhesions, partial SBBO), vagotomy owing to associations with achlorhydria, and diabetes leading to alterations in intestinal motility may predispose to SBBO.
2. Note: SBBO very unusual in children with diabetes mellitus.

SCREEN

1. Not all patients have typical symptoms of SBBO; screening required (Table 4).
2. Serum cobalamin is not a useful screen since body stores usually sufficient for 5 yr after onset of cobalamin malabsorption. Elevated folate levels may be useful.
3. Schilling test with intrinsic factor.
4. Quantitative fecal fat excretion or spot fecal fat.
5. Upper gastrointestinal series and small bowel follow-through to document intestinal strictures and anatomic reasons for delay in transit.

DIAGNOSIS

1. Duodenal biopsy: patchy enteropathic changes with increased inflammatory cells is typical. Need to rule out celiac disease (Table 5).
2. Quantitative culture from proximal small intestine establishes diagnosis; > 10^6 colony forming units bacteria that are not typical residents: abnormal. Coliforms and anaerobic colonic-type bacteria normally do not reside in mouth, stomach, or SI.
3. Can also run conjugated and deconjugated bile acid profiles in duodenal fluid (increased deconjugated bile acids in presence of bacteria).
4. Noninvasive: measure elevated urinary indican (produced by conversion of dietary tryptophan to indican by bacteria); specificity low.
5. Noninvasive: total serum bile acids often elevated in patients with SBBO and almost all is free bile acids with deoxycholate uniquely elevated (distinguishes SBBO from ileal resection).
6. Noninvasive: breath tests (Figure 2).
   a. Measurement of ^{14}C after oral ingestion of appropriate substrate; utilization by bacteria releases $^{14}CO_2$. False-negative if bacteria unable to deconjugate. False-positive in patients with mucosal inflammation affecting distal ileum. ^{13}C substrate test also can be used and is 100% sensitive and 67% specific.

TABLE 4   CLINICAL FEATURES OF SMALL BOWEL BACTERIAL OVERGROWTH

CLASSIC
Chronic diarrhea
Steatorrhea
Anemia

SYSTEMIC
Arthritis
Tenosynovitis
Vesiculopapular rash
Erythema nodosum
Raynaud phenomenon
Nephritis
Hepatitis
Hepatic steatosis

OTHERS
Weight loss
Short stature
Abdominal pain
Protein-losing enteropathy
Hypoalbuminemia
Osteomalacia
Night blindness
Ataxia

b. H$_2$ expiration level measurement now available. Mammalian cells do not produce H$_2$ whereas prokaryotic do. Provision of nonabsorbable sugar supplies substrate, resulting in increased H$_2$ expired. Shortcomings: children with diarrhea and low fecal pH may have altered flora that does not yield H$_2$. Concurrent use of medications, especially antibiotics, also affects it. End-expiratory samples most representative but difficult in young children.

TABLE 5   DIAGNOSTIC TESTS FOR SMALL BOWEL BACTERIAL OVERGROWTH

SCREENING
Sudan stain for neutral fat
72-Hour fecal fat
Schilling test with intrinsic factor
Folic acid, vitamin B$_{12}$
Barium meal with follow-through

DIAGNOSTIC
Invasive
  Duodenal aspiration for culture (aerobic, anaerobic bacteria and
    exclude known pathogens)
  Deconjugated bile salts
  Short-chain fatty acids
Noninvasive
  Indicanuria
  Serum bile acids
  Breath tests

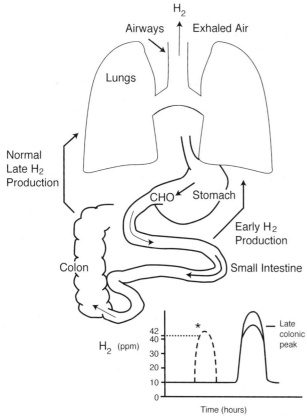

FIGURE 2   Conceptual framework for breath hydrogen testing. CHO denotes ingesting carbohydrate. *An early peak and an elevated baseline of hydrogen measured in expired breath samples are both suggestive of small bowel bacterial contamination.

TREATMENT

1. Correction of underlying disease.
2. Medical therapy:
   a. Nutritional deficits treated: easy digestible nutritional supplements low in fat. Medium-chain triglycerides may be advocated; total parenteral nutrition.
   b. Vitamin deficiencies: repleted. Especially fat-soluble. Vitamin B$_{12}$ deficiency rare because time required to deplete is long (5 yr); correctable by monthly injections. Iron supplementation as required.
   c. Antibiotics: directed to eradicate *Bacteroides* to resolve SBBO. Examples: tetracycline, Flagyl, lincomycin, and chloramphenicol. Course is 2–4 wk. If relapse, second course of same antibiotic for 4–8 wk. Culturing for sensitivity questionable since usually not just one organism responsible.
   d. Possible probiotics.

QUESTIONS

CHOOSE THE BEST ANSWER:

1. Which is not a classic characteristic of small bowel bacterial overgrowth?
   a. Abnormal bacterial colonization of the small bowel.
   b. Steatorrhea.
   c. Anemia.
   d. Abdominal pain.
   e. All of the above are classic symptoms of small bowel bacterial overgrowth.

2. Which of the following are not protective mechanisms against the development of small bowel bacterial overgrowth?
   a. Migrating motor complexes.
   b. Gastric acid.
   c. Secretory immunoglobulin A.
   d. Short chain fatty acids
   e. Mucus.

TRUE OR FALSE:

3. Vitamin B$_{12}$ malabsorption not correctable by intrinsic factor is the most consistent finding in small bowel bacterial overgrowth.
4. Bacterial overgrowth in the distal small intestine causes more symptoms than small bowel bacterial overgrowth in the proximal small intestine.
5. Erythema nodosum and Reynaud phenomenon are associated with small bowel bacterial overgrowth.
6. Small bowel bacterial overgrowth is a common feature in children with diabetes.
7. Celiac disease can present similar to small bowel bacterial overgrowth.
8. Antibiotic treatment for small bowel bacterial overgrowth should be directed at *Bacteroides*.

CHOOSE THE BEST ANSWER:

9. Which of the following is a useful screening tool for small bowel bacterial overgrowth?
    a. Serum cobalamin level.
    b. Serum folate level.
    c. Blood count.
    d. Fecal nitrogen measurement.
    e. All of the above are useful.

10. How long does it take to deplete body vitamin B_{12} stores before the serum cobalamin level is reduced?
    a. 5 d.
    b. 5 wk.
    c. 5 mo.
    d. 5 yr.
    e. None of the above.

GASTROINTESTINAL MANIFESTATIONS OF PRIMARY IMMUNODEFICIENCIES

SYNOPSIS

IMMUNE SYSTEM

1. Humoral: Generation of antibodies reactive with a given antigen. Depends on effector mechanisms that remove antigen bound to antibody either by ingestion by phagocytic cells or complement–dependent lysis of bacteria.
2. Cellular: Cell-mediated responses involving induction of specific effector cytotoxic cells or secretion of cytokines that trigger inflammation. Cells include B cells and T cells (Th1, Th2, and Tc).
    a. Th1 cells: secrete cytokines that activate other T cells.
    b. Th2 cells: secrete cytokines that activate B cells.
    c. B cells: involved in antibody production; adapted for defense against parasites.
    d. Tc (cytotoxic) cells: cause the death of viral infected cells and play a role in graft rejection.

PRIMARY IMMUNODEFICIENCIES

X-LINKED AGAMMAGLOBULINEMIA

1. Absent or very low levels of all immunoglobulin classes including secretory immunoglobulins.
2. Afflicted males usually well up until 6 months of life owing to transmitted maternal immunoglobulins. Then, severe, recurrent respiratory and meningeal infections unless prophylactic antibiotics or gammaglobulin therapy is started. Polymorphonuclear neutrophil leukocytes (PMN) function normal, but cyclic neutropenia can occur. Circulating mature B cells absent, as are lymph node and gut plasma cells. Mutations occur at the BTK gene, a B lymphocyte–specific kinase.
3. Complications: recurrent bacterial infections, *Giardia*, bacterial overgrowth, nonspecific colitis, and chronic rotavirus.

IMMUNOGLOBULIN A DEFICIENCY

1. Selective immunoglobulin (Ig) A deficiency: the most common primary immunodeficiency.
2. Most are asymptomatic but some may have frequent respiratory and gastrointestinal (GI) infections (susceptibility of infection associated with IgG2 or 4 deficiency).
3. Associated with ataxia-telangiectasia.
4. Autosomal inheritance. Linkage to 6p21.
5. Ten- to twenty-fold increased celiac disease (serum assayed antiendomysium antibodies and IgA antigliadin unhelpful; rely on IgG gliadin). *Giardia* is common. Increased prevalence among Crohn disease patients.
6. No specific treatment; aggressive treatment of infections. Intravenous (IV) administration of IgA may lead to anaphylaxis. Only extensively washed normal donor red blood cells or blood products from other IgA-deficient individuals should be administered.

HYPER IgM SYNDROME

1. Rare inherited disorder resulting from defects in the CD40 ligand and signaling pathway (present on CD4 T cells responsible for formation of memory B lymphocytes and promotes Ig isotype switching).
2. Clinical presentation: similar to that for X-linked agammaglobulinemia with recurrent pyogenic infections. Lymphoid hyperplasia often seen in hyper IgM syndrome. Serum IgA, IgG, IgE levels low; hyper IgM usually present. Chronic diarrhea and liver involvement; mouth and rectal ulcers, neutropenia, and *Pneumocystis carinii* pneumonia (PCP).
3. Association with autoimmune diseases.

TRANSIENT HYPOGAMMAGLOBULINEMIA OF INFANCY

1. Postnatally, a physiologic decrease in serum IgG with the nadir reached between 3rd and 6th month. In premature infants the nadir is even lower: the amount of transplacental Ig is less.
2. Intrinsic Ig synthesis: IgM appears first, then IgG and IgA. Transient hypogammaglobulinemia is primarily a deficiency of IgG.
3. Symptoms: recurrent respiratory infections, chronic diarrhea, and malabsorption.
4. Spontaneous resolution before age 4 yr, often between age 1 and 2 yr.

IgG SUBCLASS DEFICIENCY

1. Most with IgG2 deficiency also IgA deficient. Minority evolve toward common variable immunodeficiency (CVID).
2. Chronic diarrhea common. Nonspecific colitis frequent problem among those with deficiencies of IgA, IgG2, and IgG4.

CVID

1. One of the most frequent primary immunodeficiencies.
2. Characterized by reduced serum levels of IgG, IgA, and IgE; failure of B cells to mature into mature plasma cells as well as T cell functional abnormalities.

3. Notable clinical variability. Typically, recurrent otitis, pulmonary infections, and chronic diarrhea with malabsorption. Mild steatorrhea; small bowel biopsy showing mild–moderate villous atrophy (spectrum of abnormalities include patterns resembling graft-versus-host disease [GVHD] and inflammatory bowel disease). Gastritis can be seen in association with pernicious anemia. Nodular lymphoid hyperplasia can be seen in those who do have B cells. Malignancy frequent, including GI tumors and lymphomas. Autoimmune disease frequent. Bacterial overgrowth common. Rotavirus, *Campylobacter* infections common.

4. Treatment often requires nutritional support. Subset with excessive suppressor cell activity may benefit from cimetidine.

HYPER IgE SYNDROME AND IMMUNE DYSREGULATION, POLYENDOCRINOPATHY, ENTEROPATHY, X-LINKED SYNDROME

1. Immune dysregulation, polyendocrinopathy, enteropathy (IPEX), severe persistent diarrhea despite bowel rest, early onset of insulin-dependant diabetes mellitus, thyroid disorders, and eczema with high IgE.
2. X-linked. Affected males die of overwhelming infection.
3. Related to mutations of the *FOXP3* genes.
4. Remission observed after allogeneic bone marrow transplant. Immunosuppression may provide temporary benefit.

SEVERE COMBINED IMMUNODEFICIENCY

1. Hereditary disorder characterized by profound deficiency of both T and B lymphocyte function. Virtual absence of immune function from birth.
2. Severe life-threatening infections, chronic diarrhea, malabsorption, and failure to thrive in the first few months of life.
3. Majority of autosomal recessive cases have genetic deficiency in purine degradation enzymes (adenosine deaminase [ADA] or purine-nucleoside phosphorylase [PNP]).
4. Patients may have history of neonatal hyperpigmented rash secondary to GVHD from transplacentally acquired maternal lymphocytes or after transfusion.
5. Extreme susceptibility to viral infections, succumbing to overwhelming measles. Viral agents may cause chronic enteropathy. Susceptibility to systemic infections caused by *Candida*, PCP, and *Listeria*.
6. Histology shows blunted villi, absence of plasma cells, periodic acid–Schiff positive macrophages in lamina propria. Paucity of lymphoid tissue.
7. Omenn syndrome: lymphoid hyperplasia, hepatosplenomegaly, large numbers of oligoclonal T cells, and eosinophilia.
8. Management: antimicrobial therapy, avoidance of infection with live vaccine immunization, and avoidance of conventional blood transfusion. Treatment of choice: bone marrow transplant. ADA or PNP replacement may be helpful. Death usually by age 1–2 yr unless transplanted.

MAJOR HISTOCOMPATIBILTY COMPLEX CLASS II DEFICIENCY

1. Rare; defects in human leukocyte antigens (HLA) class II expression and lack of cellular and humoral immune responses.
2. Early onset with recurrent infection and severe diarrhea.
3. Prognosis poor; death at mean age 4 yr unless bone marrow transplant.

INTERFERON GAMMA DEFICIENCY

Associated with neonatal intractable diarrhea and weight loss secondary to *Cryptosporidium parvum*.

WISKOTT-ALDRICH SYNDROME

1. X-linked recessive syndrome, characterized by T cell dysfunction, severe eczema, thrombocytopenia, and repeated opportunistic infections. In first few months, often presents with bloody diarrhea. Later, infections with bacteria with polysaccharide capsules, and opportunistic infections.
2. Median survival < 6 yr. Specific antibodies produced poorly, but normal numbers of B lymphocytes present. T cells show decrease in number and function.
3. Optimal therapy: bone marrow transplant corrects all problems except thrombocytopenia.

ATAXIA-TELANGIECTASIA

1. Chromosomal instability disorder marked by progressive ataxia, oculocutaneous telangiectasias, and variable immunodeficiency owing to low IgA and IgG.
2. Associated with impaired organ maturation, radiograph hypersensitivity, and high incidence of neoplasia; persistent increased α-fetoprotein, and carcinoembryonic antigen production. Repeated sinopulmonary and bronchiectasis infections. GI disease not common unless accompanied by secretory IgA deficiency.
3. No treatment available.

DiGEORGE SYNDROME

1. Rare syndrome triad: hypocalcemia, congenital heart disease, and thymic hypoplasia (absent or decreased T-lymphocytes).
2. Results from failure of formation of 3rd and 4th pharyngeal pouches.
3. Defect due to deletion of large region on chromosome 22.

X-LINKED LYMPHOPROLIFERATIVE SYNDROME

1. Also known as Duncan disease or Purtilo syndrome.
2. Characterized by dysregulated immune response most commonly to Epstein-Barr virus infection. Chronic, fatal infection results in progressive hypogammaglobulinemia, aplastic anemia, or malignant B cell lymphoma.
3. Defective gene identified as *SAP-SLAM*.

DEFECTS OF PHAGOCYTIC FUNCTION

CHRONIC GRANULOMATOUS DISEASE

1. Primary immunodeficiency that affects phagocytes, causing defective oxidative burst capacity.

2. Characterized by recurrent pyogenic infections with catalase-positive organisms, multifocal abscesses at the skin and liver, lymphadenopathy, hepatosplenomegaly, chronic lung disease, and persistent diarrhea.
3. Can present with enterocolitis resembling Crohn disease; often yellow pigment in macrophages. Also can present with granulomatous narrowing of gastric antrum (gastric outlet obstruction).
4. Most common pathogen is *Staphylococcus aureus*.
5. X-linked recessive and autosomal recessive inheritance. Mutations occur in any of 4 genes that encode the subunits of NADPH oxidase.
6. Diagnosis: demonstration of absent or greatly diminished respiratory burst capacity. Nitroblue tetrazolium test can be used (no change in color in chronic granulomatous disease).
7. Management: antimicrobial therapy and drainage of abscesses. Steroids and sulfasalazine may help with intestinal inflammation, including gastric outlet obstruction (also enteral nutrition needed). Interferon-gamma increases the respiratory burst activity and is used for therapy with notable reduction in serious infections.

LEUKOCYTE ADHESION MOLECULE (CD11/CD18) DEFICIENCY
1. Characterized by inability of phagocytes to adhere to vascular endothelium and migrate into tissues.
2. Clinical manifestations: delayed umbilical cord separation and omphalitis. Stomatitis/pharyngitis (40% of cases), gingivitis (56%), perirectal abscess, and distal ileocolitis resembling Crohn disease. Bacterial septicemia common. Common bacterial infections: *S. aureus*, group A streptococcus, *Proteus*, *Pseudomonas*, and *Escherichia coli*.
3. No specific therapy. Broad-spectrum antibiotics to fight infection. Uniformly fatal in first 10 years of life. Bone marrow transplant is only effective cure.

OTHER DISORDERS OF NEUTROPHILS
1. Glycogen storage disease (GSD) type IB and Hermansky-Pudlak syndrome: nonspecific colitis that resembles inflammatory bowel disease (IBD).
2. Granulocyte colony-stimulating factor may help GSD type IB and improve neutropenia and colitis.

CHRONIC MUCOCUTANEOUS CANDIDIASIS
1. Primary defect in cell-mediated immunity to *Candida*.
2. Characterized by candidal infection involving esophageal and buccal mucosa, skin, and nails. May also present with chronic indeterminate colitis.
3. Frequently associated with endocrinopathy (Addison disease, hypoparathyroid hormone, or hypothyroidism) and pernicious anemia.
4. Use of H2 blockers reduces gastric acidity and increases esophageal candidal involvement.

AUTOIMMUNE POLYENDOCRINOPATHY CANDIDIASIS ECTODERMAL DYSTROPHY
1. Autosomal recessive disease characterized by polyendocrinopathy as well as hepatitis, chronic mucocutaneous candidiasis, dental enamel and nail dystrophy, alopecia, and keratopathy.
2. Malabsorption with steatorrhea described in one-quarter of patients.

CHÉDIAK-HIGASHI SYNDROME
1. Defective lysosomal granule formation resulting in phagocytic dysfunction, partial albinism, and mild neurologic impairment.
2. Crohn disease involvement of bowel reported.

ACRODERMATITIS ENTEROPATHICA
1. Autosomal recessive disease resulting in severe zinc deficiency.
2. Characterized by eczema, alopecia, chronic diarrhea, malabsorption, and recurrent sinopulmonary infections.

INTESTINAL LYMPHANGIECTASIA
1. Intestinal lesion resulting in lymphopenia, hypogammaglobulinemia, and protein-losing enteropathy.
2. Diagnosis: intestinal biopsy. As with other protein losing enteropathies, serum IgM tends to remain within normal limits, whereas IgG and IgA may drop to very low levels.
3. Treatment: low-fat diet, supplementation with medium-chain triglycerides (reduce lymph flow and reduce losses). Steroids may help local inflammation.

FACIAL DYSMORPHY, INTRACTABLE DIARRHEA, AND IMMUNODEFICIENCY
1. Present with diarrhea in first 6 months of life; small for gestational age, facial dysmorphism, and trichorrhexis nodosa.
2. Defective antibody responses on antigen-specific skin tests. Small bowel biopsy shows moderate or severe villous atrophy.
3. Prognosis poor.

INTESTINAL ATRESIA ASSOCIATED WITH IMMUNODEFICIENCY
1. Association between intestinal atresia and severe combined immunodeficiency.
2. Autosomal recessive. Irradiation of blood products is recommended pending evaluation of immune status in the case of multiple GI atresias.

DIAGNOSIS

TABLE 1 INITIAL LABORATORY SCREENING FOR IMMUNODEFICIENCY

CBC, WBC and differential, platelets (count and size)
Serum protein electrophoresis
Chest radiography for thymic evaluation
Quantitative serum Igs
  IgG, IgM, IgA, IgE, and IgG subclasses
Flow cytometry
  Quantitation of total T cells (CD2, CD3)
  T-cell subsets (CD4, CD8)
  B cells (CD19, CD20)
  NK cells (CD16, CD56, CD57)
  HLA-DR (to rule out bare lymphocyte syndrome)
Metabolic bursts (to rule out CGD), including NBT testing
In vitro proliferative response to mitogens (PHA, Concanavalin A)
  and antigens (MLR)
Isohemagglutinin titers
Antibody titers (to documented immunizations) (diptheria, tetanus,
  rubella, measles)
C3, C4, CH50
If indicated
  Sweat Cl⁻ (to rule out cystic fibrosis)
  α₁-Antitrypsin
  Celiac disease screening

CBC = complete blood count; CGD = chronic granulomatous disease; HLA = human leukocyte antigen; Ig = immunoglobulin; MLR = mixed leukocyte reaction; NBT = nitroblue tetrazolium; NK = natural killer; PHA = phytohemagglutinin; WBC = white blood count.

QUESTIONS

CHOOSE THE BEST ANSWER:

1. Immunoglobulin A deficiency is associated with all of the following except:
   a. Small bowel bacterial overgrowth.
   b. *Giardia*.
   c. Celiac disease.
   d. Crohn disease.
   e. None of the above.

TRUE OF FALSE:

2. Intestinal atresias may be associated with defective immune status.
3. X-linked agammaglobulinemia patients are often ill in the neonatal period.
4. Transient hypogammaglobulinemia of infancy often resolves spontaneously.
5. The most common form of significant primary immunodeficiency is common variable immunodeficiency.

CHOOSE THE BEST ANSWER:

6. The distinguishing feature between X-linked agammaglobulinemia and hyper immunoglobulin M syndrome is:
   a. Low immunoglobulin A, G, and E levels.
   b. Lymphoid hyperplasia.
   c. Recurrent pyogenic infections.
   d. Neutropenia.
   e. None of the above.

7. Common variable immunodeficiency is all of the following except:
   a. Associated with autoimmune disease and malignancy.
   b. Associated with bacterial overgrowth.
   c. Associated with nodular lymphoid hyperplasia.
   d. Associated with celiac disease.
   e. Associated with all of the above.

MATCH THE CONDITION TO ITS CHARACTERISTIC:

a. Hyper immunoglobulin E syndrome.
b. Severe combined immunodeficiency.
c. Wiskott-Aldrich syndrome.
d. Ataxia-telangiectasia.
e. DiGeorge syndrome.
f. Duncan disease.
g. CD11/CD18 deficiency.
h. Glycogen storage disease type IB.
i. Chronic mucocutaneous candidiasis.
j. Chronic granulomatous disease.
k. Chédiak-Higashi syndrome.
l. Intestinal lymphangiectasia.

8. Deficient lysosomes.
9. Gastric outlet obstruction.
10. Addison disease, hypoparathyroidism, and hypothyroidism.
11. Cerebellar ataxia and nystagmus.
12. Often fatal Epstein-Barr virus infection.
13. Eczema, thrombocytopenia, and repeated opportunistic infection.
14. Islet cell deficiency and neonatal insulin-dependent diabetes.
15. Adenosine deaminase deficiency.
16. Neonatal hyperpigmented rash with transfusion.
17. Omenn syndrome.
18. Delayed umbilical cord separation.
19. Neutropenia and colitis resembling inflammatory bowel disease.
20. Failure of formation of 3rd and 4th pharyngeal pouches

HIV AND OTHER SECONDARY IMMUNODEFICIENCIES

SYNOPSIS

HUMAN IMMUNODEFICIENCY VIRUS

1. Hallmark of human immunodeficiency virus (HIV)-1 infection is loss of cell-mediated immunity, predominantly CD4+ T cells or T helper cells (key orchestrators of the immune response). Degree of immunosuppression is determined by age-specific CD4 T-lymphocyte count and percentage.

TABLE 1   INFECTIONS OF THE GASTROINTESTINAL TRACT IN CHILDREN WITH HIV INFECTION

INFECTION TYPE	CLINICAL PRESENTATION	TREATMENT
BACTERIA		
Shigella spp	Acute/persistent diarrhea	TMP-SMX, fluoroquinolone, ceftriaxone, cefotaxime
Nontyphi *Salmonella*	Acute/persistent diarrhea, septicemia	TMP-SMX, ampicillin, fluoroquinolone, ceftriaxone
Campylobacter spp	Acute/persistent diarrhea	Erythromycin, fluoroquinolone
MAC	Persistent diarrhea, malabsorption	Macrolide, ethambutol, rifabutin
VIRUSES		
Rotavirus	Acute diarrhea	—
Adenovirus	? Ribavirin/cidofovir	
CMV	Esophagitis, colitis	Ganciclovir, foscarnet, cidofovir
HSV	Esophagitis, perianal disease	Acyclovir
PARASITES		
Cryptosporidium parvum	Acute/persistent diarrhea	Paromomycin, immunoglobulin*
Isospora belli	Acute/persistent diarrhea	TMP-SMX
Giardia intestinalis	Acute/persistent diarrhea	Metronidazole, albendazole
Microsporidia	Acute/persistent diarrhea	Albendazole
Cyclospora cayetanensis	Acute/persistent diarrhea	TMP-SMX
Strongyloides stercoralis	Acute/persistent diarrhea; hyperinfection syndrome	Thiabendazole, albendazole
FUNGI		
Candida albicans	Esophagitis	Fluconazole, itraconazole, amphotericin

CMV = cytomegalovirus; HSV = herpes simplex virus; MAC = *Mycobacterium avium-intracellulare* complex; TMP-SMX = trimethoprim-sulfamethoxazole.
These anti-infective agents should be used in standard pediatric doses except for TMP-SMX for isosporiasis or cyclosporiasis, when double the usual dose should be given, and albendazole, which should be given for 4 weeks. Only one species of microsporidian (*Encephalitozoon intestinalis*) is likely to respond well to albendazole, and very little information is available to confirm its efficacy in children.
*Anti-*Cryptosporidium* immunoglobulin is unlikely to be available outside a research setting.

2. Clinical manifestations of HIV infection related to the gastrointestinal (GI) tract in children usually attributed to infections (Table 1).

ASSOCIATED INTESTINAL AILMENTS

1. Eight organisms that infect the GI tract in HIV-infected persons are classified as acquired immunodeficiency syndrome (AIDS) defining conditions: cytomegalovirus, herpes simplex virus, *Histoplasma capsulatum*, *Isospora belli*, *Mycobacterium avium-intracellulare* complex, *Salmonella*, *Candida* (esophageal candidiasis), and cryptosporidiosis.
2. Many children with HIV/AIDS have wasting or failure to thrive during the course of their disease. Characteristics include the following:
   a. Poor energy intake secondary to infections, encephalopathy, and GI medication toxicities.
   b. Malabsorption owing to infection or HIV enteropathy.
   c. Increased energy use owing to high levels of inflammation.
   d. Psychosocial factors.
3. Increased risk for development of malignancies. In children, the most common tumors include lymphoproliferative disorders (ranging from non-Hodgkin lymphoma to mucosa-associated lymphoid tissue tumors), smooth muscle tumors (leiomyomas and leiomyosarcoma: risk is 10,000 times higher in children with HIV infection). Kaposi sarcoma uncommon in children with HIV.

EVALUATION

1. Initial evaluation involves stool examination for bacteria and enteropathogens or parasites.

2. In children with diarrhea and fever: blood for bacterial culture, mycobacterial culture, and cytomegalovirus culture and polymerase chain reaction are useful.
3. If diagnosis not established using these techniques, then endoscopy helpful, particularly in detecting *Mycobacterium avium* complex and cytomegalovirus infection.
4. Radiologic techniques to determine site and extent of disease.

TREATMENT

Prompt, aggressive control of infections. In those with acute diarrhea, replacement of fluid and electrolytes and nutritional support are important.

SECONDARY IMMUNODEFICIENCIES

1. GI manifestations are common, with an increase in opportunistic, enteric infections.
2. Children receiving chemotherapy are particularly at risk. Main problems occur with neutropenia and gram-negative bacilli infection (especially *E. coli*).
3. Parasitic infections (especially *Cryptosporidium* and *Strongyloides*) may be important causes of chronic diarrhea and GI disease.
4. In patients who have undergone a bone marrow transplant, cytomegalovirus is an important problem causing notable GI ulceration. Similarly, graft-versus-host disease is an important cause of GI disease in this population and requires endoscopic evaluation.
5. Management requires treatment of infectious agents and supportive therapy, especially nutritional.

QUESTIONS

1. The following gastrointestinal tract infections in HIV-positive patients qualify as AIDS-defining conditions except:
   a. Isosporiasis.
   b. Cryptosporidiosis.
   c. Persistent rotavirus infection.
   d. Salmonella septicemia.
   e. Cytomegalovirus colitis.

2. The following contribute to wasting and failure to thrive in HIV-infected children except:
   a. Infection.
   b. HIV enteropathy.
   c. Inflammation.
   d. Psychosocial factors.
   e. All of the above contribute.

3. Which of the following tumors are not commonly found in HIV-infected children?
   a. Kaposi sarcoma.
   b. Leiomyomas.
   c. Leiomyosarcoma.
   d. Non-Hodgkin lymphoma.
   e. Mucosa-associated lymphoid tissue tumors.

4. You are asked to see a child with chronic diarrhea who is HIV infected. The child has been able to maintain weight thus far but has been passing bloody stools. There is no history of fever. Stool evaluation has returned negative, including culture for bacteria, ova, and parasites and acid-fast stain. What should you do next?
   a. Obtain a gastrointestinal contrast radiologic study.
   b. Schedule the child for an endoscopy.
   c. Provide nutritional support.
   d. Obtain blood work, including blood culture, viral culture, and mycobacterial culture.
   e. Increase antiretroviral therapy.

SHORT BOWEL SYNDROME AND INTESTINAL TRANSPLANTATION

SYNOPSIS

CAUSES OF SHORT BOWEL

Majority of cases are a result of necrotizing enterocolitis; also may result from congenital anomalies, Crohn disease, midgut volvulus, radiation enteritis, and Hirschsprung disease.

NORMAL PHYSIOLOGY

1. Jejunum: long villi; high concentration of enzymes, transport proteins, and porous tight junctions. Site for greatest nutrient absorption in small intestine. Leaky: free, rapid flux of water and electrolytes from vascular to intraluminal space.

2. Ileum: short villi; tighter junctions and more lymphoid tissue. Efficient absorption of fluid and electrolytes but less absorptive than jejunum. Vitamin B_{12} and bile salts absorption occur through site-specific receptors. Site of gastrointestinal (GI) hormones, especially those affecting small intestinal motility: enteroglucagon, peptide YY.

3. Ileocecal valve: barrier for reflux of colonic bacteria into the small intestine. Also plays a role in regulating exit of fluid, nutrients from small bowel to colon.

CONSEQUENCES OF RESECTION

1. Malabsorption: major consequence with loss of surface area and enzymes or transporters. Bile salt depletion may occur in those with significant ileal resection with resulting malabsorption of fats and fat-soluble vitamins.

2. Motility abnormalities: following ileal resection, transit time is faster through the jejunum and stomach.

3. Hypergastrinemia: with resection, normal negative feedback for gastrin is lost with resulting hypergastrinemia and acid-peptic disease or esophagitis.

INTESTINAL ADAPTATION

1. Hyperplasia of mucosal epithelium: preceded by increased crypt cell production, increasing crypt depth, and lengthening of intestinal villi. In conjunction with dilatation of the small bowel, this results in increased surface area. Functional immaturity improves with time. Dietary substrate exposure may also cause a functional adaptive response. Ileum can develop absorptive capacity of jejunum, but not vice versa.

2. Pediatric patients with neonatal small bowel resection may not reach their full adaptive potential until beyond 5 years of life.

3. Enteral nutrition: stimulates intestinal adaptation via secretion of trophic hormones and stimulation of secretions and regeneration of mucosa following injury; important in maintaining mucosal mass. Functional workload is a major stimulus except hydrolyzed casein more trophic than whole protein. Long-chain triglycerides more trophic than medium-chain. High-fat diets reverse mucosal atrophy more than carbohydrate- and protein-rich diets (Table 1).

4. Hormones important in intestinal adaptation:
   a. Enteroglucagon: highest concentration in distal small bowel; patients with enteroglucagon tumors have massive mucosal hyperplasia. Pro-enteroglucagon peptides may have similar actions.

TABLE 1   NUTRIENTS THAT MAY STIMULATE ADAPTATION MORE THAN OTHERS

Long-chain fats
Omega-3 fatty acids
Short-chain fatty acids
Fiber
Glutamine?

Glucagon-like peptide 2 also appears to be a significant hormone for adaptation.
b. Gastrin: highly elevated after intestinal resection; trophic to stomach and proximal small intestine.
c. Epidermal growth factor: found in breast milk; stimulates proliferation in gut epithelium, especially stomach.

d. Neurotensin: found in distal small intestine, stimulating hyperplasia in the small intestine. Also regulates growth of colonic mucosa.
e. Secretin and cholecystokinin: prevent mucosal hypoplasia.
f. Insulin-like growth factor (IGF)-1: plays a role in adaptation process.

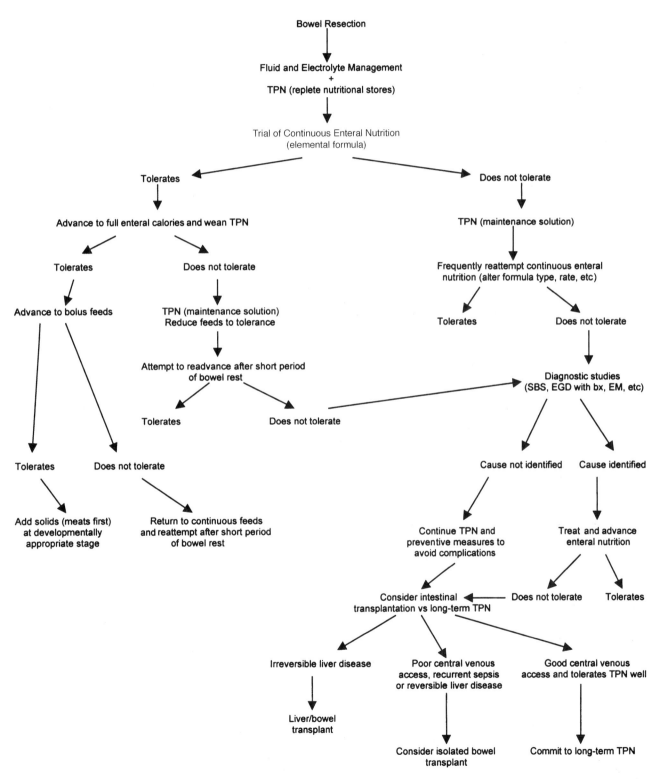

FIGURE 1 A diagram of the clinical management decisions in short-bowel syndrome. bx = biopsy; EGD = esophagogastroduodenoscopy; EM = electron microscopy; SBS = short bowel syndrome; TPN = total parenteral nutrition.

g. Peptide YY: stimulates adaptation, reduces GI motility, and increases nutrient contact.

h. Prostaglandins: may play role in regulating intestinal epithelial cell proliferation.

i. Polyamines: stimulate mucosal hyperplasia, essential for normal cell growth and differentiation.

CHRONIC COMPLICATIONS

SMALL BOWEL BACTERIAL OVERGROWTH

1. Small bowel bacterial overgrowth (SBBO) is one of the least recognized conditions in short bowel syndrome (SBS) but also one of the most treatable.

2. Not uncommon that small intestinal bacteria count $>10^5$. Motility often slowed, bowel dilated, and ileocecal valve absent. Reduction in gut-associated lymphoid tissue may impair immune response to bacteria.

3. Bacteria deconjugate bile salts, resulting in rapid reabsorption of bile acids, impaired micellar solubilization, and steatorrhea.

4. Mucosal inflammation exacerbates nutrient malabsorption. Bacteria also may compete with host for vitamin B_{12}.

5. D-Lactic acidosis and small bowel enterocolitis are SBBO complications. Bacteria make both D- and L-lactate, but only L-lactate is metabolized by humans. D-Lactic acidemia can result in neurological symptoms, ranging from disorientation to coma. Ulcerations can be quite large in colitis/ileitis seen in SBBO; can be accompanied by arthritis. Treatment: sulfasalazine and immunosuppressives often successful.

6. Diagnosis: increased bacterial small bowel counts by small bowel aspiration and culture. Also, breath hydrogen test as measured after 2 g/kg up to 50 g glucose.

7. Treatment: intermittent broad-spectrum antibiotics. Oral Flagyl 10–20 mg/kg/d alone or with Bactrim. Oral gentamicin also helpful. Daily saline enemas or lavage with polyethylene glycol solutions may be required to reduce bacterial content. Antimotility agents may exacerbate SBBO.

WATERY DIARRHEA

1. Often the result of osmotic load with large carbohydrate bolus feeds.

2. Elevated serum gastrin (often present in short gut) may be responsible for increased fluid secretion; rarely responds to H2 blocker. Somatostatin analogs used with varying results.

3. Cholestyramine binds bile acids where increased bile acids in colon cause secretion and watery diarrhea. In ileal resection: possible bile acid insufficiency; cholestyramine may exacerbate by further reducing bile acid concentration.

4. Antimotility agents may be considered; slow transit may contraindicated in SBBO.

COMMON NUTRITIONAL DEFICIENCIES IN SBS

1. Fat-soluble vitamins.
2. Trace metals: zinc and selenium.
3. Calcium and magnesium.
4. Vitamin B_{12}: especially with ileal resection.

PARENTERAL NUTRITION–INDUCED LIVER DISEASE

1. Major cause of death in children with SBS; mechanism unknown.

2. Prevention of liver disease: aggressive enteral feeds (provide at least 20–30% of total requirement), prevent catheter sepsis, prevent SBBO.

3. 20% of infants on total parenteral nutrition (TPN) may develop cholelithiasis.

BONE MINERALIZATION

Inadequate dietary calcium and phosphorus intake and poor absorption of these elements contribute to a high incidence of impaired bone mineralization in patients with SBS.

CATHETER-RELATED COMPLICATIONS

1. Common. Highest prevalence in infants aged < 1 yr.

2. Infection and thrombosis common. Catheter infections may result from poor catheter care or SBBO.

SURGICAL CONSIDERATIONS AND OPTIONS

1. Primary prevention of SBS should be a priority. Second look laparatomies to preserve bowel of "questionable viability" and avoid extensive resection. When resection performed, the goal should be to preserve all bowel possible, including the ileocecal valve.

2. At time of adjunctive surgical procedures: liver biopsy to determine extent of TPN cholestasis. Prophylactic

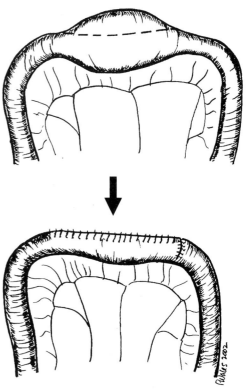

FIGURE 2 Tapering enteroplasty. The antimesenteric portion of the dilated segment of bowel is removed. A portion of the absorptive surface is lost.

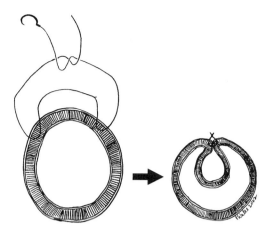

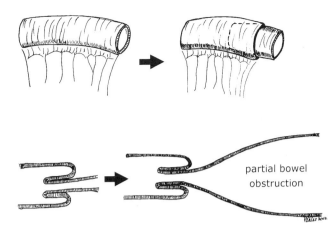

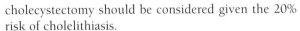

partial bowel obstruction

FIGURE 3   Intestinal plication. A portion of the dilated bowel wall is inverted into the bowel lumen and secured by seromuscular sutures.

FIGURE 4   Creation of intestinal valves. A segment of bowel is telescoped into the distal bowel and secured with sutures. This will slow transit and induce a partial bowel obstruction. The proximal bowel dilates, and an intestinal lengthening procedure becomes possible.

cholecystectomy should be considered given the 20% risk of cholelithiasis.

3. Techniques to improve intestinal function: lysis of adhesions and strictureplasty or segmental intestinal resection in cases of mechanical bowel obstruction; re-establishment of intestinal continuity (advantages: increases surface area for absorption and facilitates adaptive response in distal bowel; disadvantage: diarrhea and calcium oxalate nephrolithiasis in the case of colon continuity where oxalate is absorbed owing to delivery of bile acids to the colon preventing oxalate excretion in the stool).

4. Techniques to improve intestinal motility: intestinal tapering and plication (disadvantage: loss of some absorptive area with tapering and potential for bowel

obstruction with inversion of the bowel) (Figure 2 and 3); antiperistaltic small intestinal segments (often not done in neonates and infants because of potential for bowel growth and obstruction if such growth occurs in the reversed segment); colonic interposition (peristalsis occurs less frequently in the colon than in the small bowel); creation of intestinal valves producing a partial obstruction (limitation: risk of mechanical bowel obstruction) (Figure 4).

5. Techniques to increase absorptive surface area: the Bianchi procedure (Figure 5) with longitudinal intestinal lengthening (complications: small bowel obstruction secondary to adhesions, strictures or leaks, and

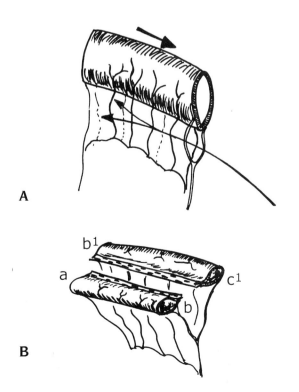

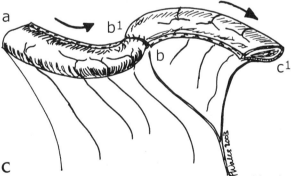

FIGURE 5   Bianchi procedure. *A,* The mesenteric blood vessels within the two leaves of the mesentery are separated under the dilated bowel segment. *B,* The dilated bowel is divided longitudinally within the mesenteric leaves to create two parallel loops of bowel half the diameter of the original loop. *C,* The two bowel segments are anastomosed end to end to create a bowel segment double the length of the original. The bowel mesentery needs to be amenable to mobilization for this to be feasible. The bowel at "a" is the most proximal portion and the bowel at "c" is the most distal. The end of the reduced loop at "b1" is anastomosed to the proximal end of the other loop at "b2" to create an isoperistaltic segment of tapered and lengthened bowel.

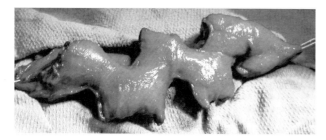

FIGURE 6 Serial transverse enteroplasty. Zigzag pattern of bowel created after sequential and opposite firings of a surgical stapler across the dilated bowel loop. The channel size is determined by the surgeon. The normal loops of bowel can be used as an internal guide. A gastrointestinal contrast study is performed on the seventh postoperative day prior to initiation of enteral feeds.

recurrent bowel dilatation); the Kimura procedure: coaptation of the antimesenteric surface of a dilated bowel segment to host organs to improve vascular supply, then longitudinal division of the bowel and anastomosis (similar to Bianchi); and serial transverse enteroplasty (the bowel is stapled into V-shapes on alternating sides, decreasing its width and increasing its length) (Figure 6).

PROGNOSIS
1. Reasonable, if > 25 cm small intestine remaining with ileocecal valve or > 40 cm small intestine remaining without ileocecal valve, in terms of coming off TPN to enteral nutrition only.
2. If on TPN > 4–5 yr, unlikely to survive without life-long TPN.

TRANSPLANTATION
Specific clinical issues to consider in small bowel transplantation as compared to other forms of organ transplantation:
1. Large volume of transplanted tissue with a large number of lymphocytes (Peyer patches) with thus a significant risk of graft-versus-host disease.
2. The small bowel allograft is contaminated with bacteria, increasing the risk of translocation when rejection develops.

Indications and Contraindications

TABLE 2   INDICATIONS FOR INTESTINAL TRANSPLANT

LIFE-THREATENING COMPLICATIONS ARISING FROM PARENTERAL NUTRITION THERAPY	TYPE OF TRANSPLANT
Impending loss of venous access, that is, when 2 of the 4 available sites have been lost in infants or 3 of 6 in older children Recurrent sepsis (especially if metastatic, eg, brain abscess or infective endocarditis, if unusually severe, resulting in multiorgan failure)	Isolated bowel transplant
Erratic fluid balance requiring hospitalization Congenital intractable epithelial disorder, eg, microvillous inclusion disease and tufting enteropathy Some cases of short-bowel syndrome	Isolated bowel transplant or combined liver and bowel transplant depending on severity of hepatic complications of parenteral nutrition
Irreversible liver disease: hyperbilirubinemia persisting beyond 3–4 mo of age and features of portal hypertension, splenomegaly, prominent superficial abdominal veins	Combined liver and intestinal transplant

Adapted from Kaufman SS, Atkinson JB, Bianchi A, et al. Indications for paediatric intestinal transplantation: a position paper of the American Society of Transplantation. Pediatr Transplant 2001;5:80–7.

TABLE 3   CONTRAINDICATIONS TO INTESTINAL TRANSPLANT

Patients with the following conditions should not normally undergo intestinal transplant because they are unlikely to derive an obvious benefit:
  Profound neurologic disabilities
  Life-threatening and other noncorrectable illnesses not directly related to the digestive system
  Severe or acquired immunodeficiency
  Nonresectable malignancies
  Multisystem autoimmune diseases
  Those with insufficient vascular patency to guarantee easy central venous access for up to 6 mo following transplant

Adapted from Kaufman SS, Atkinson JB, Bianchi A, et al. Indications for paediatric intestinal transplantation: a position paper of the American Society of Transplantation. Pediatr Transplant 2001;5:80–7.

Surgical Considerations
1. Infants requiring liver or small bowel transplants have often had prior surgery, rendering the abdominal cavity even smaller. Thus a size mismatch between recipient capacity and donor organ occurs. The reduction en bloc technique accommodates up to a 5:1 size mismatch. This is accomplished by removal of the right lobe of the donor liver en bloc with removal of the middle section of the small bowel allograft (with preservation of the distal ileum). Vascular anastomoses occur at the hepatic vein to inferior vena cava and celiac axis to infrarenal aorta.
2. In contrast, isolated small bowel transplant is more straightforward with the proximal end anastomosed to jejunum or stomach and the distal end brought out as an end stoma or connected to residual large bowel.
3. Whatever reconstruction is done, it is essential to allow exteriorization of the small bowel allograft to allow for regular biopsy for early detection of rejection.

Results
1. Liver and small bowel transplant: 50% survival > 3 yr.
2. Isolated small bowel transplant survival is slightly better.
3. Infection rate with intestinal transplant is higher than with liver transplant.

4. Early mortality occurs in first 6 weeks and is around 20%; often related to poor preoperative condition of patients who develop multiorgan failure prior to transplant.

Complications of Small Bowel Transplant

1. Technical: tend to occur in first 10 days postoperatively. Include intestinal perforation, prolonged ileus, biliary obstruction or leaks, traumatic pancreatitis, and hemorrhage. Signs may be subtle in the face of high immunosuppression.

2. Chylous ascites may also develop secondary to lacteal interruption if feeds are high in long-chain fats in the first few postoperative weeks.

3. Infections: all infections require aggressive therapy. Opportunistic infections with *Pneumocystis carinii* (PC) and vancomycin-resistant enterococcus (VRE) are important considerations. PC prophylaxis should be given, and treatment for VRE should be prompt with quinupristin-dalfopristin antibiotics. Cytomegalovirus prophylaxis should be administered given the severity of consequences. Epstein-Barr virus is associated with lymphomas with the use of tacrolimus for immunosuppression.

4. Risk factors for post-transplant lymphoproliferative disease (PTLD) include: young age, no prior immunity to Epstein-Barr virus, dependence on tacrolimus, and the donor being positive for Epstein-Barr virus. Main treatments: early detection, reduction of immunosuppression and adjuvant therapy if tumor fails to regress. Even with such therapies, mortality with PTLD is high (about 50%).

5. Acute cellular rejection: common; major cause of graft loss (Table 4). Common symptoms: malaise, fever, and increased stomal output or diarrhea, usually 1–2 wk after transplant. Diagnosis: mucosal histology. Prompt treatment with high-dose intravenous steroids and antibiotics as well as increase in tacrolimus effective.

6. Centrilobular rejection in liver: acute cellular rejection of liver allograft independent of small bowel allograft in combined recipients is unusual. Usually responds to increases in immunosuppression.

7. Chronic small bowel allograft rejection: not well understood. Often present with episodes of diarrhea alternating with episodes of obstruction ("distal ileal obstruction syndrome"); may require resection of affected bowel. Diagnosis: selective angiography (vascular phenomenon where mesenteric vessels are inflamed and have impeded blood flow).

8. Drug toxicity: Compared with isolated liver transplant, twice as much immunosuppression required for small bowel allograft tolerance. Adverse effects: usually hypertension, bone marrow toxicity, and nephrotoxicity. Effects mainly related to tacrolimus. Tacrolimus induces endothelin receptor production, resulting in arteriolar constriction in systemic circulation and kidneys; common practice to give prostaglandin infusions for up to 10 days postoperatively to reduce this risk. Also tacrolimus affects tubular handling of magnesium, resulting in hypomagnesemia, which can cause neurotoxicity (tremor and convulsions). Insulin-dependent diabetes can also result from tacrolimus (idiosyncratic). Alternative drugs include sirolimus (which acts at the TOR receptor during G1 phase of the cell cycle) and mycophenolate mofetil. Steroids used at higher doses in small bowel transplant; can result in impaired linear growth.

Postoperative Graft Function and Diet Management

1. Oral fluids introduced soon after ileus resolves with advancement to enteral feeds by day 7.

2. Typically, the allograft develops secretory diarrhea by day 5 (differential: normal recovery of allograft, sepsis, and rejection), which often lessens by day 14 to 21.

3. In regards to enteral stimulation, long-chain fats are avoided in the first 6 weeks owing to the risk of chylous ascites. Care must also be taken with carbohydrate content so as not to induce osmotic diarrhea. Enteral feeds are introduced gradually and stepwise over time.

4. In transplanted bowel, motility depends on the intrinsic nervous system and is sensitive to local factors rather than autonomic nervous control (ie, no vagally mediated postprandial suppression of motility). Thus, antimotility agents such as loperamide are needed.

TABLE 4   SMALL BOWEL ALLOGRAFT: GRADES OF ACUTE CELLULAR REJECTION

GRADE	MUCOSAL BIOPSY HISTOLOGY	CLINICAL FEATURES
1 Mild	2–5 apoptotic bodies per 10 crypts, a few inflammatory cells scattered in lamina propria	Increase in bowel frequency or ileostomy output may go up by 50%
2 Moderate	5–10 apoptotic bodies per 10 crypts, infiltration of crypts by lymphocytes, obvious increase in inflammatory cells in lamina propria	Secretory diarrhea, malaise, low-grade fever
3 Severe	Greater than 10 apoptotic bodies per 10 crypts, some loss of villi, destruction of crypts in places, ulceration may be seen, numerous inflammatory cells in lamina propria	Secretory diarrhea associated with thirst and dehydration, protein-losing enteropathy, lassitude, fever ± peripheral edema, gram-negative septicemia
4 Exfoliative	Extensive ulceration, lamina propria replaced by inflammatory cells, complete loss of crypts in places	Prostration, fever, gastrointestinal bleeding, systemic inflammatory response syndrome

Adapted from Lee RG, Nakamura K, Tsamauda ACM, et al. Pathology of human intestinal transplantation. Gastroenterology 1996; 110:1820–34, Roberts CA, Radio SJ, Markin RS, et al. Histopathologic evaluation of primary intestinal transplant recipients at autopsy: a single center experience. Transplant Proc 2000;32:1202–3 and White FV, Reyes J, Jaffe R, et al. Pathology of intestinal transplantation in children. Am J Surg Pathol 1995;19:687–98.

QUESTIONS

TRUE OR FALSE:

1. The jejunum can adapt and carry out ileal functions in the setting of an ileal resection.
2. Insulin-dependent diabetes is an idiosyncratic reaction to tacrolimus.

CHOOSE THE BEST ANSWER:

3. The ileum:
   a. Has longer villi than the jejunum.
   b. Is the main site of nutrient absorption.
   c. Is the secretion site of gastrointestinal hormones affecting gut motility.
   d. Allows rapid flux of water and electrolytes.
   e. All of the above are true.
   f. None of the above is true.

4. Intestinal adaptation:
   a. Is mainly carried out by hyperplasia of the epithelium.
   b. Can be affected by nutrient exposure.
   c. Can occur beyond 5 years after resection in the neonatal period.
   d. All of the above.
   e. None of the above.

5. Hormones involved in the adaptation of the gut include all except:
   a. Enteroglucagon.
   b. Insulin-like growth factor 1
   c. Peptide YY.
   d. Insulin.
   e. Gastrin.

6. All of the following stimulate enteral adaptation except:
   a. Long-chain fatty acids.
   b. Omega-3 fatty acids.
   c. Medium-chain fatty acids.
   d. Fiber.
   e. None of the above.

7. The following are associated with a good prognosis in terms of short gut syndrome (SGS):
   a. Still on total parenteral nutrition at 6 years of age after neonatal necrotizing enterocolitis and SGS.
   b. Patients with 20 cm small intestine with ileocecal valve.
   c. Patients with 30 cm small intestine without ileocecal valve.
   d. Patients with 45 cm small intestine without ileocecal valve.
   e. None have a good prognosis.

8. Combined liver and small bowel transplant survival at 3 years is:
   a. 10–15%.
   b. 20–30%.
   c. 30–40%.
   d. 50–60%.
   e. 70–80%.

MATCH THE PURPOSE TO THE SURGICAL PROCEDURE:

a. To improve intestinal function.
b. To improve intestinal motility.
c. To increase absorptive surface area.

9. Bianchi procedure
10. Intestinal tapering and plication
11. Kimura procedure
12. Lysis of adhesions

CHOOSE THE BEST ANSWER:

13. Risk factors for post transplant lymphoproliferative disease in transplant patients include the following except:
   a. Young age.
   b. Prior immunity to Epstein-Barr virus.
   c. A tacrolimus based immunosuppressive regimen.
   d. Epstein-Barr virus–positive donor.
   e. All of the above are true.

CROHN DISEASE

SYNOPSIS

1. Crohn disease is a chronic inflammatory disorder of the gastrointestinal (GI) tract that manifests during childhood or adolescence in up to 25% of patients (Figure 1).
2. Most prevalent in North America and northwestern Europe (especially Scandinavia and the United Kingdom). More common in white; Jewish background at increased risk.
3. Peak incidence in late adolescence and young adulthood; second peak at age 50–60 yr. Overall, more females than males by 20–30%; in childhood, more males than females.

GENETIC INFLUENCES

1. 44–58% concordance rate in monozygotic twins. Develops earlier in children of affected parents.
2. Crohn susceptibility gene: *CARD15* (previously known as *NOD2*) with polymorphisms associated with both sporadic and familial Crohn disease, especially ileal disease. *CARD15* polymorphisms explain 20% of the genetic predisposition to Crohn disease.
3. Other genes associated with susceptibility to and progression of Crohn disease include tumor necrosis factor alpha (TNF-α) gene within major histocompatibility complex class III and intercellular adhesion molecule 1.

ENVIRONMENTAL INFLUENCES

1. Most widely held theory: Crohn disease constitutes a dysregulated, exaggerated immune response to bacteria and viral antigens.

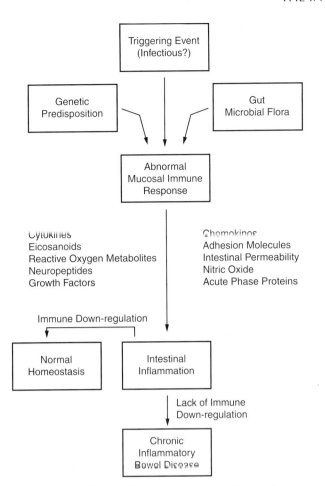

FIGURE 1 Multifactorial etiopathogenesis of Crohn disease. It is postulated that in a genetically susceptible individual, interacting environmental factors and the host intestinal microbial flora, in the presence of a yet unspecified triggering event, activate an aberrant immune response, the end result of which is chronic intestinal inflammation.

2. Events early in life may influence the risk of developing inflammatory bowel disease (IBD), including maternal or neonatal infections. Breastfeeding may reduce the risk of developing Crohn disease. Smoking is a risk factor (possibly related to potentiation of multifocal GI infarction). Risk for former smokers does not differ from those who have never smoked.

3. Oral contraceptives have also been implicated as a risk factor.

IMMUNOREGULATORY ABNORMALITIES

1. A leaky mucosal barrier or excessive permeability plays a role in perpetuating inflammation in IBD.

2. *CARD15* important in activation of nuclear factor κB (NF-κB) signaling cascade by bacterial proteins. *CARD15* mutations result in T-cell dysfunction, with Th1 responses predominating. Unrestrained intestinal Th1 activation results in tissue damage.

PATHOLOGY

1. Panenteric process. Segmental. Terminal ileum most commonly affected site; 40% ileocolic, 20% colon only, and 10% isolated ileal or jejunal involvement

2. Earliest lesion: aphthous ulcer over lymph follicles and Peyer patches.

3. Pathologic hallmark: transmural inflammation. Noncaseating granulomas (as in tuberculosis) occur more commonly in submucosa than mucosa (20–40% biopsies).

4. Histology does not directly correlate with clinical response.

CLINICAL PRESENTATION

1. Mean time between symptoms and diagnosis: 6 mo.

2. Classic presentation: abdominal pain, diarrhea, poor appetite, and weight loss. May present as short stature (alterations in growth produced by undernutrition as well as proinflammatory cytokines). Perianal disease can present in an isolated fashion. GI blood loss can contribute to iron deficiency anemia.

EXTRAINTESTINAL MANIFESTATIONS

1. Found in 25–35% of adults with IBD.

2. Two types: parallel disease and independent of disease.

3. Joints: arthritis and arthralgias. Most common extraintestinal manifestation of Crohn disease (15%). Most likely to precede GI symptoms and dominate clinical presentation. Settles without deformity with treatment of bowel disease, except for juvenile ankylosing spondylitis, which occurs more frequently in IBD (course can be independent of bowel disease and does not require presence of human leukocyte antigen B27).

4. Skin: Erythema nodosum (8–15%) and pyoderma gangrenosum (1.3%). Erythema nodosum tends to occur with disease but does not reflect severity. Pyoderma gangrenosum runs own course.

5. Eye: uveitis, episcleritis, and orbital myositis. Asymptomatic uveitis described in Crohn disease usually when only colon involved.

6. Hepatobiliary: primary sclerosing cholangitis (PSC); usually in ulcerative colitis (UC) but also Crohn colitis. PSC can precede onset in 50% of cases. Elevations in liver function tests over 6 months suggestive. Autoimmune hepatitis rare. Pancreatitis can also occur.

7. Renal complications: stones (ureteric obstruction and hydronephrosis) and ureteral obstruction. Calcium oxalate stones. (Normally, oxalate in the lumen is bound to calcium, and the poorly absorbed calcium oxalate is excreted in the feces, but when ileum is diseased or resected, increased luminal concentrations of malabsorbed fatty acids compete for calcium. Oxalate absorption and renal excretion are, therefore, increased.)

8. Hypercoagulability with increased fibrin and factors V and VII, low antithrombin III.

9. Decreased bone density: treat with calcium and vitamin D.

DISEASE COMPLICATIONS

1. Malnutrition: weight loss and emaciation are the most prevalent nutritional disturbances. Reduced intake is the major cause.

TABLE 1   FACTORS CONTRIBUTING TO GROWTH ABNORMALITIES IN CHILDREN WITH CROHN DISEASE

FACTOR	REASON
Cytokines produced by chronically inflamed intestine	Direct role of inflammatory cytokines in linear growth inhibition (IGF-1 inhibition; interference with kinetics of bone growth)
Insufficient caloric intake	Food avoidance because of exacerbation of gastrointestinal symptoms by eating; cytokine-mediated anorexia
Stool losses	Mucosal inflammation leading to protein-losing enteropathy; steatorrhea if extensive
Increased nutritional needs	Fever, chronic deficits
Corticosteroid treatment	Inhibition of IGF-1

IGF-1 = insulin-like growth factor 1.

2. Growth impairment: chronic undernutrition and growth inhibition by proinflammatory cytokines, steroids, and low insulin-like growth factor 1 levels (mediated by high interleukin [IL]-6, malnutrition, and steroids) (Table 1).

3. Perianal disease: abscesses and fistulae occur in one-third of patients, more frequently in association with colorectal disease than small intestinal disease. IBD5 risk haplotype at 5q31 associated with perianal disease.

DIAGNOSIS

1. No single test can confirm suspicion of Crohn disease. Diagnosis based on clinical presentation, radiologic assessment of small bowel, endoscopic evaluation, and exclusion of other causes of infectious bacterial pathogens.

2. Serologic techniques are important for the alternate diagnoses of *Yersinia* and amebiasis. Intestinal tuberculosis and schistosomiasis should be excluded.

3. Upper endoscopic findings: use caution in interpreting all gastric and duodenal inflammation as indicative of Crohn disease.

4. Serologic test: antineutrophil cytoplasmic antibodies (ANCAs) and anti-*Saccharomyces cerevisiae* antibody (ASCAs) have been recommended as tools to facilitate IBD screening and to differentiate UC from Crohn disease. Low sensitivities: 50–60%. Differentiation between Crohn disease and UC: problematic; perinuclear (p)ANCA is positive in up to 35% of Crohn colitis patients; ASCA less detected in these patients. Specificities of Crohn colitis serology (ASCA+ pANCA–) and UC (pANCA+ASCA–) are high and predictive values are also high in the presence of a positive test.

TREATMENT

Nutritional Support

Encourage a diet liberal in proteins with calories sufficient to maintain and restore weight and to support growth. Intensive nutritional support may be required when patients are significantly malnourished or in the setting of growth retardation.

Pharmacologic Therapy

Systemic Corticosteroids

1. Prednisone is converted to its active form prednisolone in the liver. Possibility of reduced absorption in patients with active small intestine disease.

2. Mode of action: inhibition of cell-mediated immunity and anti-inflammatory effects; inhibition of NF-κB function, reducing IL-1 and IL-2 levels. Steroids enhance sodium and water absorption and thus decrease diarrhea.

3. Steroids most useful and effective in those with small intestinal disease and in those with active disease. Little justification for use as a prophylactic agent.

4. Side effects: acne, moon facies, hirsutism, cutaneous striae, pseudotumor cerebri, psychosis, proximal myopathy, subcapsular cataracts, aseptic necrosis of the femoral head, growth reduction, and reduction in calcium absorption and increase in urine calcium excretion.

Controlled Ileal-Release Budesonide

1. High affinity for the glucocorticosteroid receptor in the intestinal mucosa with rapid transformation to inactive metabolite by liver following absorption.

2. Decreased adverse systemic effects compared with classic corticosteroids.

3. Major clinical indication: treatment of Crohn disease involving the ileum or right colon. Less effective than systemic steroids. No evidence of benefit as prophylaxis.

Sulfasalazine and 5-Aminosalicylic Acid

1. 5-Aminosalicylic acid (5-ASA) has greater role in the management of UC than in Crohn disease. Efficacious in treating colonic inflammation but not helpful in isolated ileal Crohn disease. Time-release 5-ASA preparation has been modestly helpful in patients with isolated ileitis. Little data to support sulfasalazine or 5-ASA agents use as a maintenance therapy in Crohn disease.

2. Pharmacology: 5-ASA inhibits leukotriene synthesis and myeloperoxidase activity (scavenging reactive oxygen species). Rapidly absorbed in proximal small intestine.

3. Adverse effects: sulfasalazine: 20–25% patients unable to tolerate. Dose dependent: headache, nausea and vomiting, and mild hemolysis. Glucose-6-phosphate-dehydrogenase (G6PD) contraindication to drug. Idiosyncratic reaction: fever, exanthems, Stevens-Johnson syndrome, pulmonary fibrosis, hepatotoxicity, and agranulocytosis. Reversible impairment of male fertility. Reduces folate absorption but supplementation to prevent anemia not necessary. 80–90% of patients intolerant of sulfasalazine will tolerate 5-ASA products. Pulmonary fibrosis and agranulocytosis not seen with

5-ASA. 5-ASA dose needs to be increased from sulfasalazine by 50%.

ANTIBIOTICS AND PROBIOTICS

Metronidazole
1. Well-established in the control of perianal fistulae in Crohn disease. Data support the use of Flagyl to delay recurrence after ileal resection.
2. Dose: 10–20 mg/k/d.
3. Adverse effects: peripheral predominantly sensory neuropathy. Paresthesia always resolve with discontinuation. Disulfiram-like effect with alcohol ingestion. Mutagenesis and carcinogenesis demonstrated in lab animals.

Probiotics
Most data in UC. Some data in Crohn disease are promising in the prevention of postoperative recurrence.

AZATHIOPRINE AND 6-MERCAPTOPURINE
1. Delayed onset precludes use in acute setting. Used as steroid-sparing agent, with fewer relapses, lower cumulative prednisone dosage, and better growth.
2. Azathioprine converted to 6-mercaptopurine (6-MP) via series of enzyme reactions (Figure 2). Both affect immune system including direct cytotoxicity and inhibition of cytokines. Azathioprine also releases nitroimidazoles with additional immunologic effects.
3. Adverse effects: hypersensitivity reaction (in first several weeks of therapy): fever, pancreatitis, rash, arthralgias, and nausea, vomiting, and diarrhea. Nonallergic toxicity: leukopenia, thrombocytopenia, infection, and hepatitis. No documented associations of azathioprine or 6-MP with increased risk of malignancy. Infectious complications described in 1–2%.
4. Monitoring of intracellular metabolites is recommended to adjust dosage for safety. Data are conflicting regarding levels and efficacy.

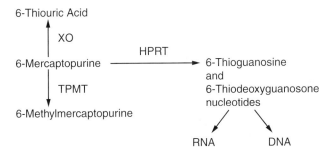

FIGURE 2 6-Mercaptopurine (6-MP) metabolism. The initial metabolism of 6-MP occurs along the competing routes catalyzed by thiopurine methyltransferase (TPMT), xanthine oxidase (XO), and hypoxanthine phosphoribosyltransferase (HPRT). Relative deficiency of TPMT or competition for XO leads to increased formation of 6-thioguanosine and 6-deoxythioguanosine nucleotides. The corporation of these nucleotides into ribonucleic acid (RNA) and deoxyribonucleic acid (DNA) induces cytotoxicity.

METHOTREXATE
1. Limited use. Inhibits conversion of folate to tetrahydrofolic acid (active form), which impairs deoxyribonucleic acid (DNA) synthesis.
2. Adverse events: minor; nausea and asymptomatic increase in liver enzymes. Hypersensitivity pneumonitis rare; not observed in IBD.
3. In placebo-controlled trial of 25 mg intramuscularly qwk for 16 wk, clinical improvement after 6 wk.

CYCLOSPORIN A
1. Suppression of IL-2. Concentrations in colon highest.
2. Most serious complication: nephrotoxicity (dose-related). Monitor drug trough and creatinine (if rises 30% above baseline, dose reduction).
3. Randomized controlled trials in Crohn disease disappointing.

INFLIXIMAB
1. Chimeric (murine-human) antibody directed against circulating and membrane-bound TNF-α (a proinflammatory cytokine markedly increased in Crohn disease). Dose 5 mg/kg; remission by 4 wk higher than with placebo. Usual time to respond: 2 wk. Effective in healing fistulous disease.
2. Side effects associated with development of antibodies to infliximab (ATI): often delayed hypersensitivity reactions with malaise, fever, and muscle ache occurring 1–12 d after infusion. Development of ATI may affect efficacy with shorter duration or loss of response. Concomitant use of 6-MP is associated with a lower incidence of ATI. Infliximab may induce anti-double-stranded DNA antibodies. Associated with increased risk for disseminated tuberculosis.

FISH OIL
Competes with arachidonic acid (AA), leading to a reduction in AA's metabolism to leukotriene B4 (an amplifier of intestinal inflammation). Compared with placebo, appears to reduce clinical relapse rate disseminated in Crohn disease.

ENTERAL NUTRITION THERAPY
1. Mode of action unknown.
2. Controversy regarding enteral therapy versus drug therapy. Randomized trials comparing steroids and sulfasalazine therapy to semielemental formula demonstrated superior outcomes in drug group. Enteral nutrition is more effective than placebo. Existing data do not support an advantage to elemental feedings versus more palatable polymeric formulation. Randomized controlled trial shows adjunctive nutritional support with partial parenteral nutrition plus an ad lib oral diet as effective as elemental liquid diets by nasogastric tube or total parenteral nutrition (TPN) with bowel rest.
3. Main limitation: tendency for prompt recurrence after cessation.
4. Benefits: linear growth (data suggest better linear growth on enteral diet therapy vs. alternate-day steroids).

5. No evidence to suggest TPN superior to enteral nutrition in the treatment of acute inflammation.

SURGERY

1. Indications: intractable symptoms, obstruction, enterovesicular fistula, intraabdominal abscess, and perforation or intractable hemorrhage.
2. Recurrence after surgery: patients undergoing ileal resection typically recur proximal to ileocolonic anastomosis; in those having colonic resection, recur on either side of anastomosis. Few reliable prognostic factors of recurrence. The length of recurrent ileal disease the same as length of ileum inflamed preoperatively. Children undergoing resection because of stenosing or fistulizing complications had delayed recrudescence of disease compared with those operated on for refractory medical therapy. Rapid return of symptoms after major resection in extensive ileocolitis suggests that medical strategies should be maintained in this group.

CLINICAL COURSE AND PROGNOSIS

1. One-third of patients have mild disease never requiring steroids, one-third remit and relapse requiring steroids, one-third have chronically active disease. 36% of patients undergo intestinal resection by 5 yrs.
2. Cancer: cumulative frequency of risk for colorectal cancer in extensive Crohn colitis: 8% after 2 decades of disease.

QUESTIONS

TRUE OR FALSE:

1. There are more affected females than males in pediatric Crohn disease.
2. Th1 responses predominate in Crohn disease.
3. Histology directly correlates with clinical response in Crohn disease.
4. Erythema nodosum runs an independent course from disease course in Crohn disease.
5. The course of pyoderma gangrenosum correlates with disease activity in Crohn disease.
6. ATI predicts reduced efficacy of infliximab in Crohn disease.
7. Bowel rest and total parenteral nutrition has not been demonstrated in studies to be more efficacious than enteral nutrition in Crohn disease.
8. 5-Aminosalicylic acid agents are as effective for treating ileal Crohn disease as for treating ulcerative colitis.
9. CARD15 explains nearly all of the genetic predisposition for Crohn disease.
10. 6-Mercaptopurine (6-MP) and azathioprine have not been found to be associated with an increased malignancy risk to date in Crohn disease patients.
11. Budesonide is effective for terminal ileal and right colonic disease in Crohn disease.
12. Agranulocytosis is not seen with exposure to 5-aminosalicylic acid agents.

ULCERATIVE COLITIS

SYNOPSIS

1. Classic definition: inflammation limited to colon and rectum.
2. Untreated ulcerative colitis (UC): distal colon most severely affected and rectum virtually always involved.
3. Inflammation: limited primarily to the mucosa with continuous involvement extending from the rectum proximally. Ulcers are typically broad and shallow. Regenerating granulation tissue and residual mucosa may form pseudopolyps. Cryptitis, crypt abscesses, mucin depletion, and surface erosions typify active inflammation, whereas chronic changes result in crypt architectural distortion with diminished goblet cells and Paneth cell metaplasia in the left colon. No granulomas or transmural inflammation are present.
4. 15% of children have isolated rectal involvement (ulcerative proctitis), 20% have left-sided disease. Pan colitis is the most common pattern.
5. UC is limited to the colon, but "backwash ileitis" with nonspecific inflammation of the ileum can occur.

EPIDEMIOLOGY

1. Bimodal distribution of age of onset with peaks at 2nd and 3rd decades and 5th and 6th decades. Highest incidence in children age 10–18 yr.
2. Common in North America and northern Europe, less prevalent elsewhere. Current incidence estimates for northern Europe and the United States: 1.5–4/100,000 children/yr.
3. Occurs equally in males and females. More common among Jewish than non-Jewish. Decreased risk of UC among smokers.

ETIOLOGY AND PATHOGENESIS

1. Unknown, but both genetic and environmental factors play a role (Table 1).
2. Current theory: disease results from an exaggerated immune response to normal constituents of mucosal microflora.

CLINICAL FEATURES

1. Cardinal symptoms: diarrhea, rectal bleeding, and abdominal pain.
2. Commonly, insidious diarrhea with later hematochezia without systemic signs. Normal physical exam.
3. 30% with moderate illness: bloody diarrhea, tenesmus, malaise, low-grade fever, anorexia with weight loss, mild anemia, and hypoalbuminemia. Physical exam with abdominal tenderness. Stool with blood and leukocytes.
4. 10% with severe illness: ≥ 5 blood stools/d, significant anemia, hypoalbuminemia, fever, tachycardia, and weight loss. Abdomen is diffusely tender or distended.

TABLE 1   ETIOLOGIC FACTORS IN THE PATHOGENESIS OF ULCERATIVE COLITIS

EVIDENCE FOR GENETIC PREDISPOSITION
Frequent positive family history (15–25%)
Higher rate of concordance in monozygotic twins than in dizygotic twins
Association with specific HLA class II genes
Association with other genetic disorders, eg, Turner syndrome

ENVIRONMENTAL FACTORS
Early childhood events, eg, diarrheal illness; may increase risk
Appendectomy at an early age; may decrease risk
Psychological stress; may cause exacerbations
Smoking tobacco; decreases risk
Drugs
    Nonsteroidal antiinflammatory drugs; may cause exacerbations
    Oral contraceptives; conflicting data
Microbial factors; important in pathogenesis

HLA = human leukocyte antigen.

5. Isolated rectal involvement unusual in children but presents with tenesmus, urgency, passage of formed or semiformed stool with blood or mucus. Limited proctitis extends to involve more proximal colon over time in one-third to one-half cases.

6. Although UC is confined to the colon, children with UC may develop gastroesophageal reflux or dyspepsia with inflammation of the upper gastrointestinal (GI) tract.

EXTRAINTESTINAL MANIFESTATIONS

1. 25–35% of patients with inflammatory bowel disease (IBD) develop extraintestinal symptoms that may occur before, during or after the development of GI symptoms.

2. Arthropathy is a frequent symptom of UC in 20–25% of patients. Can be peripheral (asymmetric, nondeforming, migratory polyarthritis of one or more large joints) or axial. Treatment of GI mucosal inflammation usually results in improvement of peripheral arthropathy but nonsteroidal anti-inflammatory drugs may be required. Sulfasalazine may have a direct effect on the arthritis as well. Axial arthropathy (ankylosing spondylitis or sacroiliitis) occurs in 1–4% and is associated with being human leukocyte antigen (HLA)-B27–positive. Ankylosing spondylitis runs a course independent of bowel disease. Patients with UC also often develop enthesopathy where there is inflammation at the tendon or ligament bony attachment sites.

3. Pyoderma gangrenosum occurs in < 1–5% of patients with UC (more common in UC than Crohn disease) and is associated with active disease. Lesions (which begin as pustules and then develop into ulcerations with well defined borders and violaceous color) tend to be multiple and below the knees at sites of trauma. Treatment involves intralesional or systemic therapy, but remission is difficult.

4. Erythema nodosum occurs less frequently in UC than Crohn disease. These are tender, warm red nodules at extensor surfaces of the lower extremities.

5. Ophthalmologic abnormalities occur in 1–3% of children with IBD. Episcleritis (hyperemia of sclera or conjunctiva without vision loss treated with topical steroids) and uveitis (acute or subacute pain eye with visual blurring, photophobia, or headache that can be asymptomatic; treated with topical or systemic steroids to avoid risk of blindness) are common.

6. Hepatic abnormalities in children with UC: transient elevations of alanine aminotransferase (ALT) in 12% related to medications or disease. Persistent ALT elevation suggests primary sclerosing cholangitis (PSC) (diagnosis based on liver biopsy and cholangiography) or autoimmune chronic active hepatitis. With PSC, medical therapy of little impact, although ursodeoxycholate may be helpful. Fatty changes of liver in IBD may be secondary to malnutrition, protein losses, anemia, or steroid use.

7. Thromboembolic disease can lead to significant morbidity in IBD in which multiple coagulation abnormalities are seen.

8. Osteopenia occurs in children with UC (less often in Crohn disease), especially in those with a history of steroid use. Chronic recurrent multifocal osteomyelitis also associated with IBD.

COMPLICATIONS

1. Toxic megacolon: life-threatening.
   a. Characterized by total or segmental nonobstructive dilatation of colon at least 6 cm in diameter associated with systemic toxicity (fever, tachycardia, hypotension, dehydration, and mental status changes). Clinical signs may be masked by high-dose steroid therapy. In toxic megacolon, severe inflammation extends beyond mucosa.
   b. Radiographs reveal colonic dilatation, usually involving transverse colon, sometimes accompanied by inflammatory changes.
   c. Risk factors: drugs that impair motility, diagnostic procedures that distend the colon, metabolic abnormalities that may compromise colonic epithelial integrity and motor function, and early discontinuation or rapid tapering of steroids or 5-aminosalicylic acid (5-ASA) agents.
   d. Patient with toxic megacolon at risk of colonic perforation, gram-negative sepsis, and massive hemorrhage.
   e. Treatment involves serial physical exams and radiographs, nasogastric decompression, prone positioning with or without rectal tube to facilitate colonic decompression, fluid and electrolyte resuscitation, total parenteral nutrition (TPN), nothing by mouth, surgical consultation, stool testing for *Clostridium difficile*, and treatment with steroids and antibiotics. Emergent colectomy may be required if such measures do not improve colonic dilatation within 48 h.

2. Massive hemorrhage may occur in UC with or without toxic megacolon. Treated with blood transfusions, aggressive therapy, and colectomy as needed.

3. Colonic strictures may occur: generally postinflammatory and fibrotic in children; may be associated with cancer in adults. Strictures usually occur in rectum and sigmoid due to smooth muscle hypertrophy.

TABLE 2   DIFFERENTIAL DIAGNOSIS OF COLITIS

INFECTIOUS ETIOLOGIES
Bacterial: *Campylobacter, Salmonella, Shigella, Escherichia coli*
    (enterohemorrhagic strains), *Yersinia, Aeromonas, Plesiomonas,*
    Clostridium difficile, Gonococcus, tuberculosis
Parasitic: *Entamoeba histolytica*
Viral: cytomegalovirus, HIV

CHRONIC IDIOPATHIC
Ulcerative colitis
Crohn disease
Behçet disease
Lymphocytic colitis
Collagenous colitis
Eosinophilic colitis

VASCULITIS
Henoch-Schönlein purpura
Hemolytic uremic syndrome

OTHER
Ischemic colitis
Allergic colitis
Enterocolitis associated with Hirschsprung disease
Diversion colitis
Chemotherapy-induced colitis
Radiation-induced colitis
Graft-versus-host disease
Necrotizing enterocolitis (in neonates)

HIV = human immunodeficiency virus.

4. Persons with long-standing UC are at markedly increased risk of colorectal cancer.
    a. Minimal risk at 8–10 yr of disease but thereafter increases by 0.5–1.0%/yr.
    b. Risk correlates to extent of disease with risk of cancer minimal in proctitis and highest in pancolitis.
    c. Surveillance colonoscopy practice is for colonoscopy every 1–2 yr after 8 yr of disease for pancolitis and after 15 years in those with left-sided colitis. Biopsies for these colonoscopies are performed in 4 quadrants at 10 cm intervals from cecum to descending colon and then at 5 cm intervals beginning at the sigmoid colon.
    d. Colectomy is recommended for cancer, high-grade dysplasia, dysplastic lesions or masses, and low-grade dysplasia.

DIAGNOSIS

1. Initial laboratory tests: complete blood count with differential, sedimentation rate or C-reactive protein, chemistries, stool for occult blood, stool cultures, and stool for *C. difficile* toxins, and a urinalysis. Serum antibodies (pANCA and ASCA) may be used to screen symptomatic children for IBD and to discriminate UC from Crohn disease (Table 2), with pANCA being more prevalent in subjects with UC (60–80%, vs 10–27% for Crohn disease). Nevertheless, such antibodies should not be used to diagnose IBD owing to suboptimal sensitivity and false-positive rates. pANCA tends to test positive in serum of patients with Crohn disease with UC features: differentiating ability of such antibody levels is also limited.
2. Plain radiographs: may detect complications. Barium enemas: provide limited information and should not be performed in setting of active colitis because of the risk of precipitating toxic megacolon. Upper GI series with small bowel follow-through: to rule out terminal ileal or more proximal GI disease suggestive of Crohn disease. Computed tomography: to identify intra-abdominal abscesses.
3. Flexible sigmoidoscopy or colonoscopy: most sensitive and specific test for intestinal inflammation. Typical gross findings: diffuse, continuous involvement of the mucosa starting at rectum (although rectal sparing has occasionally been noted) and extending proximally into the colon. Upper GI inflammation can also be seen in UC.

TREATMENT

Goals: control of symptoms, prevention of relapse, avoidance of complication, and optimizing quality of life.

MEDICATIONS

1. Aminosalicylates: 5-ASA agents act via inhibition of leukotriene B4 synthesis from arachidonic acid and scavenging of reactive oxygen metabolites.
    a. Sulfasalazine: combination of 5-ASA and sulfapyridine (bond between both split by colonic flora). Sulfapyridine responsible for many of common side effects and may cause megaloblastic anemia (interferes with folate absorption) if a folate supplement is not administered. Rare and severe hypersensitivity reactions may occur as well. 80% of adult men develop reversible sperm abnormalities. Children at risk for glucose-6-phosphate dehydrogenase deficiency should be screened prior to sulfasalazine therapy. Often, dosage of sulfasalazine gradually increased over 1 wk owing to potential for intolerance.
    b. Asacol and Pentasa contain 5-ASA in delayed-release coating to prevent proximal absorption of the drug and to ensure delivery to small intestine and colon.
    c. Olsalazine (two 5-ASAs linked by an azo bond) and balsalazine (5-ASA bonded to 4-aminobenzoyl-β-alanine).
    d. Oligospermia and folate deficiency not associated with newer 5-ASA compounds (2 and 3), compared with sulfasalazine.
    e. Topical aminosalicylates are effective in left-sided UC or proctitis. Topical agents may rarely be associated with side effects.
2. Corticosteroids: effective in the induction of remission in children with moderate or severe UC. Usually dosed for 4–6 wk with subsequent tapering of dose. If exacerbation of disease activity prevents complete withdrawal, chronic alternate-day steroid therapy may be necessary. Topical therapy may be sensible when disease is distally located. Prolonged topical therapy can also lead to systemic side effects.
3. Immunosuppressive agents administered as adjuncts to steroid therapy include 6-mercaptopurine (6-MP), azathioprine, methotrexate, mycophenolate mofetil, cyclosporine, tacrolimus, and infliximab.

a. 6-MP and azathioprine (converted to 6-MP in the liver) can reduce disease activity and allow withdrawal of steroid therapy. Time to clinical response usually 4–8 wk. Side effects include elevated transaminases or hepatitis, pancreatitis, bone marrow depression, hypersensitivity, and recurrent infections. Evaluation for thiopurine methyltransferase genetic polymorphisms can identify those at higher risk for drug toxicity. Often a high relapse rate with withdrawal of 6-MP; likely will require long-term maintenance therapy. No evidence for increased risk of cancer in long-term use of azathioprine in adults.

b. Methotrexate: alternative for those intolerant of 6-MP but less effective as therapy for UC than for Crohn disease. No published studies describing efficacy in children with UC.

c. Mycophenolate mofetil: mixed results. May have more side effects than azathioprine.

d. Cyclosporine: for severe colitis unresponsive to steroids in adults; effective generally within 7 d. Notable side effects: renal toxicity, hypertension, tremors or paresthesias, and hypertrichosis. Children on cyclosporine should receive prophylaxis for *Pneumocystis carinii* pneumonia and have careful monitoring of electrolytes, blood glucose, renal function, blood pressure, and neurologic status. Majority of patients still undergo colectomy within 1 yr.

e. Tacrolimus: can also induce remission when administered orally to children with severe active colitis. Majority of patients still undergo colectomy within 1 yr.

f. Infliximab: in open trials, clinical improvement in children and adults but in double-blind, placebo controlled studies, benefit remains unclear.

4. Antibiotics: remains controversial. Lack of evidence of effectiveness.

5. Probiotics have shown some promise for maintenance of remission in adults.

NUTRITIONAL THERAPY

The provision of adequate nutrients is essential for optimal healing of UC. Enteral nutrition is preferred to TPN when possible. Enteral nutrition is not an effective primary therapy for active UC, in contrast to Crohn disease.

SURGERY

1. Colectomy may be required for patients with severe or medically refractory disease or to prevent colon cancer.

2. Standard indications: fulminant colitis, massive hemorrhage, colonic perforation, stricture or toxic megacolon, failure of medical therapy, steroid dependency, and presence of colonic dysplasia. In children with growth retardation and delayed sexual maturity, colectomy may be considered, because catch-up growth occurs after colectomy. Except in the setting of emergent colectomy, a complete evaluation should be per-

formed to rule out Crohn disease (potential of recurrence of disease and relative contraindication for ileoanal pull-through).

3. Current standard surgery: colectomy with ileal pouch with anal anastomosis (IPAA). A 2-stage approach may be used with an initial diverting loop ileostomy to allow the pouch to heal initially followed by anastomosis and closure of the loop ileostomy. Potential complications: small bowel obstruction, pelvic sepsis, anastomotic leak, fecal incontinence, pouchitis, and strictures or fistulae. Fistula development should raise suspicion of Crohn disease.

4. In the case of emergent colectomy: 3 stages may be used.

a. Stage 1: subtotal colectomy with ileostomy and formation of rectal stump. After the first operation, the rectal mucosa is treated topically to induce healing.

b. Stage 2: the distal rectal and proximal anal mucosa is removed with formation of the ileal pouch.

c. Stage 3: ileostomy reversed.

POUCHITIS

1. Most significant complication in UC patients undergoing IPAA.

2. Symptoms: diarrhea, rectal bleeding, abdominal cramping, urgency, stool incontinence, and malaise fever. May occur more frequently in children with extraintestinal manifestations of UC, especially primary sclerosing cholangitis. Laboratory studies may show anemia and elevated erythrocyte sedimentation rate.

3. Diagnosis: flexible sigmoidoscopy with biopsies.

4. Treatment: broad-spectrum antibiotics (metronidazole most commonly used). Other options include mesalamine or steroid enemas or oral mesalamine or sulfasalazine and steroids. Probiotics may be useful for prevention or maintenance of remission.

5. Low risk of dysplasia at ileal pouch, but long-term risk of dysplasia unknown.

PROGNOSIS

1. Most children with potential for full active life with good health. 10% have only 1 episode of colitis, 50% have chronic disease, 20% have chronically active disease. Limited distal UC can extend to involve proximal colon with time.

2. The clinician should always be on the alert for signs of Crohn disease.

3. UC has no specific effect on fertility and poses no risk to the fetus. Exception: women with UC who undergo proctocolectomy with IPAA may experience reduced fertility.

4. Psychosocial aspects also need to be treated. There is an increased risk of psychiatric and behavioral issues in children with IBD. However, there is a lack of correlation between severity of illness and psychiatric and behavior issues in children with IBD. Quality-of-life scores appear to correlate more with satisfaction with social supports.

QUESTIONS

CHOOSE THE BEST ANSWER:

1. Which of the following is the most common distribution of disease in pediatric ulcerative colitis?
   a. Proctitis.
   b. Left-sided disease.
   c. Rectal sparing.
   d. Pancolitis.

2. Which of the following parallel disease activity occurs with ulcerative colitis?
   a. Pyoderma gangrenosum.
   b. Peripheral arthropathy.
   c. Axial arthropathy.
   d. Primary sclerosing cholangitis.

3. The highest incidence of ulcerative colitis occurs in which age group of children?
   a. Neonates.
   b. Toddlers.
   c. Age 5–10 yr.
   d. Age 10–18 yr.

4. Toxic megacolon is defined by persistent colonic dilatation measuring a minimal diameter of:
   a. 3 cm.
   b. 4 cm.
   c. 5 cm.
   d. 6 cm.
   e. 7 cm.

5. When should cancer surveillance begin in patients with ulcerative colitis and pancolitis?
   a. 5 years after onset of disease.
   b. 8 years after onset of disease.
   c. 12 years after onset of disease.
   d. 15 years after onset of disease.

TRUE OR FALSE:

6. Mesalamine is associated with folate deficiency.
7. Patients with ulcerative colitis have reduced fertility.

UNDETERMINED COLITIS AND OTHER INFLAMMATORY DISEASES

SYNOPSIS

EOSINOPHILIC GASTROENTEROPATHY

1. Chronic relapsing disorder in which eosinophils constitute the predominant cell type in the inflammatory infiltrate of the gastrointestinal (GI) tract.
2. Rare. Peak in 2nd and 3rd decades.
3. Two subgroups: milk sensitive and those with eosinophilic gastroenteropathy (EG).
   a. Milk sensitive: allergic histories and GI symptoms at age 5 mo, improved with milk elimination. Have immunoglobulin (Ig)G milk antibody but not raised total IgE or IgE milk.
   b. EG: average age of onset 4 yr; chronic symptoms including growth failure. 50% with no personal or family history of atopy. No response to dietary manipulation. Signs of systemic allergy and elevated IgE- and IgE milk–specific antibodies. Intermittent use of steroids necessary to control disease.
4. Eosinophilic infiltration of mucosa: small intestine, especially the jejunum, is the most commonly involved site. Inflammation of submucosa and muscularis may be prominent especially at the antrum and causes obstruction.
5. Etiology unknown. Total IgE elevated in some patients and normal in others. Inciting factor usually undetermined. Eosinophil recruitment by 3 cytokines: IL-3, granulocyte-macophage colony–stimulatin factor (GM-CSF), and IL-5.
6. Clinical symptoms: vomiting, abdominal pain, and growth failure are common. Appendiceal wall infiltration can lead to symptoms of acute appendicitis. Diarrhea may be associated with rectal bleeding. Eosinophilic esophagitis usually presents with vomiting, pain, and dysphagia (usually also accompanied by personal history of atopy). Hypoalbuminemia in 33–100% secondary to protein-losing enteropathy.
7. Peripheral eosinophilia found in 70–100%. Elevated serum food-specific IgE antibody occurs in some patients. Iron deficiency common, especially with enteric blood loss.
8. Diagnosis: strongly suggested when characteristic symptoms accompanied by blood eosinophilia. Specific food-related IgE antibodies are often not found. Radiology: narrowing, nodularity at antrum, and thickened mucosal folds at the small intestine. Esophagogastroduodenoscopy (EGD) examination of esophagus may show rings. Biopsies: increased eosinophilic density. Stomach or duodenum: may show nodularity, erythema, friability, and ulceration. Gastric biopsies: demonstrate EG more consistently than intestinal biopsies. Most with EG have > 10 eosinophils/high power field (HPF) at antral or duodenal mucosa. Allergic proctocolitis shows focal eosinophilic infiltration 15–60 eosinophils/HPF.
9. Treatment: When specific foods provoke symptoms, dietary elimination and elemental diet. When symptoms persist, steroids (1–2 mg/kg/d) and oral cromolyn (50–200 mg 4 times daily) control most symptoms. Low-dose or alternate-day steroids needed in some cases for long-term control. Inhaled steroids (fluticasone and beclomethasone) demonstrate rapid response within 1 wk. Ketotifen (H1 antihistamine) may also benefit children with EG.

HEMOLYTIC UREMIC SYNDROME

1. Development of microangiopathic hemolytic anemia, thrombocytopenia, and renal insufficiency in previously healthy persons. Several forms of disease recognized.
2. Typically occurs in children age < 5 yr. Endemic in Argentina, southern Africa, and western United States.

Epidemic form occurs in summer, with abrupt onset of diarrhea; good prognosis. Sporadic form in older children: no prodrome, seasonal influence, and higher mortality. Sibs who develop hemolytic uremic syndrom (HUS) during infancy > 1 yr apart have an autosomal recessive trait predisposing them to HUS; mortality rate 68%.

3. Most cases in Pacific Northwest preceded by infection with *Escherichia coli* O157:H7, which produce verotoxin. *E. coli* O157:H7 is disseminated through hamburger, unpasteurized milk, yogurt, unpasteurized apple cider, vegetables grown in garden fertilized with cow manure, and water and person-to-person at child daycare. Non-O157:H7 strains account for more cases in Europe than the United States.

4. Also associated with *Streptococcus pneumoniae* in absence of diarrheal disease.

5. Central lesion: vascular endothelial damage. Precipitating cause of vascular injury: release of Shiga-like toxins. Lipopolysaccharide damages endothelial cells and promotes thrombosis. Shiga-like toxin induces tumor necrosis factor (TNF) production in kidney. Vascular injury induces microangiopathic hemolytic anemia, thrombocytopenia, and local deposits of fibrin microthrombi with resulting ischemic changes.

6. Genetics: Complement regulator factor H gene *FH1* mutations found in German series in 14% patients with atypical HUS led to reduced binding of C3b/C3d to heparin and endothelium, leading to endothelial cell and microvascular damage.

7. Clinical symptoms:
   a. GI: lesions in 90–100% of children. In 70–80%, bloody diarrhea precedes recognition of HUS by 3–16 d. Other children have prodrome of abdominal pain, nonbloody diarrhea, or vomiting. Colitis may persist for 2 mo. Rectal prolapse described in up to 10% of patients with colitis. Occasionally, necrosis and perforation of the colon owing to thrombosis. Endoscopic appearance: hyperemia, edema, and petechiae. Rectal biopsies: only edema and submucosal hemorrhage with scant inflammation. Barium enema: focal diffuse bowel wall edema, thumbprinting, and colonic spasm or dilatation.
   b. Hemolytic anemia: microangiopathic hemolytic anemia in all children. Develops within 1–2 d.
   c. Thrombocytopenia: 92% owing to platelet trapping. Prothrombin time/partial thromboplastin time normal.
   d. Renal insufficiency: all cases. Oliguria 32%. Time for creatinine clearance to return to normal averages 3.7 mo. Chronic renal insufficiency persists in 9–10%.
   e. Neurologic: central nervous system (CNS) manifestations found in one-third of cases. Cerebral edema or stroke seen in up to 5% and can be fatal.
   f. Liver: transaminase, alkaline phosphatase, γ-glutamyltransferase (GGT), and 5'-nucleotidase elevations of 2–20 times are common.
   g. Elevated amylase or lipase seen in 20%. Hyperglycemia in 4–15%.

8. Diagnosis: stool specimens: yield for *E. coli* O157:H7 low if specimens sent after 1st week of diarrhea.

9. Treatment: severe GI symptoms require hospitalization and intravenous (IV) fluids. Management of fluid, electrolytes, renal insufficiency, hypertension, seizures, and hemolytic anemia. Sodium should be withheld from children with edema and hyponatremia. Potassium should not be given unless levels fall into low normal range. Nutrition important. Peritoneal dialysis employed as needed (dialysis if severe uncontrollable hyperkalemia, fluid overload, severe uremia with encephalopathy, blood urea nitrogen > 150 mg/dL, need for total parenteral nutrition, and severe CNS dysfunction) except if severe colitis or abdominal tenderness. No direct evidence that anticoagulant therapy beneficial. Transfuse for severe anemia with blood products free of T-antigen antibody. No platelets should be delivered unless severe bleed or invasive procedures since platelets lead to microthrombi. Plasma transfusions or plasmapheresis can be considered. Hypertension usually responds to short-acting calcium channel blockers.

HENOCH-SCHÖNLEIN PURPURA

1. Multisystem vasculitic disorders affecting children age < 7 yr. Characterized by urticaria or purpura, colicky abdominal pain, sometimes with hematochezia, arthralgias or arthritis, and hematuria with or without proteinuria. Symptoms persist for an average of 4 wk.

2. In 90%, upper respiratory infection or fever occurred 1–3 wk before symptoms of HUS. Seasonal variation: one-third of cases during spring. Increased frequency of *DRB1*01* and *DRB1*11* observed in patients with Henoch-Schönlein purpura (HSP).

3. Infectious agents or medications may trigger an immune response leading to IgA1 immune complex deposition in blood vessel walls. Intimal proliferation and thrombosis described in cerebral vessels in children with seizures. Vasculitis results in edema or hemorrhage in various organs.

4. Clinical symptoms:
   a. Skin: lesions in 97–100% of cases. Urticaria on extensor surfaces legs, buttocks, and arms. Children age < 2 yr present with scalp, facial, and extremity edema. Older children often show petechiae on lower extremities.
   b. GI: symptoms in 65–90%. Colicky abdominal pain associated with vomiting. Abdominal pain occurs within 8 d of rash development in 75% of patients. Hypoproteinemia with protein-losing enteropathy. GI bleeding in 25%. Rare complications: intussusception, perforation, pancreatitis, and cholecystitis. Intussusception seen in children age 5–7 yr; early surgery reduces mortality. Intussusception usually originates at ileum (90%) and jejunum (7%). EGD: coalescing purpura especially at descending duodenum, gastritis or punctuate erythema, ulcerative changes at colon. Radiologic studies at small bowel and colon show thumbprinting. Relapses of GI symptoms reported up to 7 yr after initial episode.

c. Arthritis and arthralgias: oligoarticular or nonmigratory in 65%. Ankles and knees involved more than upper extremities.

d. Renal: hematuria in 40%; two-thirds of those with hematuria also have proteinuria. Renal lesions more frequent in age < 2 yr, usually following skin and GI involvement.

e. Hepatobiliary: right upper quadrant pain in 80%. Laboratory tests revealed elevated alanine aminotransferase in 75% and GGT in 30%. Ultrasonography with hepatomegaly in 75% and gallbladder wall thickening in 25%.

f. Vasculitis of scrotum may result in findings or symptoms that must be differentiated from torsion of spermatic cord; seen in 24%.

5. Diagnosis: depends on presence of characteristic clinical features with supporting laboratory test results, endoscopy, and radiology.

a. Complete blood count: leukocytosis with left shift (10–20 K), erythrocyte sedimentation rate elevated in 75%.

b. Urinalysis may not demonstrate hematuria or proteinuria until several weeks after initial presentation.

c. High-frequency ultrasound may be helpful; thickened bowel wall.

d. Skin histology demonstrates leukocytoclastic vasculitis.

6. Management:

a. Children with severe abdominal pain: admit.

b. Supportive care, IV fluids, and nasogastric suction.

c. Steroids: GI manifestations; controversial (earlier remission but similar outcome at 72 h).

d. Surgical therapy: required rarely for GI hemorrhage, intussusception, perforation, and cholecystitis.

7. Urine should be analyzed for hematuria and proteinuria with use of antihypertensives, fluid restriction, and dialysis as necessary.

8. Relapse frequent; 40% relapse of symptoms up to 7 yr later.

BEHÇET SYNDROME

1. Multisystemic vasculitis disorder.

2. Clinical presentation similar to Crohn disease; genital ulcers, severe oral ulceration, and neurologic complications seen in Behçet syndrome.

3. Prevalence varies: most common in Japan (10/100,000); United States 0.3/100,000. Transient form may occur in neonates born to mothers with disease.

4. Genetic predisposition for those who are HLA-B51 positive. Patients tend to have positive family history.

5. Pathogenesis: unknown but genetic and immunologic factors probably contribute. Primary histopathologic lesion consists of vasculitis affecting predominantly small vessels. Endothelial proliferation and mononuclear cell infiltration. C3 and C9 in blood vessel walls, circulating immune complexes.

6. Newborn form: transient circulating IgG immune complexes and reduced complement.

7. Major symptoms:

a. Buccal ulceration: persists 1–2 wk, subsides spontaneously, and recurs days to months later.

b. Genital ulceration: 93–98% similar course as oral ulcers.

c. Uveitis: usually iritis with hypopyon and posterior uveitis (visual impairment usually bilateral); in 21–47% of affected children.

d. Skin lesions: erythema nodosum, acne, vesicles, and pustules; sterile pustule at needle trauma site in 40%.

8. Less frequent or minor symptoms:

a. GI lesions: abdominal pain, diarrhea, flatulence, vomiting, constipation, and ulcerations usually at ileocecal region (extension to serosal surface may result in perforation). No granulomas. Fistulas have been seen. Growth usually normal.

b. Vasculitis can affect both arterial and venous systems.

c. Arthritis: chronic, nonmigratory, seronegative, pauciarticular arthritis affecting knees, ankles, hips, elbows, and wrists in 50%. Usually nondestructive.

d. CNS lesions: 1–20%; transient or progressive: confusion, pyramidal signs, cranial nerve palsies, pseudotumor cerebri, and seizures.

9. Diagnosis: presence of 3 or more episodes of oral aphthous ulcers plus 2 of the following: recurrent aphthous genital ulcers, uveitis or retinal vasculitis, cutaneous vasculitis, or cutaneous hyperactivity to needle prick.

10. Treatment: mainstay therapy is steroids. Relief of symptoms occurs initially but recurrence common. Topical preparations usually effective for genital ulcers. Oral or IV administration needed for uveitis and intestinal and CNS lesions. Colchicine, azathioprine, chlorambucil, thalidomide, and cyclosporine may be effective in patients with severe disease not responsive to steroids or who cannot wean off steroids. Infliximab can also be helpful to reduce steroid dosing.

QUESTIONS

CHOOSE THE BEST ANSWER:

1. The following are true of eosinophilic gastroenteropathy except:
a. Can be responsive to dietary manipulation.
b. May not respond to dietary manipulation.
c. Most commonly involved site is the jejunum.
d. Peripheral eosinophilia common.
e. Iron deficiency is uncommon.
f. None of the above.

2. Eosinophilic gastroenteropathy:
a. Peaks in the 2nd and 3rd decades.
b. Occurs commonly at 5 months of age.
c. Occurs at an average age of 4 years.
d. All of the above.

MATCH THE ASSOCIATED FEATURES TO THE CONDITION (MAY BE MORE THAN ONE):

a. Central nervous system involvement.
b. Summer.
c. Spring.
d. Japan.
e. Immunoglobulin A immune complex.
f. C3 and C9.
g. Pseudotumor cerebri.
h. Immunosuppressive therapy.
i. Intussusception.
j. Needle prick helpful in diagnosis.
k. *Streptococcus pneumoniae*.
l. Argentina.
m. Upper respiratory prodrome.

3. Hemolytic uremic syndrome.
4. Behçet syndrome.
5. Henoch-Schönlein purpura.

NECROTIZING ENTEROCOLITIS

TABLE 1   RISK FACTORS FOR NECROTIZING ENTEROCOLITIS

PRETERM INFANT	FULL-TERM INFANT
Prematurity—immature intestine	Birth asphyxia
Ischemia	Polycythemia
Enteral feeds	Exchange transfusion
Bacterial colonization	Intrauterine growth restriction
Cyanotic congenital heart disease	
Gastroschisis	
Myelomeningocele	

TABLE 2   PRESENTING SIGNS FOR NECROTIZING ENTEROCOLITIS

Lethargy
Temperature instability
Apnea
Shock
Disseminated intravascular coagulation
Ileus
Clinitest positive stools
Heme positive stools or vomitus
Feeding intolerance

SYNOPSIS

NECROTIZING ENTERCOLITIS

1. Necrotizing enterocolitis (NEC) is an inflammatory bowel necrosis that affects primarily premature neonates (Table 1).
2. Affected full-term infants usually have risk factors for gut compromise.
3. Often presents within first days of life.

CLINICAL FEATURES

1. Affects 1–3% of all neonatal intensive care unit (NICU) admissions and 12% of premature infants weighing < 1.5 kg. No sex or race predilection.
2. Variable symptoms: abdominal distention, feeding intolerance, gastric aspirates, bilious emesis, and hematochezia (Table 2).
3. Laboratory values: leukocytosis, thrombocytopenia, electrolyte imbalance, and acidosis.
4. Pathognomonic feature: pneumatosis intestinalis on abdominal radiograph. Most common site: terminal ileum and proximal colon.
5. Sequelae: stricture, short gut syndrome, abscess formation, and disease recurrence (Table 4).

PATHOGENESIS

1. Enteral feeding: 90–95% of cases have been enterally fed. Artificial formula greater risk than breastmilk. Some breastmilk factors (polyunsaturated fatty acid) effective in reducing disease in both animal and human trials.
2. Bacterial colonization: unclear whether bacteria are a primary effector or passive participants. No specific organism linked to disease.
3. Inflammatory cascade: intestinal specimens from patients with acute NEC demonstrate increased interleukin-1, -8, and -11 and tumor necrosis factor alpha. May reflect imbalance of pro and antiinflammatory influences with favoring of proinflammatory responses among neonates predisposing to NEC.

TREATMENT

1. Mainly supportive: cessation of enteral feeds, nasogastric decompression, fluid resuscitation, broad-spectrum antibiotics, correction of anemia and thrombocytopenia, and respiratory support as needed.
2. Close monitoring necessary with repeated radiography.

TABLE 3   BELL STAGING CRITERIA

STAGE	SYSTEMIC SIGNS	INTESTINAL SIGNS	RADIOLOGIC SIGNS
Stage I: suspected NEC	Temperature instability; apnea; bradycardia; lethargy	Abdominal distention; gastric residuals; vomiting; hematochezia	Normal or mild ileus
Stage II			
Definite NEC	Same as I	Same as I plus abdominal tenderness	Pneumatosis intestinalis or portal air
Advanced NEC	Progression to shock; DIC; metabolic acidosis; thrombocytopenia; neutropenia	Peritonitis	Pneumoperitoneum

DIC = disseminated intravascular coagulation; NEC = necrotizing enterocolitis.

TABLE 4   GASTROINTESTINAL COMPLICATIONS OF
                     NECROTIZING ENTEROCOLITIS

Intestinal or colonic strictures
Enterocolic fistulae
Fluid and electrolyte imbalances
Malabsorption
Cholestasis
Anastomotic leaks and stenosis after surgery
Short-gut syndrome after surgery

3. Surgery indicated for intestinal perforation or portal
    venous gas, evidence of necrosis, abdominal wall cel-
    lulitis, fixed loop on serial abdominal radiography.

SEQUELAE

1. Most common: strictures in 10–36% of survivors.
2. Short gut syndrome when large gangrenous segments
    need to be removed. Conservative approach: proximal
    enterostomy without resection then return to operat-
    ing room in 1 wk to assess gut viability.

QUESTIONS

CHOOSE THE BEST ANSWER:

1. Risk of necrotizing enterocolitis increases with all of
    the following except:
    a. Low gestational age.
    b. Feeding.
    c. Anemia.
    d. Umbilical catheters.
    e. Gestational cocaine.

2. The following are true of necrotizing enterocolitis except:
    a. Occurs in 1–3% of all NICU admissions.
    b. There is a racial predilection.
    c. Greater risk in formula-fed infants.
    d. Most commonly occurs at ileocecal area.
    e. Associated with ischemia and infection.

3. The gastrointestinal complications of necrotizing ente-
    rocolitis include all of the following except:
    a. Enterocolic fistulae.
    b. Fluid or electrolyte imbalance.
    c. Biliary obstruction.
    d. Short gut syndrome.
    e. Malabsorption.

MATCH THE STAGE TO THE CHARACTERISTIC:

a. Stage I.
b. Stage II.
c. Stage III.

4. Temperature instability and apnea.
5. Pneumatosis intestinalis.
6. Septic shock.
7. Portal gas.
8. Pneumoperitoneum.

TRUE OR FALSE:

9. Breast-fed infants are at greater risk for necrotizing
    enterocolitis than formula-fed infants.
10. Polyunsaturated fatty acids have been shown to reduce
    the incidence of necrotizing enterocolitis in humans.

GENETIC DISACCHARIDASE DEFICIENCY

SYNOPSIS

1. Disaccharidases (membrane-bound glycoproteins)
    hydrolyze carbohydrates:
    a. Sucrase-isomaltase.
    b. Maltase-glucoamylase.
    c. Lactase-phlorhizin.
2. Maximal expression at lower and mid villus, decreased
    levels at villus tip, and minimal levels at crypts.
3. Bacterial flora salvage nondigested carbohydrates by
    fermentation to gases, lactate, and short-chain fatty
    acids, which are absorbed by the colonic mucosa.
4. Diarrhea secondary to carbohydrate malabsorption is
    more severe in children because of the more rapid
    intestinal passage of nutrients as compared to adults.
5. Diagnosis: noninvasive testing including stool and
    breath testing; invasive determination of enzyme activ-
    ities from small intestine biopsies.

SUCRASE-ISOMALTASE

1. Most abundant glycoprotein at the intestinal brush
    border membrane. Stalk domain of this protein has
    extensive O-glycosylation of serine and threonine,
    which is resistant to pancreatic proteases. Sucrase-
    isomaltase (S-I) complex itself requires pancreatic pro-
    teases to separate the two enzymes at the lumen.
2. Post-translational regulation: most common mecha-
    nism affecting physiology and expression of S-I defects
    lead to congenital sucrase-isomaltase deficiency
    (CSID).
3. CSID: most common phenotype is I followed by II; 6
    phenotypes result from point mutations.
4. Epidemiology of CSID: 0.2% in persons of European
    descent; 5% in Greenlanders. Autosomal recessive
    inheritance.
5. Sucrase hydrolyzes α-1,2 and α-1,4 glucosidic bonds;
    isomaltase cleaves α-1,6 bonds. CSID patients tolerate
    starch better than sucrose since starch has a low
    amount of α-1,6 bonds hydrolyzed by residual
    isomaltase, and colonic bacteria ferment starch in
    infants by 6 months of age.
6. Clinical features vary according to age. Chronic diarrhea
    and failure to thrive seen in infants; chronic diarrhea
    with normal growth in preschool children; irritable
    bowel and recurrent abdominal pain seen in school aged
    children; nonspecific complaints and refractory diarrhea
    in adults.

7. Diagnosis: stool pH 5–6; presence of stool-reducing substances indicative but not reliable. Rise of blood glucose < 20 mg/dL after a 2g/kg sucrose load indicates sucrose intolerance (false-positive in the setting of delayed gastric emptying or increased intestinal transit time). Breath testing shows rise of breath hydrogen > 20 ppm 90–180 min after oral load of 2 g/kg sucrose (false-negative with gastric emptying delay, acidic colonic milieu, and nonhydrogen-producing bacteria after antibiotics). Gold standard: S-I activity measurement with normal histology shows lack in sucrase activity but can have isomaltase activity.

8. Treatment: lifelong sucrose restriction depending upon patient symptoms. Diet excludes starch and glucose polymers, but tolerance to starch improves during first 3–4 yr. *Saccharomyces cerevisiae* possesses sucrase activity and low isomaltase and maltase activity and can be supplemented. Invertase produced from *S. cerevisiae* has also been useful in patients with CSID to hydrolyze sucrose.

LACTASE-PHLORHIZIN HYDROLASE

1. Integral membrane glycoprotein responsible for the hydrolysis of lactose (lactase) and digestion of β-glycosylceramides.

2. Gene located on chromosome 2. Lactase-phlorhizin hydrolase (LPH) molecule is highly N- and O-glycosylated, (crucial in the folding, maturation, and enzymatic activity of LPH). Major mechanism of regulation of LPH expression is transcription.

ADULT-TYPE HYPOLACTASIA

1. Primary type affects the majority of the world's human population: > 75% of adults show a decline in LPH levels to 5–10% of birth level. Incidence varies in different population since expression of lactase is genetically determined; 80% of blacks, Arabs, and Latinos and up to 100% of Asians and American Indians have adult-type hypolactasia.

2. Clinical symptoms: many develop signs in adolescence and adulthood. Symptoms begin briefly after milk consumption: abdominal discomfort, flatulence, and loose stools. 70% able to drink some milk; no consistent correlations between jejunal lactase levels and symptom threshold.

3. Diagnosis: laboratory assessment includes a lactose hydrogen breath test performed after 6 h overnight fast; false-positive with low gastric emptying rate, fast intestinal transit; false-negative with hydrogen nonexcreters (prior antibiotic use).

4. Therapy: calcium supplementation needs to be provided to prevent osteoporosis in lactose malabsorbers who avoid milk. In those who can tolerate small amounts, cheese and yogurt should be recommended. Lactase supplements also available.

CONGENITAL LACTASE DEFICIENCY (ALACTASIA)

1. Rare disorder; autosomal recessive. Post-translational mechanisms probably involved similar to those in CSID.

2. Symptoms start a few days after birth with onset of breast feeding/lactose formula feeding. Patients have liquid and acid diarrhea, meteorism, and severe malnutrition. Also present with hypercalcemia and nephrocalcinosis provoked by metabolic acidosis or the calcium absorption-increasing effect of lactose.

3. Diagnosis: based on low enzyme activity at small intestine biopsy in the setting of normal levels of other disaccharidases.

4. Therapy: strict lactose-free diet owing to severity of symptoms.

MALTASE-GLUCOAMYLASE

1. Digestive properties similar to isomaltase (close evolutionary relationship to S-I); contributes to digestion of α-glycosidic linkages of carbohydrates (able to hydrolyze maltose and starch but not sucrose). Maltase-glucoamylase (MGA) can compensate for lack of S-I in several CSID cases.

2. MGA plays unique role in digestion of malted dietary oligosaccharides.

3. No cleavage of mature MGA occurs in the intestinal lumen by pancreatic proteases (in contrast to S-I).

PRIMARY MGA DEFICIENCY

1. Diarrhea, abdominal distention, and bloating with introduction of starch and formula containing starch polymers in children aged 4–6 mo until 5 yr.

2. Diagnosis: starch challenge and elimination. Measure starch digestive capacity by breath testing. Stool reducing substances are inconsistently positive. Diagnosis established by low enzyme activities on duodenal biopsy with normal pancreatic amylase.

3. Treatment: elimination diet of starches and short glucose polymers.

TREHALASE

1. Another member of α-glucosidases of small intestine. Present in human serum: can be elevated in diabetes and reduced in rheumatoid arthritis.

2. Trehalose, the substrate of trehalase, is found in mushrooms, algae, insects, *Ascaris lumbricoides*, and *Artemia salina*. Trehalose is also a food additive.

TREHALASE DEFICIENCY

1. Autosomal recessive disorder found in 8% of Greenlanders.

2. Symptoms: similar to lactose intolerance.

3. Diagnosis: breath tests not reliable. Requires duodenal biopsy with enzyme activity determination.

4. Therapy: trehalose restriction.

QUESTIONS

CHOOSE THE BEST ANSWER:

1. What is the most common disaccharidase deficiency?
   a. Trehalase deficiency.
   b. Sucrase-isomaltase deficiency.

c. Primary adult-type hypolactasia.
d. Congenital lactase deficiency.

2. What does trehalase digest?
   a. Coconut.
   b. Mushroom.
   c. Wheat.
   d. Oat.
   e. None of the above.

3. The following are true of sucrase-isomaltase deficiency except:
   a. Clinical symptoms tend to improve with age.
   b. Starch restriction usually can be liberalized by age 4 yr.
   c. *Saccharomyces cerevisiae* supplementation can be helpful.
   d. Breast-fed infants are symptomatic.
   e. Greenlanders have a 5% prevalence.

4. Which of the following is false regarding primary adult-type hypolactasia:
   a. The most common form of genetically determined disaccharidase deficiency.
   b. Highly dominant phenotype in Asia.
   c. Often lactose malabsorbers can tolerate 1–2 cups of milk without difficulty.
   d. Heterozygotes are also malabsorbers.
   e. Partial resolution on lactose-free diet suggests other etiology or concomitant problem.

5. Sucrase-isomaltase deficiency:
   a. Is autosomal dominant.
   b. Produces a basic pH watery fermentative diarrhea.
   c. Increases lactate in stool.
   d. Shows elevated serum glucose with sucrose challenge.
   e. Shows decreased serum glucose with fructose or glucose challenge.

6. Disaccharidase deficiency is diagnosed by:
   a. Reducing substances in the stool.
   b. Enzyme activity measured from intestinal biopsy.
   c. Tolerance testing.
   d. Breath hydrogen testing.

CONGENITAL INTESTINAL TRANSPORT DEFECTS

SYNOPSIS

DISORDERS OF CARBOHYDRATE ABSORPTION

1. Enterocytes, renewed every 6 days, express enzymes and transporters needed for carbohydrate (CHO) digestion and absorption (Figure 1).
2. The apical brush border membrane contains:
   a. Sucrase-isomaltase enzyme digesting sucrose to glucose and fructose.

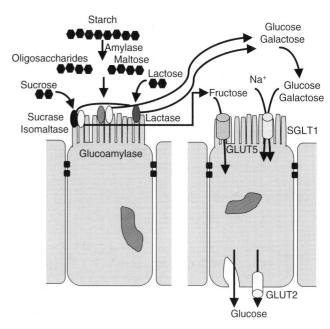

FIGURE 1 Carbohydrate assimilation. GLUT = glucose transporter; SGLT = sodium-coupled glucose transporter.

   b. Lactase-phlorhizin digesting lactose to galactose and glucose.
   c. Na$^+$-dependent glucose-galactose cotransporter (*SGLT1*)
   d. Fructose uniporter (*GLUT5*).
3. The basolateral membrane contains:
   a. Glucose-galactose-fructose uniporter (*GLUT2*).
   b. Na$^+$,K$^+$-adenosinetriphosphatase (ATPase) pump.
4. Fructose is thus passively transported across the intestine by *GLUT5* and *GLUT2*. The Na–K pump maintains the low intracellular Na.

GLUCOSE-GALACTOSE MALABSORPTION

1. Rare disorder, causes severe life-threatening diarrhea and dehydration during the neonatal period.
2. Autosomal recessive inheritance. Heterozygotes have impaired capacity to absorb glucose but asymptomatic.
3. Defect in SGLT-1 usually arises from missense mutations.
4. Clinical manifestations: majority present during the neonatal period. Diarrhea during first 2 days of life results in severe metabolic acidosis and hyperosmolar dehydration. Diarrhea results from presence of unabsorbed CHO in the gut (Figure 2).
5. Diagnosis of glucose-galactose malabsorption (GGM): three key features: elimination of glucose and galactose (lactose) from diet resulting in complete symptom resolution, a positive glucose breath hydrogen test, and normal intestinal biopsy. Stool analysis should show low pH (< 5.3) owing to CHO malabsorption and colonic bacterial fermentation with synthesis of short-chain fatty acids. Stool electrolytes demonstrate large osmotic gap (> 40 mOsm). Mucosal biopsies can also be used to assess lactase and sucrase activity to differentiate GGM from primary lactase or

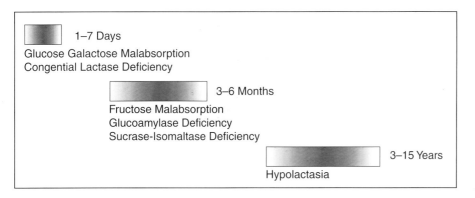

FIGURE 2 Carbohydrate assimilation: age at onset.

sucrase deficiency. Glucose breath hydrogen test useful; relies on colonic fermentation of unabsorbed CHO by bacteria that produce methane, hydrogen, and carbon dioxide; > 20 ppm for diagnosis, but patients often have levels > 100 ppm; false-negative with history of recent antibiotics and decrease of hydrogen producing bacteria.

6. Treatment: elimination diet of glucose and galactose.

FRUCTOSE MALABSORPTION

1. Implicated in both toddler's diarrhea and a rare, autosomal recessive disorder called isolated fructose malabsorption (IFM).
2. Best candidate gene for IFM: SLC2A5.
3. Clinical symptoms: malabsorption of fructose (found in fruits and fruit juices), dose-dependent, with diarrhea when daily consumption of juice > 15 cc/kg.
4. Diagnosis: fructose elimination diet or fructose breath hydrogen test. Intestinal biopsies should reveal normal histology. Malabsorption should be limited to fructose.
5. Treatment: reduce or eliminate dietary fructose. Often disease limited to early infancy; reintroduce fructose at school age.

FANCONI-BICKEL SYNDROME

1. Rare, autosomal recessive disorder.
2. Genetics: mutations at SLC2A2 (usually nonsense mutations).
3. Clinical symptoms: CHO malabsorption (usually mild feature), tubular nephropathy, hepatomegaly, abnormal glycogen accumulation, failure to thrive, fasting hypoglycemia, short stature, rickets, and osteoporosis.
4. Diagnosis: urinalysis for glycosuria, generalized aminoaciduria, and excessive urinary losses of phosphate and calcium. Histology of small bowel, liver, and kidney reveals excessive glycogen stores. Abdominal ultrasound useful to confirm enlargement of liver and kidney.
5. Treatment: supplement urinary electrolyte losses. Uncooked cornstarch to prevent hypoglycemia and minimize postprandial hyperglycemia.

DISORDERS OF AMINO ACID AND PEPTIDE ABSORPTION

PHYSIOLOGY

1. Digestion and absorption of dietary proteins requires initial hydrolysis by gastric, pancreatic, and brush bor-

FIGURE 3 Protein and amino acid assimilation in the small intestine. Various amino acid transport systems are present on the apical (B^0, $B^{0,+}$, $b^{0,+}$, y^+, IMINO) and basolateral (ASC, asc, L, y^+L, A) membrane. PEPTI = peptide cotransporter peptide transporter-1.

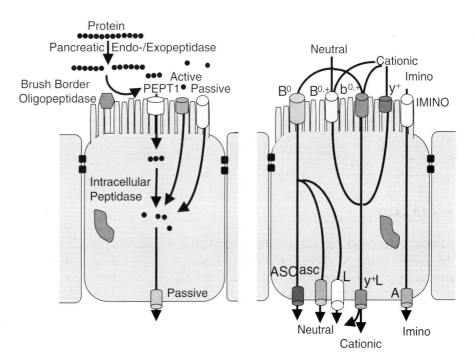

der proteases with subsequent active and passive transport of dipeptides and amino acids across the apical membrane of the enterocyte (Figure 3). Intracellular peptidases hydrolyze dipeptides to single amino acids, which are exported across the basolateral membrane via a second series of transporters.

2. Protein digestion initiated at stomach by pepsin proteases secreted by chief cells in the inactive form (pepsinogen), which is then activated by acid. Proteins that reach the intestine are further hydrolyzed by endopeptidases (trypsin, chymotrypsin, and elastase) and exopeptidases (carboxypeptidase A and B) secreted in their inactive form by the exocrine pancreas and activated by trypsin, which itself is activated by enterokinase.

3. In regards to amino acid luminal or apical transporters, there are specific transporters for neutral amino acids (B^0 and $B^{0,+}$ Na^+-dependent system), anionic and cationic amino acids (x_c^- and y^+), and cationic and neutral amino acids ($b^{0,+}$). Neutral amino acids leave the enterocyte in a size-dependent manner at the basolateral membrane (L for larger, ASC for smaller amino acids). Neutral and imino acids leave via the A system. Cationic amino acids are transported by the Na^+ dependent system y+L. The redundancy in these transport systems minimizes GI and nutritional consequences when an individual system is disrupted.

DISORDERS OF PROTEIN DIGESTION
1. Rare.
2. Enterokinase deficiency: most well characterized; children present with diarrhea, failure to thrive, and hypoproteinemic edema on a diet of intact proteins.
3. Primary trypsinogen deficiency: similar presentation as enterokinase deficiency.
4. Children with cystic fibrosis with exocrine pancreatic dysfunction: maldigestion of dietary protein, fat, and CHO.
5. Late stages of chronic pancreatitis: similar malabsorption as seen in cystic fibrosis.

LYSINURIC PROTEIN INTOLERANCE
1. Autosomal recessive disorder from mutation in *SLC7A7* gene encoding for cationic amino acid transporter y⁺LAT-1 (basolateral membrane of enterocyte and renal tubules transporting cytoplasmic dibasic amino acids [lysine, arginine, and ornithine] in exchange for Na^+ and neutral amino acids).
2. Gene encoding for y⁺LAT-1 is expressed in small intestine, kidney, and lungs. Ornithine and arginine are important urea cycle intermediates not absorbed in patients with lysinuric protein intolerance, and their relative deficiency results in hyperammonemia and alterations in mental status.
3. Main clinical symptoms: failure to thrive, diarrhea, and vomiting. Presentation: failure to thrive and self-imposed restriction of dietary protein. Distinguishing feature: ingestion of high-protein diet results in hyperammone-

mia and encephalopathy. Marked hepatosplenomegaly and frequent bone fractures. Associated with relative deficiency of total and antigen-specific immunoglobulins.
4. Diagnosis: quantitative plasma amino acids or urinary organic acids where plasma diamino acids are low with elevation of urinary lysine and orotic acid.
5. Treatment: systemic repletion of lysine (oral not tolerated). Also, citrulline supplements and dietary protein restriction.

CYSTINURIA
Transporter $b^{0,+}$ is defective in cystinuria and is selective for cationic and neutral amino acid transport across the apical membrane.

HARTNUP DISEASE
1. Autosomal recessive disorder. Defect in neutral amino acid transport. Molecular basis unknown.
2. Clinical presentation: dermatitis and neurologic delay.
3. Diagnosis: analysis of urine amino acid profiles.

IMINOGLYCINURIA
1. Autosomal recessive disorder. Defect in imino amino acid transport. Molecular basis unknown.
2. Neurologic delay.
3. Diagnosis: analysis of urine amino acid profiles.

FAT ABSORPTION PHYSIOLOGY
1. Lipolysis is initiated in the stomach by gastric lipase and concludes via the action of pancreatic lipase.
2. In early infancy, fat absorption is more dependent on gastric lipase.
3. Fatty acid and diglyceride are the products of triglyceride hydrolysis.
4. Solubilization in the lumen requires adequate levels of conjugated bile salts.

DISORDERS OF FAT ABSORPTION
1. Congenital pancreatic lipase deficiency: very rare autosomal recessive disorder leading to fat malabsorption.
2. Tangier disease: defective process (cholesterol export out of the basolateral membrane of the enterocyte occurs via ATP-binding transporter *ABCA1*) where there is a deficiency of high-density lipoproteins, predisposing persons to premature coronary artery disease despite hypocholesterolemia.
3. Sitosterolemia: associated with mutations are *ABCG5* and *ABCG8* transporters (transporters of plant sterol sitosterol).

ABETALIPOPROTEINEMIA
1. Results from failure to reassemble dietary fat in the form of β-lipoproteins, which transport triglyceride and cholesterol esters. Patients have severe deficiency in triglycerides and cholesterol esters. Disease due to an absence of microsomal triglyceride transfer protein (MTP). MTP moves lipids to newly formed and unstable apolipoprotein B proteins. In the absence of

lipoprotein assembly, lipid droplets accumulate in the endoplasmic reticulum.

2. Clinical presentation: in infants, failure to thrive, emesis, and low-volume diarrhea. Later, patients may avoid fatty meals to minimize diarrhea. Neuromuscular abnormalities develop, including loss of deep tendon reflexes from long-term vitamin E deficiency, retinitis pigmentosa, ataxia, and spinocerebellar degeneration.

3. Diagnosis: plasma triglycerides levels < 10 mg/dL with cholesterol levels 25–40 mg/dL. Acanthocytosis is seen in peripheral blood as a result of abnormal lipoproteins in the erythrocyte membrane. Esophagogastroduodenoscopy at small bowel reveals yellow discoloration. Biopsies reveal fat-laden enterocytes at upper villus.

4. Treatment: low-fat diet. Supplementation of fat-soluble vitamins, especially vitamin E.

HYPOBETALIPOPROTEINEMIA

1. Results from the formation of abnormally truncated forms of apolipoprotein B. Mutations in the *APOB* gene.

2. Primary distinction between abetalipoproteinemia (ABL) and hypobetalipoproteinemia (HBL): ABL heterozygotes have normal cholesterol and triglyceride levels, while HBL heterozygotes have low lipoprotein levels.

3. Clinically: autosomal dominant. Heterozygotes with no GI and minimal if any neuromuscular abnormalities. Homozygotes have similar symptoms as ABL.

4. Diagnosis: heterozygotes have lower cholesterol, triglyceride, and lower low-density lipoproteins than normal. Homozygotes have similar cholesterol, triglyceride, chylomicron, and very-low-density lipoprotein levels as ABL patients. Acanthocytes and fat-laden enterocytes also seen.

5. Treatment: Similar to ABL with fat restriction, supplementation of vitamin E.

CHYLOMICRON RETENTION DISEASE

1. Otherwise known as Andersen disease. Autosomal recessive disorder. Failure to secrete chylomicrons across the enterocyte at the basolateral membrane.

2. Clinical symptoms: severe diarrhea in neonates; in early adolescence, neuromuscular manifestations of vitamin E deficiency. Often retinitis pigmentosa and neuromuscular manifestations, milder than in HBL and ABL.

3. Enterocytes also fat-laden.

4. Treatment: dietary fat restriction; vitamin E supplementation.

PRIMARY BILE ACID MALABSORPTION

1. Rare autosomal recessive disorder. Impairment of bile acid reabsorption owing to a defect in the function of the ASBT transporter at cholangiocytes and ileocytes (essential role in the enterohepatic circulation of bile salts).

2. Clinical presentation in infants: diarrhea, failure to thrive, and low plasma low-density lipoprotein choles-

terol. Diarrhea attributed to steatorrhea and bile acid–stimulated secretory diarrhea.

3. Mutations found at *SLC10A2* gene.

4. Diagnosis: normal small intestine. Measure bile acid absorption by using bile acid analogue ^{75}Se-homocholate-taurine test.

5. Treatment: diarrhea should improve with a trial of cholestyramine and low-fat diet.

DISORDERS OF MINERAL AND ELECTROLYTE ABSORPTION AND SECRETION

CONGENITAL CHLORIDE DIARRHEA

1. Most common cause of congenital secretory diarrhea in the presence of normal intestinal mucosa; one-half of all cases reported in Finland.

2. Gene localized to 7q31, identified as *SLC26A3*, which encodes a Na$^+$-independent Cl-/HCO3- exchanger expressed at apical membrane of the enterocyte.

3. Clinical symptoms: may occur in utero with severe polyhydramnios and dilated loops of small bowel resembling intestinal atresia. Present during the first week of life with life-threatening secretory diarrhea. Patients may experience intestinal and colonic ulcerations perhaps secondary to lack of HCl neutralization.

4. Diagnosis: suggested if fecal chloride exceeds the concentration of cations (Na$^+$ and K$^+$). Metabolic alkalosis, hypochloremia, hypokalemia, and hyponatremia.

5. Treatment: mainstay is oral or parenteral administration of KCl. Administration of proton-pump inhibitors may improve diarrhea.

CONGENITAL SODIUM DIARRHEA

1. Exceedingly rare autosomal recessive disorder presenting with secretory diarrhea and similar characteristics in patients with congenital chloride diarrhea.

2. Impaired function of intestinal Na$^+$–H$^+$ exchanger (probably NHE-3). GI tract has 3 Na$^+$–H$^+$ exchangers (NHE-2 and NHE-3 at small intestine and NHE-4 at stomach)

3. Clinically, high-volume secretory alkaline diarrhea with high sodium concentration. Hyponatremia, low or normal excretion of urinary Na$^+$, metabolic acidosis results. Polyhydramnios from in utero diarrhea also associated.

4. Diagnosis: confirm the presence of elevated levels of fecal Na$^+$ and HCO3$^-$.

5. Treatment: maintain fluid and electrolyte balance.

ACRODERMATITIS ENTEROPATHICA

1. Rare autosomal recessive disorder of impaired intestinal zinc absorption. Genetic locus at 8q24.3 with mutations of *SLC39A4* gene, which is expressed at apical membrane at the intestine, colon, stomach, and kidney and controls zinc transport into the cytoplasm of various cells.

2. Present in early infancy with profound depletion of total body zinc. Anorexia, diarrhea, and severe failure to thrive. Dermatitis at hands, feet, and perirectal and

oral regions has a vesicobullous character. Alopecia of scalp and face. Humoral, cell-mediated immunodeficiencies may contribute to poor wound healing and infections. Mental lethargy and neurosensory abnormalities may be present.

3. Diagnosis: low levels of alkaline phosphatase (zinc-dependent metalloenzyme). Both serum and urinary zinc are significantly reduced. Radiolabeled zinc has been used to measure intestinal absorption. Histology at the small bowel: inclusion bodies at Paneth cells, enterocytes, and abnormal intracellular organelles as well as villus atrophy.

4. Treatment: large oral doses of zinc. Ability to treat with oral zinc shows that zinc transport is able to occur but may be less efficient.

CALCIUM ABSORPTION

Occurs by active and passive transport mechanisms. Passive absorption occurs paracellularly along the entire small intestine, important with abundant dietary calcium. Active calcium transport (*TRPV6* at enterocytes) occurs primarily at the duodenum and is important when the level of dietary calcium is low. Once in the cytoplasm, calcium forms a complex with calbindin. Calcium efflux out of the enterocyte takes place by Ca-ATPase (PMCA1b) or by Na^+–Ca^{2+} exchanger *SLC8A1*. Vitamin D affects the expression of *TRPV6* and calbindin. There are no inherited defects in intestinal calcium transport.

DISORDER OF MAGNESIUM TRANSPORT

Congenital primary hypomagnesemia is a rare, autosomal recessive disorder associated with impaired absorption of dietary magnesium and a renal tubular defect of magnesium transport. Hypocalcemia secondary to low parathyroid hormone and 1,25-vitamin D levels is common. Mutations in paracellin-1 lead to this disorder.

DISORDERS OF COPPER TRANSPORT

MENKES SYNDROME

1. Rare X-linked recessive disorder of copper deficiency resulting from defective synthesis of the Menkes syndrome transport protein (MNK). Transporter localized to membrane of the trans-Golgi network. MNK expressed by enterocytes and cells of placenta and central nervous system. Defects in the function of MNK result in inadequate efflux of copper from the gut to the body. Associated with hypoceruloplasminemia.

2. Presentation: failure to thrive, various neurologic symptoms, hyperpigmentation, and morphologic changes of hair. Most die by 4 years old.

3. Copper supplementation not efficacious.

WILSON DISEASE

1. Autosomal recessive disorder of copper accumulation owing to malfunctioning of the Wilson disease transporter, localized to membranes of the trans-Golgi network and limited mainly to hepatocytes. Results in failure to excrete copper to bile with liver accumulation. Hypoceruloplasminemia.

2. Presents during early adolescence with either neurologic or hepatic consequences of copper overload.

3. Therapy: chelation with D-penicillamine or ammonium tetrathiomolybdate for renal copper excretion; oral zinc inhibits dietary copper uptake; liver transplant.

DISORDERS OF IRON TRANSPORT

1. Hereditary hemochromatosis: autosomal recessive disorder characterized by excessive iron absorption by the intestine and secondary multiorgan failure owing to excessive iron deposition. Most common genetic disorder among individuals of European ancestry (carrier frequency 1 in 8). Gene at 6p. Most common form secondary to mutations in *HFE* gene: main mutations are Cys282Tyr, His63Asn, and Ser65Cys. Decreased HFE expression reduces cytoplasmic iron levels and augments transporters thus increasing iron intake. Transporters expressed primarily on duodenal enterocytes at upper villus.

2. Other proteins also linked with other forms of hemochromatosis. Mutations in ferroportin 1 found in an autosomal dominant form of hemochromatosis.

DISORDERS OF VITAMIN ABSORPTION

FOLATE MALABSORPTION

1. Congenital folate malabsorption (Figure 4): rare autosomal recessive disorder associated with clinical symptoms of diarrhea, glossitis, and seizures in the face of pancytopenia. Underlying mechanism not identified.

2. Folate deficiency results in hyperhomocysteinemia because 5-MTHF (intracellular form of folate) required for synthesis of methionine from homocysteine.

3. Associated with neural tube defects in neonates and an increased risk of cardiovascular disease in adults with elevated homocysteine levels.

4. Diagnosis: serum folate and homocysteine levels.

VITAMIN B₁₂ MALABSORPTION

1. Absorption of vitamin B_{12} (cobalamin) initiated by gastric acid that removes cobalamin from proteins and transfers it to haptocorrin (binding protein). Intrinsic factor (IF) (made by parietal cells) binds cobalamin after pancreatic proteases hydrolyze the cobalamin-haptocorrin complex in the duodenum. Ileal enterocytes express cubulin, which form a heterodimer with amnionless and forms a receptor for the cobalamin-IF complex. Amnionless then directs the receptor-vitamin complex to the endosomes. Cobalamin-IF complex cleaved within the endosome forming cobalamin-transcobalamin 2, which enters the systemic circulation.

2. Clinical consequences of folate and vitamin B_{12} deficiency overlap since cobalamin is a cofactor for methionine synthase, which uses a methyl group from 5-MTHF (intracellular folate form) to convert homocysteine to methionine. Hyperhomocysteine-

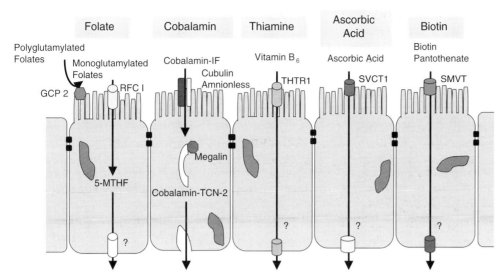

FIGURE 4 Water-soluble vitamin absorption in the small intestine. GCP = glutamate carboxypeptidase; MTHF = methyltetrahydrofolate; RFC = reduced folate transporter; SMVT = sodium multivitamin transporter; SVCT = sodium-vitamin C cotransporters; TCN = transcobalamin; THTR = thiamine transporter protein.

mia thus results from both vitamin B_{12} and folate deficiency.

3. Defects of cobalamin absorption are uniquely associated with methylmalonicacidemia.

4. Primary or secondary achlorhydria is associated with cobalamin deficiency since gastric acidity required for formation of the cobalamin-haptocorrin complex. Small bowel bacterial overgrowth may also disrupt the cobalamin-IF complex and lead to a decline in cobalamin levels. Cobalamin is exclusively in the ileum.

5. There are three rare autosomal disorders associated with congenital cobalamin deficiency.
   a. Congenital pernicious anemia associated with absence of IF, which facilitates binding of cobalamin to the cubilin-amnionless receptor.
   b. Imerslund-Graesbeck syndrome associated with mutations in the cubilin receptors in Finnish patients and in the amnionless gene in Norwegian cases.
   c. Congenital defects of transcobalamin result in inadequate levels of vitamin B_{12}, bone marrow failure, and range of neurologic deficits.

6. In order to assess vitamin B_{12} stores, measure vitamin B_{12}, homocysteine, and methylmalonic acid in serum. The Schilling test can be useful to determine the origin of cobalamin deficiency.

ABSORPTION OF VARIOUS WATER-SOLUBLE VITAMINS

1. Vitamin C is transported by the Na^+-dependent vitamin C transporter (SVCT1). Critical during the perinatal period.

2. Biotin and pantothenic acid transport occurs via the Na^+-dependent multivitamin transporter (SMVT).

3. Thiamine absorption is facilitated by the thiamine transporter protein 1 (THTR1).

4. Thiamine-responsive megaloblastic anemia syndrome: rare autosomal recessive disorder associated with megaloblastic anemia, diabetes mellitus, and deafness. Associated with mutations of THTR1.

ABSORPTION OF VARIOUS FAT-SOLUBLE VITAMINS

1. All fat-soluble vitamins are absorbed by enterocytes by passive diffusion mainly (facilitated by bile salt emulsification).

2. Retinol-binding protein deficiency: rare inherited disorder; leads to ophthalmologic findings and low serum vitamin A.

3. Selective vitamin E deficiency has been identified that occurs secondary to mutations in the tocopherol transfer protein resulting in a form of spinocerebellar ataxia and undetectable serum vitamin E levels.

QUESTIONS

MATCH THE CHARACTERISTICS AND CONDITIONS:

a. Severe watery diarrhea, metabolic acidosis, and dehydration immediately after birth.
b. Failure to thrive, steatorrhea, and loss of deep tendon reflexes in infancy.
c. Hyperammonemia with high-protein diet.
d. Hyperhomocysteinemia.

1. Imerslund-Graesbeck syndrome.
2. Congenital glucose-galactose malabsorption.
3. Abetalipoproteinemia I.
4. Lysinuric protein intolerance.

MATCH THE TRANSPORTER TO ITS SUBSTRATE:

a. *GLUT2.*
b. *SGLT1.*
c. *GLUT5.*

5. Fructose.
6. Glucose and galactose.
7. Fructose, glucose, and galactose.

MATCH THE COPPER TRANSPORTER TO ITS LOCATION:

a. Liver.

b. Enterocyte.

8. Menkes syndrome copper transporter location.
9. Wilson disease copper transporter location.

CHOOSE THE BEST ANSWER:

10. Abetalipoproteinemia:
    a. Is due to an absence of microsomal triglyceride transfer protein.
    b. Is associated with liver transaminases elevation.
    c. Is not associated with enterocyte pathology.
    d. Presents in adolescence.
    e. All of the above are true.

TRUE OR FALSE:

11. There is redundancy in the transport of amino acids at both the apical and basolateral membranes of the enterocyte.

12. Menkes syndrome is inherited in an autosomal recessive fashion.

CHOOSE THE BEST ANSWER:

13. You are consulted for a newborn infant with copious watery stool output. There was polyhydramnios in utero with distended loops in the intestine and abdominal distention at birth. Stool Na is 145 meq/L with stool Cl 90 meq/L. Stool pH is 7. What is your recommendation besides replacing stool losses and rehydration?
    a. Sodium citrate and glucose electrolyte solution.
    b. KCl and NaCl supplementation to maintain normal blood pH.
    c. Glucose- and galactose-free diet.
    d. Cholestyramine.
    e. Octreotide.

14. Acrodermatitis enteropathica is associated with:
    a. Low alkaline phosphatase levels.
    b. Vesicobullous dermatitis at the perirectal and oral regions.
    c. Autosomal recessive inheritance.
    d. All of the above.
    e. None of the above.

CONGENITAL ENTEROPATHY INVOLVING INTESTINAL MUCOSAL DEVELOPMENT

SYNOPSIS

1. Criteria for intractable diarrhea of infancy:
   a. Severe life-threatening diarrhea within first 2 yr of life requiring total parenteral nutrition (TPN).
   b. Persistent villus atrophy on multiple biopsies
   c. Resistance to bowel rest and therapeutic trials.
2. Histologically, two forms:
   a. Mononuclear cell infiltrate of lamina propria: considered to be associated with T cell activation.
   b. Villous atrophy without mononuclear cell infiltrate but with specific abnormalities involving epithelium.

MICROVILLOUS ATROPHY (MICROVILLOUS INCLUSION DISEASE)

1. Usually develop severe secretory diarrhea within days of birth (but can present later with "late-onset microvillus atrophy" with less severe diarrhea).
2. Histology reveals variable degree of villous atrophy usually without inflammatory infiltrate with accumulation of periodic acid–Schiff (PAS)-positive secretory granules at the apical cytoplasm (Figure 1). Electron microscopy of small intestinal biopsies reveal absent or grossly abnormal microvilli and numerous vesicular bodies with microvillous inclusions (Figure 2). Lesion also present in large bowel. Underlying pathogenesis unclear.
3. Autosomal recessive transmission with no candidate genes yet identified.
4. Affected children have severely reduced life expectancy especially in the congenital form with 1-year survival rate < 25%.
5. Treatment: octreotide may be helpful. Parenteral nutrition (PN), but complications limit long-term survival. Intestinal transplant is only definitive treatment.

INTESTINAL EPITHELIAL DYSPLASIA (TUFTING ENTEROPATHY)

1. More common than microvillous inclusion disease (MVID), especially in patients of Arabic, Middle Eastern, and North African origin.
2. Presentation during first weeks of life with severe watery diarrhea.
3. Most with consanguineous parents or affected sibling; suggests autosomal recessive transmission. Gene yet to be identified.
4. Diarrhea persists in spite of bowel rest but at a lower level than in microvillous atrophy (MVA) or MVID. Cases reported with phenotypic abnormalities such as choanal atresia, rectal or esophageal atresia, and punctiform keratitis.
5. On histology, villous atrophy present but variable in severity. Abnormalities localized in epithelium with

formation of tufts of extruding epithelium (Figure 3). Abnormal laminin and heparin sulfate proteoglycan deposition as well as increased desmoglein described.

6. Diagnosis difficult owing to unclear appearance of the tufts and presence of activated T cells in the lamina propria, suggesting an immune-related enteropathy. Tufting at small intestine and colon. Repeated duodenal or jejunal biopsies and strict elimination of MVID may be needed for diagnosis.

7. Treatment: requires permanent PN. Indication for intestinal transplant.

SYNDROMATIC DIARRHEA
1. No family history or consanguinity.
2. Onset: first 6 mo of life, usually age < 1 mo.
3. Symptoms: watery diarrhea (50–100 cc/kg/d). Small for gestational age. Facial dysmorphism: prominent forehead, broad nose, and hypertelorism (Figure 4). Trichorrexia nodosa (woolly hair, easily pulled out, and poor pigmentation).

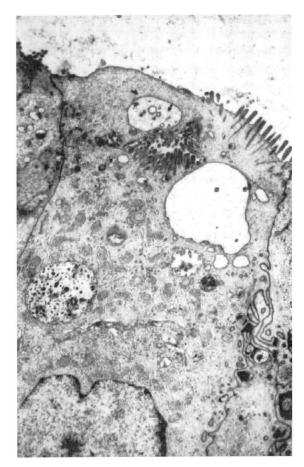

FIGURE 2 Microvillous atrophy/microvillous inclusion disease. Electron microscopy of jejunal biopsy specimen. The brush border is almost absent. The cytoplasm contains a microvillous inclusion.

4. Histology: small bowel biopsy with moderate or severe villous atrophy, variable mononuclear cell infiltration of lamina propria, and absence of epithelial abnormalities.
5. Poor prognosis: death by age 2–5 yr. Some with early-onset liver disease.
6. Laboratory test results: defective antibody responses and cytopathic responses; not fully characterized.

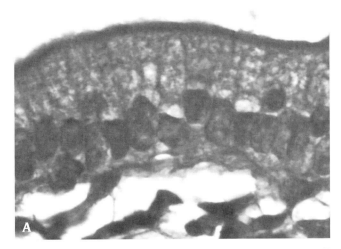
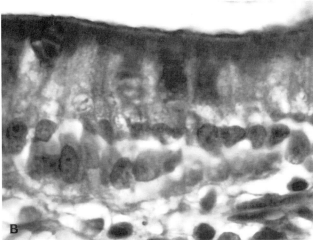

FIGURE 1 Microvillous atrophy/microvillous inclusion disease (MVA/MVID) (periodic acid–Schiff [PAS] staining; ×120 original magnification). A, Normal mucosa, normal PAS, brush border staining. B, Abnormal accumulation of PAS-positive material in the apical cytoplasm of epithelial cells in MVA/MVID.

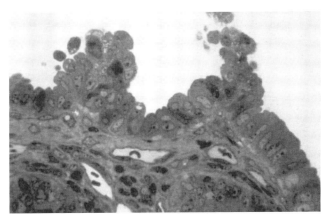

FIGURE 3 Intestinal epithelial dysplasia. Disorganization of surface epithelium showing tufts with apical rounding epithelial cells (hematoxylin and eosin; ×120 original magnification).

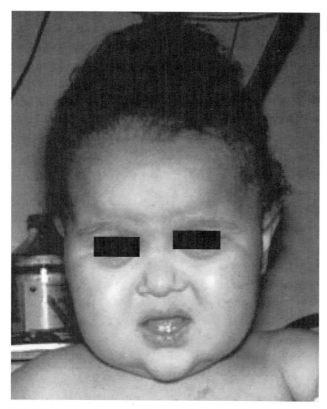

FIGURE 4 Syndromatic diarrhea. Patient with an abnormal face, a prominent forehead, a broad nose, and hypertelorism.

QUESTIONS

MATCH THE CHARACTERISTICS AND CONDITIONS:
a. Microvillous atrophy or microvillous inclusion disease.
b. Intestinal epithelial dysplasia.
c. Syndromatic diarrhea.
d. All of the above.
e. None of the above.

1. Choanal atresia and keratitis.
2. Trichorrexis nodosa.
3. Abnormal laminin and heparin sulfate deposition.
4. PAS-positive secretory granules.
5. Autosomal recessive.
6. Esophageal atresia.

CELIAC DISEASE

SYNOPSIS

1. Multifactorial disease in which environmental triggers as well as inherited factors confer susceptibility. Reaction in celiac disease is against gluten. Wheat, rye, barley, and oat contain gluten.
2. Concordance rate of monozygotic twins is 86%. Celiac disease strongly associated with human leukocyte antigen class II DQ2; 90% of cases are DQ2, 10% are DQ8. Patients usually of European ethnic origin. In white populations, 15–20% are DQ2+ and 20% DQ8+.
3. T cell–mediated chronic inflammatory bowel disorder with an autoimmune component and extraintestinal manifestations. Three prominent features:
   a. Remission highly dependent on gluten exclusion.
   b. Requires unique genetic background for antigen presentation (DQ2 or DQ8).
   c. Patients have specific circulating autoantibodies to ubiquitous transglutaminase (TG)-2 (a calcium-dependent enzyme that modifies proteins by crosslinking, transamidizing, or deamidizing specific polypeptide bound glutamines).
4. Pathogenesis model: TG-2–deamidized gluten peptides presented in the context of DQ2 or DQ8 stimulate proliferation of T cells derived from celiac patients and secretion of inflammatory cytokines, particularly interferon. B cells turn then against self TG-2 and start producing autoantibodies.

CLINICAL PRESENTATIONS

1. Typically manifests during infancy, before school age.
2. Classically, malabsorption within some months of starting a gluten-containing diet with chronic diarrhea, vomiting, and abdominal distention. Failure to thrive and proximal muscle wasting. In patients with prolonged diarrhea: hypotonia, hypoproteinemia, dehydration, hypokalemia, hypoprothrombinemia, hypocalcemia, and rickets can be seen. In older child: delayed puberty, short stature, iron deficiency anemia, and osteoporosis. Recently, later presentation with milder symptomatology seen; clinical suspicion must be high.
3. Celiac disease highly prevalent in type 1 diabetes mellitus (2–5%), in selective immunoglobulin A deficiency (10%), and Down syndrome (10%).
4. Another presentation is that of dermatitis herpetiformis (an extraintestinal manifestation). Other linked disorders include permanent-tooth enamel defects, central and peripheral nervous system involvement, liver involvement, and autoimmune diseases in general.
5. The risk for malignant complications of untreated celiac disease appears to not be as high as previously thought.

DIAGNOSTIC CRITERIA

1. Gold standard: small intestinal mucosal lesion and villous atrophy with crypt hyperplasia (Figure 1). Another characteristic is increased intraepithelial lymphocytes.

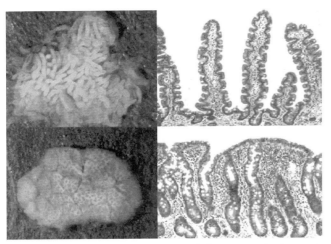

FIGURE 1 Dissection microscopic (*left*) (×50 original magnification) and histologic sections (*right*) (hematoxylin and eosin; ×280 original magnification) of small intestinal mucosal biopsy specimen with normal mucosal morphology with high villi (*upper*) and celiac disease (*lower*) (subtotal villous atrophy with crypt hyperplasia).

2. Neither repeated biopsy or gluten challenge is considered mandatory in cases with full remission with gluten withdrawal to establish the diagnosis. Individual tolerance to gluten is variable.

3. Serology (endomysial or TG-2 autoantibodies) and human leukocyte antigen (HLA)-DQ typing is helpful to diagnose celiac disease. Sensitivities and specificities of the autoantibody tests are close to 100%.

TREATMENT

A lifelong gluten-free diet is the only effective therapy. Wheat, rye, and barley products should be avoided. Oat appears not to be disease-inducing.

QUESTIONS

TRUE OR FALSE:

1. Celiac disease is frequently associated with DQ2 haplotype.
2. Small intestinal biopsy is no longer required for the diagnosis of celiac sprue.
3. Celiac disease is a T-cell–mediated inflammatory bowel disorder.
4. The most prevalent presentation of celiac disease currently is the classic presentation with severe diarrhea, malabsorption, and abdominal distention.

CHOOSE THE BEST ANSWER:

5. Celiac disease is associated with which of the following conditions:
   a. Insulin-dependent diabetes mellitus.
   b. Sjögren syndrome.
   c. Cerebral calcification.
   d. Thyroiditis.
   e. Dermatitis herpetiformis.
   f. Osteopenia.
   g. Splenic atrophy.
   h. Cow's milk sensitive enteropathy.
   i. Tooth and enamel defects.
   j. All of the above.

6. Histology associated with celiac disease includes the following:
   a. Increased villous height to crypt depth.
   b. Crypt hyperplasia.
   c. Intraepithelial lymphocyte infiltration of mucosa.
   d. All of the above.

FOOD-ALLERGIC ENTEROPATHY

SYNOPSIS

CLINICAL FEATURES

CLASSIC FOOD-SENSITIVE ENTEROPATHY

1. Most common syndrome: cow's milk enteropathy. Classic presentation: chronic diarrhea and failure to thrive. Other features: abdominal distention and perianal erythema or napkin rash. 40% also sensitive to soy, often after honeymoon toleration period of 2 weeks. Usually self-limited; most tolerate reintroduction at age 2–3 yr. Many have symptoms without immediate reactions.
2. Skin tests, immunoglobulin (Ig) E may be normal. Endoscopy: duodenal ulcer or ileal lymphoid hyperplasia.
3. Where breast milk sensitization exists, symptoms can begin very early in life. Usually failure to thrive seen in only 25%.

FOOD PROTEIN–INDUCED ENTEROCOLITIS

1. Severe, occasionally life-threatening form of mucosal food hypersensitivity. Most commonly associated with cow's milk or soy ingestion. Negative skin tests do not exclude.
2. Presentation: severe vomiting and diarrhea; also blood and mucus passage per rectum. Withdrawal of milk or soy induces remission but early rechallenge induces systemic reaction.
3. With colonoscopy, the colitis associated with food-sensitive enteropathy is milder than that seen in inflammatory bowel disease.

HISTOLOGIC FEATURES

Typically patchy, suggesting need for more than 1 biopsy. Lymphonodular hyperplasia at duodenal bulb can be found with increased intraepithelial T cells.

SPECIFIC FOODS CAUSING ENTEROPATHY SYNDROMES

1. Cow's milk, soy, hydrolysates, wheat gluten, egg, peanuts, tree nuts, and fish. Multiple food allergies have been reported.
2. One important clinical issue in the case of multiple food allergies is maintenance of a nutritionally ade-

quate diet. Pancreatic enzyme supplementation may be helpful (but should exclude cystic fibrosis first).

IMMUNOPATHOLOGY

1. Transforming growth factor β appears to be an important cytokine in preventing development of infant food allergy. Interleukin-5 and eotaxin may be important in recruitment of eosinophils.
2. At whole population level, low IgA more predictive of allergic sensitization than high IgE. Food allergy and low-grade enteropathy common in IgA-deficient adults.

DIAGNOSTIC STRATEGIES

FOOD CHALLENGE

1. Diagnostic requirement of food allergy.
    a. Response to an elimination diet.
    b. Clinically reproducible intolerance to re-exposure to food or food substance.
    c. Gold standard: double-blinded placebo-controlled food challenge (more specific for immediate allergies).
2. Challenges extended over several days in those who have delayed reactions, as in classic cow's milk–sensitive enteropathy.

SKIN PRICK TEST

1. Drop of potential antigen placed on skin and introduced into skin with lancet with positive and negative controls (histamine and saline respectively). Wheel > 3 mm indicates positive, mediated by mast cell response.
2. Atopy patch test: antigen maintained for 48 h against skin in sealed patch; skin response initially studied after 24 h. Positive test: erythema or induration mediated by T-cell response. May be more useful in measuring delayed responses.

RADIOALLERGOSORBENT TEST

1. Measures specific IgE antibodies.
2. Positive predictive value 95% for egg, milk, peanut, and fish. Tests reported on quantitative scale (0–6 with ≥ 3 predicting immediate reactions to allergen). Higher titers increase the likelihood of long-lasting sensitization.
3. Study of epitope sequences may give prognostic information with binding to linear peptide sequences predicting long-lasting allergy.

IN VITRO TESTING

Lymphocyte function tests useful only in research. Peripheral blood lymphocytes from allergic children produce a Th2 response to antigen.

MANAGEMENT OF FOOD-SENSITIVE ENTEROPATHY

1. Primary prevention: whether food allergies or food-sensitive enteropathy can be prevented by avoidance of allergies in early life is controversial.

2. Treatment of established food-sensitive enteropathy: complete exclusion of causative agent, particularly for cow's milk sensitive enteropathy (avoidance of soy also recommended).

QUESTIONS

CHOOSE THE BEST ANSWER:
1. The following is the most common food producing food-allergic enteropathy:
    a. Cow's milk.
    b. Soy.
    c. Wheat.
    d. Peanuts.
    e. Eggs.
2. The following is the gold-standard diagnostic test for food allergy:
    a. Lymphocyte function test.
    b. Skin prick test.
    c. Radioallergosorbent test.
    d. Double-blinded placebo-controlled food challenge following food elimination.
    e. None of the above.

MATCH THE AGENT TO THE ACTION:
a. Interleukin-5.
b. Transforming growth factor β.

3. Eosinophil recruitment.
4. Prevention of food allergy.

MATCH THE CELLULAR RESPONSE TO THE TEST FORMAT:
a. Mast cell response.
b. T-cell response.

5. Atopy patch testing.
6. Skin prick testing.

TRUE OR FALSE:
7. Low immunoglobulin A is more predictive of allergic food sensitization than high immunoglobulin E.
8. Peripheral blood lymphocytes from allergic children produce a Th1 response to antigen.
9. Soy protein sensitivity occurs in 75% of children with cow's milk protein sensitivity.

AUTOIMMUNE ENTEROPATHY

SYNOPSIS

THREE TYPES OF AUTOIMMUNE ENTEROPATHY

1. Autoimmune enteropathy (AIE) type 1: identical to immune dysregulation, polyendocrinopathy, enteropathy, X-linked (IPEX) syndrome.
2. AIE type 2: without extraintestinal manifestations.
3. AIE type 3: in girls.

IPEX SYNDROME

1. Rare; usually fatal during early infancy. No estimates of incidence.

2. Main clinical characteristics: combination of early-onset type 1 diabetes, severe immune-mediated enteropathy, and eczema-like dermatitis.

3. T-cell mediated disorder. Recent characterization of specific mutations in the *FOXP3* gene associated with disease.

4. Clinical presentation: IPEX is the classic, full presentation of autoimmune enteropathy. Onset of diabetes often occurs prior to gastrointestinal (GI) symptoms. Onset of diarrhea occurs within first 3 months of life. Diarrhea is usually secretory (~150 cc/kg/d) with occasional mucus or blood and stool sodium > 100 meq/L. Patients usually develop a protein-losing enteropathy with marked hypoalbuminemia. Eczema is often severe. Thyroiditis most often presents as hypothyroidism. Renal involvement described. Other involved organ systems: liver and lung.

5. Endoscopy: upper and lower endoscopies mandatory for evaluation. Entire GI tract can be involved. Endoscopic and histologic findings often do not correlate.

6. Histology: required histologic findings: combination of villous atrophy and a massive mucosal mononuclear cell infiltrate (mainly of T lymphocytes). In contrast to celiac disease, T-cell infiltration predominates in the lamina propria rather than epithelium. Mononuclear infiltrate consists mainly of CD4+ and CD25+ T lymphocytes and macrophages. Extensive GI involvement often associated with a poor outcome.

7. Laboratory findings: no pathognomonic laboratory abnormality is seen in IPEX. Clinical lab tests often in the normal range, except for signs of diabetes, protein-losing enteropathy, hypothyroidism, and cytopenia. Electrolyte disturbances seen secondary to diarrhea. Peripheral blood lymphocyte counts, T- and B-cell subsets, CD4-to-CD8 ratio, humoral immunity are normal. In contrast, IgE levels are often dramatically raised. Persistent or periodic eosinophilia frequent. Skin hypersensitivity tests are often abnormal. Autoantibodies of enterocyte or colonocyte often present, with high titers of antienterocyte, indicating poor prognosis. Indirect immunofluorescence studies demonstrate that these autoantibodies are directed against the cytoplasm of mature enterocytes with increasing intensity towards the villous tip. Antigoblet cell antibodies also seen. Also a gut- and kidney-specific antibody versus AIE75 can be seen with high specificity in IPEX patients. Multiple other circulating autoantibodies can be demonstrated (Table 1).

AIE TYPE 2: WITHOUT EXTRAINTESTINAL MANIFESTATIONS

1. Secretory diarrhea with positive antienterocyte or anticolonocyte antibodies and positive anti-AIE75 antibodies.

2. No extraintestinal manifestations.

TABLE 1   LABORATORY FINDINGS IN IPEX

BIOLOGIC PARAMETERS	FINDING IN IPEX
White blood cells	Normal; sometimes eosinophilia
CD4-to-CD8 ratio	Normal or CD4+ slightly increased
IgG, IgA, IgM	Normal
IgE	High–extremely high
Antienterocyte antibodies	Present (IgG type, sometimes IgA or IgM)
Anticolonocytes antibodies	Present (IgG type, sometimes IgA or IgM)
Antigoblet cell antibodies	Present or absent
Anti-AIE-75 antibodies	Present or absent
Anti-GAD	Present or absent
Anti-SMA	Present or absent
Anti-DNA	Present or absent
Albumin	Always (markedly) decreased
Liver enzymes	Can be increased
α_1 Antitrypsin clearance	Pathologic

AIE = autoimmune enteropathy; DNA = deoxyribonucleic acid; GAD = glutamic acid decarboxylase; Ig = immunoglobulin; IPEX = immune dysregulation, polyendocrinopathy, enteropathy, X-linked syndrome; SMA = smooth muscle antibodies.

3. *FOXP3* mutations not characteristic.

AIE TYPE 3: IN GIRLS

Rare. In most, extraintestinal autoimmune manifestations present.

DIFFERENTIAL DIAGNOSIS

1. Need to rule out primary and secondary immunodeficiencies. Thus, cellular and humoral immune functions need to be characterized.

2. IPEX has overlap with the following:
   a. Wiskott-Aldrich syndrome: eczema, thrombocytopenia, and autoimmunity. CD8+ counts are low and have a combined immune defect with recurrent bacterial infections. *WAS* gene mutations present.
   b. Autoimmune polyendocrinopathy, candidiasis, and ectodermal dystrophy (APECED) syndrome: diarrhea with malabsorption and diabetes or hypothyroidism. Symptoms occur later in life. Inherited in an autosomal recessive fashion. *AIRE* gene mutations.
   c. Omenn syndrome: erythrodermia with T-cell infiltration, lymphadenopathy, diarrhea with failure to thrive, and raised IgE with eosinophilia. B-cell counts low or zero. T-cell proliferation responses poor. Mutations in *RAG1* or *RAG2* genes.

TREATMENT AND OUTCOME

1. Mortality extremely high in IPEX. All patients initially dependent on parenteral nutrition. Currently only 2 approaches successful:
   a. Immunosuppression.
   b. Bone marrow transplant.

2. Strong immunosuppression required: steroids, tacrolimus, 6-mercaptopurine/azathioprine. Cyclosporine not entirely effective. Infliximab promising. Prophylaxis for opportunistic infections.

3. Outcome measure: cessation of secretory diarrhea, weaning from total parenteral nutrition, and restarting enteral nutrition.

QUESTIONS

TRUE OR FALSE:

1. *FOXP3* mutations are characteristic of the immune dysregulation, polyendocrinopathy, enteropathy, X-linked (IPEX) syndrome.
2. *FOXP3* mutations are not seen in autoimmune enteropathy type 2.
3. The entire gastrointestinal tract can be involved in autoimmune enteropathy.
4. In type 3 autoimmune enteropathy, extraintestinal autoimmune manifestations are not often present.
5. Cyclosporine induces remission effectively in IPEX syndrome patients.
6. Immunoglobulin A, M, and E levels are often normal in IPEX syndrome.

MATCH THE GENE TO THE SYNDROME:

a. *WAS* gene.
b. *AIRE* gene.
c. *RAG1* or *RAG2* gene.
d. *FOXP3* gene.

7. Omenn syndrome.
8. Wiskott-Aldrich syndrome.
9. Autoimmune polyendocrinopathy, candidiasis, and ectodermal dystrophy syndrome.
10. Immune dysregulation, polyendocrinopathy, enteropathy, X-linked syndrome.

INTESTINAL POLYPS AND POLYPOSIS

SYNOPSIS

POLYPS:

1. Three major presentations: bleeding, abdominal pain, and intestinal obstruction or intussusception (rarest in children).
2. Neoplastic: benign or malignant adenomas.
3. Non-neoplastic: hamartomas (juvenile), hyperplastic, and inflammatory.

JUVENILE POLYPS (COLONIC POLYPS)

1. Benign. Common during childhood, presenting with painless hematochezia during defecation. Hematochezia recurrent; present for > 3 mo in 55%.
2. Most frequent type of gastrointestinal (GI) polyp in pediatrics. Peak incidence at age 2–6 yr. Affects more males than female. Etiology unknown.
3. Gross appearance: smooth, bright red, friable surface. 90% appear pedunculated with narrow stalk. Generally 1–2 cm in diameter. Surrounding colonic chicken skin mucosa (pale yellow speckled pattern from lipid accumulation in lamina propria is seen with larger polyps at base). Microscopically: Swiss cheese appearance. Lamina propria with inflammatory cell infiltrate. No smooth muscle cells in stroma.

TABLE 1   CLASSIFICATION OF POLYPOSIS SYNDROMES

Adenomatous polyposis syndromes
  Familial adenomatous polyposis
  Gardner syndrome
  Turcot syndrome
Hamartomatous polyposis syndromes
  Juvenile polyposis
  Bannayan-Riley-Ruvalcaba syndrome
  Cowden disease
  Peutz-Jeghers syndrome
Mixed polyposis syndrome
Hyperplastic polyposis

4. Diagnosis: anorectal examination and colonoscopy. Polyps distally located (70%) and single (73%). Pancolonoscopy recommended to rule out proximal polyps.
5. Treatment: polypectomy.
6. Prognosis: recurrence rate 4–7%. Risk of cancer almost negligible. If positive family history or multiple juvenile polyps, rule out juvenile polyposis.

HYPERPLASTIC POLYPS

1. Rare in children. Single or multiple dewdrop mucosal elevations with smooth convex surface usually < 5 mm at rectosigmoid.
2. Asymptomatic.
3. Microscopically, elongated colonic crypts, papillary epithelial cell configuration, well differentiated absorptive and goblet cells.
4. No malignant potential.

ISOLATED ADENOMAS

1. Extremely rare in children.
2. Neoplastic epithelial polyps with cellular atypia, increased mitosis, and nuclear hyperchromatism. Invasive adenocarcinoma defined by extension of malignant cells through muscularis mucosa.
3. Two glandular patterns: tubular (organized glandular pattern) and villus (frond-like pattern associated with a greater risk of high-grade dysplasia and invasive cancer). If more than 75% tubular elements, then tubular adenomas; if > 75% villous, then villous adenoma.
4. Originate via gene mutation. Development of cancer requires 7–10 yr.
5. Endoscopy: dye spraying (0.5% indigo carmine) in combination with high-resolution endoscopy allows differentiation of adenomas from hyperplastic polyps. Evenly dotted or honeycomb dye pattern: hyperplastic polyp otherwise adenomatous (especially cribriform pattern).
6. Adenoma found in child: look for history of familial adenomatous polyposis and history of colorectal cancer. Requires postpolypectomy surveillance.

INFLAMMATORY POLYPS

Arise during healing phase of severe colitis after full-thickness ulceration.

TABLE 2   POLYPOSIS SYNDROMES AFFECTING CHILDREN

SYNDROME TYPE	GENE	CLINICAL FEATURE	CANCER RISK
Adenomatous			
Familial adenomatous polyposis (MIM 175100)	*APC*	GI polyposis, CHRPE	Colon 100%, periampullary thyroid, hepatoblastoma, other
Gardner syndrome	*APC*	Colon adenomas, desmoids, dental anomalies, osteomas, epidermal cysts	As for FAP above
Attenuated FAP	*APC*	Reduced adenomas number	Colon
Turcot syndrome type II (BTPS) (MIM 276300)	*APC*	GI adenomas, CNS tumors	Colon, brain
Hamartomatous			
Peutz-Jeghers syndrome (MIM 175200)	*LKB1/STK11*	GI hamartomas, mucocutaneous pigmentation	GI tract, pancreas, ovary, breast, cervix, testicle
Juvenile polyposis (MIM 174900, 601299)	*SMAD4, MPSH, BMPR1A*	Colon/stomach hamartomas, congenital heart disease, cleft lip/palatine, malrotation	Colon, stomach, duodenum, pancreas
PTEN hamartoma tumor syndromes			
Cowden disease (MIM 158350)	*PTEN*	GI hamartomas, macrocephaly, mucocutaneous pigmentation, thyroid disease, fibrocystic breast disease, endometrial fibroids, urinary/uterine abnormalities	Breast, thyroid, skin
Bannayan-Riley-Ruvalcaba syndrome (MIM 601728)	*PTEN*	GI hamartomas, macrocephaly, speckled penis	Breast, thyroid

BTPS = brain tumor polyposis syndrome; CHRPE = congenital hypertrophy of the retinal pigment epithelium; CNS = central nervous system; FAP = familial adenomatous polyposis; GI = gastrointestinal.

INHERITED ADENOMATOUS POLYPOSIS SYNDROMES

FAMILIAL ADENOMATOUS POLYPOSIS AND GARDNER SYNDROME

1. Auto dominant syndrome.
2. Progressive development of hundreds to thousands of adenomatous polyps in the colon arising from germline mutation of the adenomatous polyposis coli (*APC*) gene 5q21.
3. Average age of colorectal cancer 39 yr.
4. *APC* limits gene transcription and cell proliferation via control of the Wnt-1 signaling pathway. Mutations deregulate this pathway with initiation and promotion of tumorigenesis. Additional early activation of oncogenes synergize with *APC* mutations to trigger chromosomal instability.
5. Extracolonic manifestations: those without extracolonic manifestations have familial adenomatous polyposis, those with have Gardner syndrome (Table 3).
6. Diagnosis: presence of 100 or more adenomatous polyps. In children, if even 1 adenoma is found, workup should be performed. Also, in at-risk individuals the presence of > 3 pigmented ocular fundic lesions confirms diagnosis.
7. For at-risk individuals, if *APC* gene mutation is present, start annual colonoscopic surveillance at age 10–12 yr. If not present, start at age 25 yr. If genotyping not available, start flexible sigmoidoscopy or colonoscopy at age 10–12 yr then q2yr until age 35 yr then as per standard risk. If upper GI (UGI) polyps: esophagogastroduodenoscopy and UGI series q3-4yr. After colectomy, if retained rectum or J pouch, flexible sigmoidoscopy q6mo to 1–2 yr. Annual physical exam and routine blood testing mandatory.

TABLE 3   EXTRACOLONIC FEATURES IN FAP

CANCERS (LIFETIME RISK)	OTHER LESIONS
Duodenal (1–5%)	CHRPE
Pancreatic (2%)	Nasopharyngeal angiofibromas
Thyroid (2%)	Osteomas
Brain (medulloblastoma) (< 1%)	Radiopaque jaw lesions
Hepatoblastoma (0.7% of children < 5 yr old)	Dental abnormalities
	Lipomas, fibromas, epidermoid cysts
	Desmoid tumors
	Gastric adenomas/fundic gland polyps
	Duodenal, jejunal, ileal adenomas

CHRPE = congenital hypertrophy of the retinal pigment epithelium; FAP = familial adenomatous polyposis.
Adapted from Cruz-Correa M, Giardello FM. Diagnosis and management of hereditary colon cancer. Gastroenterol Clin North Am 2002;31:537–49.

8. Treatment: colectomy for high dysplasia, > 200 polyps, polyp size > 10 mm. Ileal pouch anal anastomosis (IPAA): risk of postoperative complications, worse functional outcome, and risk of adenomas at ileal pouch. For UGI polyps: duodenal resection. In patients with desmoid tumors, perform colectomy in one stage. Nonselective or selective COX2 inhibitors: reduces number and size of adenomas but does not prevent development; not effective for UGI polyps.

Variants of Familial Adenomatous Polyposis

1. Attenuated adenomatous polyposis coli (AAPC) characterized by multiple adenomas, late onset of cancer and frequent absence of extracolonic features. Fundic gland polyps and duodenal polyps more prominent than colonic polyps.
2. Turcot syndrome: multiple colonic adenomas associated with primary brain tumor.
   a. Type I: patients with glioblastomas and germline mutations in mismatch repair genes.
   b. Type II: more common. Germline mutations of *APC* and medulloblastoma.

HAMARTOMATOUS POLYPOSIS SYNDROMES

JUVENILE POLYPOSIS COLI

1. Most common of hamartomatous syndromes characterized by multiple GI polyps in absence of extraintestinal features. Criteria: ≥ 3 juvenile polyps of colon, polyposis involving entire GI tract. or any number of polyps in proband with known family history of juvenile polyps.
2. Autosomal dominant inheritance with variable penetrance.
3. Juvenile polyposis of stomach without intestinal polyps may be regarded as a separate clinical entity. Patients have anemia and hypoproteinemia. Most require gastrectomy; may have increased risk of gastric cancer.
4. In children, symptoms include rectal bleeding and prolapse, crampy abdominal pain, and intussusception. Most present 2–12 yrs. In most cases, polyps only in colon. Association with birth defects in 15% (malrotation, genitourinary, and cardiac defects).

5. Genetics: subsets have mutations in *PTEN* (tumor suppressor gene). *SMAD4* (transduces signals from transforming growth factor [TGF]-β ligands that regulate cell proliferation, differentiation, and death) and *BMPR1A* mutations shown to cause juvenile polyposis.
6. Malignant potential, but less than with familial adenomatous polyps. Screen first-degree relatives starting at age 10 yr if asymptomatic. Regular screenings with colonoscopy q2 yr. If unable to control symptoms or polyps too numerous, consider colectomy. Insufficient data to justify prophylactic colectomy.

PHOSPHATASE AND TENSIN HOMOLOG HAMARTOMA TUMOR SYNDROMES

1. Includes Cowden disease (CD) and Bannayan-Riley-Ruvalcaba syndrome (BRRS). Germline mutations in *PTEN* account for 80% of CD and 60% of BRRS. *PTEN* signals apoptosis and mediates cellular growth arrest, regulating cell survival pathways.
2. Cowden disease: autosomal dominant (with great variation, age-related penetrance), characterized by multiple hamartomas that affect all 3 germ layers with increased risk of breast, thyroid, and endometrial neoplasias. 10–50% familial. No increase in risk of invasive GI cancers. GI polyposis should be addressed with endoscopic surveillance. Screening for breast and thyroid cancers should begin in teenage years.
3. Bannayan-Riley-Ruvalcaba syndrome: hamartomatous polyposis associated with macrocephaly, speckled or freckled penis, delayed development in childhood, lipomatosis, and hemangiomatosis.

PEUTZ-JEGHERS SYNDROME

1. Hamartomatous GI polyposis syndrome associated with risk of GI and extraintestinal cancers.
2. Clinical presentation: skin pigmentation with small macules clustered around mouth, eyes, nostrils, perianal area, and buccal mucosa; occurs before GI polyps, often fades with age except buccal mucosa lesions persist. One-third have symptoms in first decade with 50–60% before 20 y. Commonly present with abdominal pain secondary to obstruction with polyp intussusception or GI bleeding. Peutz-Jeghers syndrome (PJS) polyps pref-

TABLE 4   SURVEILLANCE GUIDELINES FOR PEUTZ-JEGHERS SYNDROME

SITE	PROCEDURE	ONSET (YR)	INTERVAL (YR)
Stomach	Upper endoscopy	10	2
Small bowel	Small bowel follow-through	10	2*
Colon	Pancolonoscopy	10	2*
Breast	Breast examination	25	1
	Mammography	25	2–3
Testicle	Testicular examination	10	1
Ovary	Uterus pelvic examination	20	1
	Pelvic ultrasonography	12	1
Pancreas	Endoscopic ultrasonography (if available) or abdominal ultrasonography	30	1–2

*May consider lengthening interval based on clinical history.

erentially located in small intestine or equally distributed at GI tract. Polyps grow to a very large size and are often pedunculated, especially at small bowel.

3. Pathology: there is hyperplasia of the smooth muscle later in PJS polyps.
4. Genetics: germline mutations in *STK11* gene in 70% of PJS families, 50% of sporadic PJS patients. *STK11* involved in cell proliferation and apoptosis. Marked phenotypic variability of expression in PJS families.
5. Cancer risk: risk of cancer both at GI and extraintestinal sites increased in adults with PJS. Extraintestinal cancers include pancreatic, gonadal, and breast cancer.
6. Therapy: surveillance (Table 4). Polyps > 1.5 cm should be resected.

OTHER POLYPOSIS SYNDROMES

BOURNEVILLE TUBEROUS SCLEROSIS
1. Auto dominant disease with variable penetrance.
2. Mutations seen at tuberous sclerosis loci 1 and 2.
3. Classic triad of mental retardation, epilepsy, and adenoma sebaceum in the presence of hamartoma lesions. Hamartomatous polyps resembling PJS polyps and adenomatous polyps may occur, usually at distal colon.

HEREDITARY MIXED POLYPOSIS SYNDROME
Characterized by atypical juvenile polyps with mixed features of hamartomas and adenomas at colon with risk of colorectal cancer.

HYPERPLASTIC POLYPOSIS
Uncommon condition with large number of hyperplastic polyps throughout colon.

QUESTIONS

MATCH THE CHARACTERISTICS AND CONDITIONS:
a. Hamartomatous.
b. Adenomatous.

1. Gardner syndrome.
2. Bannayan-Riley-Ruvalcaba syndrome.
3. Juvenile polyposis coli.
4. Cowden disease.
5. Turcot syndrome.
6. Familial adenomatous polyposis.
7. Peutz-Jeghers syndrome.

a. *PTEN.*
b. *APC.*
c. *SMAD4.*

8. Juvenile polyposis coli.
9. Familial adenomatous polyposis.
10. Bannayan-Riley-Ruvalcaba syndrome.
11. Cowden disease.

a. Freckling at glans penis.
b. Orocutaneous freckling.
c. Follicular thyroid carcinoma.
d. Medulloblastoma.
e. Congenital hypertrophy of retinal pigment epithelium.
f. Epilepsy.
g. Glioblastoma.

12. Cowden disease.
13. Bannayan-Riley-Ruvalcaba syndrome.
14. Peutz-Jeghers syndrome.
15. Turcot syndrome type II.
16. Gardner syndrome.
17. Bourneville tuberous sclerosis.
18. Turcot syndrome type I.

OTHER NEOPLASMS

SYNOPSIS

BENIGN INTESTINAL TUMORS
Adenomas are the most common benign tumors followed by leiomyomas and lipomas.
1. Adenomas and lipomas found primarily in the colon but can also appear at small intestine. Present with lower tract bleeding or abdominal pain or intussusception.
2. Leiomyomas more common in the proximal gut, with only isolated case reports of colonic involvement.

ADENOCARCINOMA OF THE INTESTINE

CARCINOMA OF THE COLON
1. Cumulative lifetime risk 6%. In United States, more common in blacks than whites until age 60 yr (Table 1).
2. Most common primary malignant solid tumor of the intestinal tract in childhood. In children, male-to-female ratio 1.5:1. No apparent increase in juvenile colorectal cancers among children with a family history of colorectal cancer.
3. In inflammatory bowel disease, cancer is a complication. In ulcerative colitis, total duration of colitis is an important risk determinant with the risk of colorectal cancer increasing by 0.5–1%/year after the first 8–10 yr of disease. Cancer risk also proportional to disease extent (highest in pancolitis). Similar colorectal cancer predictors in Crohn disease proportional to extent of colonic involvement and duration of disease. In ulcerative colitis, cancers occur at site of active or prior inflammation, while in Crohn disease, one-third of gastrointestinal (GI) cancers occur at grossly normal bowel segments.
4. Hereditary polyposis carries a high risk for colon cancer, especially familial adenomatous polyposis and Gardner syndrome.
5. Hamartomatous polyp syndromes (eg, Peutz-Jeghers syndrome) are also associated with increased risk for colon cancer.

TABLE 1   CONDITIONS ASSOCIATED WITH COLON CARCINOMA

ENVIRONMENTAL FACTORS
Diet high in calories, fat, and cholesterol and low in fiber
Exposure to radiation or chemicals

DISEASES WITH HERITABLE COMPONENTS
Inflammatory bowel disease (ulcerative colitis, Crohn disease)
Polyposis syndromes: (familial polyposis coli, Gardner syndrome, juvenile polyposis, Peutz-Jeghers syndrome)
Hereditary syndromes without polyposis (Lynch I, Lynch II, familial predisposition to adenoma formation)

ACQUIRED DISEASES
Association with previous ureterosigmoidostomy
Bacteremia or endocarditis secondary to *Streptococcus bovis* infection

6. Autosomal dominant inheritance of a propensity towards development of colon cancer is also seen in the Lynch syndromes (hereditary nonpolyposis colorectal cancers). Two types: type I, hereditary site-specific colon cancer (increased incidence for colon cancer only), and type II, cancer family syndrome (increased risk for extracolonic and colonic adenocarcinomas).

7. Antecedent ureterosigmoidostomy associated with increased risk of colon cancer: requires annual colonoscopy beginning 5–6 yr after surgery.

8. *Streptococcus bovis* bacteremia and bacterial endocarditis associated with colon cancer in adults, but not yet reported in children.

9. Associated genetic mutations:
   a. *APC, DCC,* and *MCC. APC* and *MCC* on chromosome 5q (early role in adenoma to carcinoma sequence). *DCC* on chromosome 18q (intermediate stage of carcinogenesis).
   b. *K-ras*: plays role in intermediate stage of carcinogenesis.
   c. *TP53*: plays role in late carcinogenesis.
   d. *hMLH1, hMSH2, hPMS1, hPMS2, hMSH6, hMLH3*: mismatch repair genes.

10. Pathology: in adults, cancers more common in rectum and left colon; childhood and adolescent colon cancers are more evenly distributed through the large intestine. Mucinous (50%) and signet ring (10%) histology are found in higher proportion of pediatric cases. Cancers grow locally with regional dissemination to the lymphatics followed by distal metastasis.

11. Duke classification: A limited to mucosa, B1 extended into muscularis propria, B2 penetrated bowel wall through serosa but no lymph node involvement, C1 limited to bowel wall and lymph nodes, C2 penetration of bowel wall and lymph nodes, and D distant metastases. Younger patients tend to have more advanced carcinoma stages at diagnosis.

12. Clinical features: abdominal pain (95% of cases).

13. Diagnosis: colonoscopy, since carcinomas distributed throughout the colon. Staging requires imaging studies. Use of molecular markers (CEA and Carbohydrate 19-9 antigen) not well studied in children.

14. Treatment: primary treatment is surgery with wide resection, removal of lymphatic drainage. Resection of omentum, ovaries should be considered owing to high rate of recurrence at these sites from lymphatic spread. Adjuvant and primary chemotherapy of little benefit in young patients with colon cancer. Radiation therapy success needs further study. Overall, prognosis dismal in children: 5 yr survival rate of < 3%.

ADENOCARCINOMA OF THE SMALL INTESTINE
Adenocarcinomas of the small intestine in childhood should prompt search for underlying predisposition (eg. Peutz-Jeghers syndrome, Gardner syndrome, or small bowel Crohn disease). Contrast studies remain the primary investigative tool.

INTESTINAL LYMPHOMA

1. Lymphoma is third most common malignant neoplasm of children in United States. Primary GI lymphoma occurs in < one-half of all patients with non-Hodgkin lymphoma. In children, most common sites of involvement: distal ileum, cecum, and appendix. Male-to-female ratio 2:1 in children.

2. Childhood lymphomas have 3 main categories: small noncleaved cell (Burkitt v. non-Burkitt lymphoma), large cell, and lymphoblastic.

3. Risk factors: inherited (ataxia-telangiectasia, Wiskott-Aldrich syndrome, common variable immunodeficiency, X-linked lymphoproliferative syndrome with Epstein-Barr virus infection, or severe combined immunodeficiency) or acquired (post-transplant) immunodeficiency states.

4. In adults, T-cell lymphomas seen in celiac disease. Also reported in isolated children with celiac disease.

5. *C-myc* oncogene alterations seen in Burkitt lymphoma.

6. Clinical features: children present with abdominal pain and distention, change in bowel habits, and nausea and vomiting. Ileocecal intussusception seen given localization to the terminal ileum, cecum, and appendix. Bone marrow involvement in one-third. Mandibular and central nervous system (CNS) involvement common in endemic Burkitt lymphoma.

7. Diagnosis: biopsy for histopathology, immunophenotype, and cytogenetics. Bone marrow biopsy may be needed. Formal staging should be performed urgently in order to start therapy given the rapid progression of disease. Serum lactate dehydrogenase appears to correlate with tumor burden.

8. Treatment: Resection with associated mesentery and lymph nodes. Chemotherapy required with or without CNS therapy depending on tumor burden. Patients with large tumor burden are at risk for tumor lysis, requiring allopurinol, hydration, and urinary alkalinization.

9. Prognosis: with exclusive abdominal disease, 95% cure expected with resection or chemotherapy. Bone marrow involvement associated with poorer prognosis.

IMMUNOPROLIFERATIVE SMALL INTESTINAL DISEASE

1. Occurs in the Mediterranean basin, Iran, Pakistan, Taiwan, and South Africa.
2. Proliferation of immunoglobulin A (IgA)-secreting B lymphocytes throughout the small intestine. High levels of IgA heavy chains can be detected in serum.
3. Most occur in patients aged 10–40 yr in poor sanitation conditions. Present with malabsorption, protein-losing enteropathy, weight loss, and abdominal pain.
4. Diffuse infiltrate of plasma cells present throughout lamina propria of the small intestine. In advanced disease, a large cell lymphoma can develop.
5. Treatment: early antibiotics may induce remission. Advanced stages are treated with surgery, radiation therapy, and chemotherapy.

LEIOMYOSARCOMA

Intestinal leiomyosarcoma extremely rare in childhood. One-half of cases occur during infancy; minority of cases affect the GI tract. Slight female predominance. Presentation: intestinal bleeding, bowel obstruction, and intussusception.

QUESTIONS

TRUE OR FALSE:

1. Adenomas are the most common benign intestinal tumor.
2. Colon cancer is most common in the Caucasian population in the United States.
3. Childhood colon cancer is responsive to adjuvant chemotherapy.
4. Intestinal lymphoma occurs most commonly at the ileocecal area in children.
5. Colon cancer occurring in Crohn disease can occur at sites where there has not been intestinal inflammation.

CHOOSE THE BEST ANSWER:

6. Which of the following are associated with colon cancer development?
   a. Crohn disease.
   b. Antecedent ureterosigmoidostomy.
   c. Peutz-Jeghers syndrome.
   d. Diet low in fiber.
   e. All of the above.

7. Immunoproliferative small intestinal disease is prevalent in all of the following areas except:
   a. Taiwan.
   b. Iran.
   c. Mediterranean basin.
   d. South Africa.
   e. Mexico.

MATCH THE STAGE OF CARCINOGENESIS TO THE GENE AFFECTED AND ACTIVE IN CARCINOGENESIS DURING THAT PERIOD:

A. Early carcinogenesis.
B. Intermediate carcinogenesis.
C. Late carcinogenesis.

8. APC.
9. TP53.
10. K-ras.
11. DCC.

IDIOPATHIC CONSTIPATION

SYNOPSIS

Constipation is idiopathic when it cannot be explained by anatomic, physiologic, radiologic, or histopathologic abnormalities.

NORMAL STOOL FREQUENCY

1. First week of life: 4/d.
2. 1 yr: 2/d.
3. Normal adult: 3/d to 3/wk; generally attained by age 4 yr.

NORMAL DEFECATION

1. The internal and external anal sphincters surrounding the anal canal form an angle with the puborectalis muscle (85°–105° at rest). Stool is propelled into the anorectum during defecation, where rectal distention results in reflex relaxation of the internal anal sphincter with simultaneous external sphincter contraction until defecation is socially appropriate.
2. At the time of defecation, increased intrarectal pressure moves feces toward the anal canal, the puborectalis muscle relaxes straightening the anorectal angle, inhibiting the external anal sphincter and allowing fecal evacuation.
3. Voluntary contraction of the puborectalis muscle and external anal sphincter decreases the anorectal angle < 85°–105°, which prevents defecation.

ETIOLOGY AND PATHOGENESIS OF CONSTIPATION

1. Multiple factors: decrease in propulsive forces, impaired rectal sensation, or functional outlet obstruction.
2. Family history in 40% of cases; concordance 6 times higher in identical versus fraternal twins.
3. Believed that most childhood chronic constipation results from stool withholding. In toddlers: coercive or inappropriately early toilet training may contribute. In older children, retention initiated by situations making stooling inconvenient or uncomfortable; subsequent stretching leads to an atonic and desensitized rectum.

ENCOPRESIS

1. When large stool volumes stretch the rectum, the internal anal sphincter relaxes and anal canal is short-

ened. The external anal sphincter is eventually unable to function adequately to prevent defecation and stool leakage occurs.
2. Rarely occurs in those aged < 3 yr; often resolves spontaneously before late adolescence.

CLINICAL SIGNS AND SYMPTOMS
1. Longer intervals between bowel movements may be the only complaint.
2. Abdominal pain, anorexia, vomiting, abdominal distention, excessive flatulence, blood-streaked stools, enuresis, and recurrent urinary tract infections.

DIFFERENTIAL DIAGNOSIS
1. Hirschsprung disease (colonic aganglionosis).
2. Short-segment Hirschsprung disease can present with fecal soiling, usually much less severe than from rectal impaction.

INVESTIGATIONS
1. Plain abdominal radiograph: to establish fecal impaction.
2. Barium enema: unprepped to detect a transition zone indicative of Hirschsprung disease.
3. Anorectal manometry: detects anomalies of defecatory function and threshold for rectal sensation and internal sphincter relaxation; screens for Hirschsprung disease (see section on Hirschsprung disease) and anismus (paradoxical contraction of external anal sphincter and puborectalis during defecation).
4. Anal sphincter electromyography: performed at the time of manometry, evaluates activity of the external anal sphincter and puborectalis muscles.
5. Defecography: radiographic means of studying defecation dynamics. Owing to radiation exposure, not used routinely in children.
6. Colorectal transit studies: Hinton technique: 20 radiopaque markers ingested on first day with daily radiographs for up to 7 days until all are expelled. Most normal adults pass 80% of the markers within 5 days. Modification in this technique: 20 markers on each day for 3 days followed by radiogaphy on days 4 and 7. Upper limit of normal for total colonic transit time: 68 h in adults and 50–62 h in children. Allows differentiation of slow-transit constipation, holdup in the left colon and rectosigmoid, and those with normal colonic transit time.
7. Colonic manometry: can precisely evaluate colonic motor function.
8. Rectal biopsy: in patients in whom Hirschsprung disease strongly suspected. Also can identify intestinal neuronal dysplasia, hyperganglionosis, and hypoganglionosis.

TREATMENT
1. Infants on breast milk with infrequent stooling: if healthy, secondary to almost complete absorption of breast milk with little residue for stool formation.
2. Infants with simple, acute constipation: dietary measures (increase in fluid and carbohydrate intake). Karo syrup helpful. If anal fissure develops, treat promptly with ointment to reduce friction during stool passage. Older infants may increase sorbitol-containing fluids or be prescribed an osmotic laxative. Mineral oil–based therapies may be used in children > 6 mo without neurologic or gag deficit or history of vomiting. Senna and polyethylene glycol therapies useful.
3. Toddlers: usually respond to increased fluids and increased sorbitol and fiber intake. Explanation of stool withholding behaviors should be performed. Clean-out therapies with enemas may be necessary followed by stool softeners and establishment of a regular bowel habit. Therapy should be continued for 4–6 mo.
4. Patients with continued problems without withholding: evaluate further for organic disease, including serum calcium, thyroid function test, and antiendomysial titer evaluation. Anorectal manometry or barium enema to exclude Hirschsprung disease and defecation and anatomic abnormalities. Consider colonic manometry to exclude occult myopathy or neuropathy; magnetic resonance imaging of the lumbosacral spine to exclude occult spinal cord abnormalities.
5. Patients with emotional disturbances: should be treated by a psychiatrist or behavioralist.
6. Biofeedback: based on operant conditioning, learning through reinforcement. Sensory retraining can be done, as well as learning how to relax the external anal sphincter during defecation in those with anismus. May be effective in a subpopulation with abnormal defecation dynamics on anorectal manometry.
7. Surgical treatment: anorectal myectomy and proctocolectomy for some adults with intractable constipation with a very high complication rate. Myectomy should be reserved for those with ultrashort-segment Hirschsprung disease. The Malone appendicocecostomy for antegrade colonic enemas may be used to manage children with intractable constipation. Cecostomies may also be placed endoscopically.

PROGNOSIS
1. Long-term outcome not well established.
2. Mineral oil and close monitoring helpful in most cases.
3. Early onset of constipation, family history of constipation, and long duration of symptoms prior to referral to a gastroenterologist may predict poor outcome.

QUESTIONS

TRUE OR FALSE:
1. Straightening of the anorectal angle prevents defecation.
2. Most childhood constipation results from stool withholding behaviors.
3. Encopresis often occurs in children < 2 years old.

CHOOSE BEST ANSWER:

4. Anorectal manometry can detect the following abnormal defecation problems:
   a. Long-segment Hirschsprung disease.
   b. Short-segment Hirschsprung disease.
   c. Anismus.
   d. Poor rectal sensation.
   e. All of the above.

5. All of the following medical recommendations or therapies are correct for the treatment of idiopathic constipation in children except:
   a. In otherwise healthy breastfed infants, reassurance should be given regarding infrequent stooling.
   b. Mineral oil–based therapies are useful in children > 6 mo without neurologic problems or a history of vomiting.
   c. Toddler withholding behaviors should be explained to the family.
   d. Patients with continued problems in the absence of withholding behaviors should be reassured.
   e. All of the above are correct.

6. The following predict poor outcome for idiopathic constipation except:
   a. Late referral to a gastroenterologist.
   b. Early onset of constipation.
   c. Family history of constipation.
   d. Long duration of symptoms.
   e. All of the above are predictive of poor outcome.

DYSMOTILITIES

SYNOPSIS

1. Dysmotility diseases classification:
   a. Primary visceral myopathies.
   b. Primary visceral neuropathies.
   c. Secondary to toxic, metabolic, infectious, or systemic disorders affecting smooth muscle or the enteric or extrinsic nervous system.
2. Clinical symptoms: variable and nonspecific. Location of affected bowel is more important determinant of clinical manifestation than underlying cause. Common symptoms: abdominal distention, constipation, vomiting, failure to thrive, dyspepsia, abdominal pain, and intermittent diarrhea (secondary to bacterial overgrowth, malabsorption). Within the same family, a spectrum of symptoms may occur.
3. Intestinal dysmotilities less frequently caused by smooth muscle than by neural disorders. Symptoms more severe and prognosis worse in primary myopathies than primary neuropathies. Definitive diagnosis requires full thickness gastrointestinal (GI) wall biopsy.

PRIMARY VISCERAL MYOPATHIES

1. Five histologic phenotypes. Clinically, four types described. May begin at any age, but especially at second decade.
2. Familial visceral myopathy (FVM) type 1: autosomal dominant. Affects females more than males in frequency and severity. Characterized by dilated esophagus, elongated megaduodenum, and redundant, dilated colon. Bladder affected in one-half of cases. Most symptomatic around puberty. 10% develop pseudo-obstruction. Histology: marked thinning, degeneration, and vacuolation of smooth muscle replaced by fibrous tissue. Treatment: dietary modification and intermittent use of antibiotics to treat bacterial overgrowth; surgical therapy indicated if refractory to dietary and medical management and in pseudo-obstruction.
3. FVM type 2: mitochondrial neurogastrointestinal encephalomyopathy. Autosomal recessive. Phenotypic features: external ophthalmoplegia with ptosis and diplopia, cardiac conduction defect, mild muscular atrophy, and dilatation of the entire GI tract with scattered small intestinal diverticula. GI symptoms develop during teenage years. Skeletal muscle biopsy shows typical ragged red fibers of mitochondrial myopathies. Deficiency of cytochrome-c oxidase has been demonstrated and lactate is often elevated. Histology: similar to FVM type 1. Prognosis: poor. Treatment: most require total parenteral nutrition (TPN).
4. FVM type 3: dilatation of entire GI tract without extraintestinal manifestations. Autosomal recessive. Prognosis poor.
5. FVM type 4: characterized by gastroparesis, tubular narrow small intestine, normal esophagus, and normal colon. Symptoms occur as early as age 2 yr. Hypertrophy of circular muscle layer seen. Autosomal recessive.
6. Familial childhood visceral myopathy with diffuse abnormal muscle layering: X-linked inheritance. Present during neonatal period. Short gut and malrotation present. Striking histologic finding: extracircular muscle coat between the outer and inner layer of muscularis propria with the myenteric plexus embedded.
7. Sporadic infantile or childhood visceral myopathy: most cases sporadic. Most children develop symptoms at birth or within first year. Distal to esophagus, entire GI tract is markedly dilated. Almost all have involvement of urinary tract system with megaureters and megacystis (hollow visceral myopathy). Histology: gross fibrosis of muscularis propria and profound atrophy of smooth muscle. Prognosis poor in diffuse disease.
8. African degenerative leiomyopathy: distinctive, nonfamilial form of degenerative visceral myopathy occurring largely in Africa (southern, eastern, and central Africa). Histology: myocyte atrophy with vacuolated cytoplasm, extracellular edema, and fibrous replacement in the circular muscle layer. Presentation at mean 9.5 yr: bowel dilatation, severe constipation, and pseudo-obstruction; bladder involvement in 10%.

Therapy: neostigmine, low-residue diet, laxatives, enema, and surgical intervention.

9. Megacystic-microcolon-intestinal hypoperistalsis syndrome: most severe form of pseudo-obstruction. Female-to-male ratio 4:1. Nonobstructive bladder enlargement, dilated, aperistaltic proximal small bowel, narrowed distal small bowel, and malrotated microcolon located entirely on the left side of the abdomen, usually present after birth. Occasional megaesophagus. Intestinal length shortened to ⅓ normal. Caused by a myopathy with vacuolar degenerative changes of smooth muscle cells. Phenotype can also be a manifestation of neuropathy with hypo- or hyperganglionosis or giant ganglia. Autosomal recessive suggested but most cases sporadic. Absence of a subunit of the nicotinic acetylcholine receptor may play a role. Prognosis poor. Most die in first year owing to renal insufficiency, postoperative complications, or sepsis. Must be differentiated from prune belly sequence (disorder affects mainly males with dilated abdomen, constipation, hydronephrosis, and megacystis with malrotation but no intestinal hypoperistalsis or microcolon).

SECONDARY MYOPATHIES
Most described in adults as may take several years of disease process to damage intestinal smooth muscle.

CONNECTIVE TISSUE DISORDERS
1. Scleroderma or progressive systemic sclerosis is a systemic disease characterized by excessive collagen deposition in skin and in multiple internal organs. Associated with prominent and severe alterations of microvasculature, autonomic nervous system, and immune system. GI involvement in 50%; affects most patients with diffuse systemic sclerosis, less often patients with calcinosis, Raynaud phenomenon, esophageal dysmotility, sclerodactyly, and telangiectasias (CREST).
2. Motility abnormalities: 75–90% at esophagus, 50–70% at anorectum, and 40% at small bowel. Fecal incontinence is most common colonic presentation of systemic sclerosis. Lesions similar throughout GI tract with atrophy, fragmentation of muscularis propria, collagen infiltration, and fibrosis in late stage of disease.
3. Findings more marked in circular than longitudinal layer. Manometry in scleroderma may show complete absence of the migrating motor complex (MMC), predisposing to bacterial overgrowth and bezoar formation. In early stage, MMCs can be generated by octreotide, cisapride, or erythromycin.
4. Treatment: supportive and symptomatic.
5. GI dysmotilities also seen in patients with Ehlers-Danlos syndrome, dermatomyositis, polymyositis, and mixed connective tissue disease. Smooth muscle dysfunction with bowel dilatation can be seen in lupus and result from vasculitis.

CHRONIC ENTERIC MYOSITIS AND AUTOIMMUNE MYOPATHY
Infiltration of intestinal smooth muscle layer by lymphocytes found in Crohn disease and other forms of chronic intestinal inflammation associated with altered motility. Acquired myositis of muscularis propria and antibodies against smooth muscle reported.

MUSCULAR DYSTROPHY
1. Myotonic muscular dystrophy: progressive systemic disease with myotonia and skeletal muscle wasting. Involvement of smooth muscle of GI tract and bladder well documented. Histology of small intestine and colonic smooth muscle: muscle being replaced by fat. Motor abnormalities found in entire GI tract.
2. Duchenne muscular dystrophy (X-linked disorder with skeletal and cardiac muscle degeneration leading to progressive weakness, death from respiratory failure): myofiber degeneration and accumulation of fat and connective tissue and hypertrophy of the remaining muscle on histology. Cause: deficiency of dystrophin. Visceral smooth muscle involvement of GI tract can be detected by manometry.

DISORDERS OF THE ENTERIC AND AUTONOMOUS NERVOUS SYSTEM
1. The enteric nervous system (ENS) functions independently of the central nervous system. The myenteric plexus is located between the longitudinal and circular muscle layers and provides motor innervation. The submucosal plexus lies in the submucosa between the circular muscle layer and muscularis mucosae and is important in regulating secretory control.
2. The ENS controls segmental, propagating contractions, exocrine and endocrine secretions, microcirculation, and immune processes at the GI tract.
3. Intestinal neuronal dysplasia: describes different qualitative (immature or heterotopic ganglia) or quantitative (hypo- and hyperganglionosis) abnormalities of the ENS. Reported in all age groups. No histologic or clinical or genetic definitions; the term should be used with caution.

PRIMARY VISCERAL NEUROPATHIES

FAMILIAL VISCERAL NEUROPATHY
1. Familial visceral neuropathy (FVN) without extraintestinal manifestations: autosomal dominant disorder affecting large and distal small bowel. Symptoms develop after infancy. Main complaints: severe slow-transit constipation. Pseudo-obstructive episodes occur in one-half of cases. No evidence of extrinsic autonomic dysfunction. Histology: markedly reduced number and degeneration of argyrophilic neurons and nerves in the myenteric plexus with hypertrophy of smooth muscle. No inflammatory cells or intranuclear inclusions observed. Subtotal colectomy contraindicated as may accelerate small bowel disease.
2. FVN with neuronal intranuclear inclusions: autosomal dominant. Symptoms develop in childhood. GI symptoms: dysphagia, diarrhea, constipation, and pseudo-obstruction. Also autonomic dysfunction, ataxia, dysarthria, mental retardation, and dementia. Charac-

teristic eosinophilic intranuclear inclusions have been identified in the neurons of the degenerated myenteric plexus all along the GI tract and nerves of the central and peripheral nervous systems. Manometry: lack of phase III of the MMC and irregular, nonpropagated contractions in the small intestine. No therapy exists.

3. FVN with short bowel, malrotation, and pyloric hypertrophy: functional obstruction symptoms occur in neonatal period with most patients dying in first year of life. Abnormalities of myenteric plexus with lack of argyrophilic neurons and degenerated neurons demonstrated. Autosomal recessive and dominant patterns described. Malrotation, short bowel, and pyloric hypertrophy and abnormal ileocecal connection without an appendix have been described.

4. FVN with neurologic involvement: early childhood symptoms with neuropathic GI dysmotilities and involvement of the peripheral or central nervous system. Inheritance modality unclear. Mitochondrial involvement may be present.

5. FVN (ganglioneuromatosis) associated with multiple endocrine neoplasia (MEN) type IIB: of the MEN syndromes, MEN IIB is the only form involving the GI tract with a susceptibility gene being the RET proto-oncogene; autosomal dominant inheritance. In most, GI dysmotility is first manifestation of the disease. Characteristic pathology: increased density of ganglion cells in the submucous and myenteric plexus with penetration of hyperplastic nerves into the mucosal zone, found throughout GI tract. Acetylcholinesterase staining is increased as well. Features: colonic dysfunction with chronic constipation and bowel dilation; may be confused with Hirschsprung disease; GI symptoms often develop before other MEN IIB features recognized. Ileostomy or elective subtotal colectomy may be required for chronic constipation. Early diagnosis of MEN IIB essential to perform prophylactic thyroidectomy before medullary thyroid carcinoma and to screen for development of pheochromocytoma.

6. Visceral neuropathy (VN) associated with neurofibromatosis (von Recklinghausen disease): single or multiple neurofibromas in the small intestine occur in 10% of patients; autosomal disorder; may cause functional or mechanical obstruction.

HISTOPATHOLOGY

1. Hypoganglionosis: defined by a reduced number of ganglion cells in the myenteric plexus and submucous plexus. Requires full-thickness sample > 1 cm in length for evaluation. Hypoganglionosis can always be detected in a short segment (transitional zone) proximal to the aganglionic bowel in Hirschsprung disease. Non-Hirschsprung disease–related hypoganglionosis has been reported in many children with severe constipation. Ganglions are smaller and often infiltrated with collagen. Schwann nerve fibers are often thickened. Most disease is located in the distal colon. Clinical course varies markedly.

2. Hyperganglionosis: characterized by an excess of intestinal neurons in the myenteric plexus with or without involvement of the submucous plexus. Remember that normally infants have a higher neuronal density than older children. Severe hyperganglionosis is the hallmark of visceral neuropathy occurring in patients with MEN type IIB. Thus, patients with this finding should undergo RET gene analysis. Hyperplasia of the myenteric and submucous plexus proximal to the transition zone has been reported in Hirschsprung disease patients. RET mutation found in Hirschsprung disease leads to loss of function while MEN type IIB mutations lead to gain in function.

3. Qualitative abnormalities of ganglion cells: reported in children presenting with primary intestinal motility disorders; may be an expression of immaturity or degeneration. Clinical symptoms: nonspecific; indistinguishable from other enteric neuropathies.

SECONDARY OR ACQUIRED VISCERAL NEUROPATHIES

1. Damage of ENS is due to a known agent or secondary to a systemic disease in these entities. May manifest at any age. Occur less often in children than adults as it may take many years to accumulate damage.

2. Infectious agents: Chagas disease caused by infection with Trypanosoma cruzi is a well-known example of ENS destruction due to an autoimmune response elicited by the infection. Most common clinical presentation is achalasia followed by intestinal dysfunction and chronic intestinal pseudo-obstruction. Obstructive episodes also described during acute Lyme disease. Viral etiologies also include herpes viruses (cytomegalovirus, varicella-zoster virus, Epstein-Barr virus, and herpes simplex virus type 1) and human immunodeficiency virus (HIV).

3. Toxins: abnormal antroduodenal manometry has been described in some children with fetal alcohol syndrome.

4. Drugs: may affect GI motility as a main target organ (prokinetics or loperamide) or as unwanted side effects (opiates, macrolides, anticonvulsive, HIV medications). Nonreversible visceral neuropathy also described in adults with long-term intake of cathartics or chemotherapeutic agents.

5. Radiation therapy: damages all structures of the bowel. Acute manifestations usually subside within weeks but late complications may occur up to decades later. Most symptomatic patients are adults. Neuronal and muscular structures of the bowel are affected and contribute to motility disorder. Antroduodenal manometry shows a wide variety of abnormalities. Major features: attenuated postprandial motor response and reduced intensity of nighttime MMCs.

6. Chronic inflammation and autoimmune disease: gut dysmotility reported in patients with different noninfectious inflammatory diseases.

7. Autonomic neuropathy: autonomic nervous system interacts with the ENS and smooth muscle cells;

autonomic system disorders affect intestinal motility. One-half of children with autosomal recessive familial dysautonomia (Riley-Day syndrome) develop GI problems with attacks of severe vomiting and crises (hypertension, sweating, and erythematous blotching of the skin). Children with triple-A (alacrima-achalasia-addisonian) or Allgrove syndrome, autosomal recessive, have autonomic dysfunction, including GI dysmotility. Autonomic neuropathy in diabetes common in adults but does not reach clinical significance in childhood.

8. Endocrine disorders: several endocrine disorders may manifest with GI dysmotility symptoms. Hypothyroidism may present with severe slow-transit constipation or pseudo-obstruction, whereas hyperthyroidism may present with diarrhea with or without steatorrhea. Impaired gut contractions with dysmotility and steatorrhea observed in children with hypoparathyroidism, especially when part of a polyendocrine deficiency syndrome. Tumors producing catecholamines or vasoactive peptides (eg, pheochromocytoma, carcinoid, and gastrinoma) may present with dilated small bowel, dysmotility, and watery diarrhea.

9. Metabolic disease: several metabolic disorders with and without electrolyte disturbances may result in acute or chronic GI dysmotility including organic aciduria and end stage liver or renal disease. Storage diseases such as Fabry disease or amyloidosis may result in permanent neuromuscular damage.

10. Anorexia nervosa and bulimia: delayed gastric emptying and small bowel transit documented. Usually resolves with treatment.

11. Ogilvie syndrome (acute colonic pseudo-obstruction): severe form of adynamic ileus with massive colonic dilatation in the absence of mechanical obstruction. Occurs in hospitalized patients with a wide variety of medical and surgical conditions. Most respond to conservative therapy. Colonoscopic decompression performed to prevent ischemia and perforation. Intravenous neostigmine rapidly decompresses the colon and may be tried.

DISORDERS OF THE INTERSTITIAL CELLS OF CAJAL

1. Interstitial cells of Cajal (ICC): important modulators of communication between muscles and nerves, identified by immunoreactivity for tyrosine kinase receptor Kit.

2. Unclear whether ICC alterations are primary or secondary to disease.

QUESTIONS

TRUE OR FALSE:

1. Intestinal mucosal biopsies suffice for the diagnosis of primary visceral myopathies and neuropathies.

2. The delayed gastric emptying and small bowel transit seen in anorexia nervosa usually resolve with nutritional recuperation.

3. Autonomic neuropathy seen in association with diabetes in adults is rare in childhood diabetes.

4. RET mutation in proto-oncogene in multiple endocrine neoplasia type IIB is associated with a gain in function of the coded protein.

5. Intestinal dysmotilities are most commonly caused by smooth muscle myopathy.

6. Intestinal neuronal dysplasia is a well-defined entity.

MATCH THE CONDITIONS WITH MODE OF INHERITANCE:

a. Autosomal dominant inheritance.
b. Autosomal recessive inheritance.
c. X-linked inheritance.

7. Familial visceral neuropathy without extraintestinal manifestations.
8. Familial visceral myopathy type 1.
9. Familial visceral myopathy type 2.
10. Familial childhood visceral myopathy with diffuse abnormal muscle layering.

MATCH THE DISEASE WITH THE AFFECTED SYSTEM:

a. Autonomic nervous system.
b. Enteric nervous system.

11. Riley-Day syndrome.
12. Familial visceral neuropathy.
13. Allgrove syndrome.

HIRSCHSPRUNG DISEASE

SYNOPSIS

1. Congenital absence of the enteric nervous system extending continuously and proximally for a variable distance from the internal anal sphincter.

2. Prevalence: 1/5,000 live births. Male-to-female ratio 4:1 for short-segment disease and 1:1 as length of involved bowel increases. 7% of cases have a family history of Hirschsprung disease but family prevalence is 21% in individuals with total colonic disease.

3. Limited to rectum and sigmoid in 90%. Long segment involves colon proximal to the sigmoid colon and occurs in about 10%.

4. 15% present with at least 1 other congenital anomaly (Table 1). Chromosomal anomalies seen in 12%, with trisomy 21 found in 2–8% of persons with Hirschsprung disease.

5. Autosomal dominant or recessive. Penetrance of mutations generally low; depends on sex and extent of aganglionosis in affected family members.

PATHOGENESIS

Failure of craniocaudal migration of precursors of the enteric nervous system (ENS) from 5th to 12th week of gestation. Absence of ganglia interrupts expression of inhibitory parasympathetic fibers, inhibiting relaxation. Preganglionic parasympathetic fibers have high acetylcholinesterase.

TABLE 1   ANOMALIES ASSOCIATED WITH HIRSCHSPRUNG DISEASE

SYNDROMES	KEY FEATURES
Chromosomal*	
Down	Mental retardation with characteristic features
Syndromes requiring Hirschsprung disease	
Goldberg-Shprintzen†	Cleft palate, hypotonia, mental retardation, facial dysmorphism
Shah-Waardenburg‡	Pigmentary abnormalities (white forelock, depigmentaton of skin, premature graying, heterochromic irides), and sensorineural deafness
Hirschsprung disease with distal limb anomalies (several syndromes)	Polydactyly, brachydactyly, or nail hypoplasia with other assorted anomalies
BRESHEK	Brain abnormalities, mental retardation, ectodermal dysplasia, skeletal malformation, ear/eye anomalies, kidney dysplasia (ie, BRESHEK with Hirschsprung disease)
Syndromes with Hirschsprung disease as an occasional finding	
Mowat-Wilson	Facial dysmorphic features, mental retardation
Congenital central hypoventilation	Abnormal autonomic control of respiration
Bardet-Biedl	Pigmentary retinopathy, obesity, hypogonadism, mild mental retardation, postaxial polydactyly
Multiple endocrine neoplasia IIA	Medullary thyroid carcinoma, pheochromocytoma, parathyroid hyperplasia
Kaufman-McKusick	Hydrometrocolpos, postaxial polydactyly, congenital heart defect
Smith-Lemli-Opitz	Growth retardation, microcephaly, mental retardation, hypospadias, syndactyly of second and third toes, dymorphic features
Cartilage-hair hypoplasia	Short-limb dwarfism, metaphyseal dysplasia, transient macrocytic anemia, immunodeficiency, fine and sparse blond hair
Syndromes with a possible association with Hirschsprung disease§	
Fukuyama congenital muscular dystrophy	Muscular dystrophy, polymicrogyria, hydrocephalus, mental retardation, seizures
Clayton-Smith	Dysmorphic features, hypoplastic toes and nails, deafness, ichthyosis
Kaplan	Agenesis of the corpus callosum, adducted thumbs, ptosis, muscle weakness
Dermotrichic	Alopecia, ichthyosis, mental retardation, seizures
Okamoto	Hydrocephalus, cleft palate, agenesis of the corpus callosum, familial dysautonomia

Adapted from Chakravarti A, Lyonnet S. Hirschsprung disease. In: Scriver Cr, Beaudet Al, Sly WS, Valle D, editors. The metabolic and molecular basis of inherited disease. New York: McGraw-Hill; 2001. p. 931–42.

*Hirschsprung disease is also seen in association with the following chromosomal disorders: chromosome 2p deletion syndrome, chromosome 22q11.2 deletion, cat-eye syndrome (supernumerary dicentric chromosome 22q), chromosome 20p deletion, and deletions/duplications of chromosome 17q21-q23.

†Goldberg-Shprintzen and Mowat-Wilson syndromes may or may not be related disorders.

‡Other neurocristopathies are reported in association with Hirschsprung disease that likely share a molecular basis with Shah-Waardenburg syndrome. These include Yemenite deaf-blind hypopigmentation (Online Mendelian Inheritance in Man database [OMIM] #601706), ABCD syndrome (OMIM #600501), familial piebaldism (OMIM #172800), and congenital deafness.

§Hirschsprung disease is also reported in association with the following syndromes: Pallister-Hall, Fryns, Jeune asphyxiating thoracic, frontonasal dysplasia, osteopetrosis, Goldenhar, Lesch-Nyhan, Rubinstein-Taybi, Toriello-Carey, and spondyloepimetaphyseal dysplasia with joint laxity.

SUSCEPTIBILITY GENES

1. Identified gene mutations account for only one-half of cases.
2. *RET*: tyrosine kinase inactivation associated with Hirschsprung disease; dominant mutation with low penetrance; accounts for 50% of familial cases, especially long-segment disease. Some of same mutations of *RET* that cause Hirschsprung disease cause multiple endocrine neoplasia (MEN) type IIA. *RET*, 3q21 and 19q12 loci mutations associated with short-segment Hirschsprung disease. 78% of affected individuals in one series carried maternally derived *RET* mutation.
3. *EDNRB* (endothelin receptor B) and *EDN3* (endothelin 3) genes: cause Hirschsprung disease associated with pigmentary abnormalities and sensorineural deafness (Shah-Waardenburg syndrome). Endothelin B mutations often associated with short-segment Hirschsprung disease. Endothelin B expressed by early ENS precursors; endothelin 3 expressed by the surrounding mesenchyme. Endothelin B inhibits neuronal differentiation.
4. Endothelin-converting enzyme 1 (protease activating endothelin 3).
5. *SOX10*: transcription factor expressed in early ENS precursors, supporting their survival. Mutations cause Shah-Waardenburg syndrome. Most mutations are dominant and occur de novo. Penetrance high.
6. *ZFHX1B* (zinc finger homeobox 1B): inactivation mutations cause Mowat-Wilson syndrome (characteristic facies, microcephaly, and mental retardation, with or without Hirschsprung disease).

CLINICAL PRESENTATION

1. Neonate with Hirschsprung disease is usually full-term of normal birth weight. 94% fail to pass meconium within 24 h, 57% within 48 h. Abdominal distention, vomiting, constipation, and poor feeding often seen. Diarrhea often indicates enterocolitis.
2. Infant or child usually presents with constipation beginning in infancy responding poorly to medical management. Fecal urgency, stool withholding behaviors and fecal soiling not noted. Poor weight gain,

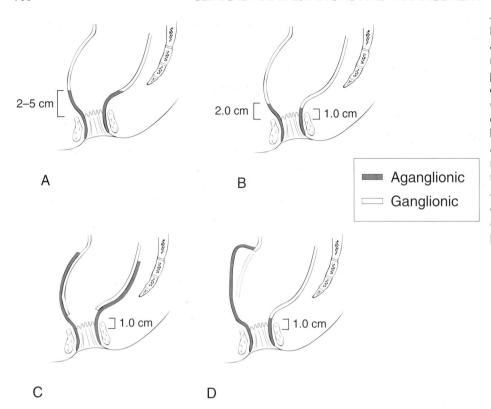

A   B

C   D

Aganglionic
Ganglionic

FIGURE 1 Summary of anorectal anatomy following the more commonly performed pull-through procedures for Hirschsprung disease: *A,* Rehbein; *B,* Swenson; *C,* Soave; and *D,* Duhamel. Reproduced with permission from Teitelbaum D, Coran AG, Weitzman J, et al. Hirschsprung's disease and related neuromuscular disorders of the intestine. In: O'Neill J, Rowe MI, Gosfeld JL, et al, editors. Pediatric surgery. 5th ed. St. Louis: Mosby-Year Book, Inc.; 1998. p. 1381–424.

anemia, hypoalbuminemia, and bouts of diarrhea common. Urinary retention may occur secondary to ureteral compression.

3. Physical exam may reveal a tympanitic distended abdomen with palpable fecal masses. Rectal exam essential to evaluate for imperforated anus, anteriorly displaced anus, anal stenosis. Digital rectal exam demonstrates a tight but patent anus with an explosion of air or liquid with removal of the examiner's finger. Patients with enterocolitis have diarrhea and appear ill with fever and lethargy.

INVESTIGATIONS

1. Radiology: absence of pelvic or rectal gas in prone infant is suggestive. Unprepared contrast enema most likely to aid in diagnosis in children aged > 1 mo. Classic findings include contracted distal colon with abrupt transition to a widely dilated proximal colon. Rectal diameter same as or smaller than diameter of sigmoid is suggestive of Hirschsprung disease. Contrast enema should not be done in patients with clinical enterocolitis or recent rectal biopsy owing to risk of perforation.

2. Anorectal manometry: measures ENS function. Technique looks for normal relaxation of the internal anal sphincter in response to balloon rectal distention. Requires patient cooperation. Technique difficult in very young infants. Anorectal manometry necessary for the diagnosis of ultrashort-segment Hirschsprung with failure of internal anal sphincter relaxation on rectal distention.

3. Rectal biopsy: gold standard for diagnosis. Diagnosis usually established by rectal suction biopsy from the

appropriate location (a segment of hypoganglionosis exists normally in the submucosal plexus just above the dentate line ranging from 3–17 mm in length). General practice is to obtain suction rectal biopsies no closer than 2 cm above dentate line. In ultrashort-segment Hirschsprung disease, rectal biopsy is normal.

4. Pathology: increase in darkly staining fibers in lamina and muscularis propria (with stain for acetylcholinesterase) and absence of ganglia at submucosa and myenteric plexi.

TREATMENT

1. Definitive therapy is surgical.
2. Medical management of enterocolitis important in stabilizing the patient and includes:
   a. Placement of rectal tube for decompression and irrigations.
   b. Intravenous antibiotics.
3. Four surgical pull-through approaches commonly used: Rehbein, Swenson, Soave, and Duhamel (Figure 1).
   a. Rehbein: leaves 3–5 cm of aganglionic colon above dentate line.
   b. Swenson: ganglion containing bowel anastomosed end to end to rectum within 2 cm of dentate line with both muscular and mucosal anastomosis.
   c. Soave (endorectal pull-through): ganglionic intestine incised and pulled through to muscular cuff and anastomosis created to submucosal–mucosal tube close to the anus. Associated with higher incidence of postoperative enterocolitis and constipation.
   d. Duhamel: position proximal ganglionic intestine posterior to the rectum with anastomosis side to side to posterior wall of aganglionic rectum.

LONG-TERM COMPLICATIONS AND RESULTS

1. Enterocolitis is major cause of morbidity and mortality. Frequently occurs after pull-through. Individuals with Down syndrome at increased risk for enterocolitis.
2. Need to rule out anorectal stenosis; some may be managed by anal dilatations; 20–30% may require anal myectomy or myotomy for relief of constipation.
3. After resection of aganglionic bowel, some patients are unable to absorb nutrients and are dependent on parenteral nutrition.
4. Dysmotility may improve with time. Intestinal neuronal dysplasia and abnormalities in interstitial cells of Cajal in the ganglionic segments of bowel have been reported.
5. Rectal fecalomas develop in a small subset of patients, associated with retention of a septum between aganglionic rectum and the pulled-through intestine following a Duhamel procedure.
5. Long-term follow-up of surgically treated patients often reveals ongoing difficulties with fecal incontinence and weight gain. With time, fecal continence improves.

GENETIC COUNSELING

1. Generalized risk to siblings is 4% and increases as the length of involved bowel increases. Prenatal diagnosis is possible if mutation is known. However, genetic testing is limited as the penetrance of single gene mutations is low (except for *SOX10* mutations).
2. Genetic testing for *RET* mutations has potential to identify significant risks for other diseases seen in persons with Hirschsprung disease, for example, MEN type IIA (medullary thyroid carcinoma, pheochromocytoma, and hyperparathyroidism). In the setting of early identification of MEN type IIA mutation, prophylactic thyroidectomy and screening for pheochromocytoma and hyperparathyroidism should be performed.

QUESTIONS

CHOOSE THE BEST ANSWER:

1. The best diagnostic test for ultrashort-segment Hirschsprung disease is:
   a. Rectal suction biopsy.
   b. Barium enema.
   c. Abdominal radiograph.
   d. Anorectal manometry.

2. The following are true of Hirschsprung disease except:
   a. Hirschsprung disease has both autosomal recessive and dominant inheritance patterns.
   b. Penetrance of *RET* mutations associated with Hirschsprung disease is high.
   c. More males than females are affected in short-segment Hirschsprung disease.
   d. Hirschsprung disease is usually limited to the rectum and sigmoid colon.

3. *RET* mutations are associated with all of the following except:
   a. Long-segment Hirschsprung disease.
   b. Short-segment Hirschsprung disease.
   c. Multiple endocrine neoplasia type IIA syndrome.
   d. All of the above are associated with *RET* mutation.
   e. None of the above are associated with *RET* mutation.

4. Aganglionosis on rectal suction biopsy is seen in all of the following except:
   a. Ultra-short segment Hirschsprung disease.
   b. Biopsy taken within 2 cm of the dentate line in a person with Hirschsprung disease.
   c. Biopsy taken more than 2 cm proximal to the dentate line in a person with Hirschsprung disease.
   d. Biopsy taken within 2 cm of the dentate line in a person without Hirschsprung disease.

CHRONIC INTESTINAL PSEUDO-OBSTRUCTION SYNDROME

SYNOPSIS

1. Rare disorder. Impaired intestinal or colonic motility leads to clinical bowel obstruction. One-half of patients never tolerate enteral feeding.
2. Neuropathic pseudo-obstruction: can be confined to extrinsic innervation, intrinsic innervation, or both. In pediatrics, most neuropathic forms of chronic intestinal pseudo-obstruction (CIP) involve intrinsic innervation. Exact mechanisms unknown.
3. Myopathic pseudo-obstruction: results from smooth muscle cell injury. May be primary or secondary to a systemic disease. Histopathology of affected muscle may be normal, and protein expression alterations may be secondary to intestinal distention, making characterization difficult. Duchenne muscular dystrophy and myotonic dystrophy are skeletal myopathies that may present with gastroparesis and CIP.
4. Mitochondrial: mitochondrial neurogastrointestinal encephalomyopathy (MNGIE) is an autosomal recessive disorder involving the enteric neuromuscular system associated with deletions and depletion of mitochondrial deoxyribonucleic acid (DNA). Characterized by a myopathy of striated muscle with ragged red fibers and mixed enteric neuromyopathy.

CLINICAL FEATURES

1. Rare condition.
2. Male-to-female ratio 1:1, but girls more frequently affected in neonatal forms.
3. Familial cases < 5%.
4. Prenatal signs in 20%, especially nonobstructive megacystis.
5. Two-thirds present within first month of life, 80% by age 1 yr.

TABLE 1   CAUSES OF SECONDARY INTESTINAL PSEUDO-OBSTRUCTION IN CHILDREN

TOXIC
Ketamine
Carbamazepine
Clonidine
Atropine, anticholinergics
Theophylline
Fludarabine
Vinblastine and other vinca alkaloids
Neuroleptics
Antidepressants
Phenothiazine
Opiates
Calcium channel blockers
Fetal alcohol syndrome

METABOLIC
Electrolyte imbalance (K^+, $\uparrow Mg^{++}$, Ca^{++})
Hypothyroidism
Hypoparathyroidism
Carnitine deficiency
Vitamin E deficiency ("brown bowel syndrome")

INFECTIOUS
Viral: CMV, EBV, herpes zoster, rotavirus
Trypanosoma cruzei (young adults)
Lyme disease

IMMUNE
Celiac disease
Systemic sclerosis
Lupus (myopathy)
Autoimmune leiomyositis
Autoimmune enteric ganglionitis (with antienteric neurons antibodies, anti PCNA antibodies)
Guillain-Barré syndrome

TUMORAL
Neural crest cell tumor: neuroblastoma, ganglioneuroblastoma
Pheochromocytoma
Thymoma (with antiacetylcholine receptor antibodies)

STRIATED MYOPATHY
Myotonic dystrophy
Duchenne muscular dystrophy
Desmin myopathy
Mitochondrial myopathy

CENTRAL OR PERIPHERAL GENERALIZED NEUROPATHY
Degenerative process: diabetes, amyloidosis (not reported in children)
Mitochondrial neurogastrointestinal encephalopathy
Familial dysautonomia
Acquired cholinergic dysautonomia or acquired pandysautonomia

MISCELLANEOUS
Angioedema
Postradiation enteropathy
Kawasaki disease

CMV = cytomegalovirus; EBV = Epstein-Barr virus; PCNA = proliferation cell nuclear antigen.

CLINICAL PRESENTATIONS

1. Prenatal or neonatal onset: severe abdominal distention with bilious emesis. Obstructed urinary system may be a presenting feature. Immaturity of intestinal motility in preterm infants may mimic CIP (migrating motor complex [MMC] does not appear until 34–35 wk).
2. Infantile or late-onset form:
   a. Major forms with acute presentation: some present with subacute or recurrent episodes of gastrointesti-
   nal (GI) obstruction depending on affected regions. Episodes may be persistent but usually are intermittent. Exacerbations can be precipitated by stress, fever, vaccines, etc. Diarrhea owing to small bowel bacterial overgrowth common. Dysphagia rare but abdominal pain is often severe enough to lead to feeding problems. Urinary tract involvement in 33–92%.
   b. Moderate forms with subacute presentation: 70% present with progressively severe constipation (< 1 stool per 7–15 days), abdominal distention, bilious emesis, and failure to thrive.
3. External ophthalmoplegia in the setting of frequent intestinal nonobstructive dilatation and dysmotility episodes should prompt evaluation for mitochondrial disease.

DIAGNOSIS

Difficult because of variable presentation and lack of specific diagnostic test. Work-up should include the following:
1. Rule out any fixed obstructive lesion.
2. Confirm abnormal motility of the GI tract.
3. Find any treatable systemic cause of secondary CIP (Table 1).

TESTS

1. Radiology: contrast studies should be performed to exclude any intraluminal or extrinsic lesion. Malrotation is frequent (up to 40% of neonates).
2. Surgery: avoid unnecessary exploratory laparotomy to avoid adhesion formation (not recommended to perform surgery only to obtain intestinal specimens for histopathology). However, emergent laparotomy may be necessary to exclude an obstructing lesion.
3. Functional motility testing: manometric studies.
   a. Esophageal manometry is abnormal in 50–90% CIP patients.
   b. The rectoanal inhibitory reflex is normal in all patients with CIP (absent only in Hirschsprung disease).
   c. Antroduodenal manometry confirms dysmotility of the upper GI tract, almost always involved in children with CIP. Allows characterization of myopathic v. neuropathic forms. In neuropathies, abnormalities include: absence of phase 3 motor complexes, abnormal configuration or propagation of phase 3, bursts of uncoordinated phasic activity, sustained periods of prolonged phasic activity dur-

TABLE 2   DIFFERENTIAL DIAGNOSIS OF CHRONIC INTESTINAL PSEUDO-OBSTRUCTION IN CHILDREN

Aerophagia
Gastroparesis
Constipation
Cyclic vomiting syndrome
Severe irritable bowel syndrome
Bacterial overgrowth of various origin
   (lactase deficiency, disaccharidase deficiency, intestinal duplication)
Aerodigestive fistula
Munchausen syndrome by proxy

ing fasting, and the inability to induce a fed motility pattern after feeding.
  d. Electrogastrography results are often nonspecific and do not differentiate between CIP and other forms of intestinal dysmotility.
  e. Nuclear medicine studies usually show delayed gastric emptying.
4. Histopathology may confirm the abnormal aspect of the enteric neuromusculature. Requires full-thickness intestinal wall biopsies > 1 cm in length.
5. Audiologic assessment is important to rule out deafness in patients with *SOX10* gene mutations.
6. Carnitine and vitamin E levels should be checked in cases of fat malabsorption or maldigestion to rule out deficiency.

TREATMENT

1. Supportive. Aims: maintain nutritional status, preserve growth, and avoid life-threatening episodes of sepsis; acceptable quality of life.
2. Symptomatic treatment: acute episodes of abdominal distention may benefit from bowel decompression by nasogastric tube or venting gastrostomy. Intravenous (IV) replacement of fluids and electrolytes should be performed. IV antibiotics may be needed for catheter sepsis, bacterial overgrowth, or infection.
3. Steroids useful in immune-mediated myositis and ganglionitis.
4. Prokinetics usually without clinical benefit. Bethanechol may be useful in some patients with megacystis.
5. Surgery: gastrostomy or jejunostomy should be performed to bypass functional obstruction and obtain decompression when attacks of obstruction are frequent or life-threatening. Note: surgery is associated with adhesion formation, which may contribute to the problem.
6. In children with genitourinary involvement, management important to avoid renal complications. Intermittent urethral catheterization is mainstay of therapy. Prophylaxis of urinary tract infection should be undertaken.
7. Only definitive cure: intestinal transplant. Isolated small bowel transplant may unmask associated esophageal and gastric dysmotilities post transplant.

OUTCOME AND PROGNOSIS

1. In secondary and acquired forms, outcome dependent on underlying disease. Most often, viral infections resolve spontaneously.
2. In primary forms, prognosis poor.

MORTALITY

1. Progress in parenteral nutrition management and use of bowel decompression have modified mortality rate from 90% to 10–25%.
2. Underlying CIP rarely cause of death except in cases with MEN type IIB and medullary carcinoma. High mortality rate usually due to iatrogenic complications (total parenteral nutrition catheter-related sepsis, liver failure, and post-transplant complications).

PROGNOSTIC FACTORS

Neonatal onset, genitourinary involvement, requirement for surgery, and myopathic disorders are more frequent in cases with a poor prognosis. The presence of phase 3 MMC on antroduodenal manometry has been reported to be a good prognostic indicator for enteral feeding tolerance and response to cisapride.

QUESTIONS

TRUE OR FALSE:
1. About one-half of patients with chronic intestinal pseudo-obstruction syndrome never tolerate enteral feeds.
2. The histopathology of muscles in myopathic pseudo-obstruction can be normal.
3. Chronic intestinal pseudo-obstruction is commonly diagnosed in preterm infants.
4. Surgery should be performed as a diagnostic procedure to obtain a full-thickness intestinal wall biopsy in cases suggestive of chronic intestinal pseudo-obstruction.

CHOOSE THE BEST ANSWER:
5. External ophthalmoplegia in the setting of frequent intestinal nonobstructive dilatation and dysmotility episodes should prompt evaluation for the following:
   a. Hirschsprung disease.
   b. Mitochondrial disorders.
   c. Dysautonomia syndromes.
   d. Medullary thyroid carcinoma.

6. Audiologic assessment is important with patients with what mutation?
   a. *RET* gene.
   b. *SOX10* gene.
   c. Endothelin 3.
   d. Endothelin receptor B.
   e. All of the above.

SECRETORY TUMORS AFFECTING THE GUT

SYNOPSIS

MULTIPLE ENDOCRINE NEOPLASIA
1. Two hit hypothesis: where two mutations are required for the syndrome to appear. Three types:
   a. I: mutations occur in tumor suppressor gene menin (11q13); parathyroid adenomas, islet cell tumors of the pancreas, and nonfunctional pituitary adenomas.
   b. IIA: mutations at RET proto-oncogene; medullary carcinoma of the thyroid, parathyroid hyperplasia, and pheochromocytoma.
   c. IIB: mutations at RET proto-oncogene; multiple mucosal, alimentary tract neuromas, medullary carcinoma of the thyroid, and pheochromocytoma.

2. Multiple endocrine neoplasia (MEN) I: major morbidity from MEN I in children is rare. Gastrinoma not seen in children age < 12 yr.
3. MEN II: IIA accounts for 75% of MEN II. IIB (Sipple syndrome): children present with gastrointestinal (GI) symptoms and have high risk of developing malignant thyroid tumors. IIB infants have feeding problems, severe constipation in first year (rectal biopsies with ganglioneuromatosis). Older patients with IIB usually with Marfanoid habitus and skeletal abnormalities. All with MEN IIB develop medullary carcinoma of the thyroid; thyroidectomy should be performed prophylactically by 4 years of age.
4. High concentrations of somatostatin receptor SSTR2.

GASTRINOMA AND ZOLLINGER-ELLISON SYNDROME

1. Age of onset: 7–90 yr of age, peak incidence at 30–50 yr; one-third of adult patients have MEN I.
2. Presentation: recurrent peptic ulcer disease or unexplained diarrhea.
3. 60% malignant. Most common sites of metastases are local lymph nodes and liver.
4. Prominent gastric folds on endoscopy. 75% have confirmed peptic ulcer disease. Multiple ulcers in unusual locations are pathognomonic of Zollinger-Ellison syndrome (ZES), but 75% of ulcers are solitary and located at the duodenal bulb.
5. Diagnosis: confirmed on biopsy.
6. Best screening test: fasting gastrin (usually < 125 pg/mL).
7. Secretin stimulation test: secretin results in at least a doubling of the gastrin level in patients with gastrinoma (usually increases by > 200 pg/mL)(Figure 1).
8. Localization: gastrinomas very small; multiple tumors are common. Typically found in gastrinoma triangle (between the cystic duct, 3rd portion of the duodenum, and neck of the pancreas). Somatostatin receptor scintigraphy (SRS) better for localization than ultrasonography, computed tomography, magnetic resonance imaging, or angiography.
9. Treatment: only potential cure, complete surgical resection. If resection not possible, embolization may be helpful. Medical management: high doses of proton pump inhibitors. Intravenous pantoprazole controls acid in > 90%. Objective: to keep acid secretions < 10 meq/h. In extensive metastatic disease, chemotherapy has been helpful with streptozocin.
10. Prognosis: 30% can be cured by resection. Otherwise, 15 yr survival rate is 83%. Poor prognosis correlates: primary pancreatic lesions, metastases to lymph nodes, liver, bone, ectopic Cushing disease, and highly exaggerated gastrin level. Those with MEN 1 can rarely be cured. A normal fasting gastrin–secretin stimulation test immediately postoperatively predicts long-term cure.

VIPOMA

1. Verner-Morrison syndrome; watery diarrhea, hypokalemia, achlorhydria syndrome (WDHA); and pancreatic cholera.

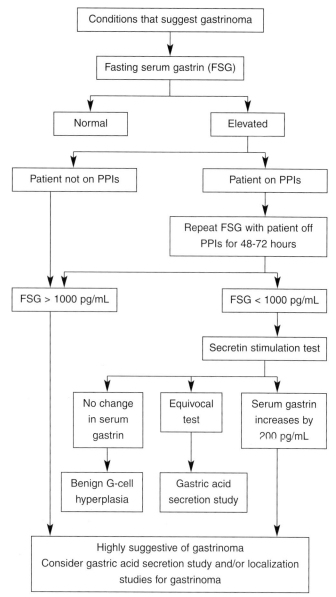

FIGURE 1 Elevated fasting gastrin level or positive secretin stimulation test in the setting of elevated basal acid secretion strongly suggests the presence of a gastrinoma. PPI = proton pump inhibitor.

2. WDHA has been reported in all age groups.
3. Virtually all present with watery diarrhea and hypokalemia. Fecal losses while fasting are at least 20 cc/kg/d; most > 50 cc/kg/d. Steatorrhea not a feature of the syndrome. Flushing is present in 20% and intermittent. Hypochlorhydria (70%), hyperglycemia (20–50%), and hypercalcemia (20–50%) also seen.
4. In children most VIPomas are ganglioneuromas or ganglioneuroblastomas at neck, thorax, or suprarenal or pelvic areas. Neuroblastomas may also secrete vasoactive intestinal polypeptide (VIP). Extrapancreatic lesions located in usual areas of neurogenic tumor occurrence (adrenal gland and paravertebral sympathetic tissues).
5. Diagnosis: verify secretory nature of diarrhea. Rule out toxigenic infectious organisms (*Clostridium difficile* or toxigenic *Escherichia coli*). If suspicious for a secretory

TABLE 1   CAUSES OF HYPERGASTRINEMIA

HYPERGASTRINEMIA WITHOUT GASTRIC HYPERSECRETION
Achlorhydria or hypochlorhydria associated with
   Pernicious anemia
   Atrophic gastritis
   Gastric ulcer
   Prior vagotomy
   Helicobacter pylori infection
   Therapy with proton pump inhibitors

HYPERGASTRINEMIA WITH GASTRIC HYPERSECRETION
Gastrinoma
Renal failure
Retained antrum
Antral G-cell hyperplasia
Pheochromocytoma
Hypercalcemia
Duodenal ulcer
Pyloric obstruction

Adapted from Spindel E, Harty RF, Leibach JR, McGuigan JE. Decision analysis in evaluation of hypergastrinemia. Am J Med 1986;80:11–7.

tumor, send for gastrin, 5-hydroxyindole acetic acid, prostaglandin E2, and serotonin levels. Chromogranin A is a standard probe for neuroendocrine tumors, including gastrinomas and carcinoid tumors. VIPomas should be considered in those with VIP levels just above the upper limit of normal.

6. Localization should be performed prior to operative resection via imaging modalities and SRS.

7. Treatment: operative resection offers only possible cure; in childhood 70–80%. Overall survival in children with neuroblastomas poor (35–40%). With successful resection, VIP levels fall to normal within hours. If resection not possible, symptomatic remission may be achieved with medication, although difficult. Prednisone can reduce diarrhea. Octreotide may be helpful.

SOMATOSTATINOMA

1. Somatostatin: potent inhibitor of the release of a variety of hormones.
2. Symptoms: diabetes, gallstones, steatorrhea, and hypochlorhydria.
3. Not found in children aged < 18 yr.

GLUCAGONOMA

1. Excessive secretion of glucagons induces a catabolic state, glucose intolerance, hypoaminoacidemia, and characteristic dermatitis.
2. Striking clinical features: weight loss, rash, and diabetes. Rash: red scaly lesions on extremities and creases and periorally that become bullous, crusty, and confluent.
3. Not described in patients aged < 18 yr.

CARCINOID SYNDROME

1. Symptoms: episodic flushing, facial swelling, palpitations, abdominal pain, and explosive diarrhea. Late symptoms: mesenteric fibrosis and endocardial or car-

diac valvular fibrosis. Caused by metastasized tumors of enterochromaffin cells. Symptoms mediated by serotonin, bradykinin, and histamine.

2. Carcinoid tumors in children usually an incidental finding at appendectomy. Appendiceal carcinoids < 1 cm treated by simple excision. Tumors > 2 cm at risk for metastasis; right hemicolectomy is recommended for tumors > 2 cm to remove regional lymph nodes.
3. Poor prognosis if multiple liver metastases, carcinoid syndrome, or high tumor level markers.
4. Diagnosis: 24 h urine collection for 5-hydroxyindoleacetic acid. SRS can be used for localization.
5. Surgical resection and embolization of liver metastases offers palliation and prolongs survival. Treatment of choice: somatostatin or octreotide. Chemotherapy for metastases.

QUESTIONS

MATCH THE MULTIPLE ENDOCRINE NEOPLASIA (MEN) SYNDROMES WITH THEIR ASSOCIATED TUMORS:

a. MEN I.
b. MEN IIA.
c. MEN IIB.

1. Medullary carcinoma of the thyroid, parathyroid hyperplasia, and pheochromocytoma.
2. Parathyroid adenomas, islet cell tumors of the pancreas, and nonfunctional adenomas of the pituitary.
3. Multiple mucosal and alimentary tract neuromas, medullary carcinoma of the thyroid, and pheochromocytoma.

CHOOSE THE BEST ANSWER:

4. Which is not associated with an elevated fasting gastrin?
   a. Gastric ulcer.
   b. Renal failure.
   c. Prior vagotomy.
   d. *Helicobacter pylori* infection.
   e. Liver failure.

5. Which is false regarding childhood VIPomas?
   a. Most VIPomas are ganglioneuromas or ganglioneuroblastomas at the neck, thorax, or suprarenal and pelvic areas.
   b. Vasoactive intestinal polypeptide (VIP) levels are often slightly above normal levels.
   c. Virtually all will present with watery diarrhea and hypokalemia
   d. Steatorrhea is a feature of this disease.
   e. All of the above are true.

6. Which is true regarding carcinoid tumors in children?
   a. Carcinoid tumors are composed of enterochromaffin cells.
   b. Symptoms are common in children.
   c. Symptoms are mediated by gastrin.

d. Treatment of choice is glucagon.

e. All of the above are false.

7. Which is not associated with mutations in the RET proto-oncogene?

a. Multiple endocrine neoplasia I.

b. Multiple endocrine neoplasia IIA.

c. Multiple endocrine neoplasia IIB.

d. Hirschsprung disease.

e. All have mutations in the RET proto-oncogene.

SYSTEMIC ENDOCRINOPATHIES

SYNOPSIS

DIABETES MELLITUS

1. Gastrointestinal (GI) manifestations well-described. (Table 1)

2. Pathogenesis: autonomic neuropathy, microangiopathy, hyperglycemia, electrolyte disturbances, and plasma hormone disturbances.

3. Gestational diabetes: fetus with increased risk of abortion, congenital malformations, macrosomia with increase in heart and liver size, intrauterine growth restriction, respiratory distress, hypoglycemia, hypocalcemia, jaundice secondary to polycythemia, cardiomyopathy, and increased perinatal mortality.

4. Neonatal small left colon: results in low obstruction of large bowel (failure to pass meconium) and bilious emesis. Etiology unclear. Treatment conservative: parenteral nutrition and nasogastric decompression. Resolves in first 1–2 wk of life.

5. Diabetic ketoacidosis: can mimic an acute abdomen. Elevations of amylase usually represent salivary amylase. Upper GI hemorrhage, gastric distention, and dysmotility secondary to hypermagnesemia reported.

6. Diabetes and GI neuropathy: neuropathic changes in the GI tract occur over prolonged periods with poor diabetic control; diabetic neuropathy rare in children. However, 25% of children with diabetes mellitus (DM) have evidence of low sensory nerve conduction and autonomic dysfunction at time of diagnosis with deterioration after 2 yr of disease. Neuropathy associated with DM appears to result from altered sympathetic function and cholinergic denervation.

7. Diabetes and the esophagus: alterations in esophageal function in diabetic children rare.

8. Diabetes and the stomach: alterations in gastric emptying among pediatric diabetics uncommon but in up to 58% of adult diabetics. Gold standard of diagnosis is scintigraphy done during a period of euglycemia. Etiology due to vagal dysfunction. Treatment: better glycemic control, dietary changes (smaller, more frequent low-residue meals), and alternative therapies including gastric pacemakers and *Clostridium botulinum* toxin injection into the pylorus to improve gastric emptying. Prokinetic pharmacotherapy useful (erythromycin domperidone). Hemorrhagic gastritis, acute or chronic gastritis, and pernicious anemia reported. Peptic ulcers seen at lower rate in diabetics than in general population owing to increased glucagon, which decreases gastric acid production.

9. Diabetes and *Helicobacter pylori*: diabetes is not a risk factor for infection.

10. Diabetes and autoimmune gastritis: 15–20% of DM adults have parietal cell antibodies; may be predisposed to gastric cancer and carcinoid tumors.

11. Diabetes and small bowel motility: delayed intestinal transit seen in up to 33% (decreases in contraction amplitude and alterations in migrating motor complex).

12. Diabetes and celiac disease: celiac disease and DM also linked to *HLA-DQ2*. Prevalence of celiac disease in type 1 DM is 10–30 times that of general population; celiac disease not increased in patients with type 2 DM. Gluten-free diet typically results in improved diabetic control in those with symptoms.

13. Diabetes and the liver: most common cause of elevated transaminase levels or hepatomegaly in DM is macrosteatosis. When inflammation results, nonalcoholic steatohepatitis may result with progression to cirrhosis. Predominant deposited lipid is triglyceride; hepatomegaly may result from increased glycogen stores. Fatty liver diagnosed in up to 17% of type 1 DM and up to 45% of type 2 DM. Degree of transaminase elevation does not correlate to degree of liver injury. Treatment: weight loss (≤ 1.6 kg/wk), better glycemic

TABLE 1   EFFECTS OF DIABETES MELLITUS ON THE GASTROINTESTINAL SYSTEM

ABNORMALITY/ASSOCIATION	GASTROINTESTINAL MANIFESTATION
Diabetic ketoacidosis	Nausea, anorexia, vomiting
Esophageal dysmotility	Dysphagia, reflux esophagitis
Esophageal candidiasis	Odynophagia, dysphagia
Gastroparesis/gastritis	Nausea, vomiting, gastric outlet obstruction
Small intestine dysmotility	Malabsorption, diarrhea, bacterial overgrowth
Impaired intestinal fluid reabsorption	Diabetic diarrhea
Celiac disease	Diarrhea, steatorrhea
Steatohepatitis	Abnormal transaminases, hepatic fibrosis
Hepatocellular carcinoma	Twofold increased risk
Cholelithiasis	Biliary sepsis

Adapted from Weber JR, Ryan JC. Effects on the gut of systemic disease and other extraintestinal conditions. In: Feldman M, Scharschmidt BF, Sleisenger M, editors. Sleisenger and Fodtran's gastrointestinal and liver disease: pathophysiology, diagnosis and management. Vol. 6. Philadelphia: WB Saunders; 1998. p. 411–38.

control, and vitamin E supplementation. Mauriac syndrome: hepatomegaly associated with increased glycogen, hypoglycemia, dwarfism, and cushingoid appearance. Results from increased serum glucose leading to hepatic glycogen accumulation and inactivation of glycogen phosphorylase with inhibition of glycogenolysis and increased glycogen stores. Treatment: insulin and better glycemic control. Among diabetics receiving peritoneal dialysis with added insulin, risk of developing subcapsular fatty changes. Hepatocellular carcinoma twice as prevalent in diabetics.

14. Diabetes and biliary function: frequency of cholecystitis, ascending cholangitis, and cholelithiasis in adult diabetics greater than in general population.

15. Diabetes and exocrine pancreas: 30% of adult DM have decreased exocrine pancreatic secretion, likely secondary to glucagons excess, malnutrition, vagal nerve dysfunction, and decreased insulin effects. Among diabetics who consume alcohol, 2–4 times the risk of pancreatic adenocarcinoma compared to general adult population.

16. Diabetic diarrhea: occurs in up to 20% with DM. Typically worse at night; more males than females. Etiology multifactorial, associated with rapid intestinal transit or defect in adrenergic stimulation of colonic water reabsorption. Clonidine and octreotide may be helpful. 50% have fecal incontinence secondary to decreased anal sphincter tone and rectal sensation. Need also consider drug, sorbitol, and small bowel bacterial overgrowth etiologies.

POLYGLANDULAR AUTOIMMUNE SYNDROME

1. Polyglandular autoimmune syndrome type I, also known as autoimmune polyendocrinopathy candidiasis ectodermal dystrophy. Autosomal recessive disease.

2. Characterized by a) failure of parathyroid, adrenal cortex, gonads, beta cells, parietal cells, and thyroid and/or hepatitis, b) chronic mucocutaneous candidiasis, c) dystrophy of dental enamel and nails, alopecia, vitiligo, or keratopathy. Number of endocrine organs involved varies: most with 4. Hypoparathyroidism most common; adrenocortical failure second most common. All have oral candidiasis; onset varies: 1 mo to 21 yr. Nail involvement in 71%. Autoimmune hepatitis 10–18%. Hepatic autoantigens: cytochrome P450 1A2, aromatic L-amino acid decarboxylase (AADC).

3. Typically affects those of Iranian, Jewish, Finnish, or Scandinavian descent.

4. One major mutation accounts for 90% cases (gene at chromosome 21q22.3: autoimmune regulator 1).

HYPERPARATHYROIDISM

1. Primary hyperparathyroidism rare, often undiagnosed. Sporadic adenomas causative. Rarely manifestation of multiple endocrine neoplasia (MEN) type I or II.

2. Identified in those with hypercalcemia, low or normal phosphate, and elevated parathyroid hormone (PTH).

3. Clinical manifestations: muscle weakness, paralysis, hyporeflexia. GI symptoms absent or nonspecific; poor appetite, weight loss, abdominal pain, nausea, constipation, vomiting, and peptic ulcer disease. Severe pancreatitis after parathyroidectomy in these patients may occur in up to 3% of patients.

HYPOPARATHYROIDISM

1. Rare among children.

2. May occur as part of other syndromes: polyglandular autoimmune syndrome, Pearson syndrome, and DiGeorge syndrome.

3. Hypocalcemia, hyperphosphatemia, and decreased PTH.

4. Clinical manifestations: neuromuscular instability; seizure, tetany, paresthesias, laryngospasm, bronchospasm, and prolonged Q-Tc. Also associated with malabsorption, pernicious anemia, and Addison disease. 11% with decreased PTH have chronic diarrhea and steatorrhea. Intestinal lymphangiectasia reported.

5. Symptoms of malabsorption may be earliest sign. Diarrhea typically ceases with vitamin D therapy. Need to rule out magnesium deficiency.

HYPOTHYROIDISM

1. Congenital hypothyroidism associated with constipation, feeding difficulties, amd prolonged neonatal jaundice.

2. Frequency of celiac disease in patients with autoimmune thyroid disease 4.3%.

3. Hypothyroid adults have an average of 3 bowel movements per week. Normal anorectal manometry shown but decreased rectal sensation. No change in whole-gut transit time.

4. Myxedema associated with decreased esophageal peristalsis and impaired lower esophageal sphincter function resulting in reflux. Hypothyroidism can also cause gastric hypomotility and secondary pseudo-obstruction.

5. Mild liver transaminitis in 50% of hypothyroid patients but histology normal. Hypothyroidism can cause exudative ascites in absence of overt liver disease.

HYPERTHYROIDISM

1. Associated with diarrhea. Anorectal manometry studies: lower maximal resting pressure, lower maximal anal squeeze pressure, and lower threshold sensation for evacuation. Accelerated small bowel and colonic transit present. Also, thyroid hormone can increase intestinal secretion via increased intracellular cyclic adenosine monophosphate.

2. Hyperthyroidism may cause myopathy or dysfunction of the striated muscles of pharynx and proximal esophagus with dysphagia or aspiration. Esophageal peristalsis increased in thyrotoxicosis.

3. Graves disease associated with ulcerative colitis.

4. Hyperthyroidism associated with minor histologic changes in liver.

PITUITARY HORMONES

1. Adrenocorticotropic hormone enhances brush border enzyme activity.

2. Thyrotropin-stimulating hormone causes thyroxine secretion with major effects on gut motility.

3. Growth hormone (GH) causes intestinal villus growth and enhances absorption.
4. Acromegaly (increased GH) associated with increased incidence of adenomatous colonic polyps, cancers of colon and stomach.

HYPOADRENOCORTICISM
1. Glucocorticoids increase absorption in the small intestine and digestive capacity of the brush border. Increased sodium absorption at the colon occurs as well.
2. Some patients with Addison disease have steatorrhea with normal jejunal histology, which resolves with hormone replacement.

DIENCEPHALIC SYNDROME
Complex of hypothalamic dysfunction.
1. Association between brain tumors of the anterior hypothalamus and severe failure to thrive almost exclusively seen in infants and young children (85% < 2 yr). Most have space-occupying lesions at region of optic chiasm.
2. Three major features: failure to thrive in spite of normal energy intake, motor hyperactivity, apparent euphoria. Autonomic disturbances may occur. Rotary nystagmus may be the only neurologic sign.
3. At diagnosis, length and head circumference are normal (except 33–58% have hydrocephalus). Vomiting occurs in 68%.
4. Etiology of extreme loss of subcutaneous fat tissue unclear. Patients may have an increase in resting energy expenditure.
6. Optimal therapy involves complete tumor resection with chemotherapy and radiation therapy as needed.

QUESTIONS

TRUE OR FALSE:
1. True pancreatitis is a common cause of elevated amylase in diabetic ketoacidosis.

2. Alterations in esophageal function are rare in diabetic children.
3. Diabetes is a risk factor for *Helicobacter pylori* infection.
4. Celiac disease has an increased prevalence among children with type 2 diabetes.
5. Fatty liver is more common among type 2 diabetics than in type 1 diabetics.
6. All patients with polyglandular autoimmune syndrome have mucocutaneous candidiasis.
7. Graves disease is associated with ulcerative colitis.

CHOOSE THE BEST ANSWER:
8. All is true about the gastrointestinal tract in hypothyroidism except:
   a. Congenital hypothyroidism associated with constipation, feeding difficulties, and prolonged neonatal jaundice.
   b. There is an increased frequency of celiac disease in patients with autoimmune thyroid disease.
   c. Hypothyroid patients have normal anal sphincter tone.
   d. Liver histology is abnormal in 50% of hypothyroid patients.
   e. Hypothyroidism can cause exudative ascites in the absence of overt liver disease.

MATCH THE FOLLOWING HORMONES WITH THEIR GASTROINTESTINAL EFFECTS:
a. Adrenocorticotropic hormone.
b. Thyroxine.
c. Growth hormone.

9. Affects motility.
10. Enhances brush border enzyme activity.
11. Causes intestinal villus growth.

ANSWERS

CONGENITAL ANOMALIES OF THE INTESTINES
1. a.
2. b.
3. a.
4. c.
5. True
6. True
7. True
8. False. Can be low or high. Look for anocutaneous fistula; if present, low.
9. False. Most are asymptomatic.
10. False. 60%.
11. False. Counterclockwise.

12. d.
13. b.
14. a.
15. d. Antimesenteric border.
16. c.

HERNIAS
1. d.
2. e.
3. c.
4. d.
5. d.
6. d.

7. True.
8. False. More common in slim persons.
9. True.

PERITONITIS

1. a.
2. d.
3. True.
4. False. It is an absolute indication.
5. False. Perforation due to ectopic gastric mucosa or ileoileal intussusception. Infection of gastric mucosa by *Helicobacter pylori* plays a minor role.
6. False. Usually localized at junction of fixed and mobile bowel segment (Treitz angle and ileocecal junction).
7. Spontaneous common bile duct perforation.

BENIGN PERIANAL LESIONS

1. a.
2. e.
3. c.
4. b.
5. d.
6. d. Occurs in more males than females.
7. c.
8. d. Associated with sphincter hypertonicity.

SURGICAL ABDOMEN

1. a.
2. d.
3. b.
4. c.
5. f.
6. e.
7. False. They do not resolve; prompt surgery required owing to high risk of incarceration.
8. True.

APPENDICITIS

1. False. Male-to-female ratio 1.4:1.
2. True.
3. False. Computed tomography with rectal contrast.
4. b.
5. c.
6. a.
7. a.
8. b, d.
9. d. Along with bowel rest and total parenteral nutrition.
10. c.
11. a.

INTESTINAL BACTERIAL INFECTIONS

1. c.
2. d.
3. d.
4. c.
5. d.
6. a.

7. a.
8. b.
9. a.
10. d.
11. False. Can worsen course and increase risk of hemolytic uremic syndrome.
12. True.
13. False. Watery without blood or pus.
14. True.
15. a.
16. c.
17. a.
18. a.
19. b.
20. e.
21. f.

FOODBORNE ILLNESS

1. a.
2. False. Once formed in food impossible to remove.
3. True.
4. j.
5. b.
6. e.
7. f.
8. h. Hypoglycin A.
9. g.
10. a.
11. c.
12. d.
13. d.
14. d.
15. d.
16. e.
17. e.
18. d. Ubiquitous; even if eradicated, recontamination likely.
19. c. Tapeworm absorbs free vitamin B_{12}.
20. b. Associated with sushi eating.
21. a.
22. e.
23. d.

VIRAL INFECTIONS

1. c.
2. a.
3. c.
4. b.
5. d.
6. f.
7. c.
8. True.
9. True.

PARASITIC AND FUNGAL INFECTIONS

1. b.
2. b. *Enterocytozoon bieneusi* can also cause sclerosing cholangitis in human immunodeficiency virus. *Encephalitozoon intestinalis* can spread to kidneys and be shed in urine.

3. b.

4. b, c.

5. b.

6. b, e. Penetrates skin, goes to lungs and trachea, then esophagus and intestines.

7. b.

8. b, f. Worms in jejunum; larvae go via lymphatics to skeletal muscle.

9. c. Only ciliate causing human disease; from pigs.

10. c.

11. b.

12. b, e. Larvae in lungs and worms in intestine.

13. b.

14. b.

15. c.

16. b, f. Cysticercosis disseminates to eye, central nervous system, skeletal muscle, and myocardium.

17. c, e. Can also cause liver abscess. Can spread to lung, brain, and kidney when abscess bursts into hepatic vein.

18. b. Can also obstruct appendix, pancreatic duct.

19. b. Also associated with B_{12} deficiency.

20. b.

21. b. Largest human fluke.

22. b.

23. c.

24. c. Can be confused with appendicitis.

25. c. Localized granulomatous masses: bilharziomas Also associated with stricture formation.

26. c, d.

27. g. Not associated with human disease.

28. b, c, e. TI and colon can rarely be involved. Usually pulmonary infection.

29. a. Only parasitic infection of stomach.

30. f.

31. l.

32. b.

33. d.

34. b.

35. h.

36. d

37. a.

38. a.

39. c.

40. f.

41. c.

42. f, g.

43. f, g.

44. f.

45. f.

46. b, d, e.

47. e.

48. i.

49. b.

SMALL BOWEL BACTERIAL OVERGROWTH

1. d.

2. d. Made by bacteria.

3. True.

4. False. Proximal is worse.

5. True.

6. False. Uncommon.

7. True. Biopsy to rule out.

8. True. If eradicate, small bowel bacterial overgrowth improved.

9. b. Elevated.

10. d.

GASTROINTESTINAL MANIFESTATIONS OF PRIMARY IMMUNODEFICIENCIES

1. e. Associated with all of the above.

2. True.

3. False. Usually well until 6 months of age owing to transplacentally transmitted maternal antibodies.

4. True. Spontaneously resolve before age 4 yr.

5. True.

6. b.

7. e.

8. k.

9. j. Secondary to granulomatous narrowing.

10. i. Associated with endocrinopathy.

11. d.

12. f. X-linked lymphoproliferative disease, also known as Purtilo syndrome.

13. c. Often present in first few months along with bloody diarrhea. Median survival 6 mo

14. a. Affected males usually die of overwhelming infection.

15. b. Autosomal recessive.

16. b.

17. b. Lymphoid hyperplasia, HSM, large numbers of oligoclonal T cells, and eosinophilia.

18. g.

19. h.

20. e. Hypoparathyroidism, anomalies great vessels, dysmorphic facies, esophageal atresia, bifid uvula, and congenital heart disease.

HIV AND OTHER SECONDARY IMMUNODEFICIENCIES

1. c.

2. e.

3. a.

4. b. To determine etiology.

SHORT BOWEL SYNDROME AND INTESTINAL TRANSPLANTATION

1. False. The ileum can carry out jejunal functions but not vice versa.

2. True.

3. c.

4. d.

5. d.

6. c.

7. d.

8. d.

9. c.

10. b.

11. c.

12. a.
13. b. No prior immunity to Epstein-Barr virus is a risk factor.

CROHN DISEASE
1. False.
2. True.
3. False.
4. False.
5. False.
6. True.
7. True.
8. False.
9. False.
10. True.
11. True.
12. True.

ULCERATIVE COLITIS
1. d.
2. b.
3. d.
4. d.
5. b.
6. False. Sulfasalazine.
7. False.

UNDETERMINED COLITIS AND OTHER INFLAMMATORY DISEASES
1. e.
2. d.
3. a, b, k, l.
4. a, d, f, g, h, j.
5. c, e, i, m.

NECROTIZING ENTEROCOLITIS
1. c.
2. b.
3. c.
4. a.
5. b.
6. c.
7. b.
8. c.
9. False.
10. True.

GENETIC DISACCHARIDASE DEFICIENCY
1. c.
2. b.
3. d. No sucrose in diet.
4. d.
5. c.
6. b. Except perhaps primary adult hypolactasia where intestinal biopsy may not be necessary.

CONGENITAL INTESTINAL TRANSPORT DEFECTS
1. d.
2. a.

3. b.
4. c.
5. c.
6. b.
7. a.
8. b.
9. a.
10. a.
11. True.
12. False. X-linked inheritance.
13. b.
14. d.

CONGENITAL ENTEROPATHY INVOLVING INTESTINAL MUCOSAL DEVELOPMENT
1. b.
2. c.
3. b.
4. a.
5. a, b.
6. b.

CELIAC DISEASE
1. True.
2. False.
3. True.
4. False.
5. j.
6. b, c. Also decreased villus to crypt depth.

FOOD-ALLERGIC ENTEROPATHY
1. a.
2. d.
3. a.
4. b.
5. b.
6. a.
7. True.
8. False. Th2.
9. False. 40%.

AUTOIMMUNE ENTEROPATHY
1. True.
2. True.
3. True.
4. False. Often extraintestinal autoimmune manifestations are present.
5. False.
6. False. IgE is dramatically elevated.
7. c.
8. a.
9. b.
10. d.

INTESTINAL POLYPS AND POLYPOSIS
1. b.
2. a.
3. a.
4. a.

5. b.
6. b.
7. a.
8. c.
9. b.
10. a.
11. a.
12. c.
13. a.
14. b.
15. d.
16. e.
17. f.
18. g.

OTHER NEOPLASMS
1. True.
2. False. More common in blacks in the United States.
3. False.
4. True.
5. True.
6. e.
7. e.
8. a.
9. c.
10. b.
11. b.

IDIOPATHIC CONSTIPATION
1. False. Straightening of the anorectal angle allows feces to be evacuated.
2. True.
3. False. Encopresis is rare in children < 3 years old.
4. e.
5. d. Patients with continued problems in the absence of withholding behaviors should have further investigations.
6. e.

DYSMOTILITIES
1. False. Requires full thickness biopsy.
2. True.
3. True.
4. True.
5. False. Intestinal dysmotilities are more commonly caused by neural versus myopathic disorders
6. False.
7. a.
8. a.
9. b.
10. c.
11. a.
12. b.
13. a.

HIRSCHSPRUNG DISEASE
1. d.
2. b.
3. d.
4. a.

CHRONIC INTESTINAL PSEUDO-OBSTRUCTION SYNDROME
1. True.
2. True.
3. False. Need to be careful about this diagnosis in preterm infants as may reflect immaturity rather than true dysfunction.
4. False. Owing to risk of adhesions, should only be performed in the setting of requirement to perform an enterostomy.
5. b.
6. b.

SECRETORY TUMORS AFFECTING THE GUT
1. b.
2. a.
3. c.
4. e.
5. d.
6. a.
7. a. Menin mutations.

SYSTEMIC ENDOCRINOPATHIES
1. False. Elevated serum amylase often secondary to salivary amylase.
2. True.
3. False.
4. False. Increased prevalence among children with type 1 diabetes.
5. True.
6. True.
7. True.
8. d. Liver histology is normal.
9. b.
10. a.
11. c.

CLINICAL MANIFESTATIONS AND MANAGEMENT:
The Liver and Metabolic Disease

NEONATAL CHOLESTASIS

SYNOPSIS

CHOLESTASIS

1. Definition: reduction in canalicular bile flow manifested as conjugated hyperbilirubinemia.
2. Development: extrahepatic biliary tree develops from an outgrowth of the ventral foregut. The intrahepatic biliary tree differentiates from the multipotent hepatoblast in a centrifugal fashion.

BILE FLOW

1. Bile acid–dependent flow: active canalicular transport of bile acids, accompanied by osmotic water flow and diffusion of other solutes.
2. Bile acid–independent flow: mediated by active transport of other anions and cations. Little contribution of this component during the neonatal period.
3. In the neonatal period: physiologic cholestasis associated with immature or altered metabolism and transport of bile acids at birth.

CHOLESTASIS IN THE NEWBORN

EXTRAHEPATIC DISORDERS

1. Extrahepatic biliary atresia (EHBA). Bile duct stricture. Choledochal cyst.
2. Anomalies of choledochopancreaticoductal junction.
3. Spontaneous perforation of the bile duct.
4. Inspissated bile.
5. Mass: intraductular: stone and rhabdomyosarcoma; extraductular: hepatoblastoma and neuroblastoma.

INTRAHEPATIC DISORDERS

1. Idiopathic neonatal hepatitis.
2. Intrahepatic cholestasis, persistent: Alagille syndrome; nonsyndromic paucity of intrahepatic ducts;

severe intrahepatic cholestasis with progressive hepatocellular disease.
3. Intrahepatic cholestasis, recurrent: benign recurrent intrahepatic cholestasis; hereditary cholestasis with lymphedema (Aagenaes syndrome).
4. Anatomic: congenital hepatic fibrosis, infantile polycystic disease (liver and kidney), and Caroli disease.
5. Disorders of amino acid metabolism (tyrosinemia).
6. Disorders of lipid metabolism: Wolman disease or cholesterol ester storage disease, Niemann-Pick disease, and Gaucher disease.
7. Disorders of carbohydrate metabolism: galactosemia, fructosemia, and glycogen storage disease type IV.
8. Disorders of bile acid metabolism, primary: 3β-hydroxysteroid Δ^5-C$_{27}$ steroid dehydrogenase/isomerase, Δ^5-3-oxosteroid 5β-reductase.
9. Disorders of bile acid metabolism, secondary: Zellweger syndrome, cerebrohepatorenal syndrome, and peroxisomal enzymopathies.
10. Disorders of bile acid transport: Rotor syndrome and Dubin-Johnson syndrome.
11. Mitochondrial hepatopathies.
12. Metabolic disease: α_1-antitrypsin deficiency, cystic fibrosis, hypopituitarism, hypothyroidism, neonatal iron storage disease, Menkes syndrome, hemophagocytic lymphohistiocytosis, and arginase deficiency.

TOXIC

Cholestasis associated with total parenteral nutrition, fetal alcohol syndrome, and other drugs.

CHOLESTASIS WITH INFECTION

Sepsis, syphilis, toxoplasmosis, *Listeria*, hepatitis A virus, human immunodeficiency virus, human parvovirus B19, *Cytomegalovirus*, herpes simplex virus, human herpesvirus 6, coxsackievirus, echovirus, rubella, hepatitis B virus, hepatitis C virus, and congenital viral infections.

GENETIC

1. Trisomy E (18), Down syndrome (trisomy 21), and trisomy 17.
2. Donahue syndrome (leprechaunism).

VASCULAR

Budd-Chiari syndrome, perinatal asphyxia, multiple hemangiomata, and cardiac insufficiency.

MISCELLANEOUS

1. Congenital disorders of glycosylation.
2. Shock and hypoperfusion.
3. Intestinal obstruction.
4. Neonatal lupus.
5. Arthrogryposis, renal tubular dysfunction, and cholestasis syndrome.

CLINICAL PRESENTATION OF CHOLESTASIS

1. Variable degrees of jaundice, dark urine, light stools, and hepatomegaly. Synthetic dysfunction and hepatocellular necrosis may be present.

TABLE 1   ESTIMATED FREQUENCY OF VARIOUS CLINICAL FORMS OF NEONATAL CHOLESTASIS

CLINICAL FORM	CUMULATIVE PERCENTAGE
"Idiopathic" neonatal hepatitis	15
Extrahepatic biliary atresia	25–30
α_1-Antitrypsin deficiency	7–10
Intrahepatic cholestasis syndromes (eg, Alagille, PFIC type I)	20
Bacterial sepsis	2
Hepatitis Cytomegalovirus	3–5
Rubella, herpes	1
Endocrine (hypothyroidism, panhypopituitarism)	1
Galactosemia	1
Inborn errors of bile acid biosynthesis	2–5

PFIC = progressive familial intrahepatic cholestasis.

2. In cases of rapid progression of hepatocellular disease, fibrosis occurs with portal hypertension.

PATHOGENESIS OF EHBA VERSUS NEONATAL HEPATITIS

1. Ductal plate malformation theory: altered embryogenesis resulting in anatomic abnormalities of the biliary tree.
2. Infantile obstructive cholangiopathy resulting from inflammation at various levels of the hepatobiliary tract. If the injury site is predominantly the bile duct epithelium, the resulting cholangitis leads to obliteration of bile duct and biliary atresia. If injury site is primarily hepatocellular, clinical picture may be that of neonatal hepatitis.

IDIOPATHIC NEONATAL HEPATITIS

1. Prolonged neonatal cholestasis associated with low birth weight. One-third have failure to thrive.
2. Majority appear well but jaundiced. > 50% develop jaundice in first week of life. Acholic stools uncommon. Liver firm and enlarged.
3. Serum bile acid levels markedly elevated. Bilirubin and aminotransferase mildly or moderately elevated (2–10 times upper limit of normal).
4. Associated anomalies unusual and should suggest other diagnoses.
5. Biopsy: stereotypical; multinucleated giant cells, hepatocellular ballooning, focal hepatic necrosis, and extramedullary hematopoiesis. Portal triad inflammation with lymphocytes and polymorphonuclear neutrophil leukocytes. Varying portal fibrosis. Bile duct proliferation and bile duct plugging absent.
6. Treatment: nutritional support, vitamins, and management of pruritus. Repeat liver biopsy for histology; electron microscopy and metabolic studies for children who do not follow a "normal" course with prolonged cholestasis (> 3.5 mo), fasting hypoglycemia, or recurrent cholestasis.
7. Prognosis: sporadic cases (classic giant cell hepatitis) more favorable than familial cases.

EXTRAHEPATIC BILIARY ATRESIA

Please see review of section on Biliary Atresia.

EVALUATION

1. No pathognomonic or prognostic biochemical feature for neonatal cholestasis (Table 2).
2. No single test reliable in differentiating neonatal hepatitis from biliary atresia.

LABORATORY DATA

1. Urine-reducing substances may produce false-negative for galactosemia if not receiving a galactose-containing formula or in case of notable vomiting (verify galactosemia instead with measurement of red blood count galactose 1-phosphate uridyltransferase, provided that there have been no recent blood transfusions).

TABLE 2   STAGED EVALUATION OF NEONATAL CHOLESTASIS

Differentiate cholestasis from physiologic breast milk jaundice and determine severity of disease
  Clinical evaluation (history, physical examination, stool color)
  Fractionated serum bilirubin (+ serum bile acids)
  Tests of hepatocellular and biliary disease (ALT, AST, alkaline phosphatase, GGT)
  Tests of hepatic function (serum albumin, prothrombin time, blood glucose, ammonia)
Exclude treatable and other specific disorders
  Bacterial cultures (blood, urine)
  VDRL test and viral serology as indicated (think HSV)
  α_1-Antitrypsin phenotype
  T_4 and TSH (rule out hypothyroidism)
  Metabolic screen: urine-reducing substances (drugs may cause false positives), urine bile acids, serum amino acids, ferritin, urine organic acids
  Sweat chloride/mutation analysis
Differentiate extrahepatic biliary obstruction from intrahepatic disorders
  Ultrasonography
  Hepatobiliary scintigraphy (not always essential)
  Liver biopsy

ALT = alanine transaminase; AST = aspartate transaminase; GGT = γ-glutamyl transpeptidase; HSV = herpes simplex virus; T_4 = thyroxine; TSH = thyroid stimulating hormone; VDRL = Venereal Disease Research Laboratory.

2. Elevated serum methionine and tyrosine levels may reflect severe liver disease and not be diagnostic of an underlying defect.
3. Phenotype is preferred in the evaluation of α_1-antitrypsin since neonates may have low levels despite normal phenotypes.
4. Toxoplasmosis, other agents, rubella, cytomegalovirus, and herpes simplex (TORCH) titers have low diagnostic yield and should be replaced by request for specific viral titers or cultures in the correct clinical setting.
5. γ-Glutamyl transpeptidase elevated in most cholestatic disorders, but normal levels seen in disorders where there is an abnormality of bile acid export or synthesis rather than bile acid–mediated injury of the canalicular membrane.
6. When considering a congenital defect in glycosylation, transferring immunoelectrophoresis should be performed.
7. Serum α-fetoprotein should be measured in tyrosinemia given increased risk of malignancy for screening and diagnostic purposes.
8. In the presence of splenomegaly, Niemann-Pick disease should be considered and addressed with a bone marrow aspirate.
9. Neurologic findings should suggest mitochondropathies and fatty acid oxidation defects.

RADIOLOGY

1. Ultrasonography: helpful for determining presence of choledochal cyst or tumor. Absence of gallbladder on a fasting study suggestive but not diagnostic of biliary atresia. Triangular cord sign may be predictive of biliary atresia in the setting of an abnormal gallbladder but operator dependent.

2. Chest radiograph: to look for situs abnormalities as well as butterfly vertebrae, rickets.
3. Radionucleotide imaging: differentiates biliary atresia from nonobstructive causes of cholestasis. Uptake of the iminodiacetic acid analogs varies: in biliary atresia, normal; in neonatal hepatitis, delayed. Pretreatment with phenobarbital enhances excretion and increases sensitivity. Nonexcretion may be related to severe intrahepatic cholestasis rather than extrahepatic obstruction. Passage of tracer into gastrointestinal tract is 100% sensitive for excluding biliary atresia, only 60% specific for biliary atresia.

LIVER BIOPSY
Most reliable and definitive procedure in the evaluation of the neonate with conjugated hyperbilirubinemia.

MEDICAL MANAGEMENT
1. Fat malabsorption: owing to decreased bile acids, low intraluminal micelles, fat absorption ineffective. Long-chain triglyceride lipolysis and absorption ineffective, but medium-chain triglycerides readily absorbed. Must also supplement essential fatty acids. Supplemental liposoluble vitamins needed (2–4 times the recommended daily amount) (Table 3).
2. Malnutrition: cholestatic infants require 130% of the caloric intake of age-matched controls; 60% should be in carbohydrate form, 20–30% in protein form.
3. Vitamin E deficiency: associated with progressive neuromuscular syndrome (areflexia, cerebellar ataxia, posterior column dysfunction, and peripheral neuropathy). Most reliable index of vitamin E status: ratio of serum vitamin E to total serum lipids. If age < 12 yr, ratio < 0.6 mg/g indicates vitamin E deficiency.
4. Pruritus: Phenobarbital (5–10 mg/kg/d): stimulates bile acid–independent flow and decreases bile acid pool size; sedative side effects. Rifampin (10mg/kg/d): inhibits hepatic uptake of bile acids. Ursodeoxycholate (UDCA) (15–30 mg/kg/d): alters bile acid composition; may be of benefit. Opioid antagonists: may alleviate but none completely abolish pruritus. In intractable pruritus unresponsive to medical therapy, partial biliary diversion has been performed.
5. Calcium: most children with cholestasis have severe osteopenia despite vitamin replacement. Calcium and magnesium supplementation advisable. Calcium sup-

plements should not be taken with UDCA as UDCA negatively affects calcium absorption.
6. Zinc deficiency more prevalent in cholestasis. Iron deficiency common in cholestasis.
7. Portal hypertension: progressive fibrosis and cirrhosis leads to portal hypertension. Restrict dietary sodium to 1–2 mg/kg/d. Diuresis with spironolactone and Lasix as needed. Therapeutic paracentesis with intravenous albumin may be necessary. Variceal management includes sclerotherapy, octreotide, and balloon tamponade.
8. Orthotopic liver transplant: an option for infants and children who progress to end-stage liver disease.

QUESTIONS

TRUE OR FALSE:
1. There is no single test reliable in differentiating neonatal hepatitis from biliary atresia.
2. Absence of a gallbladder on fasting ultrasonography is diagnostic of biliary atresia.
3. Presence of a gallbladder on fasting ultrasonography entirely rules out biliary atresia.
4. Passage of tracer on a hydroxy iminodiacetic acid scan into the gastrointestinal tract is 100% sensitive for excluding biliary atresia.

CHOOSE THE BEST ANSWER:
5. You are called to the emergency room to evaluate a 2-week-old newborn infant previously well but now presenting with a 1-week history of progressive vomiting and jaundice. After an initial evaluation, you are concerned about galactosemia but have been told that the newborn screen was negative. What further information do you need to make your recommendations?
   a. Whether the infant was being fed a lactose-containing formula at the time of newborn screen testing.
   b. Whether the infant has received a blood transfusion.
   c. Whether the infant was vomiting at the time of newborn screen testing.
   d. All of the above.
   e. None of the above.

6. Features not typical of neonatal hepatitis include all of the following except:
   a. Dysmorphic features.
   b. Acholic stools.
   c. Bile duct proliferation on liver pathology.
   d. Cholestasis lasting > 4 months.
   e. Jaundice in the first week of life.

7. A male infant presents to you at 6 weeks of age with a history of prolonged jaundice beginning in the newborn period. He was born full-term at 5 pounds and currently measures at the 5th percentile for weight, 50th percentile for length. TORCH titers are negative. Current laboratories reveal aspartate transaminase 150 U/L, alanine transaminase 100 U/L, total bilirubin 5.0 mg/dL,

TABLE 3 RECOMMENDED ORAL VITAMIN SUPPLEMENTATION

VITAMIN	PREPARATION, DOSE
Fat soluble	
Vitamin A	Aquasol A: 3,000–25,000 IU/d
Vitamin D	Cholecalciferol: 500–5,000 IU/d or 25-Hydroxycholecalciferol: 3–5 µg/kg/d
Vitamin K	Phytonadione (K1): 2.5–5 mg every other day
Vitamin E	Aquasol E: 50–400 IU/d or TPGS 15–25 IU/kg/d
Water soluble	Twice the recommended daily allowance

TPGS = d-α-tocopherol polyethylene glycol 1000 succinate.

and direct bilirubin 3.2 mg/dL. There is firm hepatomegaly on examination. You examine the diaper and find a yellow-green stool. What are you most likely to find on biopsy examination?

a. Bile duct proliferation with bile plugs.
b. Multinucleated giant cells with portal triad inflammation.
c. Lack of intrahepatic bile ducts.
d. Cirrhosis.
e. All of the above.

INTRAHEPATIC BILE DUCT DISEASE

SYNOPSIS

Development of the intrahepatic biliary tree begins during gestational weeks 5–9. Intrahepatic ducts form first with the ductal plate followed by remodeling from hepatic hilum centrifugally toward the periphery of the liver. Process continues through the first month of life ex utero.

INTRAHEPATIC BILE DUCT CYSTIC CONDITIONS

1. Important distinction between communicating and noncommunicating cysts to the biliary tree. Communicating: can cause disease (stones, cholangitis, and neoplasia). Noncommunicating: usually asymptomatic unless large (may present as abdominal mass or biliary obstruction).
2. Solitary cysts: generally unilocular cysts lined with a single layer cuboidal or columnar epithelium. Present in 4th to 6th decade with symptoms of fullness or mass. Rare in children.
3. Mesenchymal hamartomas: more common in pediatric age group. Multiple cysts with a solid component.
4. Ciliated hepatic foregut cysts: characterized by a lining of ciliated pseudostratified columnar epithelium resting on a basement membrane, surrounded by smooth muscle bundles. More common in males in 4th to 5th decade.
5. Peribiliary cysts: derived from dilatation of peribiliary glands at the hilum and large portal areas. Not reported in childhood.
6. Hepatobiliary cystadenomas: benign multilocular cystic neoplasms. Occur in middle-age women. Occur in the liver but also arise within the extrahepatic biliary tree and gallbladder. Lined by a flattened, occasionally papillary, mucin-producing columnar epithelium. In females, cysts surrounded by dense mesenchymal tissue resembling ovarian stroma.

INHERITED INTRAHEPATIC BILE DUCT CYSTIC DISEASE

1. Ductal plate malformation (DPM) seen in all major heritable conditions characterized by intrahepatic bile duct cysts. Renal cysts typically present.
2. Congenital hepatic fibrosis (CHF): characteristic hepatopathology resulting in portal hypertension and increased risk of ascending cholangitis. Characteristic lesion: DPM. Variable fibrosis: usually diffuse, occasionally confined. Firm hepatomegaly with prominent left lobe, splenomegaly, and hypersplenism. Associations: autosomal recessive polycystic kidney disease (ARPKD); cholangiocarcinoma (uncommon but serious complication); other visceral abnormalities (congenital heart disease, pulmonary hypertension and arteriovenous fistulae, berry aneurysms, and osteochondrodysplasia); phosphomannose isomerase deficiency (syndrome of intestinal lymphangiectasia and protein-losing enteropathy). Treatment: portosystemic shunting treatment of choice (low incidence of postoperative encephalopathy or hyperammonemia). Prolonged cholangitis is a major complication responsible for hepatic failure and death.
3. CHF and nephronophthisis: combination of hepatic lesions (features consistent with DPM) with severe tubulointerstitial renal disease (interstitial inflammation, fibrosis with tubular atrophy, cysts, and secondary glomerulosclerosis). Usually progressive renal failure by age 20 yr.
4. CHF and malformation syndromes: associated with DPM.
   a. Meckel-Gruber syndrome: recessively inherited lethal condition with central nervous system (occipital meningoencephalocele) abnormalities, bilateral large multicystic kidneys, CHF, and polydactyly. Gene loci: *MKS1, MKS2, MKS3*.
   b. Jeune syndrome (asphyxiating thoracic dystrophy): rare, autosomal recessive skeletal dysplasia leading to respiratory insufficiency owing to a severely constricted thoracic cage.
   c. Ivemark syndrome (renal-pancreatic-hepatic dysplasia and frequent polysplenia).
5. Controversial whether CHF and ARPKD represent single disorder or are distinct entities. Renal pathologies differ markedly: ARPKD: renal lesions diffuse and prominent; CHF: renal lesions not as evident early on and are minor.
6. Autosomal dominant polycystic kidney disease (ADPKD): most common hereditary kidney disorder; 1/1,000–1/400 worldwide. Hepatic lesions are primarily duct cysts that increase in size over time. Commonly, such cysts do not communicate with the distal biliary tree and do not contain bile. Significant number of deaths result from hepatic complications including cyst infection, cholangiocarcinoma, portal hypertension, and pressure secondary to cysts. The renal lesion consists of cysts arising from multiple areas along the nephron. Cysts can be found in many other organs (spleen, pancreas, thyroid, ovary, and epididymis). Arterial aneurysms are present in up to 30%. ADPKD results from mutations at *PKD1* and *PKD2*, the products of which are polycystin 1 and 2. *PKD3* also implicated.
7. ARPKD: spectrum of clinical and pathological manifestations. Two invariant features: DPM and fusiform dilatation of renal collecting ducts. Renal disease may vary from lethal perinatal disease to an incidental finding in older children. The liver lesion is uniform in

ARPKD with portal tract fibrous enlargement. Cysts more frequent with age. Mutations at *PKHD1*, which encodes for fibrocystin and polyductin.

8. Isolated hepatic polycystic disease: distinct entity from ADPKD. Autosomal dominant inheritance; no renal lesions. Mutations at the *PRKCSH* gene. Cysts arise from dilatation of biliary microhamartomas and peribiliary glands; age-dependent; rare in childhood. Higher prevalence of mitral valve abnormalities in this group.

9. Caroli disease: congenital dilatation of the larger intrahepatic bile ducts. Two variants: pure ductal ectasia without other hepatic pathology ("Caroli disease") and Caroli disease associated with lesions of CHF ("Caroli syndrome"). Communicating duct cysts occur in both variants. Caroli disease: very rare; not inherited. Caroli syndrome: unclear whether a variant of CHF; autosomal recessive. Controversial whether Caroli disease is associated with choledochal cyst. Caroli disease usually becomes symptomatic in adults. Children may present with Caroli syndrome owing to renal and liver abnormalities. In both, duct ectasias predispose to recurrent cholangitis, abscesses, sepsis, amyloidosis, and cholangiocarcinoma.

BILE DUCT PAUCITY

Ratio of ducts to portal tracts < 0.9 (not applicable to premature infants). Associated disorders with bile duct paucity are listed below (Table 1).

SYNDROMIC BILE DUCT PAUCITY

1. Alagille syndrome. Autosomal dominant. Mutations in *JAG1* at 20p12 (70% of individuals with Alagille syndrome), which encodes a ligand in the Notch pathway involved in cell fate determination.

2. Characterized by marked reduction in number of interlobular bile ducts and cholestasis in association with cardiovascular, skeletal, ocular, facial, renal (usually deposition of lipids at the glomeruli), and pancreatic and neurodevelopmental abnormalities (Table 2). Early infancy: duct paucity may be absent. Usually presents in first 3 months of life among those who are symptomatic. Diagnosed when characteristic or compatible liver histology accompanied by extrahepatic findings. Extreme variability in clinical manifestations; incomplete penetrance of the syndrome.

3. Diagnosis established with presence of cholestasis and 2 of 4 abnormalities (facies, murmur, vertebral anomalies, and posterior embryotoxon). Genetic testing can identify mildly affected patients (relatives). Important to distinguish from biliary atresia: Kasai procedure may lead to worsening disease. Young infants: biopsy can be nondiagnostic; may be helpful to repeat biopsy or perform operative wedge biopsy or operative cholangiogram. Laboratory tests not helpful in differentiating Alagille syndrome from other causes of extrahepatic obstruction in young patients. Older children: striking elevations in bile acid levels, serum lipids, γ-glutamyltransferase, and alkaline phosphatase; prothrombin time and measures of synthetic and metabolic functions are normal.

TABLE 1   DISORDERS ASSOCIATED WITH BILE DUCT PAUCITY IN CHILDREN

SYNDROMIC BILE DUCT PAUCITY—ALAGILLE SYNDROME
NONSYNDROMIC BILE DUCT PAUCITY
Metabolic and genetic disorders
  α$_1$-Antitrypsin deficiency
  Cystic fibrosis (rare)
  Peroxisomal disorders (rare)
  Progressive familial intrahepatic cholestasis (rare)
  Trisomy 21 (rare)
  Prune-belly syndrome (rare)
Infection
  Congenital cytomegalovirus infection (rare)
  Congenital syphilis (rare)
  Congenital rubella (rare)
Inflammatory and immune disorders
  Graft-versus-host disease
  Chronic hepatic allograft rejection
  Sclerosing cholangitis
  Sarcoidosis (rare)
Other
  Drug- or antibiotic-associated vanishing bile duct syndrome
  Familial idiopathic adulthood ductopenia
  Biliary atresia (late)
Panhypopituitarism (rare)
  Idiopathic

4. Treatment: treat fat malabsorption and fat-soluble vitamin deficiencies. Pruritus can be severe: antihistamines, cholestyramines, ursodiol, and naltrexone useful; rifampin useful in one-half of patients. Partial biliary diversion may be helpful for medically refractory cases.

5. Prognosis: variable outcome usually directly related to severity of hepatic or cardiac disease. Transplantation: careful consideration of parent as donor (can be asymptomatic with disease).

NONSYNDROMIC BILE DUCT PAUCITY

1. Graft-versus-host disease (GVHD): rare to find hepatic lesions without cutaneous lesions. Duct injury present with epithelial atypia, vacuolization, and regeneration. Endotheliitis may be useful to reflect GVHD. Duct paucity. Uncommon to find cirrhosis.

2. Liver allograft rejection: bile duct injury is significant element of rejection of hepatic allografts. Three elements needed for diagnosis: duct injury, portal inflammatory infiltrate, and endotheliitis. If severe, injury may result in duct loss and paucity. Chronic rejection (usually present between 6 wk and 6 mo after transplant) often requires retransplant owing to relentless progression of disease.

3. Cytomegalovirus: bile duct paucity may result from an obliterative cholangitis. Also seen in congenital rubella and congenital syphilis.

4. Drug-associated bile duct paucity: most frequently reported after use of antibiotics.

5. Extrahepatic biliary atresia: development of paucity described in patients both pre- and post-Kasai.

6. Primary sclerosing cholangitis: characterized by generalized beading and stenosis of the biliary tree in absence of choledocholithiasis with histologic abnor-

TABLE 2   CLINICAL MANIFESTATIONS OF ALAGILLE SYNDROME

SYSTEM	FINDINGS
Hepatic	Duct paucity, cholestasis, neonatal hepatitis, fibrosis, cirrhosis, portal hypertension, liver failure, hepatocellular carcinoma, nodular hamartoma
Cardiac	Murmur, pulmonic valvular stenosis, tetralogy of Fallot, pulmonary atresia, truncus arteriosus, ventricular septal defect complex, ventricular septal defect, atrial septal defect, anomalous venous return
Vascular	Peripheral pulmonic stenosis, pulmonic outflow stenosis, coarctation, patent ductus arteriosus, renal artery stenosis, middle aorta syndrome, moyamoya
Skeletal	Butterfly vertebrae, shortened interpedicular distance, shortened phalanges, short stature, spina bifida occulta, fusion of adjacent vertebrae, absent twelfth rib, shortened distal ulna and radius, clubbing, pathologic fractures, osteopenia, rickets
Ocular	Posterior embryotoxon, Axenfeld anomaly, Rieger anomaly, shallow anterior chamber, cataracts, strabismus, exotropia, ectopic pupil, optic disk drusen, iris stromal hypoplasia, band keratopathy, glaucoma, microcornea, keratoconus, congenital macular dystrophy, anomalous optic disks, fundic hyperpigmentation, pigmentary retinopathy, night blindness
Facial/cranial	Characteristic pediatric "particular facies," adult "particular facies," sinus abnormalities, chronic sinusitis, thinned cortical bones, deafness, large ears, high-pitched voice, macrocephaly
Renal	Neonatal renal insufficiency, adult renal failure, solitary, ectopic, or horseshoe kidney, bifid pelvis, duplicated ureter, small kidney, cystic and multicystic kidney, dysplastic kidney, infantile renal tubular acidosis, juvenile nephronophthisis, lipidosis, tubulointerstitial nephropathy, interstitial fibrosis
Central nervous system	Intracranial epidural, subdural, subarachnoid, and intraparenchymal bleeding; stroke; vascular malformation; mental retardation; developmental delay; school dysfunction; abnormal visual, auditory, and somatosensory evoked potentials
Cutaneous	Jaundice, xanthomata, pruritus, thickened, lichenified hands and feet
Growth disorders	Failure to thrive, fat-soluble vitamin deficiency, protein-calorie malnutrition, short stature
Pancreatic	Exocrine insufficiency, diabetes mellitus, pancreatic fibrosis
Other	Tracheal and bronchial stenosis, jejunal atresia, ileal atresia, malrotation, microcolon, otitis media, extrahepatic malignancies

Adapted from Alagille D, Estrada A, Hadchouel M, et al. Syndromic paucity of interlobular bile ducts (Alagille syndrome or arteriohepatic dysplasia): review of 80 cases. J Pediatr 1987;110:195–200, Emerick KM, Rand EB, Goldmuntz E, et al. Features of Alagille syndrome in 92 patients: frequency and relation to prognosis. Hepatology 1999;29:822–9, Crosnier C, Lykavieris P, Meunier-Rotival M, Hadchouel M. Alagille syndrome. The widening spectrum of ateriohepatic dysplasia. Clin Liver Dis 2000;4:765–78, Lykavieris P, Hadchouel M, Chardot C, Bernard O. Outcome of liver disease in children with Alagille syndrome: a study of 163 patients. Gut 2001;49:431–5, and Hashida Y, Yunis EJ. Syndromatic paucity of interlobular bile ducts: hepatic histopathology of the early and endstage liver. Pediatr Pathol 1988;8:1–15

malities of the bile ducts. Progressive obliteration of intra- and extrahepatic bile ducts may occur.

QUESTIONS

TRUE OR FALSE:
1. Noncommunicating cysts at the biliary tree are usually asymptomatic.
2. Ductal plate malformation seen exclusively in autosomal recessive polycystic kidney disease.

MATCH THE CHARACTERISTICS TO THE DISEASE:
a. Asphyxiating thoracic dystrophy.
b. Occipital meningoencephalocele, polydactyly, bilateral multicystic kidneys, congenital hepatic fibrosis.
c. Intestinal lymphangiectasia, congenital hepatic fibrosis.
d. Renal-pancreatic-hepatic dysplasia with frequent polysplenia.

3. Meckel-Gruber syndrome.
4. Jeune syndrome.
5. Ivemark syndrome.
6. Phosphomannose isomerase deficiency.

MATCH THE IMPLICATED GENE TO THE CONDITION:
a. *JAG1*.
b. *PKHD1*.
c. *PKD1*, *PKD2*, and *PKD3*.

7. Alagille syndrome.
8. Autosomal recessive polycystic kidney disease.
9. Autosomal dominant polycystic kidney disease.

EXTRAHEPATIC BILE DUCT DISEASE

SYNOPSIS

DEVELOPMENT
Extrahepatic bile ducts develop from the cephalic portion of the hepatic diverticulum during 4th to 6th week of gestation.

EXTRAHEPATIC BILIARY ATRESIA
1. Progressive fibroinflammatory cholangiopathy resulting in complete obliteration of portions of or entire extrahepatic biliary tree within weeks of birth. Obstruction leads to secondary cirrhosis. Usually gallbladder involved with only fibrous remnant remaining. Most common cause of prolonged conjugated hyperbilirubinemia in neonates. Most frequent indication for liver transplantation in children (40–50%).
2. Epidemiology: 1/15,000 to 1/8,000 live births. Higher incidence in nonwhite populations: African-American, French Polynesian, Chinese.
3. Two groups:
   a. Perinatal, isolated extrahepatic biliary atresia (EHBA): no other congenital anomalies. Usually variable jaundice-free period after birth, appropriate for gestational age.
   b. Embryonic form: 10–20%; situs inversus, polysplenia, and complete EHBA. Bilateral left sidedness usually with bilobed lungs, abdominal heterotaxia, situs ambiguous, and polysplenia. Gastrointestinal (GI) malformations (50–70%): tracheoesophageal fistula, esophageal atresia, atresias, malrotation, annular pancreas, and midline liver. Azygous inferior vena cava, preduodenal portal vein, hepatic artery anomalies, and congenital heart disease. Slight female predominance. Earlier onset of disease with no jaundice-free interval and low weight.

CLINICAL COURSE
1. Well at birth, usually full term. Weight gain initially normal, becomes suboptimal with development of disease. Direct bilirubin usually < 7 mg/dL (total 6–12). Hepatomegaly and splenomegaly present early, reflects degree of portal hypertension and hepatic fibrosis. Cardiac anomalies present with polysplenia. Any neonate with conjugated bilirubin > 2 mg/dL or 15% conjugated bilirubin needs work-up to rule out EHBA. γ-Glutamyltransferase (GGT) markedly elevated.
2. Three types:
   a. Type I: common bile duct atresia and patent proximal system.
   b. Type II: involving hepatic duct but patent proximal system.
   c. Type III: involving right and left hepatic duct at porta hepatis.
3. Pathogenesis theories: defect in morphogenesis of the biliary tract, defect in fetal or prenatal circulation, environmental toxin exposure, viral infection, or immunologic or inflammatory dysregulation.

DIAGNOSIS
1. Radiologic studies:
   a. Ultrasonography: useful to rule out choledochal cyst and other congenital malformations. Absence of gallbladder is suggestive of EHBA, but presence does not rule it out. Triangular cord is suggestive with a negative predictive value of > 95% for neonatal hepatitis.
   b. Scintigraphy: measures hepatic uptake and excretion of analogs of iminodiacetic acid into the intestine. Phenobarbital 5 mg/kg/d for 5 days prior to study increases discrimination of test.
   c. Aspiration of duodenal fluid: if bile-stained fluid present in a 24 h collection, EHBA unlikely.
   d. Endoscopic retrograde cholangiography: requires an experienced endoscopist for examination in the neonate.
2. Liver biopsy: demonstrates bile plugging, proliferated ducts, edema, and fibrosis.
3. Exploratory laparotomy with cholangiography: when liver biopsy suggestive or diagnostic work-up inconclusive, cholangiography can be helpful. Poor filling of intrahepatic bile ducts may suggest Alagille syndrome.

TREATMENT
1. Kasai procedure: Roux en Y jejunostomy. Major complications: failure to drain bile and ascending cholangitis (50–100%). Results dramatically better if done before 60 d. Single most predictive factor of long-term results: resolution of jaundice. Successful biliary drainage in 40–60% of infants. Untreated patients: mean lifespan 11 mo.
2. Postoperative care:
   a. To improve drainage - ursodeoxycholate 20 mg/kg/d (few studies show efficacy).
   b. To reduce bile duct inflammation - steroids (varying success).
   c. To decrease cholangitis risk - perioperative and postoperative antibiotic prophylaxis (no conclusive reduction in risk of cholangitis however).
   d. Nutritional support, especially if cholestasis remains - requires fat soluble vitamin supplementation.
3. If cholestasis persists, surgical revision of the portoenterostomy should be considered. Long-term outcome predicted by serum bilirubin 3 mo from surgery. In infants with serum bilirubin levels < 1 mg/dL: 53% normal growth without esophageal varices.
4. Cholangitis can occur postoperatively with good drainage. Usually present with fever, acholic stools and increased serum bilirubin. Treat with broad-spectrum antibiotics.
5. Hepatic fibrosis may continue even with low serum bilirubin. Significant portal hypertension in 34–76%.
6. Hepatopulmonary syndrome: intrapulmonary vascular dilatation. Treatable only with liver transplant.
7. Cystic dilatation of intrahepatic bile ducts and hepatocellular carcinoma: rare developments.

8. Liver transplantation: most frequent indication for orthotopic liver transplantation in children. Post-transplant survival up to 95% at 1 yr, 91% at 2 yr. Indications:
   a. Persistent cholestasis with malnutrition or growth failure and hepatocellular dysfunction.
   b. Decompensated cirrhosis.
   c. Primary therapy for children diagnosed beyond 90–120 d with established cirrhosis.

CHOLEDOCHAL CYST

1. Five types:
   a. Type I: congenital cystic dilatation of common bile duct (CBD) without intrahepatic involvement. Most common type (75–85%).
   b. Type II: diverticular malformation of the CBD; 2–3%.
   c. Type III: choledochocele associated with ampullary obstruction; 3.5%.
   d. Type IV: multiple cysts of the extrahepatic or both intrahepatic and extrahepatic ducts.
   e. Type V: single or multiple intrahepatic cysts: Caroli disease.
2. Incidence: varies; high among Asian populations. Female-to-male ratio 4:1. Usually isolated anomaly; not associated with other organ malformation.
3. Etiology: congenital or acquired. Congenital theory: unequal epithelial cell proliferation. Acquired: secondary to anomalous arrangement of distal pancreaticobiliary tree with reflux of pancreatic enzymes, inflammation, localized weakness, and dilatation.
4. Diagnosis: ultrasonography (diagnosis in 80–100%), hepatobiliary scans, computed tomography or magnetic resonance imaging, percutaneous transhepatic cholangiography, and endoscopic retrograde cholangiopancreatography (ERCP). ERCP allows definition of anatomy and sampling to rule out malignancy.
5. Histologically: fibrous wall with or without mononuclear inflammation. Generally, no epithelium lining the cysts (most common associated malignancies: adenocarcinoma of the bile duct or gallbladder). In general, total cyst excision significantly decreases malignancy development.
6. Choledochal cysts: associated with pain, abdominal mass, and jaundice. Triad present in 13–63%. Intermittent biliary stasis can result in ascending cholangitis, cholelithiasis, pancreatitis, cyst rupture, progressive biliary cirrhosis, portal hypertension, hepatic failure, and malignant transformation of the cyst itself.
7. Laboratory tests: γ-glutamyltransferase (GGT) and alkaline phosphatase elevated in 70% of patients; conjugated hyperbilirubinemia in 56%. Elevated amylase and lipase suggest associated pancreatitis and ductal obstruction. Mild transaminitis in 70%. Secondary biliary cirrhosis in 30% and can result in liver compromise.
8. Therapy: complete surgical removal. Incidence of cancer in adults as high as 18–28%, 50% if initial surgery had enteric drainage procedure. One-half of cancers are intrahepatic, so excision does not eliminate risk of cancer. If cancer occurs, poor prognosis.

ACCESSORY BILE DUCTS

1. Extranumerary ducts usually arise at right lobe of liver, entering one of normal extrahepatic ducts or cystic duct. Other accessory ducts may allow communication between other portions of the biliary tree (right and left hepatic ducts).
2. Cholecystohepatic ducts: ducts of Luschka. Abnormal duct elements arise in liver and end up at wall of gallbladder; may pass through wall to enter normal extrahepatic duct elements.
3. Accessory ducts are common; no physiologic significance.
4. In common bile duct duplication, one duct usually drains right liver, other drains left liver.

CONGENITAL BRONCHOBILIARY FISTULA

Usually between right mainstem bronchus and bile duct system within left lobe of liver.

SHORT CHOLEDOCHUS SYNDROME

Abnormal insertion of the bile duct high at duodenum. Gastritis or duodenal ulcer may occur. Malignancy may occur.

ISOLATED STRICTURE OR STENOSIS OF EXTRAHEPATIC BILE DUCTS

1. Strictures occur less commonly in children than adults. They may occur secondary to trauma, surgery, or inflammation with or without stones. Usually occurs at bifurcation of hepatic ducts. May also occur at ampulla of Vater. Sometimes secondary to relapsing pancreatitis.
2. Treatment: sphincterotomy or sphincteroplasty; choledochoenterostomy if cannot do proximal repair.

PHRYGIAN CAP

Congenital deformity of no significance where fundus of gallbladder is kinked.

PERFORATION OF THE BILE DUCTS

1. Spontaneous perforation: rare; occurs within first few months of life. Most common site: junction of cystic and common hepatic ducts (Note: Perforation secondary to pigment gallstones also occurs at junction of cystic duct and hepatic duct; supports hypothesis of intrinsic weakness of duct wall at that site). Bile may leak into peritoneum and cause sterile bile peritonitis. At surgery: common to find sac adjacent to perforation; should not be confused with choledochal cyst.
2. Clinical symptoms: infants usually asymptomatic in first few weeks of life, then progressive abdominal distention, vomiting, jaundice, discolored stools, and failure to thrive. Mild conjugated hyperbilirubinemia with minimal transaminitis and acholic stools are suggestive.

3. Ultrasonography: ascites. Radionuclide scan: Diisopropyl iminodiacetic acid tracer in peritoneum. Can also diagnose via paracentesis for bile fluid.
4. Treatment: surgical repair is primary; choledochoenterostomy if distal obstruction.

NEONATAL SCLEROSING CHOLANGITIS

1. Irregular narrowing of either intra- or extrahepatic ducts resulting from inflammation and fibrosis. Obliteration of bile ducts results in biliary cirrhosis. Cause unknown.
2. Jaundice, cholestasis, and acholic stools observed within first weeks of life. In all cases, jaundice resolves in first year of life but progresses to cirrhosis.
3. Transplantation has been used to treat some cases with no report of recurrence of disease. Role of medical therapy unknown.

PRIMARY SCLEROSING CHOLANGITIS

1. Chronic hepatobiliary disorder with inflammation of the intra- and extrahepatic bile ducts. Pathogenesis: etiology unknown.
2. Diagnosis: cholangiography (irregular narrowing, structuring, or beading of hepatic or common bile ducts) or histology (classic presentation: onion skin appearance).
3. Associations: in children, inflammatory bowel disease; in adults, autoimmune diseases including diabetes, pancreatitis, and thyroid diseases.
4. Clinically: gradual onset. Many children asymptomatic; detect with screening laboratory tests. No pathognomonic laboratory findings. In adults, elevated alkaline phosphatase. Elevated GGT more sensitive in children.
5. Treatment: no large randomized controlled trials of any therapeutic agents. Ursodeoxycholic acid has been used in children with significant reductions in alkaline phosphatase and GGT. Surgical options used primarily for biliary obstruction. Transplantation in those progressing to cirrhosis, but recurrence common.
6. Prognosis: true rate unknown. In large pediatric series, one-third of children died, secondary to cirrhosis and portal hypertension; one-third listed for transplant or transplanted.

QUESTIONS

TRUE OR FALSE:

1. Absence of a gallbladder is diagnostic of extrahepatic biliary atresia.
2. An intraoperative cholangiography is unnecessary during a planned Kasai procedure for extrahepatic biliary atresia demonstrated by liver biopsy.
3. Good bile flow after Kasai procedure is predictive of resolution of jaundice in patients with extrahepatic biliary atresia.
4. The incidence of choledochal cysts is higher in Asian populations.
5. Choledochal cysts are more common in boys.

6. The triad of pain, abdominal mass, and jaundice is a universal presentation of choledochal cyst.
7. Risk of cancer is reduced to normal with complete resection of a choledochal cyst.

CHOOSE THE BEST ANWER:

8. Congenital bronchobiliary fistulae usually arise from which mainstem bronchus?
   a. Right.
   b. Left.
   c. Both equally.

9. Which of the following is true of spontaneous perforation of the bile ducts?
   a. It is often associated with a choledochal cyst.
   b. Ultrasonography is diagnostic.
   c. It occurs most commonly at the junction of the right and left hepatic ducts.
   d. Patients are symptomatic at birth.
   e. It occurs within first few months of life.

TRUE OR FALSE:

10. There are no pathognomonic laboratory findings for primary sclerosing cholangitis.
11. Ursodeoxycholic acid has been shown in a randomized, controlled trial to improve the course of primary sclerosing cholangitis.

VIRAL HEPATITIS

SYNOPSIS

HEPATITIS A VIRUS

1. Ribonucleic acid (RNA) picornavirus. Nonenveloped. Only 1 serotype. Human strains: 4 genotypes.
2. Found in blood and stool for 2–3 wk before clinical symptoms; stool excretion then persists for an additional 2 wk. Transmission fecal-oral.
3. Endemic in developing countries: children infected in first years of life.
4. Outbreaks in homosexual men and day care centers described.
5. Virus-specific immune mechanisms in hepatic injury.

DIAGNOSIS

Serologic: detection of immunoglobulin (Ig)M anti–hepatitis A virus (HAV) 5–10 d after exposure; peak levels during acute or early convalescence with disappearance by 3–4 mo.

CLINICAL FEATURES

1. Mean incubation period 30 d.
2. Infants and young children: asymptomatic or nonspecific acute gastroenteritis; jaundice rare.
3. Older children and adults: prodrome usually 7 d; fever, headache, and malaise; then jaundice, abdominal pain, nausea and vomiting, and anorexia. Jaundice

peaks over several days; systemic symptoms wane. Symptoms resolve by 2–3 wk.

4. Most prominent finding: tender hepatomegaly; peak bilirubin usually 10 mg/dL (usually normalizes within 4 wk), peak alanine aminotransferase (ALT) usually 3,000 IU/L (normalizes within 2–3 wk).

FOUR ATYPICAL MANIFESTATIONS

1. Cholestatic hepatitis: jaundice persists for > 12 wk, accompanied by severe pruritis; usually resolves by 20–24 wk.
2. Relapsing hepatitis: multiple courses of acute hepatitis; persistence of IgM anti-HAV in serum; recurrence of fecal HAV excretion.
3. Immune-complex disorders: cutaneous vasculitis, arthritis, and cryoglobulinemia.
4. Autoimmune hepatitis: trigger of autoimmune hepatitis in susceptible individuals.

PROGNOSIS AND TREATMENT

1. Generally self-resolving with supportive measures.
2. Cholestatic hepatitis: resolution may be hastened by steroids.
3. Relapsing hepatitis: does not result in chronic hepatitis.
4. Progression to fulminant hepatitis rare. Most cases resolve spontaneously and fully. No specific therapy needed.

IMMUNOPROPHYLAXIS

1. Standard dose of immune serum globulin (ISG) before travel to endemic area: 0.02 cc/kg; 0.06 mL/kg for stays > 3 mo.
2. Postexposure prophylaxis: 0.02 cc/kg ISG within 2 wk.
3. Two HAV vaccines (inactivated virus); one in combo with hepatitis B virus (HBV) vaccine.

TARGET GROUPS FOR ACTIVE IMMUNIZATION

1. Children and employees at day care centers.
2. Travelers to endemic areas.
3. Clients and employees at residential institutions.
4. Chronic liver disease patients.
5. Native Americans on reservations.
6. Residents in community experiencing HAV outbreak.
7. Prison inmates.

8. Users of illicit drugs.
9. Homosexual men.
10. Food handlers.
11. Military personnel.

HEPATITIS B VIRUS

1. Partially double-stranded, closed circle deoxyribonucleic acid (DNA) virus. Hepadnavirus.
2. Intact viral particles: Dane particles. four major serotypes (Table 1).
3. Transmission: parenteral (needle sharing, blood transfusion), sexual and vertical (mother to fetus). Breastfeeding is not documented as a mode of HBV transmission.
4. Not directly cytopathic; hepatic injury mediated by host immune response.
5. Replication occurs via reverse transcriptase of RNA intermediate to DNA.

CLINICAL FEATURES

1. Incubation period 30–180 d. Individuals may develop prodrome: malaise, fatigue, nausea, low-grade fever, and serum sickness (arthralgias or arthritis, urticaria or angioedema, and maculopapular rash). Arthritis migratory and symmetric and subsides when jaundice begins (within 1–2 weeks.) (Figure 1).
2. Papular acrodermatitis of childhood: Gianotti-Crosti syndrome; may be major or only manifestation of HBV in infants or young children (lymphadenopathy and characteristic papular rash on face, extremities, and trunk).
3. Chronic HBV: usually asymptomatic; children grow well and are active. Liver damage mild during childhood with mild inflammation or fibrosis on biopsy. Occasionally may present with membranoproliferative glomerulonephritis, vasculitis, periarteritis nodosa, aplastic anemia, essential mixed cryoglobulinemia, and hepatocellular carcinoma (HCC). Development of HCC and cirrhosis rare in childhood; if they develop, child is usually anti-HBe positive. Major risk factor for development of chronic HBV infection is age. Risk of chronicity: 5% adults, 20% young children, and 90% neonates (Figure 2).

TABLE 1   CLINICAL INTERPRETATION OF HEPATITIS B VIRUS SEROLOGY AND VIROLOGY

CLINICAL INTERPRETATION	HBAG	ANTI-HBC	ANTI-HBS	HBAG	ANTI-HBE	HBV DNA
Chronic infection	+ > 6 mo					
"Window period" of resolved HBV infection, HBsAg lost but anti-HBs yet to develop	−	+* (IgM)	−			
Highly infectious (high viral replication)	+			+	−	+
HbsAg carrier at low risk of transmitting HBV (inactive replication)	+			−	±	−
Possible mutant				−	±	+
Possible escape mutant (eg, on lamivudine)				±	±	↑
Immune following vaccination	−	−	+			

*IgG from current or previous infection. IgM highly specific for acute infection in older children and adults, and forms about 8 weeks following infection.
Anti-HBc = anti-hepatitis B core antigen antibody; Anti-HBs = anti-hepatitis B surface antigen antibody; Anti-HBe = anti-hepatitis B e antigen antibody; HBeAg = hepatitis B e antigen; HBsAg = hepatitis B surface antigen; HBV DNA = hepatitis B virus DNA; IgG=immunoglobulin G; IgM = immunoglobulin M.

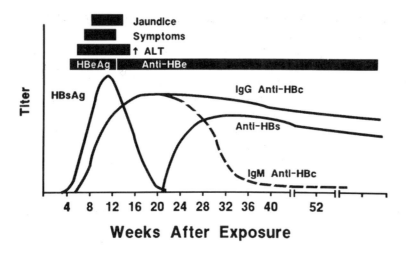

FIGURE 1 In this schematic illustration of the serologic events of acute hepatitis B, hepatitis B surface antigen (HBsAg) appears before the development of increased serum alanine aminotransferase (ALT) levels, symptoms of hepatitis, or jaundice. The sequential appearance and disappearance of hepatitis B e antigen (HBeAg) and immunoglobulin M (IgM) anti-hepatitis B core antigen antibody (anti-HBc) and the late appearance of anti-hepatitis B surface antigen antibody (anti-HBs) are depicted. Reproduced with permission from Seeff LB, editor. Current perspectives in hepatology, New York: Plenum Press; 1989.

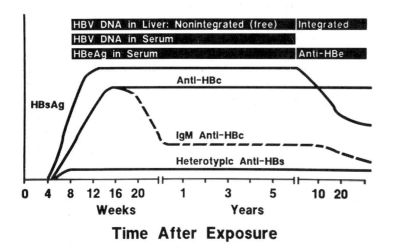

FIGURE 2 Hepatitis B surface antigen (HBsAg) remains detectable for a prolonged period in persistent hepatitis B virus (HBV) infection. Anti-hepatitis B core antigen antibody (anti-HBc) is present and hepatitis B e antigen (HBeAg) may remain detectable during the phase of active HBV replication, which is marked by the presence of HBV DNA in serum and liver (in a free, nonintegrated form). Subsequently HBV replication diminishes and HBV DNA becomes integrated into the DNA of the infected hepatocyte. Low levels of heterotypic anti-hepatitis B surface antigen antibody (anti-HBs) may be found. Reproduced with permission from Seeff LB, editor. Current perspectives in hepatology, New York: Plenum Press; 1989.

4. About 65% of pediatric patients with fulminant hepatitis B present in infancy with maternal transmission as the most important route of transmission. Very high mortality rate: 55–70% without transplant and 30–50% with transplant. Those who survive usually recover without sequelae.

Seroconversion

1. Spontaneous clearance of serum hepatitis B e antigen (HBeAg) is often preceded by elevation of aminotransferases (with 40% clearance within 1 yr after elevated ALT).
2. Another factor affecting HBe seroconversion is maternal hepatitis B surface antigen (HbsAg): those with HBsAg carrier mothers have lower HBeAg clearance rate.

3. Rate HBeAg clearance before age 3 yr < 2%/yr, after age 3 yr 5%/yr. HBeAg seroconversion usually occurs in those aged 15–30 yr.
4. Rate of hepatitis B surface antigen (HBsAg) clearance low among chronic hepatitis B patients: in carrier children < 1% and usually after HBeAg clearance. After HBsAg clearance, anti-hepatitis B surface antigen antibody (anti-HBs) is often low or undetectable. HBV vaccination is not helpful in this situation.

Virologic Factors Affecting Clinical Course

1. HBV mutations: precore G to A stop codon mutation at 1896 associated with fulminant hepatic failure (FHF), acute hepatitis, chronic hepatitis with exacerbation, HCC, and cirrhosis in adults.

TABLE 2   PHASES OF CHRONIC HEPATITIS B

PHASE	HBV DNA TITER	HBEAG/ANTI-HBE STATUS	HEPATIC INFLAMMATION
Immunotolerant	High	HBeAg positive	Minimal
Active	Low	Seroconvert from HBeAg to anti-HBe positive	Significant
Inactive	None or minimal	Anti-HBe positive	None (but subsequent cirrhosis possible)

Anti-HBe = anti-hepatitis B e antigen antibody; DNA = deoxyribonucleic acid; HBeAg = hepatitis B e antigen; HBV = hepatitis B virus.
Chance of reverting from (3) → (2): approximately 10–15% during lifetime.

2. Hepatitis B core antigen (HBcAg) is the target of cytolytic T lymphocytes. Mutation of this antigen may allow the infected hepatocytes to escape host detection.

3. Genotypes associated with clinical outcome. Genotype C associated with cirrhosis, HCC; genotype B associated with slower progression of liver fibrosis with earlier HBeAg seroconversion.

4. Core gene mutations associated with hepatoma formation in children and may induce persistent host attacks and increased risk for HCC.

5. In persons infected after vaccination, mutations in S gene or pre-S genes found, which encode envelope protein. Cause infection where HBsAg undetectable but HBeAg and HBV DNA found.

TREATMENT

Mainstays of therapy are interferon (IFN) and lamivudine. However, neither are effective in chronic HBV with normal transaminase levels. In cases where transaminases are only slightly irregular, can consider pretreatment with steroids before IFN to increase response rate.

IFN

1. IFN dose for children: 0.1 MU/kg or 3–6 MU/m^2 thrice weekly for 4–6 mo. Pegylated IFN safety and efficacy not reported in children.

2. Treatment of adults with elevated aminotransferases with recombinant IFN-α, either alone or after prednisone pretreatment, association with loss of HBeAg and normalization of aminotransferases 20–40% higher in treatment group of adults. Similar outcomes in children.

3. Factors predictive for positive response: high pretreatment levels of aminotransferases (> twice normal), HBeAg positive, low pretreatment HBV DNA (< 100 pg/mL), hepatocellular inflammation (active inflammation on liver biopsy), female sex, and late HBV acquisition. IFN not effective for HBeAg seroconversion in carrier children with normal liver enzymes.

4. Transient increase in ALT usually > twice baseline can occur during 2nd or 3rd month of treatment, more often in individuals who eventually respond to IFN. Monitor carefully for decompensation during this period. Do not use in decompensated liver disease.

5. Treatment benefits: HBV clearance, reduction of HCC, and prolonged survival.

6 Side effects: flu-like symptoms, usually short-lived. Thrombocytopenia and leukopenia occur commonly and frequently; requires transient or permanent dose reduction. Development of autoantibodies or autoimmune thyroid disease not uncommon. Less common side effects: alopecia, prolonged fatigue, and depression.

7. Therapy with IFN-α not always effective.

Lamivudine

1. Nucleoside analogue that inhibits DNA synthesis by terminating proviral DNA chain and interferes with reverse transcriptase. Good oral absorption and bioavailability (68% in children and infants).

2. Recommended dose: adults, 100 mg/d; children, 3 mg/kg/d up to 100 mg/d.

3. Candidates: age 2–17 yr, HBsAg positive > 6 mo, elevated aminotransferases for 3 mo. Mild to moderate elevation of ALT < 300 IU/L and HBV DNA positive.

4. Liver histology before and 1 year after provides data on benefit of lamivudine.

5. Stop lamivudine if any related adverse reaction. After 2 yr of lamivudine consider cessation although replication of HBV may resume with cessation. Interruption of lamivudine is not indicated on detection of mutant (YMDD) strains. However, development of resistant mutant may limit effectiveness as single agent.

6. During lamivudine theapry, monitor serum HBV, liver function tests, complete blood count, amylase and lipase, blood urea nitrogen, and creatinine for adverse events.

LIVER TRANSPLANTATION

Orthotopic Liver Transplantation (OLT):

1. Almost universally complicated by recurrent infection with severe liver disease if no prevention measures taken (see point 4).

2. Some post OLT patients develop rapid severe unresponsive form of fibrosing cholestatic hepatitis or fibrosing cytolytic hepatitis unique to HBV infection.

3. In persons with fulminant HBV or those with hepatitis D virus (HDV) coinfection, there is less HBV recurrence after OLT. In one series, better outcome of transplantation in patients with both HBV and HDV than those infected with only HBV.

4. If prophylaxis is used to prevent reinfection (high-dose HB immunoglobulin perioperatively and long-term antiviral therapy), OLT can be successful.

Immunoprophylaxis

1. Passive and active methods available.

2. Passive: HBIg prepared by fractionation of pooled plasma from donors seropositive for anti-HBs, which has high titers of this antibody. Efficacious for 3–6 mo in postexposure passive prophylaxis in 4 clinical settings: accidental needle-stick, sexual contact, perinatal exposure, and recurrence of HBV after liver transplantation.

3. Active: vaccine. Made from recombinant purified HBsAg particles from *Saccharomyces* with plasmid. Three injections over 4–6 mo provides protective antibody (anti-HBs ≥ 10 mIU/mL) in 90–95% of adults and 95% of children.

   a. Premature infants can respond to vaccine and should receive HBIg and vaccine at birth according to schedule. If mother is HBsAg negative, initiation of vaccine can be delayed until discharge or infant weight reaches 1700 g.

   b. Infants of untested women should receive vaccine only within 12 h.

   c. Children vaccinated at birth have high-level protection for at least 5 yr, adults at least 9 yr.

   d. Risk factors for failure of immunoprophylaxis: high maternal HBV DNA, low-level maternal anti-hepatitis

B core antigen antibody (anti-HBc), and uterine contractions and placental leakage during delivery.

HCC

1. Single strongest risk factor for development of HCC in chronic HBV-infected patients is family history of HCC regardless of HBV replication status. Usually detected after 20 yr of chronic HBV infection.
2. Older age and active liver disease increases risk somewhat.
3. Adult onset lower risk than infant or neonate onset.

HEPATITIS C VIRUS

1. Small, lipid-enveloped positive-sense-single-stranded RNA flavivirus.
2. Replication via RNA-dependent RNA polymerase-creating double-stranded RNA intermediate.
3. Most variability at 5' end of E2 gene (hypervariable region). Genetically heterogeneity secondary to lack of proofreading ability by RNA-dependent RNA polymerase.
4. Six major genotypes (number) with subtypes (letters): 1 and 2: worldwide; 3: Australia; 4, 5, and 6: sub-Saharan Africa. Hepatitis C virus (HCV) genotype 1 associated with higher serum HCV RNA and poorer response to current antiviral regimens than genotypes 2 or 3.
5. Worldwide prevalence: 3%. United States prevalence: 2% (among incarcerated as high as 82%, juvenile incarcerated 2%, international adoptees < 1%, 50–95% pooled plasma recipients, and 18–52% among hemodialysis and cancer survivors). Perinatal transmission about 5–6%; about 16% in human immunodeficiency virus (HIV)-coinfected mothers. No increased risk of HCV transmission by breast milk. Factors most commonly associated with hepatitis C virus (HCV) infection in 17–59-year-olds: illicit drug abuse, high-risk sexual behavior, age at first sexual encounter, and marijuana use.

CLINICAL MANIFESTATIONS

1. Mean incubation period posttransfusion 7–8 wk (6–12 wk).
2. Acute HCV usually anicteric or subclinical and only one-third will develop jaundice or symptoms. FHF very rare. In adults, 85% exposed to HCV will develop chronic infection.
3. Alcohol ingestion and immunodeficiency accelerate progression of disease.
4. Biochemical markers tend to fluctuate; necroinflammatory activity typically mild on histology. Usually aminotransferase levels 1.5 to 10 times normal. Normal ALT does not necessarily indicate absence of hepatitis.
5. In child hemophiliacs, histology mild; in adult hemophiliacs, HCV infection is associated with the development of HCC. Iron overload and HCV infection are independent risk factors for the progression of liver fibrosis.
6. Autoantibodies frequently detected in chronic HCV. Essential mixed cryoglobulinemia reported in adults, not children.
7. Type II autoimmune hepatitis (AIH) is associated with being anti-HCV positive and probably reflects autoim-

mune disorder triggered by chronic HCV. Anti-GOR (HCV-specific autoepitope) is found in majority of these patients; unique to HCV-associated type II AIH (use as confirmatory test). Seropositive HCV common in type I AIH but rarely confirmed by more definitive testing; probably represents false-positive (Table 3).

8. Porphyria cutanea tarda: chronic dermatologic condition due to reduced hepatic uroporphyrinogen decarboxylase. Two forms described: familial and sporadic. HCV found in 75%.
9. Associated with diabetes mellitus.
10. Associated with HCC. HCV is independent risk factor for HCC, usually accompanied by cirrhosis.
11. HCV chronic liver disease: leading indication for liver transplant in adults. Recurrent HCV infection nearly universal after OLT. In children with de novo infection after OLT, the course of HCV liver disease is aggressive with 23% mortality rate.
12. HCV-HIV coinfection is common. HCV infection in immunosuppressed HIV positive patients is severe, and HCV-HIV coinfected patients have more fibrosis than HCV only infected patients, even those with lower immunosuppression. Maternal-fetal transmission of HCV is highest in women who are HIV positive.

DIAGNOSIS

1. Detection of antibody directed against several viral antigens by enzyme immunoassay (EIA) or recombinant immunoblot assay (RIBA) or by detection of HCV RNA using nucleic acid tests (NATs) (Table 4).
2. RIBA less sensitive but more specific than EIA; thus, RIBA used for confirmation and EIA used for screening. CDC advises that EIA should be verified by supplemental testing.
3. NAT directly detects circulating virus - useful in certain scenarios: to diagnose HCV infection before anti-HCV antibodies appear, to detect HCV in infants born to infected mothers, and to monitor response to treatment in those with active viremia.

HISTOLOGY

Portal lymphoid follicles, lobular inflammation, steatosis, and injury to bile duct epithelium.

TABLE 3   SEROLOGIC DIFFERENTIATION OF CHRONIC HEPATITIS C VIRUS (HCV)AND AUTOIMMUNE HEPATITIS (AIH)

TEST	CHRONIC HCV	AIH TYPE 1	AIH TYPE 2
Anti-HCV ELISA	+	±	±
Anti-HCV RIBA	+	−	+ if true HCV+; otherwise negative
ANA	±	+	−
ASMA	− except in isolated cases	+	−
Anti-LKM1	±	−	+
Anti-GOR	±	−	+ if true HCV+

ANA = antinuclear antibodies; ASMA = anti-smooth muscle antibody ; ELISA = enzyme-linked immunosorbent assay; LKM1 = liver kidney microsomal 1 antibody; RIBA = recombinant immunoblot assay.

TABLE 4   SENSITIVITY AND PREDICTED VALUE OF SEROLOGIC TESTS FOR HCV INFECTION

ASSAY	SENSITIVITY (%)	POSITIVE PREDICTIVE VALUE (%)		TIME TO POSITIVE AFTER INFECTION (WK)
		LOW-PREVALENCE GROUPS	HIGH-PREVALENCE GROUPS	
EIA-1	70–80	30–50	70–85	16
EIA-2	92–95	50–60	88–95	10
EIA-3	97	25	98	7–8

Adapted with permission from Davis GL. Hepatitis C. In: Schiff ER, Sorrell MF, Maddrey WC, editors. Schiff's diseases of the liver. Vol. 1, 9th ed. Philadelphia: Lippincott, Williams and Wilkins; 2003. p. 819.
EIA = enzyme immunoassay; HCV = hepatitis C virus.

GENERAL CARE GUIDELINES

Periodic examination recommended for those with chronic HCV infection; lack of consensus on what to monitor and how frequently. Adolescents need to understand the negative impact of alcohol. Avoidance of high-risk behavior must be discussed, as well as discouragement of sharing personal items. HAV and HBV vaccination should be offered.

TREATMENT

1. Natural history of HCV in children not well understood.
2. Factors present known to be associated with favorable response to treatment in adults: short duration of infection, young age, and mild histology or no cirrhosis. Other favorable factors: HCV genotype other than I, elevated ALT, and low pretreatment serum HCV.
3. IFN: treatment in adults results in normalization of transaminases and clearance of HCV RNA in 40–50% with a notable relapse rate; sustained rates 8–35%. Better sustained responses (30–40%) with ribavirin. With pegylated IFN, rates 50–60%, especially with ribavirin. Similar rates shown in children with IFN and ribavirin 15 mg/kg/d. Pegylated IFN therapy not yet evaluated in children.
4. Adverse events to IFN: see HBV section. Do not use in very young patients.
5. Adverse events to ribavirin: anemia in nearly all patients by 4–8 wk. Associated with fetal malformations; pregnancy should be avoided during therapy and up to 6 months after completion.
6. HCV chronic liver disease: leading indication for liver transplant in adults. Recurrent HCV infection nearly universal after OLT. In children with de novo infection after OLT, the course of HCV liver disease is aggressive with 23% mortality rate.

PROPHYLAXIS

1. Anti-HCV is not a neutralizing antibody.
2. CDC does not advocate condom use in stable marriages if one partner is HCV positive; advocates testing.

HEPATITIS D VIRUS

1. Single-stranded circular RNA with core antigen (HDV Ag) and envelope from host cell membrane and all 3 HBV surface antigen proteins. Three genotypes.
2. Epidemiology parallels HBV since HBV infection is required for HDV infection. Sex transmission less efficient than HBV. Perinatal transmission can occur but is uncommon because HBV and HDV carrier mothers are usually anti-HBe positive and thus less infectious.
3. Highest endemicity seen in poorest South America and Africa, as well as Romania.
4. Subpopulations with high HBV but virtually no HDV: Native Americans, Alaskan natives, and residents of some Asian countries.
5. Risk of FHF higher in HDV–HBV coinfection than HBV alone.

PATHOGENESIS

1. Controversial.
2. Histology: in vitro evidence for direct cytopathic effects; but usually cytopathic viruses have no carrier states (as is seen with asymptomatic HDV carriers).

DIAGNOSIS

1. Coinfection: acute. Anti-HDV IgM during acute illness persists for 2–6 wk. Subsequent IgG anti-HDV develops but diminishes to undetectable when HBV infection resolves.

TABLE 5   PATTERNS OF HEPATITIS D INFECTION

	HDV CO-INFECTION (WITH ACUTE HBV)	HDV SUPERINFECTION (OF CHRONIC HBV)	CHRONIC HBV AND HDV INFECTION
HBsAg	+	+	+
IgM anti-HBc	+	−	−
anti-HBc	+	+	+
IgM anti-HDV	+	+	+
IgG anti-HDV	−	+	+
IgA anti-HDV	−	Not known	+
Presentation	Acute or fulminant hepatitis	Acute or fulminant hepatitis	Chronic liver disease
Course	Resolution	Chronic liver disease	Cirrhosis common

HDV = hepatitis D virus; HBsAg = hepatitis B surface antigen; anti-HDV = antibody to HDV; anti-HBC = antibody to hepatitis B core antigen; IgM, IgG, IgA = immunoglobulin M, G, A; HBV = hepatitis B virus.

2. Superinfection: Acute. Anti-HDV IgM without anti-HBc IgM but HBsAg positive. In chronic HBV and HDV, IgA anti-HDV present.

TREATMENT

1. Only treatment with beneficial effect is IFN-α. Treatment with moderately high dose (9 MU thrice weekly or 5 MU/d) normalizes aminotransferase; disappearance or decrease in HDV RNA and improvement in hepatic inflammation in 50%. However, majority relapse after therapy. Prolonged response in patients who become HBsAg negative.
2. No predictors of response identified.
3. Prognosis in nonresponders and in patients with relapse poor.
4. No recommendations for use of IFN in children.
5. In one series of patients with HDV and HBV who had OLT, better outcome of transplantation in patients with both HBV and HDV than those infected with only HBV.

PROPHYLAXIS

Immunoprophylaxis not available (passive or active). Antibody not neutralizing. Prevention of HBV will prevent HDV.

HEPATITIS E VIRUS

1. Single-stranded non-enveloped RNA virus. One serotype. Endemic in subtropical and tropical parts of the world. Secondary spread uncommon; secondary infection usually milder.
2. Usually contracted through contaminated water, spread via fecal-oral route. Highest attack rate in those aged 15–40 yr.
3. Pathogenesis: not elucidated.
4. Clinical features: acute, self-limited illness. Incubation period 2–9 wk. Most infections recognized by jaundice. Resolution of jaundice and transaminitis seen within 1–6 wk. High mortality rate in pregnant women in third trimester (20%) owing to submassive hepatic necrosis. High rate of disseminated intravascular coagulation in fatal cases. No chronic hepatitis E virus (HEV) reported.
5. Diagnosis: rests on detection of anti–HEV IgM; positive for 2–3 mo. Anti-HEV IgG persists long-term in one-half of patients. Enzyme-linked immunosorbent assay (ELISA) tests have high false-positive rate in population with low risk; confirmatory testing recommended. Can be detected in stool using electron microscopy.
6. Immunoprophylaxis: none.

HEPATITIS G VIRUS

1. RNA virus; parenterally transmitted agent; can be transmitted perinatally. Flaviviridae with 25% homology with HCV.
2. Clinical significance uncertain. Majority of infected patients without liver disease. Liver histology normal despite evidence of hepatitis G virus (HGV) infection in hepatocytes.
3. Coinfection: HGV–HIV slows progression of HIV; HGV–HCV does not worsen liver disease.

TRANSFUSION TRANSMISSION VIRUS

1. Single stranded DNA virus.
2. Parenteral and nonparenteral routes of transmission.
3. No significant role for transfusion transmission virus in non-A–E hepatitis in children.

SEN VIRUS

1. Single-stranded DNA virus.
2. Prevalence increase with increased volume of transfused blood.
3. Some evidence as an agent of hepatitis in a minority of cases.

CYTOMEGALOVIRUS

1. Herpes DNA virus.
2. By age 15 yr, 20% of the general population infected. By 25–30 years, 50–60% of the general population.
3. Clinically usually asymptomatic but can result in syndrome similar to Epstein-Barr virus (EBV) mononucleosis: fever, malaise, cervical lymphadenopathy, and splenomegaly. Overt jaundice rare.
4. Incubation period 3–12 wk. Maximum elevation in transaminases usually < 200, peaking 2–3 wk after disease onset, with normalization by 5th wk. Rarely, cytomegalovirus (CMV) causes massive hepatocellular necrosis. Can infect and replicate in both hepatocytes and cholangiocytes. Lifelong latent phase, but can be reactivated when immunocompromised.
5. Diagnosis: anti-cytomegalovirus (CMV) IgM or serum CMV ag or CMV urine culture. In normal host, typical viral CMV cells rare, but frequently detected in liver biopsy of transplant patients with CMV.

EPSTEIN-BARR VIRUS

1. Herpes DNA virus. Incorporates into B cells resulting in lifelong latent infection.
2. Primary infection usually asymptomatic. Infection in adolescents: classic infectious mononucleosis syndrome with fever, cervical lymphadenopathy, sore throat, fatigue, and splenomegaly. Usually anicteric hepatitis, but 5–10% can have jaundice. 1/3,000 cases can have fulminant hepatitis, bone marrow failure, or acute respiratory distress syndrome. Ubiquitous, infected > 80% of the general population by adulthood.
3. Diagnose by anti-viral capsid antigen IgM in serum.

THERAPIES FOR CHRONIC VIRAL HEPATITIS

1. IFN: antiviral and immunomodulatory proteins (Table 6). Produces antiviral proteins, inhibits RNA synthesis, and enhances human leukocyte antigen (HLA) expression to allow recognition of infected hepatocytes by cytotoxic T lymphs.
2. Nucleoside analogues: lamivudine and famciclovir. Ribavirin (enters eukaryotic cells rapidly) monotherapy does not affect HCV but has synergism with IFN (Tables 6 and 7).
3. Gene therapy: antisense oligonucleotide can inhibit viral gene expression.

TABLE 6   THERAPIES FOR CHRONIC VIRAL HEPATITIS

1. Interferon

2. Antiviral agents
   a. Nucleoside analogues (lamivudine 3TC), adefovir, penciclovir, and ribavirin
   b. Gene therapies: antisense oligonucleotide, ribozyme, interfering proteins and particles

3. Immune modulatory therapies
   a. Thymosin
   b. Deoxyribonucleic acid (DNA) vaccine

4. Combination therapy (ribavirin and interferon)

TABLE 7   CONTRAINDICATIONS TO THERAPY

INTERFERON	RIBAVIRIN
Severe depression	Marked anemia
Neuropsychiatric symptoms	Renal dysfunction
Active alcohol or substance abuse	Coronary artery disease or cerebrovascular disease
Poorly controlled autoimmune disease	Inability to practice birth control
Bone marrow compromise	
Inability to practice birth control	

TABLE 8   ADVERSE EFFECTS OF INTERFERON, LAMIVUDINE, AND RIBAVIRIN

AGENT	ADVERSE EFFECTS
Interferon	Flu-like symptoms, depression, anorexia, weight loss, hair loss, bone marrow suppression, autoantibody induction
Lamivudine	ENT problems, gastrointestinal symptoms, malaise, fatigue, lower respiratory symptoms pancreatitis, neutropenia, elevation of liver enzyme
Ribavirin	Mild anemia, hemolytic anemia, leukopenia, unconjugated hyperbilirubinemia, nausea, dyspnea, rash

ENT = ear, nose, throat

4. Immunotherapy: thymosin-α triggers lymphocyte maturation and augments T cell function and promotes reconstitution of immune defects.

QUESTIONS

MATCH THE CHARACTERISTIC TO THE VIRUS:

a. Coinfection with another virus required.
b. Disseminated intravascular coagulation often seen.
c. RNA.
d. DNA.

1. Hepatitis A virus.
2. Hepatitis B virus.
3. Hepatitis C virus.
4. Hepatitis D virus.
5. Hepatitis E virus.

CHOOSE THE BEST ANSWER:

6. Atypical clinical forms of hepatitis A virus include:
   a. Immune complex vasculitis.
   b. Multiple courses of hepatitis.
   c. Autoimmune hepatitis.
   d. Severe prolonged cholestasis.
   e. All of the above.

7. Which of the following viruses is definitely linked with hepatitis in humans?
   a. Transfusion transmission virus.
   b. SEN virus.
   c. Hepatitis D virus.
   d. Hepatitis G virus.
   e. All of the above.

TRUE OR FALSE:

8. Hepatitis B virus can be transmitted via breastfeeding.
9. Hepatitis B virus can infect the spleen, pancreas, and bone marrow.
10. Risk of chronic hepatitis B virus infection in neonates is 10%.

MATCH THE SEROLOGIC FINDINGS TO THE TYPE OF HEPATITIS B INFECTION STATE:

a. Chronic hepatitis B infection.
b. Acute hepatitis B infection.
c. Acute hepatitis B infection, resolved.
d. Vaccine protected against hepatitis B infection.

11. Anti-HBc IgM.
12. Anti-HBc IgG.
13. Anti-HBs IgG.
14. Anti-HBc IgG and HBsAg.
15. HBeAg.

MATCH THE CHARACTERISTIC TO THE VIRUS:

a. Flavivirus
b. Picornavirus.
c. Closed circular configuration.
d. Partial double-stranded DNA.
e. 25% homology with hepatitis C virus.
f. Secondary infection mild.

16. Hepatitis G virus.
17. Hepatitis B virus.
18. Hepatitis A virus.
19. Hepatitis E virus.

MATCH THE INCUBATION PERIODS TO THE VIRUS:

a. 1–6 months.
b. 1 month.
c. 2–9 weeks.
d. 6–12 weeks.

20. Hepatitis B virus.
21. Hepatitis E virus.
22. Hepatitis C virus.
23. Hepatitis A virus.

MATCH THE VIRUS WITH ITS CHARACTERISTICS OR ASSOCIATIONS:

a.   Hepatitis B virus.

b.   Hepatitis C virus.

c.   Both.

24. Six major genotypes.

25. Anti-GOR autoimmune hepatitis.

26. Gianotti-Crosti syndrome.

27. Porphyria cutanea tarda.

28. Parenteral transmission.

29. Hepatitis D coinfection.

CHOOSE THE BEST ANSWER:

30. HBeAg seroconversion:

   a. Improves as age of infected child increases.

   b. Is highest in the newborn period.

   c. Improves in infant if mother is a carrier for HBsAg.

   d. Is 96% by age 4 years.

31. Which of the following is not a predictor of improved hepatitis B virus seroconversion with interferon therapy?

   a. Normal alanine aminotransferase.

   b. Low hepatitis B virus DNA.

   c. Recent acquisition of virus.

   d. Active hepatitis histologically.

   e. All of the above are predictors.

32. Which factor is not an important criterion for treatment with lamivudine for the treatment of hepatitis B virus?

   a. Elevated alanine aminotransferase > 3 months.

   b. Low levels of hepatitis B virus DNA.

   c. Low iron content.

   d. HBsAg positive after 6 months.

33. Which of the following is not a predictor for good response to interferon therapy in hepatitis C virus?

   a. Normal alanine aminotransferase.

   b. Low viral load.

   c. Low iron load.

   d. Normal immunity.

TRUE OR FALSE:

34. HIV infection does not alter the course of HCV liver disease.

35. Maternal-fetal transmission of hepatitis C is increased in a mother with both HIV and HCV.

BACTERIAL, PARASITIC, AND OTHER INFECTIONS

SYNOPSIS

PYOGENIC ABSCESS OF THE LIVER

1. Uncommon infection in children. Pyogenic bacteria reach the liver via the portal vein or hepatic artery or from adjacent structures.

2. In developing countries, malnutrition and helminthic infestations are major risk factors associated with liver abscess in children. In developed countries, most frequent in immunocompromised. Liver abscess in neonates associated with umbilical venous catheterization, prematurity, and necrotizing enterocolitis requiring surgery.

3. Most common organisms: *Staphylococcus aureus*, *Escherichia coli*, *Pseudomonas*, and *Klebsiella*. S. aureus is most likely organism in children with liver abscess following bacteremia or in immunocompromised. Gram-negative enteric organisms and anaerobes likely when infection spreads from gastrointestinal (GI) tract via portal venous system. Fungal liver abscesses may occur in immunocompromised. Acquired immunodeficiency syndrome (AIDS) patients at increased risk for mycobacterial abscesses.

4. Clinically nonspecific. Most common presenting symptoms are fever and abdominal pain. Hepatomegaly seen in 50–73% with right upper quadrant tenderness in 40%.

5. Diagnosis: routine laboratory tests of little value. Anemia and leukocytosis typically seen. Hepatic transaminases usually normal or mildly elevated. Elevation in alkaline phosphatase and bilirubin seen in cases with biliary obstruction. Yield of blood cultures variable. Radiologic assessment: most important tool for diagnosis. Ultrasonography (US): study of choice. Computed tomography (CT) if sonogram negative and clinical suspicion high. Magnetic resonance imaging (MRI) no advantage over US or CT.

6. Treatment: antibiotic therapy with drainage of pus is mainstay of therapy. Multiple hepatic microabscesses not amenable to drainage: successfully treated with prolonged antibiotic therapy. In patients with chronic granulomatous disease, surgical drainage of large abscesses (> 5 cm) crucial for survival with or without interferon-gamma.

7. Early diagnosis and prompt therapy are important determinants of survival.

TYPHOID FEVER

1. Acute systemic illness usually caused by *Salmonella typhi*. Major health problem in tropical and developing countries; uncommon in developed countries. Presenting symptoms: fever, diarrhea, vomiting, abdominal pain, and anorexia. Hepatomegaly (52%) and splenomegaly (23%). Mild elevation of serum hepatic transaminases but clinical jaundice uncommon. Other

complications include: encephalopathy, seizures, myocarditis, and circulatory failure.

2. Histology on liver biopsy nonspecific with focal necrosis, portal inflammation, and hyperplasia of Kupffer cells.

3. Diagnosis by positive blood culture, deoxyribonucleic acid (DNA) probes, and polymerase chain reaction (PCR).

4. Therapy: antibiotics. Multidrug resistance: ciprofloxacin; ceftriaxone in tropical countries. Chronic carrier state via persistent gallbladder or liver infection.

BRUCELLOSIS

1. Zoonotic infection by *Brucella melitensis, Brucella abortus*, or *Brucella suis*. Transmitted via direct animal contact or consumption of infected unpasteurized milk products.

2. Nonspecific symptoms. Common symptoms: fever, malaise, arthralgia, weight loss, and anorexia. Hepatomegaly (28%) with splenomegaly (35%).

3. Complications: osteomyelitis, pneumonitis, meningitis, and endocarditis. Hepatosplenic abscess is a rare complication.

4. Common laboratory features: leukocytosis, elevated erythrocyte sedimentation rate (ESR), elevated hepatic transaminases, and elevated alkaline phosphatase in 58%. Histopathology of liver variable.

5. Diagnosis suspected with history of exposure; diagnosis confirmed by blood or bone marrow cultures. Presumptive diagnosis made if titers of *Brucella* antibodies are high or rising. Responds well to antibiotics (tetracycline or trimethoprim-sulfamethoxazole for 3 weeks after initial gentamicin) with an excellent prognosis.

PERIHEPATITIS (FITZ-HUGH–CURTIS SYNDROME)

1. Occurs as a complication of pelvic inflammatory disease in young adolescent females. Classic cause; *Neisseria gonorrhoeae*, also described with *Chlamydia trachomatis*.

2. Clinically, acute sharp right upper quadrant pain with or without fever, mimicking acute cholecystitis. Hepatomegaly, right upper quadrant tenderness, and friction rub over the liver may be detected. Serum hepatic transaminases, bilirubin normal. Cervical or urethral culture confirms diagnosis. Laparoscopic findings include classic "violin string" adhesions from the liver to the right costal wall.

3. Treatment: antibiotics.

CAT-SCRATCH DISEASE

1. Caused by gram-negative bacillus *Bartonella hensalae*. Highest incidence is among children aged < 10 yr.

2. Transmitted via cats/kittens: Following inoculation, a papule occurs locally which vesiculates and encrusts; followed by regional lymphadenopathy. Illness generally mild with generalized myalgias, malaise, anorexia, fever, and abdominal pain. Unusual manifestations include preauricular lymphadenopathy with conjunctivitis (Parinaud oculoglandular syndrome), pneumonia, erythema nodosum, encephalitis, and granulomatous hepatitis. Can also present as fever of unknown origin.

3. Serum transaminases, alkaline phosphatase, and bilirubin normal with elevated ESR. Abdominal imaging may reveal multiple small hypoechogenic lesions in the liver and spleen with mild hepatosplenomegaly. Liver histology shows epithelioid granulomas with central necrosis and chronic inflammation. Warthin-Starry stained bacilli may be found. Diagnosis: indirect fluorescence antibody test is rapid and reliable.

4. Self-limiting: complete resolution without therapy reported. Antibiotics used in severe cases.

SPIROCHETAL INFECTIONS

LEPTOSPIROSIS

1. Caused by *Leptospira interrogans*. Acquired by exposure to urine or other infected body fluids from animals.

2. Biphasic illness with initial septicemic phase (4–7 d) with fever, chills, headache, anorexia, abdominal pain, rash, and lymphadenopathy, followed by immune phase with lower-grade fever, hepatitis, jaundice, renal dysfunction, thrombocytopenia, and meningitis. Weil syndrome: rare, severe form associated with hepatic dysfunction, renal failure, hemorrhagic manifestations, and pulmonary involvement with high mortality. Histology reveals multinucleated cells, Kupffer cell proliferation, erythrophagocytosis, and cholestasis. Severe hepatic necrosis unusual; complete recovery of liver function seen in survivors.

3. Diagnosis requires high index of suspicion, confirmed by isolating the organism from body fluids. Fourfold titer increase establishes diagnosis.

4. Treat with penicillin or ampicillin. Childhood mortality 2% secondary to pulmonary hemorrhage.

LYME DISEASE

1. Multisystem infection caused by *Borrelia burgdorferi*. Transmitted to humans via deer tick bite. Most common vector-borne disease among children in the United States.

2. Clinical presentation includes nonspecific fever, malaise, and headache associated with a characteristic annular erythematous rash (erythema chronicum migrans) present in 68% of infected children.

3. Complications: arthritis, facial palsy, aseptic meningitis, and carditis. Rarely, can present as acute hepatitis.

4. Diagnosis should be suspected with a history of a tick bite with the classic rash on exam. Serologic testing is diagnostic.

5. Treatment: tetracycline unless age < 9 yr (then use cefuroxime, amoxicillin, or erythromycin).

6. Prognosis excellent in those adequately treated; no long-term morbidity.

RICKETTSIAL INFECTIONS

ROCKY MOUNTAIN SPOTTED FEVER

1. Disease caused by *Rickettsia rickettsii* with ticks as transmission vectors.

2. Clinical syndrome characterized by fever, headache, and classic maculopapular rash that begins peripherally and spreads to entire body. Hepatomegaly, jaundice, and variable elevations of transaminases and alkaline phosphatase.

3. Diagnosis requires high index of suspicion. Disease confirmed by demonstrating a fourfold rise in antibody titers by second to third week of illness using a complement fixation serologic test. 70–80% will have a positive Weil-Felix reaction, but test is nonspecific.

4. Treatment with tetracycline or chloramphenicol most effective. Untreated infection can lead to severe illness and fatality.

Q FEVER

1. Febrile illness caused by *Coxiella burnetii*. Transmission via inhalation. Animal hosts include cattle, sheep, and goats.

2. Acute, chronic forms. Hepatic involvement common in acute form with fever, headache, malaise, vomiting, abdominal pain, and respiratory symptoms. Rare fulminant hepatic failure reported.

3. Liver histology reveals fatty change with diffuse granulomatous lesions. Classic histopathologic finding: fibrin ring granuloma with a central clear space. Diagnosis confirmed by serologic testing (Figure 1).

4. Treatment: tetracycline, but most recover without therapy.

PARASITIC INFECTIONS

AMEBIASIS

1. Caused by *Entamoeba histolytica* (enteric pathogen in trophozoite or cyst form). Endemic in southern and western Africa, Far East, South and Central America, and Indian subcontinent. Prevalence 4%. Risk factors: lower socioeconomic status, crowding, poor sanitation, immigration from an endemic area, and young age. Transmission by fecal-oral route via cyst ingestion.

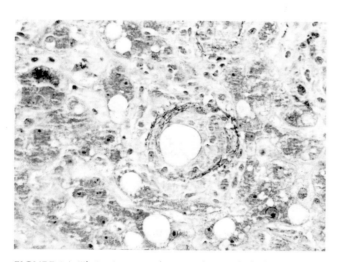

FIGURE 1 Fibrin ring granuloma with a central clear space in a patient with Q fever (hematoxylin and eosin; ×400 original magnification). Courtesy of Dr. F. A. Mitros, University of Iowa Hospital, Iowa City, IA.

Trophozoites may invade the colonic epithelium leading to colitis. Liver invasion via the portal venous system.

2. Fever and right upper quadrant pain most common symptoms of hepatic amebic abscess. Clinical jaundice uncommon. May rupture into pleura, peritoneum, and pericardium with dramatic presentation (respiratory distress, acute abdomen, and shock respectively). Anemia and leukocytosis seen in > 90%.

3. Diagnosis: stool examinations positive in minority. On ultrasonograpy, amebic abscess likely to be solitary, in the right hepatic lobe, and have a better defined margin with a peripheral halo. If diagnosis cannot be made on serology and clinical features, needle abscess aspiration can exclude pyogenic abscess (usually amoebae not recovered and pus sterile). Serologic tests for diagnosis of amebiasis include indirect immunofluorescence, indirect hemagglutination, and enzyme-linked immunosorbent assay (ELISA), but may not be reliable in infants. Use of at least 2 serologic tests is recommended.

4. Treatment: antibiotics alone without drainage. Metronidazole (30–50 mg/kg/d divided tid for 10 days) is treatment of choice. Intestinal amebicides should be given after metronidazole to eradicate intraluminal infection. Therapeutic needle aspiration recommended if clinical response is not seen within 48 h or if abscess > 7 cm or in left lobe, owing to higher risk for pericardial involvement. Surgical intervention necessary for ruptured abscess. Prognosis for uncomplicated abscess usually good, except in infancy where clinical course can be fulminant with high mortality rate.

MALARIA

1. Caused by *Plasmodium vivax*, *Plasmodium falciparum*, *Plasmodium ovale*, and *Plasmodium malariae*. Important cause of morbidity and mortality in tropical and subtropical countries. Acquired from female anopheline mosquito bite.

2. Symptoms: fever, abdominal pain, vomiting, and diarrhea. Fevers and chills may be periodic or occur daily. On examination, tender hepatosplenomegaly common. Jaundice and mild transaminitis may be seen.

3. Diagnosis established by detection of parasites on thick and thin peripheral blood smears using Giemsa stains.

4. Drug of choice is chloroquine, except for *P. falciparum*. For severe, complicated malaria, intravenous quinine is drug of choice. For chloroquine-resistant strains (ie, *P. falciparum*), quinine or mefloquine may be used.

ASCARIASIS

1. Caused by *Ascaris lumbricoides*. Most prevalent helminthic infection in the world. Endemic to areas with poor sanitation; transmitted via ingestion of eggs. Most common in childhood.

2. Clinical manifestations depend on location in GI tract. Worms may obstruct intestine, may invade ampullary orifice, and can induce biliary colic, obstruction, or acute pancreatitis.

3. Diagnosis is made by identification of ova in stools or by a history of passing worms. Elevation of liver enzymes and serum bilirubin may be seen in biliary ascariasis. Ultrasonography useful in diagnosing complications, especially those involving the biliary tree. Endoscopic retrograde cholangiopancreatography (ERCP) may also diagnose and remove worms in the biliary tree.

4. Treatment is with mebendazole or piperazine salts. Surgery may be required for obstruction.

ECHINOCOCCOSIS

1. *Echinococcus granulosus* found throughout the world, endemic in sheep and cattle raising areas. Small tapeworms that inhabit the intestine of the host (usually dogs); humans acquire infection by ingestion of ova.

2. Parasites may lodge in the liver or lungs leading to hydatid cyst formation. Although infection is acquired in childhood, symptoms may not occur for many years owing to slow cyst growth (1 cm/yr). Clinical presentation depends on size of cyst and complications owing to cyst formation. Common symptoms: abdominal pain, abdominal mass, fever, and anorexia. Portal hypertension or obstructive jaundice owing to cyst compression of the venous system or biliary tract. Cysts may rupture and cause anaphylaxis.

3. Definitive diagnosis made by positive serology and demonstrating the presence of scoleces in cystic fluid.

4. Therapy: albendazole alone or with percutaneous drainage successful.

LIVER FLUKE INFECTION

CLONORCHIASIS

1. Caused by *Clonorchis sinensis*, endemic in Far East. Infection via consumption of raw infected fish (one of the intermediate hosts, along with snails). Parasite migrates from the duodenum into the biliary tree where it matures. Injury to bile ducts manifests as adenomatous proliferation and goblet cell metaplasia. Secondary infection commonly occurs; results in recurrent pyogenic cholangitis resulting in stricture, periductal fibrosis, and hepatic abscess.

2. Patients with mild disease may be asymptomatic; severe cases present with recurrent cholangitis, biliary duct obstruction, and portal hypertension. Cholangiocarcinoma reported in adults with long-standing infection.

3. Diagnosis made by stool or duodenal aspirate examination for eggs.

4. Treatment of choice: praziquantel.

FASCIOLIASIS

1. Caused by *Fasciola hepatica*. Infection acquired by ingestion of infected watercress or water. Parasites penetrate duodenal wall, traverse peritoneum, and penetrate the hepatic capsule to reach the bile ducts.

2. Two phases of disease: acute invasive (migrating through liver) and chronic (at biliary tree). Acute manifestation: prolonged fever, abdominal pain, tender hepatomegaly with significant eosinophilia, raised ESR, and elevated alkaline phosphatase with mild or no transaminase elevation. CT may show abscess-like nodular lesions or multiple hypodense areas in the liver. Liver biopsy findings include eosinophilic abscess and coagulative necrosis. Chronic fascioliasis can cause biliary colic, jaundice, cholangitis, and pancreatitis.

3. Diagnosis by serologic testing or by finding ova in stool.

4. Triclabendazole highly effective and recommended to treat children.

SCHISTOSOMIASIS

1. Important cause of morbidity and mortality in tropical countries. Hepatic schistosomiasis caused by *Schistosoma mansoni* and *Schistosoma japonicum*. *Schistosoma mansoni* endemic in Africa, Middle East, and South America; *Schistosoma japonicum* endemic in Central and Southeast Asia. Human infection occurs when schistosoma penetrate human skin, migrate to the liver, enter the portal venous system, and reside in mesenteric veins.

2. Acute schistosomiasis (Katayama fever) results from host immunologic response to worms and eggs after 4–6 wk of exposure. Fever, cough, edema, lymphadenopathy, and eosinophilia can be seen. Untreated acute disease becomes chronic disease. Upper GI bleeding may result from esophageal varies secondary to portal hypertension which occurs secondary to fibrosis from granulomatous hepatic lesions which occur as host response to ova. Other complications: myocarditis, and transverse myelitis.

3. Laboratory features may reflect hypersplenism and pancytopenia. Liver transaminases usually normal. US detects and grades degree of portal hypertension.

5. Serologic studies are helpful for diagnosis. Diagnosis confirmed by detecting eggs in stool or in rectal biopsy tissue sample.

6. Treatment of choice: praziquantel; eradication in 90% and reversal of periportal fibrosis in some children.

FUNGAL INFECTIONS

CANDIDIASIS

1. Most frequently encountered systemic fungal infection. Liver infection consequence of hematogenous seeding. Occurs in immunocompromised patients. Other risk factors for hepatosplenic candidiasis include neutropenia, recent chemotherapy, and use of broad-spectrum antibiotics.

2. Clinical symptoms usually include fever and abdominal pain. Serum hepatic transaminases, alkaline phosphatase, and bilirubin often elevated.

3. Abdominal US and CT feature liver enlargement with multiple well-circumscribed low-density areas. Appearance of candidal abscesses usually distinct from bacterial abscesses (larger and fewer). Percutaneous liver biopsy

confirms diagnosis in 70%. Grossly, liver surface studded with yellow-to-white nodules. Histologically, candidal abscess shows fungal elements in the necrotic center surrounded by inflammatory cells and a ring of fibrosis.

4. Treatment of choice: antifungal agents including amphotericin B, 5-fluorouracil (5-FU), and fluconazole. Treatment for several months may be required. Outcome poor, with mortality rates as high as 20%.

OTHER FUNGAL LIVER INFECTIONS

1. *Histoplasma capsulatum*, *Aspergillus*, *Cryptococcus neoformans*, and *Coccidioides immitis* may also infect the liver. Usually occur in immunocompromised patients, especially those on chemotherapy.
2. Hepatic involvement may manifest as hepatomegaly, elevated serum hepatic transaminases, hyperbilirubinemia, and liver abscess formation.
3. Histology findings in the liver include granuloma, inflammatory cells, and fungal organisms. Diagnosis by serology or isolation of organisms from tissue or body fluids.
4. Therapy: antifungal agents.

QUESTIONS

CHOOSE THE BEST ANSWER:

1. You are asked to consult on a 13-year-old boy with a history of leukemia receiving chemotherapy. Over the past week, he has developed notable fevers and abdominal pain. He has a leukocytosis up to 20K but all cultures have been negative. A liver sonogram reveals a solitary 6 cm hepatic cyst with a honeycomb appearance. What are your recommendations?
   a. Broad-spectrum parenteral antibiotics; monitor for clinical improvement.
   b. Percutaneous drainage of cyst.
   c. Both a and b.
   d. Surgical resection.

2. You are asked to evaluate a 15-year-old girl with a history of multiple sexual partners and acute sharp right upper quadrant pain without fever. Physical exam reveals hepatomegaly, right upper quadrant pain, and cervical motion tenderness. Abdominal sonogram reveals absence of gallbladder disease and biliary tree abnormalities; hepatomegaly can be demonstrated. Laboratories reveal normal hepatic transaminases and bilirubin. Cervical culture reveals *Neisseria gonorrhoeae*. Treatment with appropriate antibiotics has already been started. Is further work-up necessary?
   a. Yes. Laparoscopic confirmation is required.
   b. No. No further work-up is necessary.
   c. Yes. Liver biopsy should be performed for definitive diagnosis.
   d. Yes. Peritoneal lavage should be performed.

3. The following liver infections are transmitted fecal-orally except:
   a. Amebiasis.
   b. Ascariasis.
   c. Echinococcosis.
   d. Schistosomiasis.

MATCH THE MEANS OF TRANSMISSION TO THE INFECTION:

a. Unpasteurized milk.
b. Infected raw fish.
c. Contaminated watercress.
d. Tick bite.
e. Inhalation.
f. Contaminated animal urine.

4. Leptospirosis.
5. Brucellosis.
6. Q fever.
7. Rocky Mountain Spotted fever.
8. Clonorchiasis.
9. Fascioliasis.

TRUE OR FALSE:

10. Cat-scratch disease will not resolve without antibiotics.
11. Antibiotics are of significant benefit even in late-presenting or severe forms of leptospirosis.
12. *Plasmodium falciparum* should always be treated with chloroquine.
13. Stool parasite examination is often of low yield in cases of amebic hepatic abscess.

THE LIVER, AIDS, AND OTHER IMMUNE DISORDERS

SYNOPSIS

1. Gastrointestinal (GI) symptoms typical in patients with human immunodeficiency virus (HIV). Liver commonly involved. Acute hepatitis can be first manifestation of disease (Figure 1). Liver synthetic dysfunction and portal hypertension rare. Mortality from end-stage liver disease among adult HIV patients on the rise with chronic coinfections (most commonly hepatitis B virus [HBV] and hepatitis C virus [HCV]).

2. Liver damage caused by antiretroviral drugs and medications used for prophylaxis against opportunistic infections and tumors. Although HIV directly infects hepatocytes, Kupffer cells, and endothelial cells, unclear whether HIV directly damages the liver.

3. Biliary disease in HIV-infected patients, particularly in those with acquired immunodeficiency syndrome (AIDS). Four distinct cholangiographic patterns described: papillary stenosis in 15–20%, sclerosing cholangitis in 20%, combination of both in 50%, and bile duct strictures in 15%.

HIV COINFECTIONS

1. Hepatitis B: similar transmission routes as HIV. 50% of HIV coinfected patients develop chronic HBV infection. Aggressive treatment of HIV important in the control of HBV. HIV-positive–HBV-positive patients have higher HBV DNA levels, increased hepatitis B e antigen titers with lower serum transaminases, and less histologic damage but greater risk of progression to cirrhosis and development of hepatocellular carcinoma. Suboptimal response to interferon therapy as compared to HIV-negative response. Lamivudine may significantly lower HBV DNA and transaminases and may result in seroconversion, but reactivation may occur following withdrawal. Vaccination recommended but HIV reduces vaccine efficacy.

2. Hepatitis C: 5 times more widespread than HIV infection. End-stage liver disease frequent complication in those coinfected. Sensitivity of the enzyme-linked immunosorbent assay (ELISA) 3 for HCV is > 99%, regardless of HIV status. False-negative HCV serology associated with CD4 counts < 200 cells/mcL in HIV-infected. No data on the natural history of HCV in HIV-infected children. HCV infection in adults more aggressive in HIV-positive patients; liver disease is due to direct HCV viral damage. Antiretroviral therapy has no effect on HCV. Monotherapy with interferon (IFN): poor sustained response. Pegylated IFN: sustained viral response 30–45%. IFN-ribavirin: long-term success (about 28%).

3. Hepatitis A, E, and G: prevalence, morbidity, and mortality of hepatitis A virus (HAV) infection not altered by HIV infection. Vaccination with HAV vaccine may be less effective in HIV-infected patients. Hepatitis E virus (HEV) infection self-limited in HIV infection. Hepatitis G virus (HGV) in 20–40% of HIV-positive patients but does not alter transaminases, CD4 count, or HIV levels.

4. Adenovirus: in HIV-infected persons, gallbladder ulcerations linked with adenoviral infection. Adenoviral infections usually more severe in HIV-infected. Fulminant multiorgan involvement typical; progression to liver failure not uncommon. Diagnosis made by viral isolation or histology. No effective treatment.

5. Herpes simplex virus (HSV): in HIV-positive patients, significant dissemination more common in primary infection but also seen in reactivation. Fulminant liver disease may be only presenting symptom as mucocutaneous lesions may be absent in up to 50%. Notable histologic feature is absence of inflammatory cell response in portal area or parenchyma. Viral cultures usually positive. Prompt initiation of acyclovir and discontinuation of all hepatotoxic medications is recommended.

6. Varicella-zoster virus (VZV): dissemination in HIV-positive patients may occur with primary infection or with reactivation. In contrast to HSV, VZV typically accompanied by classic skin and mucous membrane lesions. Fulminant hepatitis rare. Coagulopathy and multiorgan system failure typical of severe VZV. Immediate administration of VZV immunoglobulin (Ig) is recommended within 96 h of exposure. Prophylactic acyclovir should be prescribed; intravenous acyclovir to those who have clinical signs of VZV. Among HIV-positive patients, only asymptomatic, nonimmunosuppressed patients should be vaccinated against VZV.

7. Epstein-Barr virus (EBV): implicated in pathogenesis of non-Hodgkin lymphoma (isolated liver involvement in 14%), leiomyomas, and leimyosarcomas of the liver in children with AIDS. Elevated serum alkaline phosphatase is very sensitive marker of liver involvement in non-Hodgkin lymphoma.

8. Human herpesvirus 6: severe disseminated infection can occur in immunocompromised patients with primary infection and cause fulminant hepatitis. In vitro susceptibility to ganciclovir described, but indications for therapy not clearly defined.

9. Human herpesvirus 8: associated with Kaposi sarcoma in HIV-positive patients with liver involvement as part of a disseminated process. Patients rarely symptomatic of liver disease. Histologically, Kaposi sarcoma: dark red-purple nodules in portal regions filled with spindle-shaped endothelial cells.

OPPORTUNISTIC INFECTIONS

1. Cytomegalovirus (CMV): 33–44% of all HIV-positive patients. Presentation of CMV hepatitis usually mild. Intranuclear and intracytoplasmic inclusion bodies surrounded by clear halo ("owl-eye") with giant cells on the biopsy. CMV may affect the biliary tree. Diagnosis may be difficult as a positive urine culture may

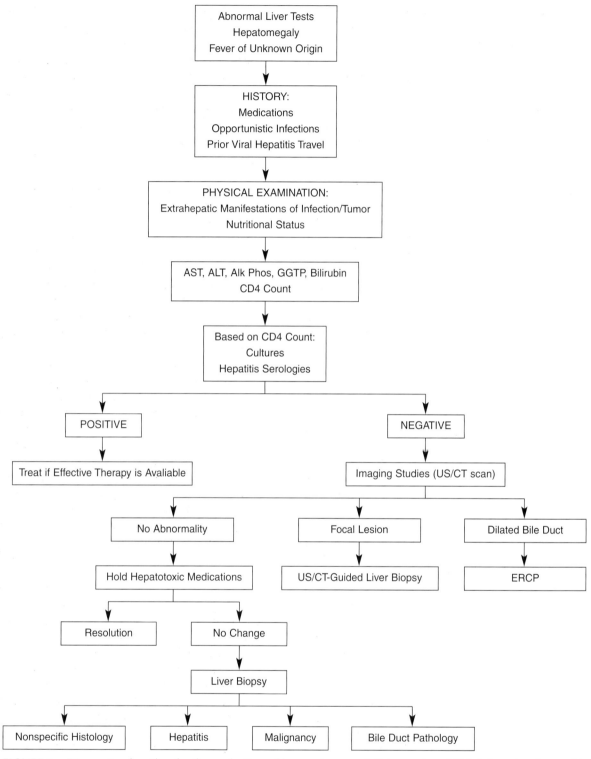

FIGURE 1 Diagnostic algorithm for the evaluation of human immunodeficiency virus (HIV)–infected patients with hepatobiliary disease. Note: risk of bleeding after liver biopsy much increased in AIDS patients, even with normal coagulation studies. Alk phos = alkaline phosphatase; ALT = alanine transaminase; AST = aspartate transaminase; CD4 count = CD4 count lymphocyte cell count; CT = computed tomography; ERCP = endoscopic retrograde cholangiopancreatography; GGTP = γ-glutamyl transpeptidase; US = ultrasonography.

represent asymptomatic shedding. CMV viremia much better predictor of active disease. No controlled trials addressing the use of foscarnet or ganciclovir in the setting of CMV hepatitis.

2. *Pneumocystis carinii*: most common protozoal pathogen among AIDS patients. Incidence decreased dramatically.

In regards to liver involvement: clinically, mild abdominal pain with variable transaminitis. Computed tomography: diffuse punctuate liver calcifications. Pathology: eosinophilic exudates with organisms on silver stain.

3. *Cryptosporidium*: most commonly identified cause of AIDS-related cholangitis (20–62%).

4. Microsporidia: less common cause of AIDS cholangitis (< 10%). Two microsporidia most commonly associated with disease: *Enterocytozoon bieneusi* and *Enterocytozoon intestinalis*. Jaundice present in only 10%. Diagnosis based on detection of organism in stool or bile aspirates.

5. Fungi: involve the liver only in disseminated disease. Imaging studies demonstrate diffuse irregularity of liver parenchyma or formed fungal abscess. Liver biopsy demonstrates poorly formed granulomata with minimal inflammation. Response to prolonged antifungal therapy variable.

6. Mycobacteria: *Mycobacterium avium* and *Mycobacterium intracellulare* are small, gram-positive, acid-fast bacilli; most common opportunistic pathogens found in AIDS patients. With decreased CD4 (< 200 cells/mcL), HIV-postive patients become at risk for disseminated *Mycobacterium avium* complex. Clinical presentation nonspecific. Unique feature in HIV-positive patients is marked elevation of alkaline phosphatase (20–40 times normal) with little transaminitis, hyperbilirubinemia, or other parameters of hepatic function. Histology of liver reveals diffuse, poorly formed granulomata; in AIDS patients, granulomas do not contain multinuclear giant cells. Diagnosis based on cultivation from liver tissue.

7. *Mycobacterium tuberculosis* found in patients less immunosuppressed (CD4 > 200 cells/mcL). Clinical presentation nonspecific. Liver biopsy reveals well-formed caseating granulomas. Current initial treatment: clarithromycin, azithromycin, ethambutol, and rifabutin.

PRIMARY IMMUNODEFICIENCIES

1. Chronic granulomatous disease (CGD): characterized by the inability of phagocytic cells to create active oxygen metabolites for efficient intracellular microbicidal activity. Inherited in an X-linked or autosomal recessive manner. Most frequent infections include pneumonia, osteomyelitis, and skin, soft tissue, or liver abscesses. Susceptibility limited to bacteria and fungi that are catalase positive and do not themselves produce reduced oxygen metabolites. *Staphylococcus aureus* and *Pseudomonas aeruginosa* are the two most common isolates from liver abscesses in patients with CGD. Antibiotic therapy should always include penicillinase-resistant penicillins. Use of interferon-γ appears to decrease the incidence of serious infections.

2. Shwachman syndrome: affects the endocrine pancreas, bone marrow, and skeleton. Most prominent features: neutropenia, pancreatic insufficiency, and short stature. Hepatomegaly and elevated transaminases reported with biopsy demonstrating steatosis and mild fibrosis. Progression of liver disease uncommon.

3. X-linked agammaglobulinemia: presents with recurrent infections in male infants after 9 months of age. Failure to synthesize all classes of immunoglobulins. Recurrent otitis, sinusitis, pneumonias, and diarrhea typical. There is an association with sclerosing cholangitis. Unusual syndrome of severe enteroviral infections, especially echovirus type 11, described with progressive, usually fatal, meningoencephalitis.

4. Common variable immunodeficiency: uncommon disorder with > 95% presenting with sinopulmonary infections. Liver affected by a granulomatous process. Most with liver involvement develop portal hypertension.

5. Severe combined immunodeficiency (SCID): group of genetic disorders characterized by block in T-lymphocyte differentiation; may be associated with other lymphocyte abnormalities. Characterized by lymphocytopenia, absence of lymph nodes or tonsil tissue, low serum immunoglobulins, and absent B and T lymphocyte responses. Frequent severe infections caused by opportunistic organisms common; may include the liver.

   a. Adenosine deaminase deficiency (ADA): systemic metabolic disorder with accumulation of deoxyadenosine triphosphate, which is toxic to lymphocytes. 85–90% present with picture consistent with severe combined immunodeficiency. Profound failure to thrive frequently present. Cupping and flaring of rib ends on radiograph associated specifically with ADA deficiency. Elevated hepatic transaminases not uncommon but usually idiopathic.

   b. Omenn syndrome: another variant of SCID. T-lymphocyte infiltration of the skin and gut is the hallmark of this condition. Present with erythroderma, alopecia, protein-losing enteropathy, and failure to thrive. Life-threatening infections common. Marked hepatosplenomegaly and lymphadenopathy may be present within first weeks of life. Laboratory evaluation demonstrates leukocytosis with elevated eosinophil counts, increased IgE, and hypogammaglobulinemia. Severe liver disease with T-cell infiltration associated with this condition.

6. X-linked lymphoproliferative syndrome: linked to vulnerability to EBV infection (often fatal), with explosive proliferation of B cells after EBV exposure. Liver involvement prominent with progression to multiorgan system failure often resulting in death. 24% will acquire malignant lymphoproliferative disorder if survive initial infection with B-cell neoplasms. Majority of non-Hodgkin lymphomas occur in the intestinal region especially at the ileocecal area.

INFECTIONS IN TRANSPLANT RECIPIENTS

1. Infectious complications after solid organ transplant divided into 3 time periods:

   a. Early post-transplant (first 4 weeks): characterized by nosocomial bacterial and fungal infections. Only significant viral infection observed is recurrent HSV.

   b. 1–6 months post-transplant: infections related to the use of immunosuppressive agents. CMV is dominant pathogen. Other pathogens include *Cryptococcus*, *Candida*, tuberculosis, HBV, HCV, and EBV.

   c. > 6 months post-transplant: usually due to effect of chronic viral infection acquired earlier or chronic graft dysfunction requiring repeated immunosuppression courses.

2. In bone marrow transplant, 3 infectious periods:
   a. Early phase (2–4 wk post-transplant): predominant risk factors: profound neutropenia and mucosal damage. Invasive fungal and bacterial infections predominate.
   b. 15–20 wk post-transplant: infections with opportunistic pathogens predominate. Major predisposing factors: immunosuppression by acute graft-versus-host disease (GVHD) and its treatment.
   c. 4–6 months post-transplant: serious infections seen predominantly in patients with chronic GVHD. Liver infections rare; most common is EBV.

3. In regards to CMV infection, primary infection more likely associated with disease than reactivation. Severity of immunosuppression is determining factor of disease severity. Clinically, mononucleosis-type syndrome. Liver disease rarely severe. Interstitial pneumonitis may be life-threatening. CMV infection in liver transplant patients may be associated with a high risk of acute rejection, possibly an increased incidence of hepatic artery thrombosis.

4. EBV: major concern in solid organ transplant recipients: post-transplant lymphoproliferative disorder (PTLD). Acute infection leads to polyclonal B cell activation. T-cell targeted immunosuppression puts allograft recipients at risk for PTLD. Primary EBV infection, young age, receiving an EBV-positive donor are predisposing factors especially in children. Sites of involvement: small bowel, intraabdominal lymph nodes, tonsils, and liver. Fever, weight loss, lymphadenopathy, hepatosplenomegaly, and abdominal pain are typical presentations. Quantitative EBV PCR techniques monitor EBV infection and reactivation.

5. HBV: more aggressive in immunosuppressed patients. Fibrosing cholestatic hepatitis is a rare, early severe complication of renal transplant in HBV-infected recipients characterized by cholestasis and rapid deterioration in liver function. Use of HBV immunoglobulin during and after transplant decreases the incidence of the recurrence rate in up to 80% of HBV-infected patients receiving liver transplant owing to severe disease. Lamivudine and adefovir also successfully used to prevent HBV recurrence. Booster vaccinations should be given to subjects who are hepatitis B surface antigen (HBsAg) negative if titers < 10 mIU/mL. Allografts from HBsAg positive donors should not be used.

6. HCV: HCV RNA positive donor organs most likely to transmit infection. Virtually all liver transplant recipients who are HCV viremic at time of transplant will be reinfected. Factors associated with more rapid progression of disease after transplant: degree of immunusuppression and coinfection with CMV or HCV genotype 1b. In bone marrow transplant patients, HCV is major cause of post-transplant cirrhosis. Clear association with veno-occlusive disease. Fibrosing cholestatic hepatitis is only early but serious complication of HCV infection observed in transplant patients. Diagnosis by detection of HCV RNA; serology is a poor marker of HCV infection. Liver biopsy important to confirm diagnosis and delineate severity of disease. Treatment: interferon with or without ribavirin usually used. Interferon associated with graft rejection in renal but not liver transplant recipients. Response rates to treatment lower than in immunocompetent patients.

7. Invasive candidiasis major cause of mortality and morbidity in patients with hematologic malignancies. Hepatosplenic involvement typical (alkaline phosphatase substantially elevated; CT identifies lesions in 90% with small round, low-attenuation lesions). Risk factors: presence of acute leukemia, prolonged neutropenia, intravascular catheters, mucosal barrier disruption, and broad-spectrum antibiotic administration. Diagnosis requires high index of suspicion. Open liver biopsy most reliable way to diagnose. Management includes antifungals (fluconazole is drug of choice).

QUESTIONS

TRUE OR FALSE:

1. HIV–hepatitis B virus (HBV) coinfection has a higher rate of chronic HBV infection.
2. Liver disease in HIV–hepatitis C virus (HCV) coinfected patients results from direct cytopathic effect by HCV.
3. Prevalence and morbidity of hepatitis A virus infection are altered by HIV.
4. Mucocutaneous lesions may be absent in up to 50% of herpes simplex virus infection among HIV-positive patients.
5. Microsporidia is the most common cause of AIDS-related cholangitis.
6. Human herpesvirus 8 is associated with Kaposi sarcoma in HIV-positive patients.
7. Fibrosing cholestatic hepatitis occurs in transplant patients with hepatitis B or C virus infection.

MATCH THE CONDITION TO THE CHARACTERISTICS:

a. Chronic granulomatous disease.
b. Common variable immunodeficiency.
c. Omenn syndrome.
d. X-linked lymphoproliferative syndrome.
e. Adenosine deaminase deficiency.

8. *Staphylococcus aureus* and *Pseudomonas aeruginosa* liver abscesses.
9. Granulomatous process in the liver, portal hypertension.
10. Variant of severe combined immunodeficiency associated with T-lymphocyte infiltration of the skin and gut.
11. Accumulation of deoxyadenosine triphosphate resulting in lymphocyte depletion.
12. Vulnerability to Epstein-Barr virus infection.

AUTOIMMUNE LIVER DISEASE

SYNOPSIS

1. Inflammatory liver disorders characterized histologically by a dense mononuclear infiltrate in portal tract and serologically by liver-specific autoantibodies and elevated globulin levels.
2. Three disorders: autoimmune hepatitis, autoimmune sclerosing cholangitis, and de novo autoimmune hepatitis after liver transplant.

AUTOIMMUNE HEPATITIS

1. Two types (Figure 1) :
   a. Characterized by antinuclear antibodies (ANA) positive or smooth muscle antibodies (SMA) positive
   b. Characterized by anti-liver kidney microsomal type 1 antibody (ALKM1) positive.
2. Targets:
   a. SMA: actin of smooth muscle
   b. ALKM1: cytochrome P4502D6 (CYP2D6)
3. Predominance of girls: about 75%.
4. ALKM1 positive type presents earlier (7.4 yr vs 10.5 yr)
5. Three clinical patterns of disease:

   a. Acute viral hepatitis (50% ANA or SMA positive, 65% ALKM1 positive, with more ALKM1 positive presenting in fulminant disease),
   b. Insidious (38% ANA or SMA positive, 25% ALKM1 positive),
   c. Portal hypertension
6. Frequency of associated human leukocyte antigens (HLA) higher in ANA positive and SMA positive. Patients with autoimmune hepatitis (AIH) have isolated partial deficiency of HLA class III component C4 (C4AQ0). Possession of HLA haplotype DR3 associated with predisposition to develop AIH type I, and possession of DR7 predisposes to AIH type II.
7. Severity of portal tract inflammation similar, although cirrhosis more common on initial biopsy among ANA and SMA positive.
8. T lymphocytes predominate among invading cells, and majority are CD4 positive. There is evidence that children with AIH have low levels of CD8 positive T lymphocytes. Some evidence that Th1 response active in causing liver damage with Th2 cytokines predominating during remission.
9. Recent studies show homology between hepatitis C virus (HCV) polyprotein and CYP2D6; implicates potential molecular mimicry mechanism.
10. Titers to liver-specific lipoprotein (LSP) correlate with biochemical and histologic severity of AIH.

Autoimmune hepatitis

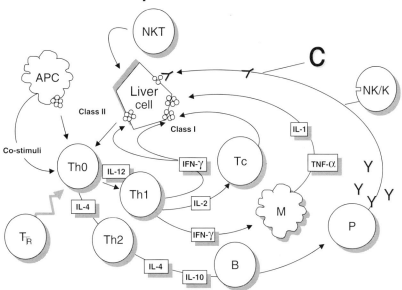

FIGURE 1 Autoimmune attack on the liver. A specific autoantigenic peptide is presented to an uncommitted T helper (Th0) lymphocyte within the human leukocyte antigen (HLA) class II molecule of an antigen-presenting cell (APC). Th0 cells become activated and, according to the presence in the microenvironment of interleukin (IL)-12 or IL-4 and nature of antigen, differentiate into Th1 or Th2 and initiate a series of immune reactions determined by the cytokines they produce: Th2 secrete mainly IL-4 and IL-10 and direct autoantibody production by B lymphocytes; Th1 secrete IL-2 and interferon-γ (IFN-γ), which stimulate T cytotoxic (Tc) lymphocytes, enhance expression of class I and induce expression of class II HLA molecules on hepatocytes and activate macrophages; activated macrophages release IL-1 and tumour necrosis factor-alpha (TNF-α). If T "regulatory" (T_R) lymphocytes do not oppose, a variety of effector mechanisms are triggered: liver cell destruction could derive from the action of Tc lymphocytes; cytokines released by Th1 and recruited macrophages; complement (C) activation or engagement of killer (NK/K) lymphocytes by the autoantibody (Y) bound to the hepatocyte surface. Natural killer T cells (NKT), cells with markers of both natural killer and T cells, are involved in liver damage in an animal model of autoimmune hepatitis. Adapted from Vergani D, Chodhuri K, Bogdanos DP, Mieli-Vergani G. Pathogenesis of autoimmune hepatitis. Clin Liver Dis 2002;6:439–49.

11. Treatment: immunosuppression, unless acute liver failure (requires transplantation).
    a. Treat with 2 mg/kg/d prednisone (maximum 60 mg/d); dose gradually decreased over 4–8 wk. If normalized, then maintain on low level prednisone (5 mg/d) to maintain normal transaminases.
    b. If not normal or requires too high a dose prednisone: azathioprine at 0.5 mg/kg/d increased to 2 mg/kg/d as needed. Owing to hepatotoxicity, azathioprine should not used as first-line therapy.
    c. Complete normalization of laboratory results may take months. Relapse rate 40%. Risk is higher if steroids are taken every other day (ie, the schedule makes relapse a higher risk). If liver biopsy normal or minimal inflammation after 1 year of normal liver function tests, stop therapy.
    d. In most children with AIH, especially if ALKM1 positive, lifelong therapy required.
    e. Cyclosporin used with good results but long-term toxicity unclear. Mycophenolate mofetil can be helpful where patients do not tolerate or respond to azathioprine.

AUTOIMMUNE SCLEROSING CHOLANGITIS

1. In childhood: may occur as isolated disease or in association with histiocytosis, immunodeficiency, psoriasis, cystic fibrosis, or inflammatory bowel disease. There is also an overlapping syndrome with AIH and autoimmune sclerosing cholangitis (ASC).
2. Liver-specific antibodies including ANA or SMA and ALKM1.
3. In Mieli-Vergani cohort (often with autoimmune features): majority respond to prednisone with or without azathioprine (in contrast to adult studies and other pediatric studies).

DE NOVO AIH AFTER LIVER TRANSPLANTATION

Treat similarly as AIH.

RECURRENCE OF DISEASE AFTER LIVER TRANSPLANTATION

1. AIH: reported in 30% of patients. Possession of HLA DR3 may confer predisposition. Discontinuation of steroid therapy may increase risk for recurrence.
2. Primary sclerosing cholangitis (PSC): reported in 6–20%; but difficult to prove as most have Roux-en-Y anastomosis with increased risk for biliary obstruction; difficult to distinguish secondary from recurrent disease. Also, radiologic and histologic features of PSC can result from ischemic biliary complications.

QUESTIONS

CHOOSE THE BEST ANSWER:

1. The following are true of autoimmune hepatitis except:
   a. Girls are predominantly affected.
   b. If ALKM1 positive, more likely to present earlier.
   c. If ALKM1 positive, less likely to present with fulminant picture.
   d. If ALKM1 positive, more likely to require lifelong therapy.
   e. Has isolated partial deficiency of human leukocyte antigens (HLA) C4AQ0.
   f. If antinuclear antibodies (ANA) positive or smooth muscle antibodies (SMA) positive, higher frequency of human leukocyte antigens (HLA).

2. The following therapies are indicated in autoimmune hepatitis except:
   a. Prednisone 2 mg/kg/d as initial therapy for insidious presentation.
   b. If not respond to prednisone, then start azathioprine.
   c. Liver transplantation if present with fulminant hepatic failure.
   d. Discontinuation of therapy after 1 year of normal laboratory results in the setting of a normal biopsy.
   e. High-dose steroids until laboratory results normalize.

TRUE OR FALSE

3. Titers to liver-specific lipoprotein correlate with histologic severity of autoimmune hepatitis.
4. There is homology between hepatitis C virus polyprotein and CYP2D6 indicating molecular mimicry as a mechanism for liver injury in autoimmune hepatitis.

CHOOSE THE BEST ANSWER:

5. Autoimmune sclerosing cholangitis is associated with all of the following except:
   a. Histiocytosis.
   b. Immunodeficiencies.
   c. Celiac disease.
   d. Inflammatory bowel disease.
   e. Cystic fibrosis.
   f. Psoriasis.

DRUG-INDUCED LIVER INJURY

SYNOPSIS

1. Hepatic drug metabolism: activation (phase I) and detoxification (phase II). Product of a phase I reaction: unstable and reactive metabolite, more polar chemical. Phase II: transforms hydrophobic chemical to hydrophilic one to allow excretion.

2. Cytochrome P450 enzymes carry out most phase I reactions. CYP2A6 and CYP3A4: reductive metabolism; CYP2A6 and CYP2E1: oxidative pathway.

3. Polymorphisms result in differences in the rate of enzyme action. Poor metabolizer phenotype is associated with absence of CYP2D6.

4. Most drug-induced liver disease is cytotoxic, some cholestatic (Table 1). Zone 3: highest metabolizing enzyme concentration for forming toxic intermediates.

5. Intrinsic hepatotoxin: predictable damage. Toxicity is dose related.

6. Idiosyncratic hepatotoxin: unpredictable, sporadic. If systemic features (fever, rash, and eosinophilia): idiosyncratic hypersensitivity reaction.

7. Autoantibodies may be elaborated against specific cytochromes (eg, tienilic acid: CYP2C9; dihydralazine: CYP1A2; halothane CYP2E1).

ACETAMINOPHEN

1. Mechanism: formation of toxic metabolite. Usually metabolized by sulfation and glucuronidation. If sufficient amount taken, these pathways become saturated and minor P450 pathway becomes important. Product of minor P450 pathway: toxic N-acetyl-p-benzoquinoneimine (NAPQI), which is conjugated by glutathione to nontoxic form. NAPQI causes cell damage and death. Fasting decreases glutathione and increases toxicity. Liver biopsy shows necrosis at zone 3.

2. Clinical course: immediate nausea or vomiting, then asymptomatic phase before hepatotoxicity. In adults poor outcome predicted by serum creatinine > 300 μmol/L, prothrombin time (PT) > 100 seconds, and international normalized ratio (INR) > 7, and grade 3 or 4 encephalopathy, or a standalone finding of arterial pH < 7.3.

3. Treatment: N-acetyl cysteine (NAC) most effective within 10 hr. Charcoal helpful within 1 hr. Hemodialysis: use early with high levels. 72 hr oral NAC regimen; 20 hr intravenous (IV) NAC. Best predictor in children for low risk of liver toxicity is normal PT and normal levels of aspartate transaminase (AST) and alanine aminotransferase (ALT) at 48 hr after ingestion.

4. Younger children resistant to hepatotoxicity. Sulfation is the predominant drug metabolism process as compared to glucuronidation in children < 12 years old as compared to adolescents and adults.

5. Problem of chronic high-dose ingestion: if acetaminophen in blood > 24 h after last dose, treat with NAC as soon as possible.

6. Chronic alcoholics more sensitive to acetaminophen, via induction of CYP2E1, which metabolizes acetaminophen.

PHENYTOIN

1. Severe hepatic necrosis and liver failure. Presents as part of systemic illness with fever, rash, Stevens-Johnson syndrome, toxic epidermolysis, lymphadenopathy, and eosinophilia.

2. Histopathology: spotty necrosis of hepatocytes; features similar to viral hepatitis.

3. Drug sensitivity reaction: may result from abnormal handling of toxic metabolite of phenytoin. In vitro studies show that if unable to detoxify phenytoin correctly, phenobarbital is also problematic; phenobarbital may potentiate damage.

4. Treatment with IV prednisolone 2mg/kg/d helpful in some persons.

CARBAMAZEPINE

1. Hepatotoxicity relatively uncommon. In adults: granulomatous hepatitis with right upper quadrant pain, and fever, similar to cholangitis. In children: hepatitis picture, sometimes drug-sensitivity picture. Carbamazepine may also be metabolized by arene oxides; thus, patient may also be sensitive to phenytoin or phenobarbital.

2. Liver biopsy: fibrosis at portal area, ductular proliferation, and mild chronic inflammation. Swollen hepatocytes in zones 2 and 3 with bridging necrosis in zone 3.

TABLE 1   SPECTRUM OF DRUG-INDUCED LIVER DISEASE

TYPE	EXAMPLES
Acute hepatitis	Methyldopa, isoniazid, halothane, phenytoin
Hepatitis-cholestasis	Erythromycin, chlorpromazine, azathioprine, nitrofurantoin, cimetidine
Zonal liver cell necrosis	Acetaminophen
Bland cholestasis	Estrogens, cyclosporines
Steatonecrosis (like alcoholic hepatitis)	Perhexiline, amiodarone
Phospholipidosis	Amiodarone
Microvesicular steatosis	Valproic acid, tetracycline
Granulomatosis	Sulfonamides, phenylbutazone, carbamazepine
Biliary cirrhosis	Practolol, chlorpropamide
Sclerosing cholangitis	Floxuridine via hepatic artery
Hepatic vascular changes	
Peliosis	Estrogens, androgens
Hepatic vein thrombosis	Estrogens (oral contraceptives)
Veno-occlusive disease	Thioguanine, busulfan, pyrrolizidine (Senecio) alkaloids
Noncirrhotic portal hypertension	Vinyl chloride, arsenic
Liver cell adenoma	Estrogens (oral contraceptives), anabolic steroids
Malignant tumors	Estrogens, anabolic steroids, vinyl chloride
Porphyria	2,3,7,8-Tetrachlorodibenzo-p-dioxin, chloroquine

PHENOBARBITAL

1. Hepatitis: rare complication; part of multisystemic drug hypersensitivity reaction. In most cases, jaundice within 1–8 wk of starting drug with rash and fever.
2. Mechanism unclear.
3. Persons who develop hepatotoxicity from phenobarbital also cannot detoxify other barbiturates, carbamazepine, or phenytoin.

LAMOTRIGINE

May cause hepatotoxicity with a typical anticonvulsant hypersensitivity syndrome clinically.

VALPROIC ACID

1. Chemically very different from other anticonvulsants.
2. Hepatotoxicity mild or severe. 11% develop abnormal liver function tests (LFTs) within short time of starting therapy; return to normal after dose decreased or discontinued. Rarely, progressive liver failure: Reye syndrome (coagulopathy early, death is frequent outcome). Time from initiating treatment and onset of liver disease usually < 4 mo. Hepatotoxicity more common in children than adults. Identifiable risk factors: age < 2 yr, use of multiple anticonvulsants, and coexisting medical problems such as mental retardation, developmental delay, and congenital abnormalities. Hyperammonemia, not associated with liver failure, is another metabolic adverse effect.
3. Mechanism of severe hepatotoxicity: generation of toxic metabolite plus idiosyncrasy. Target organelle appears to be mitochondrion. Value of carnitine repletion unproven.

SULFONAMIDES

1. Liver abnormality may be manifested only by elevated serum aminotransferases or granulomatous hepatitis, but hepatic dysfunction may be severe enough to cause hepatic failure. In general, part of a multisystemic hypersensitivity reaction. Sulfa hepatotoxicity: metabolic idiosyncrasy, not just allergy.
2. Mechanism: due to elaboration of electrophilic toxic metabolite. Persons with severe adverse reactions are slow acetylators, unable to detoxify this reactive metabolite. Reactive metabolite probably acts as hapten to initiate immune response given multisystemic hypersensitivity.

ERYTHROMYCIN

1. All forms of erythromycin potentially hepatotoxic.
2. Hepatomegaly with occasional splenomegaly frequent in children.
3. Histology: prominent cholestasis in zone 3, focal necrosis (most in zone 3), and eosinophils in portal infiltrates and sinusoids.
4. Mechanism: unclear.

PROPYLTHIOURACIL

1. Tends to occur in girls.
2. Clinical picture: nonspecific hepatitis. Rare complication. Serum aminotransferases moderately elevated. Symptoms start within 2–3 mo of starting therapy.
3. Histology: mild to severe hepatocellular necrosis.

ASPIRIN

1. Hepatotoxicity with high-dose aspirin. May be more frequent in girls. Dose-dependent. Preponderance of cases with rheumatologic diseases.
2. Presentation: anorexia, nausea and vomiting, abdominal pain, and elevated transaminases. Hepatomegaly usually present. Progressive signs of liver damage rare. Laboratory results abnormalities resolve when aspirin stopped. Rechallenge may lead to recurrent hepatotoxicity.
3. Histology: nonspecific picture; focal hepatocellular necrosis.

METHOTREXATE

1. Hepatotoxicity similar in children and adults. Chronic low-dose regimens can cause hepatic fibrosis with steatosis. Cirrhosis can develop. Increased risk in adults: obesity, diabetes mellitus, chronic alcoholism, older age, and large cumulative dose. In children, risk factor limited to obesity.
2. Children on methotrexate should have LFT check every 1–2 mo; if elevated AST or ALT on ≥ 40% tests for more than 1 yr, liver biopsy is indicated.
3. Mechanism: unknown. Chronic intermittent administration of methotrexate may lead to recurrent hepatocellular damage superimposed on partial repair or regeneration.

ANTINEOPLASTIC DRUGS

1. L-Asparaginase associated with severe steatosis, hepatocellular necrosis, and fibrosis; usually reversible with drug cessation.
2. Dactinomycin exceptionally associated with severe liver damage; resolves with drug cessation. Mechanism unknown.
3. Mithramycin associated with acute hepatic necrosis.
4. Thioguanine, cytosine arabinoside, busulfan, dacarbazine, and carmustine associated with veno-occlusive disease (VOD). VOD usually develops after allogeneic bone marrow transplantation. Presents acutely with enlarged tender liver, ascites or unexplained weight gain, and jaundice. LFTs may be elevated. Radiation therapy can lead to VOD. Patients with chronic hepatitis prior to bone marrow transplant at increased risk for VOD.
5. In dacarbazine VOD, damage to endothelium through toxic metabolites. Treatment with NAC may reverse.

CYCLOSPORINE

1. Lipophilic; metabolized by CYP3A4.
2. More common hepatic abnormality: cholestasis without hepatocellular damage. Cyclosporine inhibits bile salt excretory pump directly.

PEMOLINE

1. Significant hepatotoxicity: asymptomatic elevated aminotransferase levels, hepatitis with jaundice, and acute liver failure.
2. Monitor LFTs during therapy. If elevated aminotransferases, discontinue.

3. Mechanism unknown; do not use with other hepato-toxic drugs or if history of liver disease.

RISPERIDONE
Serum elevations in aminotransferases and bilirubin described in children (need to monitor).

ISONIAZID
1. Clinically: asymptomatic with elevated aminotrans-ferases.
2. Hepatitis illness ominous: on histology looks like acute viral hepatitis. Incidence of symptomatic isoni-azid (INH) hepatitis in children 0.1–7%.
3. Frequent monitoring of aminotransferase important in first 10–12 wk of therapy. Stop INH if anorexia or nau-sea and vomiting develop.
4. Due to toxic metabolite. Susceptibility to hepatotoxic-ity greater in rapid acetylators. Rifampicin enhances INH toxicity by inducing certain cytochromes P450. Children with simultaneous treatment with rifampicin, phenytoin, or phenobarbital may be at increased risk.

HALOTHANE
1. Two major clinical patterns: hepatitis in 1st–2nd wk after exposure and severe hepatitis with extensive necrosis and liver failure. 1/200,000 to 1/80,000 chil-dren, versus 1/30,000 to 1/7,000 in adults.
2. Metabolized by various cytochromes P450. Both oxi-dation and reduction occurs with oxidative pathway predominant in humans.

PENICILLINS
1. Semisynthetic derivative of penicillin may cause liver damage. Amoxicillin-clavulanate associated with cholestasis or mixed hepatitis-cholestasis reaction.
2. With prolonged cholestasis, bile duct paucity observed in adults. Small bile duct paucity seen with amoxicillin alone but amoxicillin-clavulanate more toxic.

MINOCYCLINE
1. Associated with hepatotoxicity: jaundice, elevated LFTs, and antinuclear antibodies (ANA) positive com-mon. Some with autoimmune hepatitis features.
2. In many, liver damage resolved with discontinuation of drug. Careful monitoring of LFTs indicated when used chronically.

HERBALS
Herbals known to be hepatotoxic: bush teas with pyrrolizidine alkaloids, comfrey, germander, chaparral, kava-kava, jin bu huan, and ma huang.

ECSTASY
1. Zone 3 necrosis. Interindividual variation in suscep-tibility.
2. Hyperthermia, rhabdomyolysis, cardiac arrhythmias, and acute renal failure.

ORAL CONTRACEPTIVE PILL
1. Cholestasis.
2. Budd-Chiari syndrome.
3. Liver cell adenoma; may progress to hepatocellular carcinoma.
4. Peliosis hepatis.

HALOPERIDOL
Cholestasis.

KETOCONAZOLE
1. Fulminant hepatitis. Hepatocellular necrosis, usually centrilobular but can be mixed with cholestasis.
2. Thought to be idiosyncratic.

RETINOIDS
Vitamin A excess: change in Ito cells; steatosis and fibrosis. Hepatitic pattern.

NONSTEROIDAL ANTIINFLAMMATORY DRUGS
Usually not hepatotoxic, except sulindac. Sulindac causes hepatitic-cholestatic reaction; can be accompanied by fever and rash.

THERAPY
1. Most drug injury resolves spontaneously with removal of drug. Severe chronic changes do not regress.
2. Some require antidotes (eg, NAC for acetaminophen).
3. Steroids beneficial when severe acute hepatitis domi-nates multisystemic hypersensitivity reaction, as with phenytoin, carbamazepine, and phenobarbital, but controversial.
4. High index of suspicion necessary for diagnosis. Liver biopsy with electron microscopy exam may be diagnostic. In vitro challenge of lymphocytes with generated toxic metabolites usually provides corroborative evidence.

QUESTIONS

CHOOSE THE BEST ANSWER:
1. The following are true of acetaminophen toxicity except:
   a. Occurs via metabolism along P450 pathway.
   b. Occurs when sulfation and glucuronidation path-ways are saturated.
   c. Occurs via exposure to N-actyl-p-benzoquinoneimine.
   d. Fasting decreases toxicity.
   e. Potentiated by chronic alcohol ingestion.
   f. Histologic damage mainly in zone 3.

2. In adults, poor outcome in acetominophen toxicity is predicted by all of the following except:
   a. Grade 3 encephalopathy.
   b. Prothrombin time > 100 s.
   c. Serum creatinine > 300 µmol/L.
   d. Grade 4 encephalopathy.
   e. Venous pH < 7.3.

3. The following drugs have the same mechanism behind their associated hepatotoxicity except:
   a. Phenobarbital.
   b. Valproic acid.
   c. Carbamazepine.
   d. Phenytoin.
   e. All of the above have the same mechanism.

4. The following are true of sulfonamide drug injury to the liver except:
   a. Increased risk for hepatotoxicity with slow acetylators.
   b. Increased risk for hepatotoxicity with fast acetylators.
   c. Hepatotoxicity represents metabolic idiosyncrasy .
   d. Hepatotoxicity represents allergy.
   e. None of the above.

5. The following are true of valproic acid induced injury to the liver except:
   a. Present within 4 months of starting therapy.
   b. More common in adults than children.
   c. Associated with multiple anticonvulsant exposure.
   d. More common in patients with developmental delay and congenital abnormalities.
   e. Also associated with hyperammonemia without liver failure.
   f. In severe hepatotoxicity, coagulopathy occurs early.

MATCH THE TREATMENT TO THE CHARACTERISTICS:

a. Erythromycin.
b. L-Asparaginase.
c. Methotrexate.
d. Mithramycin.
e. Radiation.
f. Isoniazid.
g. Halothane.
h. Penicillins.
i. Minocycline.

6. Obesity risk factor for hepatotoxicity.
7. Prominent cholestasis in zone 3.
8. Associated with being antinuclear antibodies positive.
9. Susceptibility with rapid acetylation.
10. Damage via both reductive and oxidative pathways.
11. Acute hepatic necrosis.
12. Vaso-occlusive disease.
13. Associated with small bile duct paucity.

LIVER TUMORS

SYNOPSIS

CLINICAL MANIFESTATIONS

1. Majority first detected as abdominal mass. Upper abdominal pain next most frequent complaint.
2. Vascular tumors may display signs of congestive heart failure.
3. Tumors obstructing bile flow may present with pruritus and frank jaundice (obstruction in children suggests rhabdomyosarcoma at the biliary tree).
4. Precocious puberty in males seen with hepatoblastoma and hepatocellular carcinoma (HCC) owing to ectopic gonadotropin.
5. For HCC, male-to-female ratio 8–10:1 in adults, 2:1 in children.
6. Laboratory abnormalities: hypercalcemia (not due to ectopic parathyroid hormone production) can occur in hepatoblastoma, HCC, and sarcoma. Hyperlipidemia can be seen with hepatoblastoma; when present, associated with early fatality. Thrombocytosis (HCC and hepatoblastoma) and polycythemia (HCC) also seen.

ETIOLOGY

1. Hepatitis B virus responsible for more malignancy than any other environmental agent, particularly for HCC.
2. Underlying genetic diseases: polyposis (hepatoblastoma), familial cholestatic cirrhosis (HCC), glycogen storage disease types I, III, and IV (HCC) and trisomy 2 and 20 (hepatoblastoma).
3. Estrogens in oral contraceptives are associated with hepatic adenoma development.
4. Oncogene expression: c-Ki-ras, c-Ha-ras, c-myc, fos, c-met for HCC. For hepatoblastoma: insulin-like growth factor 2, BRCA2 (Table 1).

IMAGING

1. Ultrasonography detects early liver lesions.
2. Magnetic resonance imaging and computed tomography with contrast useful for detecting extent of disease.
3. Scintigraphy with radiolabeled sulfur colloids distinguish lesions with Kupffer cells from those without.

LABORATORY TESTS

1. Serum α-fetoprotein is the most useful marker of malignant liver tumors. 80–90% of hepatoblastoma patients and 60–90% of HCC patients have elevations at diagnosis. Small cell undifferentiated hepatoblastomas and rhabdoid tumors do not make α-fetoprotein. α-Fetoprotein is elevated in hereditary tyrosinemia and ataxia-telangiectasia without presence of malignancy. Monitoring of α-fetoprotein levels can be helpful to follow recurrences of tumor.

TABLE 1   MOLECULAR GENETICS OF HEPATOCELLULAR NEOPLASMS

GENE OR LOCUS	ABNORMALITY	TUMOR TYPE	TUMORS AFFECTED (%)
HIC1 (17p13.3)	Hypermethylation, LOH, ↓ expression	HCC	90
CDK4 (12q13–15)	↑ Expression	HB	88
Telomerase (3q26.3)	↑ Expression	HCC	74
Cyclin D$_1$ (11q13)	↑ Expression	HB	70
TP53 (17p13)	Codon 249 mutation	HCC	67 in aflatoxin regions, < 15 elsewhere
FAS (CD95L)	↓ Expression	HCC	64
IGF2 (11p15.5)	LOH or LOI	HB	64
E-cadherin (16q22.1)	Hypermethylation ↓ Expression	HCC	58
TGF-β (2p13)	↑ Expression	HCC	54
β-catenin (3p22–p21.3)	↑ Expression	HB	48
RB (13q14)	LOH	HCC	47

HB = hepatoblastoma; HCC = hepatocellular carcinoma; IGF = insulin-like growth factor; LOH = loss of heterozygosity; LOI = loss of imprinting; RB = retinoblastoma; TGF = transforming growth factor.

2. Serum carcinoembryonic antigen (CEA) and neurotensin may indicate fibrolamellar type of HCC. Urine pseudouridine and plasma transcobalamin I also used as markers.

TUMORS

HEPATOBLASTOMA
1. Embryonal tumor. 90% present by age 4 yr.
2. Staging:
   a. I: complete resection.
   b. II: microscopic residual tumor. A, inside liver; B, outside liver.
   c. III: gross residual tumor. A, surgical spillage or gross nodal involvement; B, incomplete resection or node involvement.
   d. IV: metastatic disease. A, primary completely resected; B, primary not completely resected.
3. Ploidy of tumor associated with better survival with diploid versus aneuploid tumors.
4. Small cell undifferentiated histology associated with worse prognosis.

HEPATOCARCINOMA
1. Frequency of cirrhosis in children much less than in adults.
2. HCC has higher frequency of multiple nodules than hepatoblastoma; HCC more likely to disseminate via the intrahepatic portal vein and lymphatics, than hepatoblastoma at the time of diagnosis.
3. Fibrolamellar carcinoma (FLC) type rarely associated with cirrhosis, rarely produces α-fetoprotein, and tends to affect young persons (90% of cases age < 25 yr). However, children with FLC do not have a favorable prognosis and do not respond any differently to therapy than as for typical HCC.
4. Children with initially resectable HCC have a good prognosis (75% disease-free for 5 yr), but those with advanced-stage disease do poorly.

ADENOMA AND FOCAL NODULAR HYPERPLASIA
1. Both adenomas and focal nodular hyperplasia observed in patients with glycogen storage disease and women using oral contraceptives (only adenoma causally linked with oral contraceptives).
2. Both usually solitary and expansile, but adenoma more often multiple and encapsulated.
3. Both consist of well-differentiated hepatocytes arranged in cords or plates but without normal lobular pattern.
4. Adenomas lack bile duct and portal tracts, while focal nodular hyperplasia has septa radiating from a central scar in which ducts can be numerous.

VASCULAR TUMORS
1. Hemangioendotheliomas of infancy are the most common benign tumors of the liver.
   a. Can cause high-output congestive heart failure. May rupture and cause intraperitoneal hemorrhage.
   b. Two types: type I, definite vessels with few mitoses, no nuclear atypia, and frequent calcification; type II, can disseminate on occasion, with frequent mitoses.
   c. Most cases regress spontaneously or respond well to steroids.
2. Hepatic angiomyolipomas seen in 24% children with tuberous sclerosis.

MESENCHYMAL TUMORS
1. Mesenchymal hamartomas of infancy can be present at birth, grow to an enormous size, and cause heart failure because of arteriovenous shunting. 90% manifest at infancy. Usually multiple large cystic spaces with a flat endothelial or biliary epithelial lining and serous fluid content. Associated with translocation 19q13.4. Can lead to development of embryonal hepatic sarcoma.
2. Malignant mesenchymomas: contain myxoid, chondroid, muscular, bony, and fibrous tissues.
3. Embryonal undifferentiated sarcoma tends to be large, unresectable at presentation. Microscopically undifferentiated with huge bizarre cells with prominent glycoprotein inclusions and abundant myxoid stroma. Prognosis generally very poor but may respond to intensive chemotherapy.
4. Rhabdomyosarcomas of the biliary tract tend to obstruct bile flow. Cells are primitive embryonal forms.

BILE DUCT EPITHELIAL TUMORS

1. Biliary cystadenomas with mesenchymal stroma are benign tumors in young women.
2. Carcinomas observed in the remnants of choledochal cysts.

TERATOMAS

1. Rare; usually affect females.
2. When yolk sac tissue is present (as in endodermal sinus tumor) α-fetoprotein can be very elevated.
3. Treatment is surgical.

INFLAMMATORY MYOFIBROBLASTIC TUMOR, LYMPHOMA, AND LEUKEMIA

1. Inflammatory myofibroblastic tumor has histology showing dense plasma cell infiltrates associated with active fibroplasias. Etiology unknown. Some tumors regress with steroids. Some rearrangements of the *ALK* gene have been observed.
2. Primary lymphomas of the liver in children are very rare. Have monomorphous infiltrates without fibrosis.
3. Involvement of the liver in leukemia common but of rare clinical significance, except megakaryoblastic leukemia, which can present with hepatomegaly and abnormal liver function tests (LFTs). Liver biopsy in megakaryoblastic leukemia shows diffuse infiltration of sinusoids by blast cells with diffuse scarring (immunostaining with platelet glycoprotein 2b).

SECONDARY NEOPLASIA

Neuroblastoma is most common solid tumor liver metastasis in children. Other malignancies that spread to the liver include Wilms' tumor, rhabdomyosarcoma, Ewing's sarcoma, intra-abdominal small cell desmoplastic tumor, and ovarian germ cell tumors.

TREATMENT

1. Primary goal in treating liver neoplasms is complete surgical removal. Benign lesions may respond to medical management or arterial embolization.
2. Vigorous efforts are made to reach a diagnosis preoperatively or intraoperatively given different approaches (benign lesions may not need to be resected).
3. When initial surgery for cancer is too risky, preoperative chemotherapy has proven effective in shrinking tumors to allow resection. Some centers may also use radiation therapy. HCCs are resectable only 10–20% of the time.
4. Liver transplant has been used for the treatment of HCC and hepatoblastoma. In general, success is better predicted if HCCs are not multicentric, not larger than 5 cm, and do not exhibit vascular invasion, metastasis, or positive margins at surgery.

QUESTIONS

CHOOSE THE BEST ANSWER

1. The following are presentations of liver tumors except:
   a. Abdominal pain.
   b. Abdominal mass.
   c. Hypercalcemia.
   d. Precocious puberty.
   e. Hypoglycemia.

2. Which of the following is the most common etiologic agent for development of hepatocellular carcinoma?
   a. Hepatitis B virus.
   b. Glycogen storage disease.
   c. Tyrosinemia.
   d. Extreme prematurity.
   e. Birth control pills.

3. Which of the following is not a marker of hepatic malignancy?
   a. α-Fetoprotein.
   b. Carcinoembryonic antigen.
   c. Plasma transcobalamin.
   d. Urine pseudouridine.
   e. Alkaline phosphatase.

4. Which of the following is the most common benign tumor of the liver in children?
   a. Focal nodular hyperplasia.
   b. Hepatic adenomas.
   c. Mesenchymal hamartomas.
   d. Hemangioendotheliomas.
   e. Hepatic angiomyolipomas.

5. Which of the following are not at increased risk for primary liver malignancy?
   a. An 8-year-old boy with chronic hepatitis B virus infection.
   b. A 5-year-old girl with tyrosinemia.
   c. A 1-year-old boy who has tuberous sclerosis.
   d. An 18-year-old girl with a history of oral contraceptive use.
   e. A 2-year-old girl with glycogen storage disease type II.

6. Which of the following is the most common tumor metastasis to the liver?
   a. Neuroblastoma.
   b. Wilms tumor.
   c. Rhabdomyosarcoma.
   d. Lymphoma.
   e. Ewing sarcoma.

CARBOHYDRATE METABOLISM DISORDERS

SYNOPSIS

Note: disorders that block formation of sugar phosphate often do not have as severe clinical outcomes as defects that block pathway after formation of sugar phosphate.

GLYCOGEN METABOLISM ERRORS

VON GIERKE DISEASE (GLYCOGEN STORAGE DISEASE TYPE I)

1. Four types:
   a. Ia: glucose 6-phosphatase deficiency.
   b. Ib: glucose 6-phosphate transporter defect.
   c. Ic: phosphate transporter defect.
   d. Id: glucose transporter.
2. Usual presentation: infant with massive hepatomegaly, doll's facies with big cheeks owing to subcutaneous fat deposition, growth failure, hypoglycemia 3–4 h after meals. Severe metabolic decompensation with hypoglycemia, lactic acidosis, uricemia, and hypertriglyceridemia usually >10–11 mmol/L (300–400 mg/dL). Renal dysfunction is heralded by microalbuminuria, which may progress to frank proteinuria. Renal failure at 3rd to 4th decade. Excessive bleeding and bruising owing to platelet dysfunction with hyperlipidemia.
3. Liver biopsy: swollen hepatocytes owing to stored glycogen, which stains with periodic acid–Schiff stain and is digested by diastase.
4. Glycogen storage disease (GSD) type Ib: neutropenia, recurrent infections. Treat with granulocyte colony-stimulating factor.

5. Long-term problem: hepatic nodule development; need to rule out adenoma versus carcinoma.
6. Treatment: frequent enteral feeds, total parenteral nutrition (TPN) or continuous nasogastric (NG) tube feedings. Uncooked cornstarch acts as a slow-release form of glucose. Avoidance of fructose and galactose since these are converted to glucose 6-phosphate. Also allopurinol for hyperuricemia, to prevent renal urate stones. Liver transplant treats multiple adenomas, fear of malignant change, and metabolic control but does not help renal disease.

FORBES OR CORI DISEASE (GSD III): DEBRANCHER DEFICIENCY

1. Debranching enzyme deficiency. Autosomal recessive. Defect in translation of single gene at 1p21 responsible for liver and muscle isoforms of the debrancher enzyme.
2. Presents usually in early infancy with massive enlarged hepatomegaly and hypoglycemia 4–6 h after meals (improves with increasing age). Growth retardation common as well as hyperlipidemia. Lactic acidosis absent. Hypoglycemia and hyperlipidemia less severe than in GSD I. In muscle debrancher deficiency, elevated creatine kinase (CK) and progressive myopathy, cardiac failure can occur by 3rd–4th decade.
3. Liver biopsy shows glycogenosis; less steatosis but more fibrosis than in GSD I. Adenomas reported but hepatocellular carcinoma only seen with cirrhosis.
4. Two types: IIIa: liver involvement with later muscle involvement; IIIb: only liver involvement (15% of GSD III)
5. Identified in all races, but more frequent in Faroe islanders, North African Jews.
6. Diagnosis by liver enzymology. Differentiation of IIIa and IIIb requires muscle biopsy.

TABLE 1   DIAGNOSTIC INVESTIGATIONS

DISEASE	TISSUE FOR ENZYME STUDIES	ROUTINE DNA TESTING AVAILABLE	HUMAN GENE LOCUS
GSD Ia	Liver	Yes	17q21
Ib	Liver	Yes	11q23
III	Liver and muscle (ie, GSD IIIb)	Exon 3 mutations only	1q21
IV	Liver and other affected tissues	No	3p12
VI	Liver	No	14q21–22
IX	Liver, erythrocytes, leukocytes, other affected tissues	No	Product of multiple genes
Glycogen synthase deficiency	Liver	No	12p12.2
Fanconi-Bickel syndrome	Liver, kidney	No	3q26.1–26.3
Fructosuria	Liver	No	2p23.3–23.2
Hereditary fructose intolerance	Liver	No	9q22.3
Fructose 1,6-bisphosphatase deficiency	Liver	No	9q22.2–22.3
D-Glyceric acid	Liver?	No	Unknown
Galactokinase deficiency	Erythrocytes	No	17q24
Galactose 6-phosphate uridyl transferase deficiency	Erythrocytes	Yes	9p13
UDP galactose 4-epimerase deficiency	Erythrocytes	No	1p36-35
Pyruvate carboxylase deficiency	Fibroblasts	No	11q13.4–13.5
Phosphoenolpyruvate carboxykinase deficiency	Liver?	No	20q13.31 (soluble) Unknown (mitochondrial)

GSD = glycogen storage disease; UDP = uridine diphosphate.
Tissues primarily tested for enzyme activity in defects of hepatic carbohydrate metabolism. Few of these conditions can presently be diagnosed routinely by deoxyribonucleic acid (DNA) analysis, although the loci for most genes are known.

7. Treatment: frequent feeds, nighttime NG feeds, and introduction of cornstarch when older. High-protein diet may be helpful as amino acids can act as gluconeogenic precursor.

ANDERSEN DISEASE (GSD IV)
1. Branching enzyme deficiency. Gene localized to chromosome 3p12. Least common type of GSD.
2. Normal at birth, but present with failure to thrive, hepatosplenomegaly, then cirrhosis, portal hypertension in infancy. Fasting hypoglycemia generally absent. Death usually occurs between 2–5 yr without liver transplant.
3. Liver histology with interstitial and portal fibrosis leading to micronodular cirrhosis. Liver glycogen not increased.
4. No specific treatment. Liver transplant has been effective but progressive cardiomyopathy may occur post-transplant.

HERS DISEASE (GSD VI)
1. Phosphorylase deficiency. Usually benign condition only affecting the liver.
2. Hypoglycemia rare, ketosis, hyperlipidemia minimal. No lactic acidosis or elevated urate. Hepatomegaly and poor growth most notable features.
3. Usually treatment not required.
4. Excellent prognosis. Normal growth can be expected after first few years of life.

GSD IX
1. Phosphorylase kinase deficiency. Enzyme with α and β subunits. Those with α subunits (X-chromosome) have benign hepatic form of disease; those with β subunit defects (on chromosome 16) have muscle involvement and cirrhosis.
2. Common presentation: young child with protuberant abdomen (hepatomegaly which improves with age) and moderate growth retardation.
3. Elevated transaminases, modest elevation in cholesterol, triglycerides, and fasting ketosis. Hypoglycemia uncommon.
4. Liver biopsy with mild inflammation, some fibrosis, and glycogen deposition.
5. Generally benign.

FANCONI-BICKEL SYNDROME
1. Presentation usually in first year with failure to thrive, vomiting, diarrhea, rickets, polyuria, and protuberant abdomen. Glycosuria, aminoaciduria, phosphaturia, and calciuria with renal tubular acidosis. Increased alkaline phosphatase, mild–moderate fasting hypoglycemia, and hyperlipidemia. Normal lactate and urate levels.
2. Postprandial hyperglycemia and hypergalactosemia.
3. GLUT2 (facultative glucose transporter responsible for transport of glucose or galactose into hepatocytes after feeding and export of glucose out of hepatocytes during fasting): defect.

4. Treatment: management of renal Fanconi syndrome; management of deranged glucose homeostasis.
5. Prognosis good, but adults are usually of short stature and develop bone problems (rickets and osteomalacia).

GLYCOGEN SYNTHETASE DEFICIENCY
1. Very rare.
2. Usually presents in infancy with fasting ketotic hypoglycemia with low alanine, lactate levels, and postprandial hyperglycemia with increased lactate.
3. No glycogen storage in the liver; no hepatomegaly. No hyperlipidemia.
4. Liver biopsy required for enzymologic diagnosis. Gene locus 12p12.2.
5. Prognosis good with avoidance of symptomatic hypoglycemia.

FRUCTOSE METABOLISM ERRORS

FRUCTOKINASE DEFICIENCY (BENIGN ESSENTIAL FRUCTOSURIA)
1. Autosomal recessive.
2. Benign. Ingestion of fructose or sucrose leads to appearance of fructose in urine (positive-reducing substances that is not glucose).

FRUCTOSE 1-PHOSPHATE ALDOLASE DEFICIENCY (HEREDITARY FRUCTOSE INTOLERANCE)
1. Rare, recessively inherited disorder. Aldolase B (fructose 1,6-bisphosphate aldolase) deficiency at liver, kidney, and small intestine.
2. Patients healthy provided that they do not ingest significant amounts of fructose or sucrose. Symptoms include poor feeding, vomiting, failure to thrive, and abdominal pain. If ingestion persists, acute hypoglycemia, bleeding, hepatomegaly, and trembling can occur. With acute illness, laboratory findings consistent with liver failure, lactic acidosis, hyperuricemia, and proximal renal tubular dysfunction seen. Potentially life-threatening illness.
3. Diagnosis: fructose tolerance test and or enzyme assay on liver biopsy or mutational analysis.
4. Treatment: removal of all dietary fructose, sucrose, and sorbitol from the diet. Hypoglycemia can be reversed by galactose infusion. Glucagon not helpful for hypoglycemia.

FRUCTOSE-1,6-BISPHOSPHATASE DEFICIENCY
1. Autosomal recessive.
2. Affected persons may present with neonatal jaundice. More commonly present with episodic hyperventilation at time of milk weaning. Hallmark is ketotic hypoglycemia, lactic acidosis on fasting, and elevated urate. Life-threatening illness provoked by fasting.
3. Liver biopsy shows steatosis but no fibrosis.
4. Diagnosis: enzyme assay in liver biopsy.
5. Treatment: intravenous glucose for acute episode and avoidance of fasting. Limitation of fructose ingestion.

D-GLYCERICACIDURIA

1. Extremely rare. Absence of D-glycerate kinase.
2. Presence of D-glyceric acid in urine with hyperglycinemia, metabolic acidosis, and neurologic features.
3. Treatment: dietary restriction of fructose.

INBORN ERRORS OF GALACTOSE METABOLISM

GALACTOKINASE DEFICIENCY

1. Autosomal recessive. Causes only cataracts.
2. Mechanism: elevated galactose in lens leads to accumulation of galactitol, which increases osmotic pressure in lens.
3. Diagnosis: following ingestion of galactose, galactose can be detected in urine as non–glucose-reducing sugar.
4. Treatment: elimination of galactose in diet.

GALACTOSE 1-PHOSPHATE URIDYLTRANSFERASE DEFICIENCY (GALACTOSEMIA)

1. Usually presents during first several days of life after milk feedings with lactose.
2. Vomiting, diarrhea, irritability, lethargy, and hypotonia. Can have acute metabolic collapse with liver and kidney failure. Also chronic course seen with poor feeding and progressive liver disease. Mental retardation universal as well as ovarian dysfunction in females and growth failure. Cataracts common in those on unrestricted diet.
3. High incidence bacterial septicemia, especially *Escherichia coli*.
4. Diagnosis frequently made on neonatal screen. Need follow up with assay of red blood cell galactose 1-phosphate uridyltransferase activity. Galactosuria: non–glucose-reducing sugar in urine.
5. Treatment: dietary galactose restriction.

INBORN ERRORS OF PYRUVATE METABOLISM

PYRUVATE CARBOXYLASE DEFICIENCY

1. Autosomal recessive.
2. Three phenotypes:
   a. Infancy: lactic acidosis, organic aciduria, elevated pyruvate, alanine, and severe mental retardation (Canadian Aboriginals).
   b. Severe neonatal form: macrocephaly, intractable lactic academia, elevated lactate-to-pyruvate ratios, hyperammonemia, hypercitrullinemia, and hepatomegaly. Death within 3 mo.
   c. Childhood: intermittent acidosis; normal development.

PHOSPHOENOLPYRUVATE CARBOXYKINASE DEFICIENCY

1. Cytosolic and mitochondrial forms of enzyme. Deficiency rare.
2. Infantile hypoglycemia, fatty infiltration of the liver and kidneys, and liver failure.

QUESTIONS

TRUE FALSE:

1 Disorders blocking carbohydrate metabolism pathways after formation of the sugar phosphate are often clinically worse than those that block formation of the sugar phosphate.

MATCH THE CHARACTERISTICS TO THE DISORDER:

a. Only cataracts
b. Hepatic adenomas.
c. Episodic hyperventilation with milk weaning.
d. Massive hepatomegaly with hypoglycemia 4–6 h after meals.
e. Lactic acidosis and severe mental retardation in Canadian Aboriginals.
f. Glycosuria, aminoaciduria, phosphaturia, and calciuria with renal tubular acidosis.
g. Neutropenia.
h. *Escherichia coli* septicemia.
i. Asymptomatic; fructose in urine.
j. Young child with hepatomegaly and growth retardation.

2. Galactose 1-phosphate uridyltransferase deficiency.
3. Glucose 6-phosphatase deficiency.
4. Fructokinase deficiency.
5. Pyruvate carboxylase deficiency.
6. Galactokinase deficiency.
7. Fructose-1,6-diphosphatase deficiency.
8. Glycogen storage disease type Ib.
9. Fanconi-Bickel syndrome.
10. Phosphorylase kinase deficiency.

AMINO ACID METABOLISM DISORDERS

SYNOPSIS

DISORDERS OF AROMATIC AMINO ACIDS

HEREDITARY TYROSINEMIA

1. 1/100,000. Common in French-Canadians.
2. Deficiency of fumarylacetoacetate hydrolase (FAH) results in accumulation of succinylacetoacetate and succinylacetone, which inhibits δ-aminolevunic acid hydratase precipitating acute neurologic episodes (excruciating pain and posturing associated with weakness and paralysis).
3. Clinically, 2 main groups:
   a. Age < 6 mo: severe liver involvement and coagulopathy.
   b. Age > 6 mo: mild liver or renal involvement (renal involvement involves generalized aminoaciduria, phosphate loss, and renal tubular acidosis), growth failure, and rickets.

TABLE 1 COMPARATIVE FEATURES OF THE MOST COMMON DISORDERS OF AMINO ACID METABOLISM

DIAGNOSIS	PHENOTYPE	CLINICAL FEATURES	SERUM GLUCOSE	SERUM AMMONIA	METABOLIC ACIDOSIS	URINE KETONES	SERUM AMINO ACIDS	URINE AMINO ACIDS	URINE ORGANIC ACIDS	DIAGNOSIS
Tyrosinemia type 1	Acute chronic	Acute liver failure or renal Fanconi syndrome with rickets	Normal	Normal	Absent or mild	None	Elevated methionine and tyrosine	Elevated methionine and tyrosine	Succinylacetone	Succinylacetone in urine or plasma
Maple syrup urine disease	Classic	Neonatal encephalopathy; "maple syrup" urine odor	Sometimes low	Normal	Prominent	Elevated	Markedly increased alloisoleucine, BCAAs	Elevated BCAAs	Elevated BCKAs	BCKD activity in cultured fibroblasts or lymphocytes < 2%
	Intermediate	Developmental delay, seizures	Normal	Normal	Prominent during symptoms	Elevated	Same as above	Same as above	Same as above	3–30%
	Intermittent	Episodic ataxia and lethargy	Normal	Normal	Prominent during symptoms	Elevated during symptoms	Elevated BCAA during symptoms	Elevated BCAA during symptoms	Elevated BCAA during symptoms	5–20%
Isovalericaciduria, propionicaciduria, methylmalonicaciduria	Same as above	Same as above; dehydration, hepatomegaly; "sweaty feet" odor in IVA	Variable	Elevated	Prominent	Elevated	Nonspecific elevations of glycine	Nonspecific elevations	Specific OA patterns	Cultured fibroblast enzyme activity
Ornithine transcarbamylase deficiency	Classic	Lethargy, poor feeding, coma, seizures, developmental delay	Normal	Elevated	Absent	None		Nonspecific elevation	Orotic acid elevation	Small intestine or liver biopsy enzyme activity
Carbamyl phosphate synthetase deficiency	Same as above	Same as above	Normal	Elevated	Absent	None	Absent citrulline	Nonspecific elevation	Nonspecific elevation	Same as above
Citrullinemia	Same as above	Same as above	Normal	Elevated	Absent	None	Elevated citrulline	Elevated citrulline	Nonspecific elevation	Cultured fibroblast or lymphocyte enzyme activity
Argininosuccinicaciduria	Neonatal	Same as above; fragile hair	Normal	Elevated	Absent	None	Elevation of glutamine and argininosuccinic acid	Elevated arginine-succinate	Nonspecific elevation	Cultured fibroblast or erythrocyte enzyme activity
	Late onset	Developmental delay, hepatomegaly, fragile hair	Normal	Episodically elevated	Absent	None	Same as above	Same as above	Nonspecific elevation	Same as above
Arginase		Developmental delay, spasticity	Normal	Moderately elevated	Absent	None	Elevated arginine	Elevated lysine, arginine, ornithine, cystine	Orotic acid elevation	Erythrocyte enzyme activity

BCAA = branched-chain amino acid; BCKA = branched-chain α-keto acids; BCKD = branched-chain α-keto dehydrogenase; IVA = isovalericaciduria; OA = organic acid.

4. Marked elevated α-fetoprotein averages 160,000 ng/mL at the time of diagnosis.
5. Detection of urine succinylacetone useful in diagnosis. Boiled cabbage or rotten mushroom odor to urine. Measurement of FAH in cultured skin fibroblasts used as a confirmatory test.
6. Treatment: NTBC [2-(2-nitro-4-trifluoromethylbenzol)-1,3-cyclohexanedione], which prevents substrate from the FAH enzyme. In addition, tyrosine- and phenylalanine-restricted diet and nitisinone, which blocks p-hydroxyphenylpyruvate oxidase (can cause tyrosine accumulation).
7. Hepatocellular carcinoma (HCC) is a frequent complication and regular monitoring is essential with annual imaging (magnetic resonance imaging or computed tomography) and monitoring of α-fetoprotein.
8. Liver transplant is an option for therapy.

DISORDERS OF BRANCHED-CHAIN AMINO ACIDS

MAPLE SYRUP URINE DISEASE (BRANCHED-CHAIN KETOACIDURIA)

1. Autosomal recessive. Deficiency in mitochondrial branched-chain α-keto acid dehydrogenase (BCKD) resulting in accumulation of branched-chain amino acids (BCAA) and branched-chain ketoacids (BCKA).
2. BCKD is an enzyme complex coded for by separate genes leading to wide genetic heterogenicity in the phenotype.
3. Clinical phenotypes:
   a. Classic: most common, most severe. Characterized by onset of encephalopathy in neonatal period with high levels of BCAA. Ketosis and maple syrup odor to urine becomes apparent in early life. If untreated, death in first months of life.
   b. Intermediate: rare. Spared neurologic crises but elevated BCAAs. Neurologic impairment still a risk. BCKD activity 3–30% of normal.
   c. Intermittent: presents between 5 mo and 2 yr. Metabolic decompensation with infection. Plasma BCAAs normal during nonstressed times, with elevated plasma BCAAs and BCKAs during symptomatic periods. BCKD activity 5–20% of normal.
4. Diagnosis: detection of elevated BCKAs by mass spectroscopy or gas chromatography analysis of urine and elevated BCAAs in the blood. Presence of alloisoleucine pathognomonic for maple syrup urine disease (MSUD). Definitive diagnosis: low activity of BCKD in cultured lymphocytes or fibroblasts. Prenatal diagnosis: measure BCKD activity from cultured cells obtained via amniocentesis and chorionic villus sampling.
5. Treatment: initially, removal of toxic metabolites, minimizing catabolism (hemodialysis and continuous venous-venous hemoperfusion) and promoting anabolism. Dietary therapy is the mainstay and BCAAs (leucine, isoleucine, valine) are eliminated. Thiamine for 3 wk may improve BCAA-tolerance and biochemical stability. In severe cases, liver transplant has been successful.

ISOVALERICACIDURIA, PROPIONICACIDURIA, AND METHYLMALONICACIDURIA

1. Isovalericaciduria: "sweaty feet" or "cheese" odor. Autosomal recessive. Deficiency in mitochondrial flavoprotein isovaleryl-CoA dehydrogenase apoprotein results in accumulation of isovaleryl-CoA derivatives. Glycine and carnitine can be used to aid in isovaleric acid excretion.
2. Propionicaciduria: autosomal recessive disorder caused by deficiency of proprionyl-CoA carboxylase.
3. Methylmalonicaciduria: autosomal recessive disorder (1/100,000 live births). Deficiency in vitamin B_{12}-dependent methylmalonyl-CoA mutase apoenzyme results in elevated methylmalonyl CoA and methylmalonic acid. Vitamin B_{12} deficiency must be ruled out.
4. Clinical features: similar to MSUD. Moderate hepatomegaly; frequently dehydrated. Metabolic acidosis from hyperlactacidemia, elevated anion gap, and ketonuria. Hyperammonemia uniformly present. Moderate hypocalcemia and variable glucose levels common as well as cytopenias.
5. Diagnosis: based on detection of elevated organic acids in plasma or urine in the pattern specific for the different disorders. Prenatal diagnosis possible by 12–14 weeks gestation by measuring metabolites in the amniotic fluid and direct enzyme analysis from chorionic villous sampling or amniocentesis cells.
6. Treatment: protein restriction (specifically BCAAs) required. In the case of isovalericaciduria, leucine restriction required; oral L-glycine and intravenous (IV) L-carnitine may help with toxin removal. In propionicaciduria, administration of biotin may help. In acute metabolic crisis, hemodialysis or continuous venous-venous hemoperfusion is effective.

DISORDERS OF THE UREA CYCLE

The urea cycle (only in the liver) converts ammonia into nontoxic, excretable urea (Figure 1). Defects result in significant hyperammonemia and neurologic compromise. Presentation at time of high-protein intake or metabolic stress. Mainstay of therapy: protein restriction and pharmacologic interventions; nevertheless, many have repeated hyperammonemia and mental deficiency. Liver transplant treatment has been successful.

ORNITHINE TRANSCARBAMOYLASE DEFICIENCY

1. Enzyme located in mitochondrial matrix exclusively in the liver. Most common urea cycle enzyme deficiency.
2. X-linked inheritance (the only urea cycle defect inherited this way). Carrier female with spectrum of involvement.
3. Symptoms: Males: death of 75% in first months of life. Within hours or days of birth, feeding difficulties, lethargy, tachypnea or labored breathing, seizures, coma, and cerebral edema and, without treatment, death. A milder variant may present at a later age with protein challenge and infection. Females: vomiting, feeding difficulties, headache, and tiredness after a protein meal. Onset in first decade.

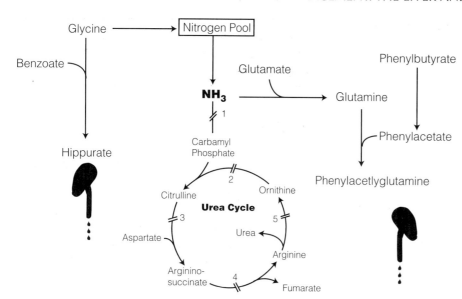

FIGURE 1 Alternative routes of waste N$_2$ excretion. 1 = carbamyl phosphate synthetase; 2 = ornithine transcarbamylase; 3 = argininosuccinate synthetase; 4 = argininosuccinase; 5 = arginase; 6 = N-acetylglutamate synthetase.

4. Laboratory results: hyperammonemia without acidosis. Oroticaciduria and absence of plasma citrulline diagnostic. Enzyme analysis from duodenal or rectal mucosal biopsy or liver will confirm the diagnosis.

5. Treatment hyperammonemic crisis: reduce NH$_4$ as soon as possible; dialysis, dietary protein restriction, and calories to reverse catabolic state. IV administration of arginine or citrulline replenishes arginine for protein synthesis. IV sodium benzolate and phenylbutyrate reduces NH$_4$ by removing glycine and glutamine from the nitrogen pool.

CARBAMYL PHOSPHATE SYNTHETASE DEFICIENCY

1. Carbamyl phosphate synthetase (CPS) I deficiency: liver mitochondrial enzyme catalyzing the formation of carbamyl phosphate from ammonia, the first step in the urea cycle.

2. Rare, autosomal recessive mutation.

3. Present in first days of life after feeds with poor feeding, lethargy, vomiting, change in tone, seizures, hypothermia, and coma. Death results in first 2–18 mo without therapy. Partial deficiency is seen in older children with high-protein intake or catabolic states.

4. Suspect in young infant with hyperammonemia without acidosis, low levels of orotic acid, citrulline, and arginine. Confirm diagnosis with enzyme activity measured from liver biopsy or small intestinal or rectal biopsy.

5. Treatment: same as that for ornithine transcarbamoylase (OTC) deficiency.

CITRULLINEMIA

1. Autosomal recessive. Deficiency of argininosuccinate synthetase, which catalyzes the formation of argininosuccinic acid.

2. Clinical presentation heterogeneous owing to widespread distribution of enzyme. Majority present in infancy with classic neonatal form (similar to OTC deficiency) or during first year with subacute form (with failure to thrive, recurrent emesis, ataxia, and seizures).

3. Suspect diagnosis in hyperammonemia without acidosis and elevation of plasma or urine citrulline. Confirm diagnosis by level of enzyme activity from cultured fibroblasts and lymphocytes. Prenatal diagnosis available by analyzing amniotic fluid for citrulline or enzyme assay from amniocytes.

4. Therapy: similar as for OTC deficiency. Arginine can dramatically lower level of ammonia.

ARGININOSUCCINICACIDURIA

1. Autosomal recessive. Results from defect in argininosuccinate lyase.

2. Clinical presentations:
   a. Neonatal: rare, similar to OTC deficiency with hepatomegaly and abnormally fragile hair.
   b. Infantile: failure to thrive, feeding difficulties, seizures, and psychomotor retardation.
   c. Late onset: most common form. In second year of life, developmental delay, feeding difficulties, irritability, and seizures secondary to hyperammonemia provoked by infection and increased protein. Hepatomegaly and fragile hair (trichorrhexis nodosa) seen.

3. Diagnosis: excess of argininosuccinate in urine or plasma. Confirm diagnosis by enzyme assay in red blood count. Prenatal diagnosis available.

4. Treatment: similar to that for citrullinemia. Sodium benzoate and phenylacetate not generally needed.

N-ACETYLGLUTAMATE SYNTHETASE DEFICIENCY

Clinical phenotype and treatment similar to that for CPS deficiency.

ARGININEMIA

1. Least common of urea cycle defects. Autosomal recessive. Deficiency of arginase.

2. Infancy onset with irritability, poor feeding, vomiting, lethargy, seizures, and coma. Survivors have spasticity or opisthotonos with developmental delay; may be thought to have cerebral palsy. Degree of hyperammonemia not as dramatic as other urea cycle defects.

3. Elevated plasma arginine diagnostic with enzyme assay confirmation in red blood cells.
4. Treatment: restrict arginine from the diet with further reductions during illness or infection.

QUESTIONS

TRUE OR FALSE:

1. Ornithine transcarbamoylase deficiency is the only inherited defect in ureagenesis that does not have autosomal recessive inheritance.
2. Oroticaciduria and absence of plasma citrulline is typically seen in laboratory evaluation of females heterozygous for ornithine transcarbamoylase deficiency.
3. Argininemia may be confused with cerebral palsy.

MATCH CONDITION TO THE CHARACTERISTIC:

a. Ornithine transcarbamoylase deficiency.
b. Argininosuccinic aciduria.
c. Argininemia.
d. N-acetylglutamate synthetase deficiency.
e. Citrullinemia.

4. Trichorrhexis nodosa.
5. Spastic diplegia.
6. Females variably affected.

a. Hereditary tyrosinemia.
b. Isovaleric acidemia.
c. Branched-chain α–keto acid dehydrogenase.

7. Boiled cabbage odor.
8. Maple syrup odor.
9. Sweaty feet odor.

INHERITED ABNORMALITIES IN MITOCHONDRIAL FATTY ACID OXIDATION

SYNOPSIS

Mitochondrial fatty acid oxidation (FAO) provides as much as 80% of the energy for heart and liver functions at all times. In the liver, FAO fuels the synthesis of ketone bodies, which are an alternative energy source. In situations of increased energy requirements (fever, exercise, and fasting), a defect in the FAO pathway leads to energy depletion in tissues of high energy demands (liver, heart, skeletal muscle, and brain).

BIOCHEMISTRY OF MITOCHONDRIAL FATTY ACID METABOLISM

1. Short- and medium-chain fatty acids passively cross mitochondrial membranes while long-chain fatty acids are actively transported and require carnitine (Figure 1).
2. Carnitine is synthesized only at the kidney, liver, and brain.
3. Substrates for mitochondrial β–oxidation are fatty acyl-CoA esters, which undergo 4 chain-shortening steps, each removing a 2 carbon acetyl group. Four enzyme types are involved with specificities for chain length: short (soluble), medium (soluble), long (membrane-associated), and very long (membrane-associated). For long-chain fatty acids, 3 of these enzymes are associated together as trifunctional protein (long-chain enoyl-CoA hydratase, long-chain

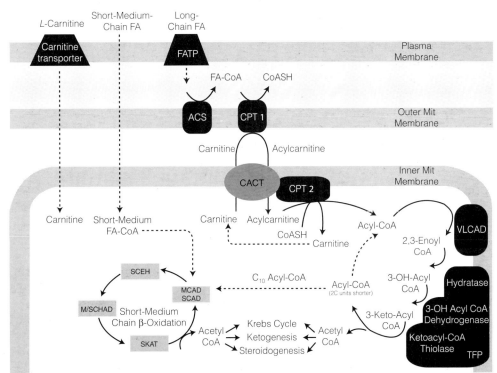

FIGURE 1 Overview of fatty acid import and metabolism. ACS = acyl-CoA synthetase; CACT = carnitine acylcarnitine translocase; CoA = coenzyme A; CoASH = unacylated coenzyme A; CPT1 = carnitine palmitoyltransferase 1; CPT2 = carnitine palmitoyltransferase 2; FA = fatty acid; FA-CoA = fatty acyl CoA; FATP = fatty acid transport protein; MCAD = medium-chain acyl-CoA dehydrogenase; Mit = mitochondrial; M/SCHAD = medium-/short-chain 3-hydroxyacyl-CoA dehydrogenase; SCAD = short-chain acyl-CoA dehydrogenase; SCEH = short-chain enoyl-CoA hydratase; SKAT = short-chain ketoacyl-CoA thiolase; TFP = trifunctional protein; VLCAD = very-long-chain acyl-CoA dehydrogenase.

3-hydroxyacyl-CoA dehydrogenase, and long-chain ketoacyl-CoA thiolase).

4. Acetyl CoA generated by fatty acid β-oxidation is then converted into acetoacetate (ketone body) via the actions of β-ketothiolase, hydroxymethylglutaryl (HMG)-CoA synthase, and HMG-CoA lyase. Acetoacetate is interconverted by 3HB dehydrogenase into 3-hydroxybutyrate, another ketone body. Acetone, the third ketone body, is formed from the decarboxylation of acetoacetate and is responsible for the fruity smell of ketoacidotic individuals.

5. Biochemical hallmark of FAO defects is hypoketotic or nonketotic hypoglycemia resulting from glucose depletion and secondary impairment of gluconeogenesis owing to lack of reducing equivalents. Resulting fat storage in liver and muscle is explained by incorporation of nonmetabolized free fatty acids into triglycerides. Intracellular toxicity is triggered by accumulation of acyl-CoA intermediates and secondary depletion of carnitine and CoA.

6. Women carrying long-chain 3-hydroxyacyl-CoA dehydrogenase (LCHAD)-deficient fetuses have been found to have preeclampsia, HELLP (hemolysis, elevated liver enzymes, low platelets), and acute fatty liver of pregnancy and placental floor infarction. May result from the placenta (which shares the same genetics as the fetus), which produces and accumulates abnormal fatty acid metabolites that then pass into the maternal circulation and overwhelm β-oxidation capacity of the heterozygous mother (worsened in the third trimester with shift of maternal metabolism toward ketogenesis).

APPROACH TO DIAGNOSIS

1. Patient's clinical history of decompensation with fever, exercise, infection, pregnancy; and family history (sudden death) may provide clues regarding a potential FAO disorder.

2. Most useful laboratory specimens for evaluation are acquired during periods of metabolic decompensation, including blood gases, electrolytes, glucose, ammonia, uric acid, liver function tests, creatine kinase, ratio of lactate to pyruvate, 3-hydroxybutyrate and acetoacetate, and urinalysis.

3. Further fatty acid analyses: urine organic acids, acyl-CoA intermediates, and resulting dicarboxylic acids (acylglycine and acylcarnitine species) help determine the type of FAO defect. Free and total carnitine analysis useful in the diagnosis of primary carnitine deficiency and to determine whether L-carnitine supplementation will be useful. Plasma fatty acid profiles can also be helpful.

4. Direct enzyme assays for the diagnosis of most FAO disorders are also available. Molecular genetic studies useful only for relatively common mutations.

SCREENING

Newborn screening via acylcarnitine quantification. Postmortem screening: histochemical and biochemical analyses of liver specimens, organic and fatty acid analyses of urine and plasma, acylcarnitine profiles in blood and bile, and determination of FAO rates using cultured skin fibroblasts.

DISORDERS OF PLASMA MEMBRANE FUNCTIONS

1. Long-chain fatty acid transport and binding defect: biochemical phenotype nonspecific. Reduced C14 to C18 intracellular fatty acid concentrations. Reduced cellular oxidation of palmitate and oleate.

2. Carnitine uptake defect: only cause of primary carnitine deficiency. Due to defective plasma membrane, carnitine transporter at both kidney and intestine. Tissue depletion of carnitine results with impairment of long-chain fatty acid transport. Patients present with progressive cardiomyopathy, hypoketotic hypoglycemia, encephalopathy, and hepatomegaly. Skeletal myopathy common. Plasma carnitine < 10% normal. Increased urinary carnitine excretion found. Diagnosis via determination of carnitine uptake in fibroblasts or analysis of the SLC22A5 gene (genotype-phenotype correlation not apparent).

DISORDERS OF THE CARNITINE CYCLE

1. Carnitine palmitoyltransferase 1 (CPT1) deficiency: 2 tissue-specific isoforms: hepatic type (CPT1A) and muscle type (CPT1B). The hepatic type (CPT1A deficiency) characterized by nonketotic hypoglycemia liver dysfunction, and encephalopathy as in Reye syndrome. No CPT1B deficiencies reported to date. In contrast to other FAO defects, CPT1A deficiency associated with elevated plasma carnitine, especially free carnitine. Diagnosis confirmed by enzyme assay in fibroblasts and molecular genetic analysis of the CPT1A gene (G710E mutation common in Hutterite). Treatment based on strict avoidance of fasting, low-fat diet supplemented with medium-chain triglycerides (MCTs).

2. Carnitine-acylcarnitine translocase (CACT) deficiency: typically present in neonatal period with hypoketotic hypoglycemia, liver failure, or hypertrophic cardiomyopathy. Treatment: frequent low-fat feedings with MCTs is mainstay. Most patients die following development of cardiac arrhythmias. Autopsy shows fatty infiltration in liver, kidney, and muscle; hypertrophic cardiomyopathy. CACT deficiency identifiable through expanded newborn screening with elevated C16, C18 and long-chain acylcarnitines (similar to CPT2 deficiency). In order to differentiate CACT and CPT2 deficiency, necessary to analyze CACT gene.

3. CPT2 deficiency: 3 types:
   a. Type 1: most severe. Presents in neonatal period; affects liver, skeletal, and cardiac muscle. Associated with congenital brain and kidney abnormalities.
   b. Type 2: involves liver, skeletal, and cardiac muscle; presents in first few years of life.
   c. Type 3: affects skeletal muscle; presents in early adulthood.
   d. Myoglobinuria, markedly elevated serum creatine phosphokinase levels are hallmarks of CPT2 deficiency. Several patients demonstrate malignant hyperthermia during surgery.

e. Acylcarnitine profiles abnormal, identical to CACT deficiency. More specific enzyme assays or molecular genetic testing needed to verify the diagnosis. Most common mutation in type 3: S113L, 413delAG mutation common in Ashkenazi Jewish population.

DISORDERS OF LONG-CHAIN FATTY ACID METABOLISM

1. Very-long-chain acyl-CoA dehydrogenase (VLCAD) deficiency: VLCAD catalyzes first step of the fatty acid β-oxidation cycle. Most severe phenotype manifests early in life, associated with nonsense mutations and complete loss of enzyme activity, with involvement of multiple organ systems especially liver and heart. Phenotype in those with mutations allowing some enzyme activity switch from hepatic presentation (metabolic crises) to muscle weakness as patients become older. Laboratory hallmarks: hypoketotic hypoglycemia and creatine phosphokinase elevations. Urine organic acid analysis nonspecific. Acylcarnitine analysis with elevated C14–C18 carnitine esters (mainly C14:1). Diagnosis confirmed by specific enzyme assay, FAO probing in fibroblast cultures, or VLCAD gene analysis

2. Trifunctional protein (TFP) and LCHAD deficiency: in TFP, α subunit harbors long-chain enoyl-coA hydratase and LCHAD enzyme activities, with β subunit harboring long-chain ketoacyl-coA thiolase enzyme activity. Mutations in either α or β subunits may result in complete TFP deficiency; a few α mutations may cause isolated LCHAD deficiency (most common mutation is 1528G→C mutation). Phenotype typical of those expected in a FAO disorder, but patients with LCHAD and TFP deficiencies can also develop pigmentary retinitis and peripheral neuropathy; many patients are born premature and small for gestational age.

3. Women carrying LCHAD-deficient fetuses have preeclampsia, HELLP, and acute fatty liver of pregnancy and placental floor infarction. May result from the placenta (which shares the same genetics as the fetus), which produces and accumulates abnormal fatty acid metabolites that then pass into the maternal circulation and overwhelm β-oxidation capacity of the heterozygous mother (worsened in the third trimester with shift of maternal metabolism toward ketogenesis).

DISORDERS OF MEDIU[...] METABOLISM

1. Medium-chain acyl-Co[...] ciency: MCAD responsib[...] of acyl CoAs with chain [...] carbon atoms. Best-known [...] sense mutations 985A→G; [...] of Northern European descen[...] been observed in all popul[...] MCAD defect leads to fasting-i[...] accumulation of plasma C6 t[...] [...]itine species with prominent octanoy[...] [...]e. Affected individuals may develop secondary carnitine deficiency. Thus, urine acylglycine analysis should be pursued in carnitine-deficiency patients. Diagnosis confirmed by measurement of MCAD enzyme activity and by molecular genetic testing of the *ACADM* gene.

2. Medium/short chain L-3-hydroxyacyl-CoA dehydrogenase (M/SCHAD) deficiency: 3 different phenotypes: cardiomyopathy and recurrent rhabdomyolysis; ketotic hypoglycemia; and hepatic involvement and steatosis. Specific laboratory findings: various chain-length dicarboxylic and 3-hydroxydicarboxylicaciduria. Plasma acylcarnitine analysis: normal or show elevated concentration of 3-hydroxybutyryl carnitine.

3. Medium-chain 3-ketoacyl-CoA thiolase (MCKAT) deficiency: only one patient described to date with emesis, dehydration, liver dysfunction, and terminal rhabdomyolysis. Urine organic acid analysis showed ketotic lacticaciduria, C6 to C12 dicarboxylicaciduria with prominent C10 and C12 species.

DISORDERS OF SHORT-CHAIN FATTY ACID METABOLISM

Short-chain acyl-CoA dehydrogenase (SCAD) deficiency: most common symptoms include developmental delay and muscle hypotonia. Biochemical markers of SCAD deficiency include an increased concentration of butyrylcarnitine in blood and ethylmalonic acid (EMA) in the urine. SCAD gene variants R147W and G185S may confer susceptibility to disease.

DISORDERS OF KETOGENESIS OR KETOLYSIS

1. HMG-CoA synthase deficiency: (Table 1) present with recurrent hypoketotic hypoglycemic episodes leading to coma; usually triggered by prolonged fasting. Nonspecific biochemical phenotype: hypoketotic hypo-

TABLE 1   DISORDERS OF KETONE BODY METABOLISM AND CHARACTERISTIC BIOCHEMICAL ABNORMALITIES

DISORDER	KETOSIS	ACIDOSIS	BLOOD GLUCOSE	BLOOD AMMONIA	PLASMA LACTATE
KETOGENESIS					
HMG-CoA synthase deficiency	–	–	↓	N	N
HMG-CoA lyase deficiency	–	+	↓	N	↑
KETOLYSIS					
SCOT deficiency	+++	+	N/↓	N	N
β-Ketothiolase deficiency	+++	+	↑/N/↓	N	N

HMG-CoA = 3-hydroxy-3-methylglutaryl coenzyme A; N = normal; SCOT = succinyl-CoA:3=oxoacid transferase; ↓ = reduced; ↑ = elevated.

...oxylicaciduria, normal blood acylcar-
...e, and elevated free fatty acids. Genetic
...of *HMGCS2* gene helpful for diagnosis.
...G-CoA lyase deficiency: Second mitochondrial enzyme mediating ketogenesis from fatty acids. Presents with acute, often lethal episodes of hypoketotic hypoglycemia and acidosis. Central nervous system particularly vulnerable. Urine organic acid profile characteristic: abnormal excretion of 3-hydroxy-3-methylglutaric, 3-methylglutaconia, 3-methylglutaric, and 3-hydroxyisovaleric acids. Acylcarnitine analysis: elevated 3-methylglutarylcarnitine. Confirm diagnosis by measuring enzyme activity in fibroblasts and genetic testing. Defect frequent in Saudi Arabia: accounts for 16% of inherited metabolic diseases.

3. Succinyl-CoA:3-oxoacid-CoA transferase (SCOT) deficiency: succinyl-CoA:3-oxoacid-CoA transferase is first step of ketone body use in extrahepatic tissues (brain, heart, and kidney). Typical presentation includes recurrent episodes of severe ketoacidosis with persistent ketonuria and hyperketonemia during the fed state. Onset in first year of life.

4. Mitochondrial β-ketothiolase deficiency: β-ketothiolase is ketogenic and ketolytic enzyme that also is involved in isoleucine catabolism. Most present with acute ketoacidosis during infections and vomiting. Asymptomatic affected individuals also described. Urine organic acid analysis diagnostic with large excretion of 2-methyl-3-hydroxybutyric acid and tiglylglycine reflecting a block in isoleucine catabolism.

OTHER

1. Glutaric acidemia type II: primary defects of electron transfer flavoprotein (ETF) or ETF- ubiquinone oxidoreductase (QO) (proteins involved in electron transfer). Also known as multiple acyl-CoA dehydrogenase deficiency since reoxidation of several mitochondrial dehydrogenases impaired. Clinical phenotype variable with early onset, severe form with or without congenital anomalies, and a milder, later-onset form. Severe neonatal onset: with congenital anomalies: patients often premature, present with overwhelming illness within 2 days of birth, die shortly thereafter. Early neonatal onset without congenital abnormalities: hypotonia, acidosis, hypoglycemia, tachypnea, hepatomegaly, and sweaty feet odor seen with death often due to severe cardiomyopathy. Milder, late-onset: presentation variable; episodic vomiting, hypoglycemia, and acidosis. Mutations in ETF-QO but not ETF associated with renal cysts. Characteristic biochemical phenotype seen with glutaric academia type II includes accumulation of EMA, glutaric acid, and 2-hydroxyglutaric acid in the urine organic acid profiles. Urinary acylglycine analysis reveals markedly elevated isovalerylglycine and hexanoylglycine accumulation, as well as elevated levels of butyrylcarnitine, isovalerylcarnitine, glutarylcarnitine and several other medium and long-chain acylcarnitine species.

2. 2,4-dienoyl-CoA reductase deficiency: only one case reported. Notable physical features: microcephaly, large face, small arms, feet, fingers, and small trunk. Biochemical profile: hyperlysinemia, carnitine deficiency, and normal urinary organic acid profile. Acylcarnitine analysis: abnormal C10:2 in blood and urine.

GENERAL APPROACH

1. Avoidance of fasting via frequent feedings (in infants every 3–4 h, in older patients uncooked cornstarch supplementation will allow longer feeding intervals and prolonged nighttime rest). In severe cases, continuous overnight administration of carbohydrates by nasogastric or gastrostomy-tube may be required.

2. Restriction of fat intake with a dietary regimen of fat restriction (25–30% total calories from fat) and high carbohydrates. In patients with long-chain FAO defects, MCTs may be substituted as lipid substrate. Supplementation of essential fatty acids at 1–2% of total energy intake suggested to avoid essential fatty acid deficiencies and pigmentary retinopathy. Fat-soluble vitamins should be supplemented.

3. Carnitine supplementation: lifesaving and essential in primary carnitine deficiency with oral doses of 100 mg/kg/d and higher required.

4. Riboflavin sometimes prescribed for SCAD and ETF or ETF-dehydrogenase deficiencies in order to boost enzyme activity (no efficacy data available).

5. Triheptanoin may be helpful in VLCAD deficiency with normalization of the acylcarnitine profile, some clinical symptoms. Fibrates may increase enzyme activity.

6. Management during intercurrent illness: reversal of catabolism by provision of energy in the form of glucose.

QUESTIONS

MATCH THE CHARACTERISTICS WITH THE DISEASE:

a. Glutaric acidemia type II.
b. Carnitine palmitoyltransferase 2 deficiency.
c. Hydroxymethylglutaryl-CoA lyase deficiency.
d. Carnitine uptake defect.
e. Isolated long-chain hydroxyacyl-CoA dehydrogenase deficiency.
f. Liver carnitine palmitoyltransferase 1 deficiency.
g. Succinyl-CoA:3-oxoacid-CoA transferase deficiency.
h. Short-chain acyl-CoA dehydrogenase deficiency.

1. Sweaty feet odor.
2. Malignant hyperthermia.
3. Reye syndrome like encephalopathy.
4. Low plasma carnitine level.
5. HELLP syndrome in pregnancy.
6. Prevalent in Saudi Arabia.
7. Ketonuria and ketonemia during fed state.

TRUE OR FALSE:

8. Acylcarnitine profiles of carnitine palmitoyltransferase 2 deficiency and carnitine-acylcarnitine translocase deficiency are identical.
9. Decreased plasma carnitine is a characteristic of carnitine palmitoyltransferase 1 (liver subtype) deficiency.
10. Short- and medium-chain fatty acids do not rely on the carnitine shuttle to enter into the mitochondrial matrix.
11. Carnitine supplementation is lifesaving in all types of fatty acid oxidation defects.

BILE ACID SYNTHESIS AND METABOLISM DISORDERS

SYNOPSIS

1. Primary bile acids: cholic acid and chenodeoxycholic acid. Conjugated to amino acids taurine and glycine.
2. Bile acid functions:
   a. Catabolic pathway for elimination of cholesterol from the body.
   b. Primary driving force for secretion of bile and for biliary excretion of endogenous and exogenous toxic substances.
   c. Within the intestinal lumen, bile acids facilitate absorption of fats and fat-soluble vitamins.
3. Efficient enterohepatic recycling: reabsorption from small intestine; effective extraction from portal venous circulation (< 5% bile acid pool lost each day in stool).

BILE ACID SYNTHESIS

1. Conversion of cholesterol C27 sterol to the 2 primary bile acids:
   a. Introduction of hydroxyl groups at C7 (for both chenodeoxycholate and cholate) and C12 for cholate only.
   b. Epimerization of 3β-hydroxyl group.
   c. Reduction of the Δ^5 bond.
   d. Reduction in length of side chain from C8 to C5 with formation of terminal carboxylic acid.
   e. Conjugation to amino acids glycine and taurine.
2. Two pathways responsible for bile acid synthesis from cholesterol:
   a. 7α Hydroxylation: "neutral" pathway.
   b. 27-Hydroxylation: "acidic" pathway.
3. Neutral pathway considered major pathway for primary bile acid synthesis with cholesterol 7α-hydroxylase as the rate-limiting enzyme.

NEWBORN INFANTS

1. First few days of life excrete significant amounts 3-oxo-Δ^4 bile acids: indicative of immaturity of bile acid synthesis.
2. Secondary bile acids in small proportions: consistent with lack of bacterial flora and maternal–fetal placental transport of secondary bile acids

3. Principal bile acid conjugation reaction of fetal liver is amidation with taurine. In fetal bile, 85% of total bile acids are taurine conjugates. In adult, glycine-to-taurine ratio is 3:1.

SECONDARY METABOLIC DEFECTS

1. Zellweger syndrome and other peroxisomal disorders.
2. Mutations in genes encoding organic anion transport proteins.
3. Smith-Lemli-Opitz syndrome with reduced cholesterol synthesis (thus resulting in reduced bile acid synthesis).

PRIMARY ENZYME DEFECTS

1. Hepatic synthesis of primary bile acids is critical because of the role of bile acids in promoting bile secretion. In patients with impaired primary bile acid synthesis, progressive cholestatic liver disease results.
2. Biochemical presentation includes markedly reduced or lack of primary bile acids in serum, bile, and urine.

CEREBROTENDINOUS XANTHOMATOSIS

1. Rare lipid storage disease caused by mutations in mitochondrial sterol 27-hydroxylase gene. Prevalence 1/70,000.
2. Progressive neurologic dysfunction, dementia, ataxia, cataracts, and xanthomatous lesions at brain and tendons.
3. Distinguish from other xanthomatous deposit diseases:
   a. Significantly reduced primary bile acid synthesis.
   b. Elevations in biliary, urinary, and fecal excretion of bile alcohol glucuronides.
   c. Low plasma cholesterol with deposition of cholesterol and cholestanol in tissues.
   d. Marked elevations in cholestanol.
4. Point mutation in chromosome 2.
5. Treatable with primary bile acids.

3β-HYDROXY-C27-STEROID OXIDOREDUCTASE DEFICIENCY

1. Most common bile acid synthetic defect described thus far. Expressed in liver and fibroblasts.
2. Heterogenous clinical presentation but all present with progressive jaundice, elevated transaminases, and conjugated hyperbilirubinemia. Clinical features include hepatomegaly with or without splenomegaly, fat-soluble vitamin malabsorption, and mild steatorrhea. Pruritis usually absent.
3. Liver histology: generalized hepatitis, giant cells, and cholestasis.
4. Serum bile acid concentrations: normal or low when conventionally measured but elevated with more specific techniques (spectrometry). Normal γ-glutamyltransferase (GGT).
5. Primary bile acids can be found in small amounts in bile because of bacterial 3β-hydroxysteroid dehydrogenase/isomerase during enterohepatic recycling.
6. Treatable by primary bile acid therapy.

Δ^4 3-Oxosteroid 5β-Reductase Deficiency

1. Exclusively of hepatic origin.
2. Clinical presentation: similar to 3β-hydroxy-C_{27}-steroid dehydrogenase/isomerase, except GGT elevated and patients often younger at diagnosis.
3. Liver function tests: serum transaminitis, marked conjugated hyperbilirubinemia, and coagulopathy.
4. Liver biopsy: marked lobular disarray; giant cell transformation, bile stasis, and extramedullary hematopoiesis.
5. Diagnosis via mass spectrometric analysis of the urine. Urinary bile acid excretion generally elevated, consistent with cholestasis. Δ^4-3-oxo bile acids comprise > 75% of total urinary bile acids. Note: increased Δ^4-3-oxo bile acids also occurs in patients with severe liver disease and in infants in the first few weeks of life.
6. Repeat analysis of urine in suspected cases important: on rare occasions liver disease resolves.
7. Treatable by primary bile acid therapy.

Oxysterol 7α-Hydroxylase Deficiency

1. More important than cholesterol 7α-hydroxylase for bile acid synthesis in early life; "acidic" pathway.
2. Severe progressive cholestatic liver disease. Normal GGT.
3. Untreatable by primary bile acid therapy.

2-Methylacyl-CoA Racemase Deficiency

1. Crucial enzyme responsible for the racemization of trihydroxycholestanoic acid (THCA) to its enantiomer and responsible for the same reaction on branched-chain fatty acid pristanoyl-CoA), resulting in profound effects on bile acid and fatty acid pathways.
2. Presents with severe fat-soluble vitamin deficiencies, neuropathies, and cholestasis.
3. Mass spectrum analysis of urine, serum, and bile are similar to peroxisomal disorders. High-performance liquid chromatography (HPLC) analysis will require quantification of THCA enantiomers. Diagnosis confirmed using fibroblast enzyme studies.
4. Primary bile acid therapy with cholate effective in normalizing liver enzymes. Dietary restriction of phytanic and pristanic acid prevents neurologic symptoms.

THCA-CoA Oxidase Deficiency

1. Unique presentation: neurologic disease; main clinical feature (ataxia) without liver disease.
2. Normal very-long-chain fatty acids and other peroxisomal enzyme markers.

Bile Acid CoA Ligase Deficiency and Defective Amidation

1. Involved in final step in bile acid synthesis: conjugation with taurine and glycine.
2. Conjugated hyperbilirubinemia, mild transaminitis or normal transaminases, and normal GGT. Severe fat-soluble vitamin malabsorption.
3. Lack of glycine and taurine conjugated bile acids.

4. No cholestasis since synthesis of unconjugated cholate provides sufficient stimulus for bile flow.
5. Treat with primary conjugated bile acids.

Cholesterol 7α-Hydroxylase Deficiency

1. Bile acid synthesis reduced with up-regulation of the alternative sterol 27-hydroxylase pathway.
2. Abnormal lipids (markedly elevated total and low-density lipoprotein cholesterol with premature gallstones); no evidence of abnormal liver function. Hypercholesterolemia unresponsive to hydroxy-methylglutaryl-CoA reductase inhibitor therapy.
3. Mutations in *CYP7A1* gene.

SECONDARY BILE ACID EFFECTS

Disorders of Peroxisomal Function

1. Two main groups:
   a. Impairment in number of peroxisomes or undetectable: Zellweger syndrome, infantile Refsum disease, neonatal adrenoleukodystrophy, and rhizomelic chondrodysplasia punctata. Severe hypotonia, psychomotor retardation, hepatomegaly, simian crease, craniofacial dysmorphism, and failure to thrive.
   b. Single enzyme defect, normal number of peroxisomes: pseudo-adrenoleukodystrophy and X-linked adrenoleukodystrophy.
2. Only those with generalized peroxisomal dysfunction (except pseudo-Zellweger syndrome) have abnormal bile acid synthesis and accumulation of bile acid precursors. Thus, high long-chain C27 bile acid precursor levels (THCA and dihydroxycoprostanoic acid [DHCA]) found in Zellweger syndrome, pseudo-Zellweger syndrome, and infantile Refsum neonatal adrenoleukodystrophy. Not found in rhizomelic chondrodysplasia punctata; reason unknown.

Defects in Canalicular Bile Acid Transport Proteins

1. Byler disease: *ATP8B1* mutation, autosomal recessive familial progressive intrahepatic cholestasis. Gene encodes P-type adenosinetriphosphatase (ATPase).
2. Low GGT.
3. Synthesize primary bile acids but at suboptimal levels.
4. Negligible chenodeoxycholate present in bile suggests impaired canalicular secretion of this dihydroxy bile acid.

Smith Lemli Opitz Syndrome

1. Autosomal recessive disease. 1/40,000 to 1/20,000.
2. Variable characteristics: dysmorphism, microcephaly, poor growth, limb abnormalities, renal, cardiac and endocrine abnormalities, cataracts, mental retardation, and early death.
3. Markedly reduced plasma cholesterol and elevated 7-dehydrocholesterol and iso-dehydrocholesterol (major neutral sterols of tissue, plasma, and feces).
4. Impacts bile acid synthesis since available supply of cholesterol reduced.

DIAGNOSIS

1. Gas chromatography (GC) and mass spectrometry (MS): principal confirmatory analysis tool.
2. In healthy persons, urinary bile acid excretion negligible, but in cholestasis, urine bile acids are increased and can be analyzed.
3. Electrospray ionization MS may be used for rapid screening with detection in blood and possible neonatal diagnosis, but GC-MS necessary for definitive diagnosis.
4. Early diagnosis important; if untreated, fatal.

TREATMENT

1. Primary bile acids, rationale:
   a. Stimulus for bile flow.
   b. Down-regulate cholesterol 7α-hydroxylase to limit production and accumulation of hepatotoxic atypical bile acids.
   c. Facilitate absorption of fats and fat-soluble vitamins.
2. Concern with chenodeoxycholate therapy in persons with preexisting liver disease: increases transaminases and diarrhea.
3. Oral bile acid therapy can help with peroxisomal disorder–associated liver disease but hampered by multiorgan involvement in these diseases. Notable failure of oral bile acid therapy in those with oxysterol 7α-hydrolase deficiency.
4. In those with bile acid conjugation defect, conjugated bile acids should be used.

QUESTIONS

MATCH THE COMPOUNDS TO THEIR CATEGORIES:

a. Chenodeoxycholate and cholate.
b. Linoleic acid.
c. Cholestanol.
d. Cholesterol 7α-hydroxylase.
e. 27-Hydroxylase.

1. Primary bile acids.
2. Neutral pathway for bile acid synthesis.
3. Acidic pathway for bile acid synthesis.

TRUE OR FALSE:

4. The acidic pathway is the predominant pathway for bile acid synthesis in adults.
5. The bile acid synthesis pathway is fully functional at birth.
6. Steatorrhea and rickets can be a manifestation of a bile acid synthesis defect.
7. Bile acids in newborns are primarily conjugated with taurine.

CHOOSE THE BEST ANSWER:

8. The following are treatable with primary bile acids except:
   a. Oxysterol 7α-hydroxylase deficiency.
   b. Cerebrotendinous xanthomatosis.
   c. 3β-Hydroxy-C_{27}-steroid dehydrogenase/isomerase deficiency.

d. Δ^4 3-oxosteroid 5β-reductase.
e. All are treatable.

9. An infant presents with progressive jaundice, elevated transaminases, and conjugated hyperbilirubinemia. Examination reveals hepatosplenomegaly and mild steatorrhea. No pruritus is present. GGT is elevated. Gas chromatography and mass spectrometry of urine reveals increased Δ^4 3-oxo bile acids (>75% of urine bile acids). What do you recommend?

   a. Primary bile acid therapy.
   b. Secondary bile acid therapy.
   c. Liver transplantation.
   d. Both a and b.
   e. None of the above.

BILIRUBIN METABOLISM DISORDERS

SYNOPSIS

CLEARANCE OF BILIRUBIN

1. Albumin-bound bilirubin passes into space of Disse between endothelium and hepatocyte (facilitated by lack of basal laminae).
2. Bilirubin dissociates from albumin and can enter hepatocyte via membrane receptor carrier and by passive diffusion. Bilirubin is transported in the cell by glutathione S-tranferase (GST).
3. Bilirubin then undergoes microsomal glucuronidation, by part of bilirubin uridine diphosphate (UDP) glucuronosyltransferase superfamily of enzymes (encoded by *UGT1* gene complex on chromosome 2)
4. Conjugated bilirubin then is complexed with glutathione and transported within cytosol by GST.
5. Secreted out of apical canalicular membrane via canalicular multispecific organic anion transporter *ABCC2* (cMOAT/MRP2), which is adenosine triphosphate–dependent (Figure 1).

PHYSIOLOGIC JAUNDICE

1. Phase I: first 5 days: rapid rise in unconjugated bilirubin. Peak 6–7 mg/dL by day of life (DOL) 3. In premature infant: mean peak 10–12 mg/dL by DOL 5–7.
2. Phase II: starts DOL 5. Characterized by stable indirect bilirubin, which persists until second week. Duration in premature infant may be 1 mo or more.

BREASTMILK JAUNDICE

1. Early onset: about 12% of breastfed babies. Onset in first 3 days. May be related to caloric deprivation and dehydration.
2. Late onset: 0.5 to 3% of healthy newborns. Bilirubin rises rapidly after DOL 4. Peaks at end of second week. Severe 15 mg/dL in 2%. Not associated with kernicterus. Cessation of breastfeeding for 24–48 h drops bilirubin. Breastmilk increases enterohepatic circulation of bilirubin.

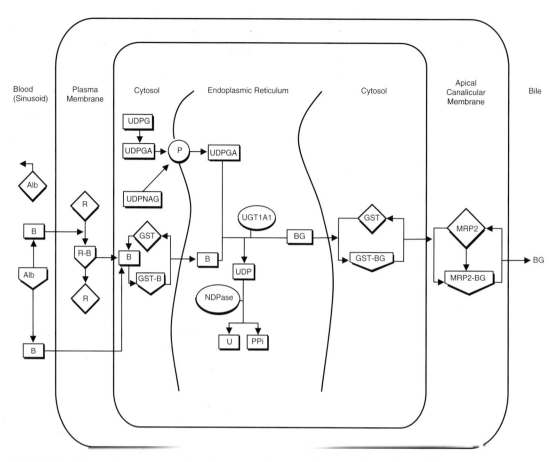

FIGURE 1   Schematic representation of hepatic bilirubin (B) metabolism. Alb = albumin; BG = bilirubin glucuronides (mono- and di-); GST = glutathione *S*-transferase (ligandin); MRP2 = multidrug resistance–associated protein 2; NDPase = nucleoside diphosphatase; P = permease; PPi = inorganic pyrophosphate; R = membrane carrier; U = uridine; UDPG = uridine diphosphate glucose; UDPGA = uridine diphosphate glucuronic acid; UDPNAG = uridine diphosphate *N*-acetylglucosamine; UGT1A1 = bilirubin uridine diphosphate glucuronosyltransferase 1A1, the isoform responsible for bilirubin conjugation.

GILBERT SYNDROME

1. Heterogenous group of disorders with ≥ 50% decrease in hepatic UDP-glucuronosyltransferase activity (Table 1). Poor correlation between measured enzyme activity and serum bilirubin concentration.
2. Prevalence 6%. *UGT1A1* gene mutants on chromosome 2. In Caucasian populations, additional TA repeat in promoter region (TATA box).
3. Autodominant or recessive inheritance.
4. Mild jaundice during fasting. Rarely diagnosed before puberty. Females clear bilirubin better than male subjects, and thus males with Gilbert syndrome (GS) have higher bilirubin levels. Hyperbilirubinemia after transplant of prior healthy donor liver may be sign that donor had GS.
5. Unconjugated serum bilirubin usually 1–4 mg/dL. No hemolysis, normal liver function tests.
6. Diagnosis: deliver intravenous nicotinic acid (adults 50 mg over 30 s) and measure unconjugated bilirubin every 30–60 min for 4–5 h. Usual rise in serum unconjugated bilirubin in normal subjects; in GS, bilirubin rise is higher and clearance delayed. (Nicotinic acid increases hemolysis).

7. Treatment: phenobarbital or clofibrate to lower bilirubin levels. Benign prognosis.

CRIGLER-NAJJAR SYNDROME

1. Two types. Autosomal recessive inheritance. Mutations to *UGT1A1* gene (see Table 1).
2. Evaluation usually in first few days life when serum bilirubin > 20 mg/dL, all elevated unconjugated bilirubin. Need to rule out other causes: hemolysis, jaundice, hypothyroidism, and breastmilk (trial of formula).
3. Type I:
   a. Complete absence of functional *UGT1A1* activity.
   b. Requires phototherapy until orthotopic liver transplantation. No response to phenobarbital.
   c. Oral agents that bind bilirubin can be helpful: agar, cholestyramine, and calcium phosphate. Plasmapheresis helpful after first year (but not peritoneal dialysis or exchange transfusion). Tin protoporphyrin (heme oxygenase inhibitor blocking bilirubin formation) may be helpful but experimental.
   d. Liver transplant provides cure.
4. Type II:
   a. *UGT1A1* activity markedly reduced but not absent.

TABLE 1   COMPARISON OF DISORDERS OF UNCONJUGATED HYPERBILIRUBINEMIA

	GILBERT SYNDROME	CRIGLER-NAJJAR TYPE 1	CRIGLER-NAJJAR TYPE II
Prevalence	3%	Rare	Rare
Inheritance	Autosomal dominant or recessive	Autosomal recessive	Autosomal recessive, rarely dominant
Genetic defect	*UGT1A1* gene	*UGT1A1* gene	*UGT1A1* gene
Hepatocyte defect site	Microsomes ± plasma membrane	Microsomes	Microsomes
Deficient hepatocyte function	Glucuronidation ± uptake	Glucuronidation	Glucuronidation
BUGT activity	5–53% of controls	Severely decreased	2–23% of controls
Hepatocyte uptake	Decreased in 20–30%	Normal	Normal
Serum total bilirubin level (mg/dL)	0.8–4.3	15–45	8–25
Serum bilirubin decrease with phenobarbital (%)	70	0	77
HPLC serum bilirubin composition:			
Fraction (Normal %)			
Unconjugated (92.6)	98.8	~ 100	99.1
Diglucuronide (6.2)	1.1	0	0.6
Monoglucuronide (0.5)	0	0	0
Bile bilirubin conjugates:			
Fraction (Normal %)			
Diglucuronide (~ 80)	60	0 to trace	5–10
Monoglucuronide (~ 15)	30	Predominant if measurable	90–95
Other routine liver function tests	Normal	Normal	Normal
Prognosis	Benign	Kernicterus common	Occasional kernicterus

BUGT = bilirubin uridine diphosphate glucuronosyltransferase; HPLC = high-performance liquid chromatography.

TABLE 2   COMPARISON OF DISORDERS OF CONJUGATED HYPERBILIRUBINEMIA

	ROTOR SYNDROME	DUBIN-JOHNSON SYNDROME
Prevalence	Rare	Rare
Inheritance	Autosomal recessive	Autosomal recessive
Genetic defect	Unknown	*MRP2* (*cMOAT*) gene
ABCC2		
Hepatocyte defect site	GST	Apical canalicular membrane
Deficient hepatocyte function	Intracellular binding of bilirubin and conjugates	Canalicular secretion of bilirubin conjugates
Brown-black liver	No	Yes
Serum total bilirubin level (mg/dL)	2–7	1.5–6.0
Serum conjugated bilirubin (%)	> 50	> 50
Other routine liver function tests	Normal	Normal
Oral cholecystogram	Usually visualizes	Usually does not visualize
99mTc- HIDA cholescintigraphy		
Liver	Poor to no visualization	Intense, prolonged visualization
Gallbladder	Poor to no visualization	Delayed or nonvisualization
Sulfobromophthalein clearance test	Serum sulfobromophthalein levels elevated (delayed clearance)	Serum sulfobromophthalein levels normal at 45 min but elevated at 90–120 min
Indocyanine green clearance test	Delayed clearance	Normal
Response to estrogens or pregnancy	No change	Increased jaundice
Total urinary coproporphyrin excretion (isomers I + III)	2.5–5 times increased	Normal
Urinary coproporphyrin isomer I composition (%) (normal = 25%)	Usually < 80% of total	> 80% of total
Prognosis	Benign (asymptomatic)	Benign (occasional abdominal complaints; probably incidental)

ABCC2 = ATP-binding cassette, subfamily C (CFTR/MRP), member 2 (cMOAT); cMOAT = canalicular multispecific organic anion transporter; GST = glutathione *S*-transferase; MRP2 = multidrug resistance–associated protein 2; 99m Tc-HIDA = technetium 99m hepatobiliary iminodiacetic acid.

b. Requires phototherapy 6–12 h daily to keep bilirubin < 20.

c. Phenobarbital (4 mg/kg/d) decreases bilirubin within 48 h with excretion of bilirubin di- and monoglucuronides. Despite decreased bilirubin response to phenobarbital, still significant hyperbilirubinemia (5–15 mg/dL).

ROTOR SYNDROME

1. Familial disorder: chronic elevation of both conjugated and unconjugated bilirubin. Usually ≥ 50% conjugated (Table 2).
2. Liver function tests and histology normal.
3. Autosomal recessive inheritance.
4. Primary abnormality: deficiency in intracellular storage capacity of liver for binding anions. Impaired

uptake of bilirubin within cytosol and leakage of bilirubin conjugates back into circulation. Patients have a deficiency of hepatic glutathione.

5. Urinary coproporphyrin values markedly increased with < 80% of total as isomer I.

6. Diagnosis: measure urinary coproporphyrin (2.5–5 times higher with isomer I < 80%).

7. Asymptomatic; no therapy required. No morbidity.

DUBIN-JOHNSON SYNDROME

1. Elevation of both conjugated and unconjugated bilirubin (≥ 50% conjugated bilirubin) (see Table 2).

2. Vague abdominal complaints. Occasional hepatomegaly but liver function tests normal.

3. More males than females. Iranian Jews increased incidence. Usually diagnosed after puberty but reported in neonates.

4. Autosomal recessive. Heterozygotes with normal serum bilirubin levels. More common than Rotor syndrome.

5. Jaundice can be worsened by pregnancy and oral contraception. Brown to black liver.

6. Defect: deficiency hepatic excretion of non–bile salt organic anions at canalicular membrane (cMOAT/MRP2).

7. Increased urinary coproporphyrin I with decrease in excretion of III. Total normal or slightly increased urinary coproporphyrins but > 80% isomer I.

8. Diagnosis: urinary coproporphyrins and isomer measurements. Need to exclude congenital erythropoietic porphyria and arsenic poisoning.

9. Cholescintigraphy with prolonged liver visualization, delayed gallbladder appearance, or nonvisualization of the biliary tree. Normal sonogram.

10. No treatment; no morbidity or mortality. Avoidance of oral contraception recommended.

QUESTIONS

CHOOSE THE BEST ANSWER:

1. A 14-year-old girl of Iranian and Jewish descent on oral contraceptives presents with vague abdominal complaints and jaundice. T bili is 6.0 with D bili 3.5. Other associated test results would include all of the following except:
   a. Technetium hepatobiliary iminodiacetic acid: intense uptake at liver with nonvisualization of gallbladder.
   b. Normal prothrombin time/partial thromboplastin time.
   c. Normal transaminases.
   d. Increased urinary coproporphyrins with > 80% type I coproporphyrin.
   e. All of the above.

2. An otherwise healthy infant presents to your office for his general pediatric visit at 2 weeks. He is notably jaundiced. His stools are colored. Weight gain is adequate. There are no signs of dehydration or infection. The infant is exclusively breastfeeding. Which of the following should not be recommended?
   a. Blood testing for serum total bilirubin and fractionation of serum bilirubin.
   b. Cessation of breastfeeding for 24–48 h with reevaluation.
   c. Blood testing for complete blood counts and peripheral blood smear.
   d. Phenobarbital.
   e. All of the above should be recommended.

TRUE OR FALSE:

3. Dubin-Johnson syndrome female patients should avoid birth control pills.

4. Gilbert syndrome is more common in males.

5. Measured enzymatic activity of bilirubin uridine diphosphate glucuronosyltransferase correlates well with serum bilirubin concentrations in Gilbert syndrome.

6. Liver biopsy is unremarkable in Crigler-Najjar syndrome type I.

MATCH THE AFFECTED GENE TO THE SYNDROME:
a. ABCC2.
b. UGT1A1.
c. Neither.

7. Gilbert syndrome.
8. Crigler-Najjar syndrome type I.
9. Crigler-Najjar syndrome type II.
10. Dubin-Johnson syndrome.

MATCH THE INHERITANCE PATTERN TO THE SYNDROME:
a. Autosomal recessive inheritance.
b. Autosomal dominant inheritance.
c. Both.
d. Neither.

11. Crigler-Najjar syndrome type I.
12. Gilbert syndrome.
13. Dubin-Johnson syndrome.
14. Rotor syndrome.

MATCH THE DEFECT TO THE SYNDROME:
a. Glucuronidation.
b. Deficient hepatic excretion of organic anions.
c. Deficient storage of binding anions.

15. Crigler-Najjar syndrome type II.
16. Dubin-Johnson syndrome.
17. Rotor syndrome.

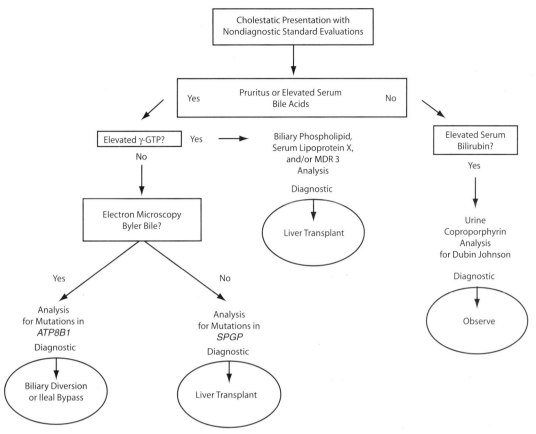

FIGURE 1 Diagnostic and therapeutic algorithm for complex cholestasis. GTP = γ-glutamyl transpeptidase; MDR = multidrug resistance; *SPGP* = sister of P-glycoprotein.

BILIRUBIN TRANSPORT DISORDERS

SYNOPSIS

BILE FLOW

1. Dependent on series of vectorial transport proteins arrayed on basolateral and canalicular membranes of hepatocytes.
2. Three different transporters involved in basolateral transport of bile acids:
   a. Na-dependent taurocholate cotransporting polypeptide.
   b. Organic anion transport protein.
   c. Microsomal epoxide hydrolase.
3. Mechanisms involved in transcellular movement of bile components not well understood.
4. Canalicular transport of bile components is rate limiting for bile flow. Many of transport processes are adenosine triphosphate–dependent.
   a. Bile salt export pump (BSEP)–sister of P-glycoprotein (SPGP): bile acid transport.
   b. Multidrug resistance-associated protein 2 (MRP2)–canalicular multispecific organic anion transporter (cMOAT): organic anion transport.
   c. Multidrug resistance protein 3 (MDR3): phospholipids transport.

DEFECTS IN CANALICULAR BILE ACID TRANSPORT: BSEP–SPGP DEFECT

1. Clinical presentation: presents with pruritus and jaundice early in life, usually before 1 yr. Clinical progression of liver disease is rapid.
2. Biochemical findings: progressive intrahepatic cholestasis; markedly elevated serum bile salts and variable elevations in serum bilirubin and aminotransferases.
3. Normal γ-glutamyltransferase (GGT) and cholesterol.
4. Liver biopsies in first 2 yr show giant cell hepatitis and cholestasis.
5. Electron microscopy (EM): distinct from Byler disease.
6. Responds well to liver transplant.

DEFECTS IN CANALICULAR PHOSPHOLIPID TRANSPORT: MDR3 DEFECT

1. Jaundice and hepatosplenomegaly. Progressive unremitting disease leading to end-stage liver disease within first decade of life.
2. Propensity for development of cholestasis of pregnancy. Consider in any child or adult with high GGT and cholestasis.
3. Elevated alanine transaminase (ALT) and GGT and markedly elevated serum bile acid levels.
4. Liver biopsy: portal inflammation, biliary fibrosis, and cirrhosis. Patent extrahepatic biliary tree. Absent serum lipoprotein X.

5. Neither ursodeoxycholic acid or ileal bypass effective for pruritus.
6. Liver transplant should be curative since tissue distribution of MDR3 protein is liver specific.

DEFECTS IN CANALICULAR ORGANIC ANION TRANSPORT

DUBIN JOHNSON SYNDROME
1. Benign direct hyperbilirubinemia.
2. Urine with elevated coproporphyrin isomer I.
3. Liver biopsy: normal except for characteristic melanin-like pigment in hepatocytes.
4. Sulfobromphthalein test shows normal hepatic uptake, delayed canalicular excretion, and a secondary peak owing to presumed reflux of dye into plasma.
5. Two phases:
   a. Cholestatic jaundice in infancy with resolution except of pruritis.
   b. End-stage liver disease with associated recurrent jaundice manifest at end of first decade or some time into second decade.
6. *MRP2/cMOAT* gene mutation.

BYLER DISEASE
1. Severe relatively unremitting pruritus.
2. Consider in patient with cholestasis; characterized by severe pruritus and markedly elevated serum bile salts with normal cholesterol and GGT.
3. Amish descent suggestive but not diagnostic.
4. Slower clinical progression than in BSEP–SPGP.
5. Histology:
   a. Early: minimal giant cell hepatitis with mild portal inflammation.
   b. Fibrosis progressive and bile duct proliferation may be noted.
   c. Characteristic EM appearance: coarsely particulate, amorphous granular biliary material.
6. Defect in gene *ATP8B1* also causes benign recurrent intrahepatic cholestasis. Function of *ATP8B1* unknown.
7. Therapy: approaches that deplete bile salt pool effective including partial biliary diversion and partial ileal bypass.

SEPSIS
Canalicular transport of bile acids and organic anions impaired via down-regulation of MRP2–cMOAT and BSEP.

LIPOPROTEIN X
Forms in cholestatic liver disease, especially when secondary to bile duct obstruction.

AAGENAES SYNDROME
Inherited cholestasis disorder that consists of periods of severe pruritus with lower extremity lymphedema.

QUESTIONS

MATCH THE CONDITION WITH THE CHARACTERISTICS:
a. Bile salt export pump (BSEP)–sister of P-glycoprotein (SPGP) defect.
b. Multidrug resistance protein 3 defect.
c. Dubin-Johnson syndrome.
d. Byler disease.

1. Rapid progression of liver disease.
2. Elevated coproporphyrin isomer I.
3. Melanin-like pigment at hepatocytes.
4. Cholestasis of pregnancy.

a. Lymphedema.
b. Amish descent.
c. Sepsis.

5. Bile salt export pump (BSEP)–sister of P-glycoprotein (SPGP) and multidrug resistance-associated protein 2 down-regulated.
6. Aagenaes syndrome.
7. Byler disease.

MATCH THE TREATMENT TO THE DISEASE
a. No therapy.
b. Liver transplantation.
c. Ileal bypass.

8. Multidrug resistance protein 3 deficiency.
9. Dubin-Johnson syndrome.
10. Byler disease.
11. BSEP–SPGP deficiency.

α_1-ANTITRYPSIN DEFICIENCY

SYNOPSIS
1. Most common metabolic disease for which children undergo liver transplantation.
2. Especially affects Caucasians of northern European ancestry.
3. Usually destructive lung disease and emphysema do not occur until adulthood.
4. α_1-antitrypsin (AT) protein encoded by 14q31-32.3
5. Variants:
   a. Most common normal variant of α_1-AT termed M1: 65–70% Caucasians in the United States. Normal M3 allele: 10% of population; differs from M1 by single base change. M2: 15–20%; additional base change from M3.
   b. Null variants: where α_1-AT not detectable, associated with premature development of emphysema.
   c. Dysfunctional variants: decrease in concentration and functional activity.
   d. Deficiency variants: reduction in concentrations.
   e. Some variants not associated with clinical disease (S variant).

f. Z variant: single base substitution from M1, resulting in substitution of Lys for Glu 342. Abnormal protein accumulation in endoplasmic reticulum (ER). Reduces stability in monomeric form and increases likelihood of polymer formation.

FUNCTION OF α_1-AT

Inhibitor of serine proteases. Most important targets: neutrophil elastase, cathepsin G, and proteinase 3 (proteases released by activated neutrophils).

SYNTHESIS

1. Predominant site of synthesis of plasma α_1-AT is the liver. Also synthesized and secreted by monocytes and macrophages.
2. Plasma levels increase 3–5-fold during inflammation. Acute phase reactant with increased levels with bacterial endotoxin exposure, IL-6 secretion from macrophages and elastase secretion from neutrophils.
3. Fecal α_1-AT concentrations correlate with inflammatory lesions of bowel. Fecal α_1-AT clearance higher in patients with homozygous deficiency than normal persons, possibly derived from sloughed enterocytes and increased α_1-AT per cell owing to intracellular accumulation.

PATHOPHYSIOLOGY

1. Substitution of Glu342 by Lys in the Z variant reduces the stability of the molecule and increases the likelihood of forming polymers.
2. Liver injury:
   a. Immune theory: liver damage results from abnormal immune response to liver antigens.
   b. Accumulation theory: liver damage caused by accumulation of mutant α_1-AT in ER of liver cells (more widely accepted [Figure 1]). Null α_1-AT gene: no accumulation and no damage.
   c. Mitochondrial autophagy and injury are marked in liver of PiZ transgenic mouse. Cyclosporin prevents mitochondrial damage.

LIVER DISEASE

1. Often first noted at 1–2 mo with persistent jaundice. Conjugated bilirubin and serum transaminases mild to moderately elevated. Alkaline phosphatase and γ-glutamyltransferase (GGT) may also be elevated. Liver may be enlarged. Occasional liver synthetic dysfunction, with even smaller percentage having fulminant liver failure in infancy. Some present with pruritus and hypercholesterolemia.
2. No evidence that MZ phenotype causes liver disease in children.
3. Children with SZ phenotype are affected by liver injury similar to PiZZ phenotype children.
4. Histology for PiZZ: periodic acid–Schiff-positive, diastase-resistant globules of hepatocytes in ER. Suggestive but not diagnostic. Inclusions are eosinophilic: most prominent in periportal hepatocytes. Variable necrosis, inflammation, periportal fibrosis, and cirrhosis. Occasional paucity of intrahepatic bile ducts.

DIAGNOSIS

1. Established by serum phenotype determination. Important in neonatal period to determine since may be difficult to distinguish from those with extrahepatic biliary atresia. Not uncommon for α_1-AT patients with PiZZ to have no excretion on hepatobiliary iminodiacetic acid (HIDA) scan.
2. Restriction fragment length polymorphism allows prenatal diagnosis of α_1-AT deficiency.

LUNG DISEASE

1. Autopsy studies: 60–65% with PiZZ develop clinically significant lung injury.
2. Typical person with lung disease is male and a smoker; 50% have cough and recurrent lung infection. Disease progresses to limitation in air flow. Chest radiograph: hyperinflation.
3. Rare for emphysema to develop during childhood. Emphysema extremely rare in those aged < 25 yr.

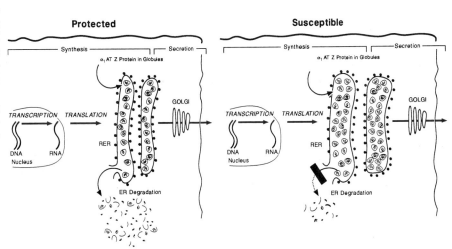

FIGURE 1 Difference in endoplasmic reticulum (ER) degradation of α_1-ATZ protein in protected and susceptible hosts. The block in ER degradation in susceptible hosts is represented by the small dark bar. Adapted from Teckman JH, Perlmutter DH. Conceptual advances in the pathogenesis and treatment of childhood metabolic liver disease. Gastroenterology 1995;108:1263–79.

4. Cigarette smoking reduces median survival by over 20 yr in α_1-AT–deficient persons.

TREATMENT
1. Most important principle: avoid cigarette smoking.
2. No specific therapy.
3. Progressive liver dysfunction and liver failure. Orthotopic liver transplantation:1 yr survival 90%; 5 yr survival 80%.
4. Rare specific clinical situations: for severe portal hypertension portacaval or splenorenal shunt may be considered.
5. Protein replacement therapy designed only for individuals with established, progressive emphysema, not individuals with liver disease.
6. Lung transplantation for severe emphysema: 5 yr survival 50%.
7. Danazol increases α_1-AT levels in serum in only 50% of deficient patients, and magnitude of effect is small.
8. Castanospermine (glucosidase inhibitor) may increase secretion of α_1-AT Z variant that is functionally active.
9. Chemical chaperones, including glycerol and 4-phenylbutyric acid (used safely in children with urea cycle disorders), may reverse misfolding of mutant proteins. Awaiting trials.
10. Possible gene replacement therapy.
11. Possible transplanted hepatocytes.

QUESTIONS

CHOOSE THE BEST ANSWER:
1. A 6-week-old girl presents with hyperbilirubinemia and acholic stools. She is otherwise well. Work-up should include all of the following except:
   a. HIDA scan for excretion of bile.
   b. Ultrasonography.
   c. Percutaneous liver biopsy.
   d. α_1-Antitrypsin serum protein level.
   e. Fractionation of serum bilirubin.

2. α_1-Antitrypsin deficiency is associated with which of the following?
   a. Emphysema in childhood.
   b. Childhood liver disease in those with the SZ phenotype.
   c. Childhood liver disease in those with the MZ phenotype.
   d. No change in median survival in smokers.
   e. None of the above.

3. The following are true of the α_1-antitrypsin protein except:
   a. In α_1-antitrypsin deficiency, there is abnormal α_1-antitrypsin accumulation in the lysosomes.
   b. The Z variant results from a single site mutation resulting in a single amino acid change.
   c. Encoded by a gene located at chromosome 14q.

d. Inhibits serine proteases.
   e. M1 variant found in 65–70% of Caucasians in the United States.

TRUE OF FALSE:
4. The most important principle in α_1-antitrypsin deficiency is avoidance of cigarette smoking.
5. No other surgical therapies except for orthotopic liver transplantation should be considered in patients with liver disease and α_1-antitrypsin deficiency.
6. α_1-Antitrypsin deficiency can be clinically confused with extrahepatic biliary atresia in early infancy.

ZELLWEGER SYNDROME AND OTHER DISORDERS

SYNOPSIS
1. Hepatocytes and renal tubular cells have greatest abundance of peroxisomes.
2. Metabolic pathways of the peroxisomes:
   a. β-oxidation of very-long-chain fatty acids (VLCFAs) and 2-methyl branched-chain fatty acids.
   b. Synthesis of sterols and bile acids.
   c. Synthesis of plasmalogens.
   d. α-oxidation of phytanic acid.
   e. Oxidase-mediated metabolism of amino acids.
   f. Catalytic and peroxidative decomposition of hydrogen peroxide.
   g. May have a role in cholesterol synthesis.

ZELLWEGER SYNDROME
1. Lethal or potentially lethal liver disease universal in Zellweger syndrome (Table 1) in those who survive neonatal period. By age 6 mo: advanced cirrhosis (Figure 1).

TABLE 1   MAJOR CLINICAL CHARACTERISTICS OF ZELLWEGER SYNDROME

Craniofacial	Midface hypoplasia resemblance to Down syndrome Hypertelorism, narrow papebral fissures Inner epicanthal folds, anteverted nares High narrow forehead, large fontanels, micrognathia
Skeletal	Clinodactyly, camptodactyly Equinovarus deformity, joint contractures
Neurologic	Severe hypotonia; absent Moro reflex, suck, grasp Complex seizure disorder (often neonatal) Profound psychomotor retardation Degenerative neurologic disease
Sensory	Optic atrophy, pigmentary retinopathy Cataracts, glaucoma, Brushfield spots Blindness (often congenital), nystagmus Sensorineural deafness
Hepatic	Hepatomegaly ± splenomegaly Prolonged or persistent jaundice Signs of portal hypertension Coagulopathy, biliary cirrhosis
Other	Cryptorchidism, hypospadias Patent ductus arteriosis, septal defects Single palmar creases

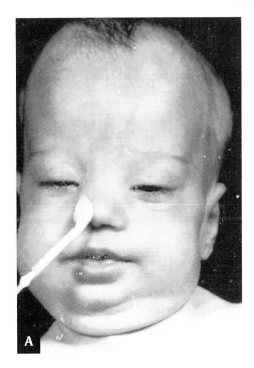
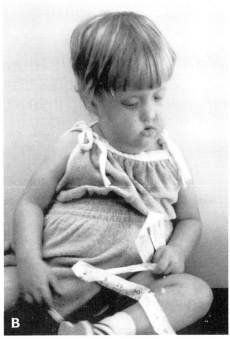

FIGURE 1 Facial appearance of two patients with Zellweger syndrome. *A*, At birth; *B*, at 3 years. Note in *B* the postural evidence of severe hypotonia.

2. Biopsy: electron microscopy, absent peroxisomes. Abnormal mitochondria with tubular cristae and paracrystalline inclusions and scattered lipid-storage macrophages with angulate lysosomes found (Figure 2).
3. Three biochemical abnormalities have special importance in evolution of liver disease in Zellweger syndrome (Table 2):
   a. Many abnormal bile acids accumulate and cause injury.

b. Severe deficiency of docosahexaenoic acid and essential polyunsaturated fatty acids.
c. Severely depressed plasmalogens.

INFANTILE REFSUM DISEASE

1. Syndrome of developmental retardation, pigmentary retinopathy, sensorineural hearing loss, and mild to moderately increased plasma phytanic acid.

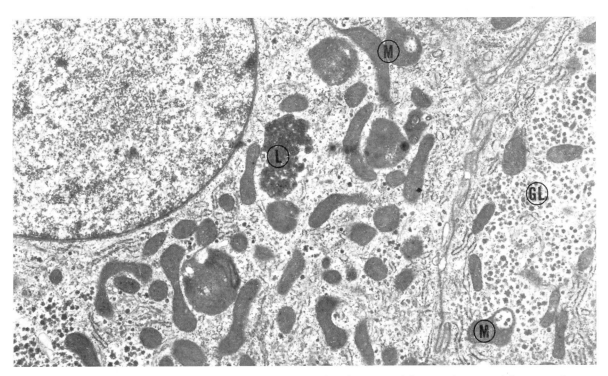

FIGURE 2 Liver ultrastructure in Zellweger syndrome. Mitochondria (M) with bizarre shapes and dense matrices are seen, together with normal lysosomes (L) and glycogen (GL). The mitochondrial abnormalities are most likely secondary phenomena because many patients with Zellweger syndrome have normal-appearing mitochondria. Courtesy of Sydney Goldfischer, MD.

TABLE 2   LABORATORY ABNORMALITES COMMON IN ZELLWEGER SYNDROME

ABNORMALITIES OF PEROXISOMAL METABOLISM
Increased levels of
  Very-long-chain fatty acids (p, u, t)
  Di- and trihydroxycholestanoic acids (p, u)
  Pipecolic and hydroxypipecolic acids (p, u)
  Phytanic and pristanic acids (p, t)
  Dicarboxylic and epoxydicarboxylic acids (p, u)
Decreased levels of
  Plasmalogens, platelet activating factor (p, t)
  Phytanic acid β-oxidation (t)
  Peroxisomal fatty acid β-oxidation (t)
  Particulate catalase (t)
  Normal bile acids (p, u)
  Docosahexaenoic and related acids (p, t)

SECONDARY OR UNEXPLAINED BIOCHEMICAL ABNORMALITIES
Increased levels of
  Serum transaminases, bilirubin
  Serum iron and iron saturation (early months)
  Cerebrospinal fluid protein (variable, late)
  Threonine (p, u)
  Urinary amino acids (generalized aminoaciduria)
  4-Hydroxyphenyllactate (u)
Decreased levels of
  Cholesterol (p)
  Prothrombin, other coagulation factors (p)

p = plasma; t = tissues/fibroblasts; u = urine.

2. Mild form of Zellweger syndrome. Hypotonia less severe. Zellweger patients rarely achieve any psychomotor development but Refsum patients have learned to walk and some language (Table 3). Most are blind and deaf.
3. Liver disease much less prominent. Hepatomegaly less common. Progressive fibrosis common.
4.   On biopsy, catalase-positive microperoxisomes, if any present. Hepatocytes and Kupffer cells have lipid vacuoles similar to X-linked and neonatal adrenoleukodystrophy (ALD).

5. In addition to full spectrum of peroxisomal biochemical abnormalities, Refsum patients have persistent low cholesterol and α- and β-lipoproteins.

NEONATAL ADRENOLEUKODYSTROPHY

1. As in Zellweger syndrome: severe hypotonia and myoclonic seizures (see Table 3).
2. Dysmorphic features: midfacial hypoplasia, epicanthal folds, and simian creases. Psychomotor retardation; few achieve mental age > 2 yr. Moderate to severe growth retardation. Nystagmus, pigmentary retinopathy, and optic atrophy. Renal cysts and punctate cartilage calcification absent in neonatal ALD
3. Unlike Zellweger patients, most neonatal ALD patients have silent or very mild liver disease. On biopsy, peroxisomes severely reduced in number and size but are detectable (unlike Zellweger syndrome and Refsum disease).
4. Plasma levels of VLCFA are lower in neonatal ALD than Zellweger syndrome.

CHILDHOOD X-LINKED ADRENOLEUKODYSTROPHY

1. Variable presentation: from early childhood to late adulthood.
2. Onset age 5–10 yr: begins with behavioral, gait, and auditory disturbances; ends fatally after several years of neurologic degeneration with or without adrenal insufficiency. Adult-onset: milder form (adrenomyeloneuropathy); peripheral nerve dysfunction and adrenal insufficiency predominate over mild central nervous system (CNS) disturbances. In both child and adult onset, neurologic and endocrine problems are acquired.
3. In both cases, elevations of VLCFA are present at birth.
4.   X-linked disease. Milder in female carriers.

TABLE 3   CLINICAL AND PATHOLOGIC CHARACTERISTICS OF THE PEROXISOMAL DISORDERS OF INFANCY AND EARLY CHILDHOOD

CHARACTERISTIC	ZELLWEGER SYNDROME	INFANTILE REFSUM DISEASE	NEONATAL ADRENOLEUKO-DYSTROPHY	ACYL COA OXIDASE DEFICIENCY	BIFUNCTIONAL ENZYME DEFICIENCY	3-KETOACYL COA THIOLASE DEFICIENCY	RHIZOMELIC CHONDRODYSPLASIA PUNCTATA
Abnormal facies	+++	+	+	−	±	+++	+++
Congenital hypotonia	+++	++	++	+++	+++	+++	−
Neonatal seizures	+++	+	++	+	+	++	+
Psychomotor retardation	+++	++	++	++	+++	+++	+++
Pigmentary retinopathy	++	+++	+++	++	++	+++	−
Sensorineural deafness	++	++	++	++	++	++	−
Absent or diminished hepatic peroxisomes	+++	+++	+	−	−	−	−
Hepatic fibrosis/cirrhosis	+++	+	+	−	±	±	−
Coagulopathy	+++	++	++	−	−	−	−
Adrenal lipid inclusions and/or atrophy	+	+	++	+++	+++	++	−
Polycystic kidneys	+++	±	±	−	±	+	−
Epiphyseal/apophyseal calcific stippling	++	−	−	−	−	+	+++
Growth retardation	+++	++	++	−	+	+	+++
Mean survival (yr)	0.6	> 5	3	4	1	0.9	1

− = absent; + = mild or occasional; ++ = moderate or common; +++ = severe or universal.

PSEUDOADRENOLEUKODYSTROPHY (ACYL-COA OXIDASE DEFICIENCY)

1. Single enzyme defect.
2. Clinically: slow development, sensorineural deafness, adrenal insufficiency, and pigmentary retinopathy (see Table 3). No clinical or biochemical liver disease. Liver histology with some increased peroxisomal size and lipoid deposits.
3. Elevated VLCFA in plasma but all other peroxisomal tests normal, including bile acid intermediates normal.

PEROXISOMAL MULTIFUNCTIONAL ENZYME 2 DEFICIENCY

1. Single enzyme defect; most common of the 3 single enzyme defects. Disorder dominated by abnormal CNS symptoms.
2. At birth, severely hypotonic, macrocephalic, neurologically depressed without hepatosplenomegaly or skeletal disease (see Table 3). Neonatal seizures common. Usually severe CNS disease leads to death within 1 year.
3. Variable degrees of hepatic fibrosis.
4. Laboratory results: increased VLCFA and increased bile acid intermediates.

PSEUDO-ZELLWEGER SYNDROME (PEROXISOMAL 3-KETOACYL-COA-THIOLASE DEFICIENCY)

1. Single enzyme defect.
2. Many clinical, anatomic, and histologic characteristics of Zellweger syndrome, but on liver biopsy found to have abundant normal to larger-than-normal peroxisomes (see Table 3).
3. Laboratory results: deficiency of peroxisomal β-oxidation (increased VLCFA and bile acid precursors).

D-SPECIFIC ACYL-COA OXIDASE DEFICIENCY

1. Initial step in β-oxidation cleavage of cholesterol side chain.
2. Similar to Zellweger syndrome with progressive cholestatic liver disease.
3. Elevated phytanic acid.

RHIZOMELIC CHONDRODYSPLASIA PUNCTATA

1. Autosomal recessive, multiple congenital malformation syndrome with major nonskeletal abnormalities in CNS (seizures, neuronal migration, and deafness), eyes (corneal defects or cataracts), and skin (ichthyosis) (see Table 3). Severe rhizomelic dwarfism and diffuse epiphyseal and epiphyseal/apophyseal punctate calcification. Most die within 1 year.
2. Disease affecting multiple peroxisomal enzymes.
3. Laboratory results: plasmalogen synthesis and phytanic acid oxidation severely deficient. Usually phytanic acid levels higher than in Zellweger patients. Intermediates of phytanic acid not increased. Plasma pipecolic acid, VLCFA, and bile acids normal.

ADULT REFSUM DISEASE (HEREDOPATHIA ATACTICA POLYNEURITIFORMIS)

1. One of rarest inborn errors of metabolism. Usually not present until age 10–30 yr. Abnormalities all acquired and progressive: pigmentary retinopathy, sensorineural deafness, cerebellar ataxia, polyneuritis, ichthyosis, and cardiac conduction abnormalities. Clinical hepatic disease absent; increased lipofuscin, lipoid accumulation. Mild proximal renal tubular insufficiency.
2. Laboratory results: increased phytanic acid (free and esterified) in blood and tissues; absent phytanic acid oxidase activity (deficiency of phytanoyl-CoA α-hydroxylase). All other peroxisomal functions normal. Phytanic acid levels > 1000 μg/mL versus 10–200 μg/mL in Zellweger syndrome.
3. Treatment: dietary phytanic acid restriction for symptom stabilization and reversal; plasmapheresis for elimination of accumulated phytanic acid.

PRIMARY HYPEROXALURIA (ALANINE–GLYOXYLATE TRANSAMINASE DEFICIENCY)

1. Type 1 hyperoxaluria. Excessive oxalate synthesis, precipitation of calcium oxalate in kidneys, and progressive nephrocalcinosis. Renal insufficiency in first decade of life, followed by extrarenal calcification of joints and myocardium.
2. Alanine-gyoxylate transaminase–deficient liver is major source of oxalate; kidney is target organ. Most oxalate made by liver, but no damage to liver. Hepatic and peroxisomal structure normal.
3. Treatment is liver–kidney transplantation.

ACATALASEMIA

Rare autosomal recessive disorder. Only pathology: oral gangrene. Catalase in other tissues presumably partially active.

DIAGNOSIS

1. Delay in diagnosis of peroxisomal disorder is common (Table 4); initial presentation may be similar to birth asphyxia. Similarly, salt-and-pepper retinopathy and psychomotor retardation may look like congenital rubella, etc.
2. Plasma VLCFA: good screening test for peroxisomal biogenesis disorder, X-linked ALD, and single enzyme peroxisomal β-oxidation defects. Most important: absolute level of C26:0 VLCFA and ratio of C26:0 to C22:0 VLCFA; both are markedly elevated in Zellweger syndrome. If VLCFA elevated, measure other metabolites, including pipecolic acid, phytanic acid, bile acid

TABLE 4   DIAGNOSTIC TESTS FOR PEROXISOMAL DISORDERS

Plasma	VLCFAs, phytanic acid, pipecolic acid, bile acid intermediates, essential fatty acids
Erythrocytes	Plasmalogens
Urine	Pipecolic acid; long-chain, odd-carbon, and epoxy dicarboxylic acids; bile acids
Fibroblasts, tissues	VLCFA levels, VLCFA β-oxidation, phytanic acid oxidation, plasmalogen levels and biosynthesis, DHAP acyl-transferase activity, alkyl-DHAP synthase activity, sedimentable catalase, peroxisomal size and abundance

DHAP = dihydroxyacetone phosphate; VLCFA = very-long-chain fatty acid.

metabolites, and plasmalogens. If all abnormal: then diagnosis may be Zellweger syndrome, neonatal ALD, or infantile Refsum disease. If pipecolic acid and plasmalogens normal: single enzyme defects are likely diagnoses. If considering rhizomelic chondrocysplasia punctata, measure plasma phytanic acid and plasmalogen levels in red blood cell membranes.

3. Liver biopsy: peroxisomal ultrastructure and specific staining may be helpful.
4. Adrenal insufficiency usually not clinically evident: need for stimulation test to diagnose.
5. Except for X-linked ALD, all are autosomal recessive diseases. Can diagnose future pregnancies with chorionic villous sampling or amniocyte culture.

TREATMENT

1. Mainly supportive, in 4 areas: nutrition, neurologic, progressive liver disease, and sensory and communication defects.
2. Note: ketogenic diet increases plasma VLCFA levels; generally not well-tolerated.
3. Apnea common to Zellweger and common cause of death.
4. In adult Refsum disease: phytanic acid restriction; similar diets not helpful in other disorders. Recent report of docosahexaenoic acid treatment in children with peroxisomal biogenesis disorders with good results.

QUESTIONS

MATCH THE DISORDER TO THE CHARACTERISTICS (MORE THAN ONE ANSWER POSSIBLE):
a. Zellweger syndrome.
b. Infantile Refsum disease.
c. X-linked adrenoleukodystrophy.
d. Pseudoadrenoleukodystrophy.
e. Peroxisomal multifunctional enzyme 2 deficiency.
f. Pseudo-Zellweger syndrome.
g. Rhizomelic chondrodysplasia punctata.
h. Adult Refsum disease.
i. Acatalasemia.
j. Neonatal adrenoleukodystrophy.
k. Primary hyperoxaluria.

1. Lethal liver disease.
2. Undetectable peroxisomes.
3. Laboratory results show only elevated plasma very-long-chain fatty acids; all other tests normal.
4. Increased very-long-chain fatty acids and increased bile acid intermediates, but normal pipecolic acid and plasmalogen levels.
5. Phytanic acid levels > 1000 µg/mL.
6. Requires liver and kidney transplantation.
7. Oral gangrene.
8. Very-long-chain fatty acids, pipecolic acid, phytanic acid, bile acid metabolites, and plasmalogens all abnormal.

9. Put in decreasing order the following list according to severity of liver disease:
   i. Zellweger syndrome.
   ii. Neonatal adrenoleukodystrophy.
   iii. Infantile Refsum disease.

   a. i, ii, iii.
   b. i, iii, ii.
   c. ii, iii, i.
   d. iii, ii, i.
   e. ii, i, iii.

10. All of the following are inherited in an autosomal recessive fashion except:
    a. Zellweger syndrome.
    b. Infantile Refsum disease.
    c. Adult Refsum disease.
    d. Childhood adrenoleukodystrophy.
    e. Neonatal adrenoleukodystrophy.

LYSOSOMAL ACID LIPASE DEFICIENCIES

SYNOPSIS

WOLMAN DISEASE

1. Clinical course: presents within first month of life with vomiting, diarrhea, hepatosplenomegaly, abdominal distention, inanition, pyrexia, adrenal cortical insufficiency, and severe failure to thrive. Intractable to medical interventions.
2. Physical exam: hepatosplenomegaly.
3. Abdominal radiograph showing massive enlargement and adrenal gland calcification.
4. No specific routine blood chemical abnormalities but anemia and abnormal liver function studies referable to severe malnutrition.
5. Infiltration of jejunum with lipid-laden macrophages.
6. Death by 3–7 mo.

CHOLESTERYL ESTER STORAGE DISEASE

1. Clinical spectrum: can present in ages 3–4 yr through adulthood (50–70 yr). Variable manifestations: isolated hepatomegaly, cirrhosis, pulmonary hypertension, adrenal calcification, and failure to thrive.
2. Intestinal abnormalities on biopsy seen but may be asymptomatic of abdominal problems.
3. Should suspect in patients with vacuolization of liver, steatosis, hepatomegaly, or uncharacterized or type IIb hyperlipidemia.
4. Hyperlipidemia is most consistent chemical abnormality in cholesteryl ester storage disease (CESD) patients.

PATHOLOGY

1. Liver:
   a. Characteristically enlarged (> 2-fold) in Wolman disease. Fibrosis in portal spaces may result in cirrhosis. Fibrosis associated with marked accumulation of triglyceride and cholesteryl esters in hepatic lysosomes and Kupffer cells and macrophages.
   b. In CESD, hepatocytes contain cytoplasmic vacuoles of variable size resembling nonalcoholic steatosis with septal fibrosis. Acid phosphatase activity abnormally high in hepatocytes. Cholesteryl ester liver content much higher in CESD than Wolman disease. Portal fibrosis and cirrhosis occur.
2. Adrenal:
   a. In Wolman disease, adrenal glands are 2–3 times normal weight with yellow color.
   b. Zona reticularis with broad infiltrations by large vacuolated cells. Areas of necrosis and calcification.
3. Small intestine:
   a. In Wolman disease, severe infiltration of lamina propria by foamy lipid-laden macrophages. Accumulation of lipid in the epithelium is also seen.
   b. In CESD, proximal small intestinal epithelium normal. Macrophages and extracellular space of the lamina propria have abundant lipids, with cholesteryl ester crystals and villi tip macrophages with autofluorescent material suggestive of ceroid-lipofuscin.

BIOCHEMICAL PATHOLOGY

1. Blood laboratory tests: Plasma triglyceride, cholesterol levels normal in Wolman disease. In CESD, patients with hypercholesterolemia with increases of low- and very-low-density lipoproteins cholesterol levels.
2. Tissue pathology: Total absence of LAL in Wolman disease may explain why both cholesteryl esters and triglycerides accumulate while remaining small amounts of LAL in CESD may explain why only cholesteryl esters accumulate in CESD.

LYSOSOMAL ACID LIPASE

1. Lysosomal acid lipase (LAL) itself is a lysosomal hydrolase synthesized in the rough endoplasmic reticulum that is cotranslationally glycosylated. Central role in modulation of cholesterol metabolism. Cleaves cholesteryl esters and triglycerides to cholesterol and fatty acids, which then exit the lysosome to cytosol.
2. In LAL deficiency, cholesteryl esters and triglycerides cannot be cleaved and thus cannot leave the lysosome. Cells detect cytosolic cholesterol deficiency and thus cholesterol biosynthesis is up-regulated. This leads to more cholesteryl ester formation.

DIAGNOSIS

LAL enzyme assay: gene mutation analysis.

TREATMENT

1. No specific treatment. Supportive therapies for Wolman disease inadequate. Enteral nutrition may be impossible; total parenteral nutrition may be required.
2. Statins may be used for theapy to counteract the upregulation of cholesterol biosynthesis. In CESD, adjunctive therapy with statins and other suppressors of hydroxymethylglutaryl-CoA reductase has been useful for decreasing heart but not liver disease or adrenal insufficiency. Supplementation with fat-soluble vitamins may be required owing to intestinal involvement.

QUESTIONS

MATCH THE DISEASE TO THE CHARACTERISTICS:
a. Wolman disease.
b. Cholesteryl ester storage disease.

1. Lipid in intestinal epithelium.
2. Normal intestinal epithelium.
3. Death by 3–7 months.
4. Variable clinical presentation.
5. Hydroxymethylglutaryl-CoA reductase inhibitor therapy useful.
6. Type IIb hyperlipidemia.
7. Accumulation of cholesteryl esters and triglycerides in tissues.
8. Accumulation of cholesteryl esters in tissues.

WILSON DISEASE

SYNOPSIS

1. Rare autosomal recessive disorder of copper metabolism. Excessive accumulation of copper in liver, central nervous system (CNS), kidneys, cornea, skeletal system, and other organs; 1/30,000.
2. Average copper (Cu) intake in American diet: 1 mg/d. Normally 50% unabsorbed, 30% lost through skin. Negligible amount excreted via urine. 20% excreted via bile. Cu is absorbed in upper intestine where it binds to proteins. Most Cu transported to liver via portal system; enters hepatocyte. Once inside hepatocyte, Wilson adenosinetriphosphatase (ATPase) 7B transports copper from endoplasmic reticulum (ER) to Golgi apparatus and ultimately facilitates transfer of copper into ceruloplasmin. In Wilson disease, mutant ATPase 7B fails to leave ER.
3. Molecular defect: > 60 disease mutations of Wilson protein ATPase 7B identified (Figure 1). Most common mutation: His 1069 Glu (H1069Q); represents 30–60% of cases in North American, Austrian, Russian, and Swedish patients.

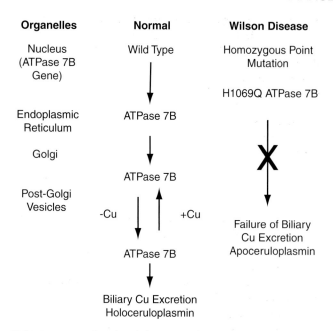

FIGURE 1 Molecular defect in Wilson disease. Under normal conditions, adenosine triphosphatase (ATPase) 7B is a transmembrane protein that traffics from the endoplasmic reticulum to the Golgi apparatus, where it is localized under basal conditions. ATPase 7B is responsible for the movement of copper into the Golgi, where ceruloplasmin probably acquires its copper. When copper is abundant, ATPase 7B traffics to a post-Golgi compartment, where it delivers copper to biliary excretory pathways that are thought to involve transfer to lysosomes and then to bile by a canalicular membrane transporter. In Wilson disease, the mutant protein fails to leave the endoplasmic reticulum and therefore is unable to transfer copper in the Golgi or facilitate copper excretion in bile. Reproduced with permission of Lippincott, Williams and Wilkins from Schilsky M. Inherited metabolic disease. Curr Opin Gastroenterol 1999;15:200–7.

4. In pediatric population, common to have hepatic manifestation precede neurologic manifestation of Wilson disease.
5. Hepatic manifestations: may present as acute self-limited hepatitis. Fulminant hepatic failure accompanied by hemolysis is more common in females (hypothesized to be secondary to sex hormone influence) and is associated with a particularly poor outcome. Lastly, chronic liver failure and cirrhosis may be the presenting syndrome with complications of portal hypertension.
6. CNS involvement: seen in children as young as age 6 yr; usual onset 10–30 yr. CNS damage limited almost exclusively to motor system. Common first symptoms: tremor, incoordination, dystonia, and difficulty with fine motor tasks. Diagnosis: computed tomography (CT) (73% ventricular dilatation, 63% cortical atrophy, 55% brainstem atrophy), but CT abnormality severities do not correlate with clinical symptoms and are of little prognostic value.
7. Psychiatric: poor school performance, anxiety, depression, phobias, and neurosis. Affected patients are fre-

quently labeled with erroneous psychiatric diagnoses before correct diagnosis of Wilson disease is made.
8. Ophthalmologic: slit lamp examination for Kayser-Fleischer (KF) ring: bulk of copper deposition at stromal layer, but no color change seen in any layers except Descemet membrane. KF rings usually present in patients with neurologic findings but frequently present in patients with hepatic symptoms. KF rings not specific for Wilson disease (Table 1). Sunflower cataracts are also seen but are less frequent than KF ring and resolve with therapy.
9. Cardiac manifestations: electrocardiogram (ECG) abnormalities seen in about one-third.
10. Renal manifestations: characterized by proximal tubular dysfunction (amino aciduria, glycosuria, increased excretion of uric acid and calcium, decreased glomerular filtration rate, and effective renal blood flow). Renal stones common; may predate diagnosis. Acidification defect (distal tubular dysfunction: unable to acidify < pH 5.2). Renal acidification defects can cause renal K wasting and recurrent hypokalemia. Renal function may improve with penicillamine therapy.
11. Skeletal: osteoporosis, rickets, spontaneous fracture, and osteoarthritis. Bone demineralization common (secondary to renal hypercalciuria, hyperphosphaturia with resulting hypocalcemia, and hypophosphatemia).
12. Other: hemolysis is a recognized complication (exact mechanism unknown but may occur secondary to oxidative injury from excess copper). Also, cholelithiasis, as a consequence of hemolysis.

LIVER PATHOLOGY
1. Fat deposition: one of earliest changes; increases until steatosis.
2. Electron microscopy: shows mitochondria of varying shapes. Peroxisomes enlarged with granular, flocculent matrix.
3. With hepatic lesion progression: collagen deposition and fibrosis.
4. Histologic features indistinguishable from autoimmune hepatitis may develop.
5. High Cu normal in fetal and neonatal liver. Cause unknown but may reflect immaturity of bile excretion. Cu may be stained with orcein. Between 3rd and 6th mo of life, hepatic Cu levels fall to within normal adult range. In children age > 6 mo, orcein-positive granules indicate elevated hepatic Cu. Elevated hepatic Cu seen in various conditions (Table 2). In early stages of Wilson disease, when liver Cu highest, Cu distributed

TABLE 1   CONDITIONS ASSOCIATED WITH KAYSER-FLEISCHER RINGS

Wilson disease
Chronic active hepatitis
Primary biliary cirrhosis
Cryptogenic cirrhosis
Intrahepatic cholestasis with cirrhosis

TABLE 2   CONDITIONS ASSOCIATED WITH ELEVATED HEPATIC COPPER CONCENTRATION

Normal infant younger than 6 mo of age
Cholestasis syndromes
  Biliary atresia
  Paucity of intrahepatic ducts
Sclerosing cholangitis
Primary biliary cirrhosis
Indian childhood cirrhosis
Primary hepatic tumors
Wilson disease

TABLE 4   CONDITIONS ASSOCIATED WITH ELEVATED URINARY COPPER EXCRETION

Wilson disease
Primary biliary cirrhosis
Chronic active hepatitis
Fulminant hepatic failure
Cholestasis syndromes
  Biliary atresia
  Paucity of intrahepatic ducts
Sclerosing cholangitis

diffusely in cytoplasm and absent from lysosomes (not stainable). In contrast to Wilson disease, orcein-positive granules seen in periphery of liver lobules. In Wilson disease, granules widespread in some lobules but may be absent in others.

DIAGNOSIS

1. Classic triad: hepatic disease, neurologic involvement, and KF rings. No single test 100% accurate.
2. First diagnostic test: serum ceruloplasmin (low in 75% with hepatic presentation) (Table 3).
3. Serum/plasma copper: decreased with low ceruloplasmin levels.
4. Serum copper: not useful diagnostically; necessary for assessment of adherence to therapy.
5. Urine copper: normally < 40 µg/d. In Wilson disease: usually > 100 µg/d (Table 4).
6. Penicillamine-stimulated copper excretion: controversial; can be used to follow chelation treatment.
7. KF ring evaluation: present in 50% with hepatic symptoms, 95% in those with neurologic or psychiatric symptoms.
8. Liver biopsy: quantification of hepatic Cu will establish the diagnosis in the absence of obstructive liver disease. Normal < 50 µg/g of liver. In Wilson disease > 250 µg/g liver. Heterozygotes about 150–200 µg/g liver.
9. If diagnosis still uncertain: measure rate of incorporation of radiocopper in ceruloplasmin. After fast of 8 h, dose of 2 mg radioCu administered orally. Serum radioCu measured at 1, 2, 4, 24, and 48 h later.

RadioCu rises in 1 and 2 h samples, then falls. Normally, serum concentration of radioCu rises in 24 or 48 h sample, representing incorporation into ceruloplasmin; in Wilson disease, second rise does not occur. However, overlapping results with heterozygotes.
10. Screening: see Table 5.
11. Natural history:
    a. Stage I: progressive accumulation copper in cytosol of hepatocytes.
    b. Stage II: copper redistributed to lysosomes and released from liver (if gradual release, asymptomatic; if rapid, hepatic necrosis (possibly fulminant hepatic failure or hemolytic anemia).
    c. Stage III: fibrosis and cirrhosis. Accumulation of copper in brain, cornea, kidney, and skeleton.
    d. Stage IV: CNS disease.
    e. Stage V: if treated, cupriuresis leads to reductions in Cu, repair of tissue injury, and clinical improvement.

TREATMENT

1. Penicillamine (Table 6): chelates Cu and is excreted in urine. Start with small dose and increase gradually. Administer orally on empty stomach in 4 divided doses, 30–45 min before meals and nighttime sleep or > 2 h after eating. Children: 20 mg/kg; adults, 1 g/d. Also, 25 mg pyridoxine thrice weekly. If no improvement, increase daily dose by 1.5–2 g/d. Higher dose: higher side effects (may worsen neurologic symptoms or initiate neurologic Wilson

TABLE 3   CONDITIONS ASSOCIATED WITH ALTERED CERULOPLASMIN CONCENTRATIONS

DECREASED
Malnutrition
Protein-losing enteropathy
Nephrotic syndrome
Hepatic insufficiency
Hereditary hypoceruloplasminemia
Neonates
Menkes syndrome
Wilson disease
Heterozygosity for Wilson disease

ELEVATED
Estrogen therapy
Infection/inflammation
Pregnancy

TABLE 5   SCREENING OF ASYMPTOMATIC RELATIVES OF PATIENTS WITH WILSON DISEASE

MANDATORY
History and physical examination
Ophthalmologic slit-lamp examination
Serum ceruloplasmin and copper concentrations
Hepatic transaminase levels
24-Hour urinary copper excretion

ADDITIONAL
Blood smear for hemolysis
Reticulocyte count and haptoglobin
Urinary calcium level
Genetic analysis

If any of the above is abnormal, liver biopsy becomes mandatory with examination of histology and measurement of quantitative liver copper content.

TABLE 6   TREATMENT OF WILSON DISEASE

Dietary restriction of copper
D-Penicillamine (with pyridoxine)
Triethylene tetramine (trientine)
Ammonium tetrathiomolybdate
Zinc
Liver transplant

TABLE 7   INDICATIONS FOR ORTHOTOPIC LIVER TRANSPLANT IN WILSON DISEASE

Fulminant hepatic failure
Cirrhosis with decompensation
Progression of hepatic dysfunction despite treatment
Exacerbation after discontinuation of therapy
Progressive and irreversible neurologic disease

symptoms). Adherence to therapy: best assessed with serial 24 h urine copper; can also use total serum Cu (µg/dL) and ceruloplasmin (mg/dL). Multiply ceruloplasmin by 3, then subtract from serum Cu: if < 20, then compliant.

Side effects: 20% of cases experience side effects within first 3 weeks. Fever, skin rash, lymphadenopathy, granulocytopenia, thrombocytopenia, nephrotoxicity, lupus, Goodpasture syndrome, elastosis perforans, pemphigoid, and dermatopathy. Penicillamine interferes with cross-linking of collagen and elastin, leading to weakening of subcutaneous tissue, so bleeding may occur with slight trauma. Reports of connective tissue defects in offspring of pregnant women taking penicillamine. If reaction occurs, stop penicillamine; may also pretreat with prednisone 0.5 mg/kg/d for 2–3 d before restarting penicillamine at lower dose and gradually increasing. Success of therapy may be limited by renal failure.

Death: described within 8 mo to 1 yr of stopping penicillamine. Possible penicillamine forms nontoxic complex with Cu: when suddenly stopped, sudden dissociation of complex and massive amounts of Cu released, which may explain rapid hepatic decomposition in sudden noncompliance. Need to follow serum transaminases as first sign of relapse when stopping penicillamine. Urine Cu rarely > 1,000 µg/d in patients taking penicillamine regularly.

2. Triethylene tetramine dihydrochloride (Trientine): alternative chelating agent; similar cupriuresis as with penicillamine. Safe during pregnancy. Given orally in divided doses of 1–1.5 g/d 1 h before and 2 h after meals. In children age < 10 yr, 0.5 g/d recommended.

3. Zinc: antagonist of Cu absorption. Cu mainly observed in proximal small bowel: absorption increased by chelating agents and high-protein diet. Fiber, bile, ascorbic acid, and zinc inhibit absorption. Once Cu crosses brush border, binds to metallothionein in cytosol of enterocytes. Zinc, Cu, glucagons, glucocorticoids, and bacteria infections induce synthesis of metallothionein. Cu that is metallothionein-bound cannot pass serosa, but is sloughed with cells into lumen and excreted in stool. Since 1–2 wk is required to induce metallothionein (slower rate of decoppering), zinc not practical for initial treatment for those with symptoms. Adult dose 50 mg zinc thrice daily, before or after food intake by 1 h; children and pregnant women, 25 mg thrice daily. Monitor treatment by 24 h urine copper: if > 125 µg copper/day, then noncompliance. Long-term effects unknown.

4. Ammonium tetrathiomolybdate: two anticopper mechanisms. It complexes ingested Cu, preventing absorption. Also forms complexes with Cu and albumin in blood, making Cu unavailable for cell uptake. Also anti-inflammatory and antifibrotic effects. Low complications. Experimental.

5. Antioxidants: may have a role in treatment of Wilson disease.

6. Liver transplantation (Table 7): clinical and laboratory results abnormalities normalize with transplant.

QUESTIONS

TRUE OR FALSE:

1. The main excretion route of copper is via bile.
2. Copper absorption is efficient.
3. In children, it is more common to present first with hepatic versus neurologic manifestation of Wilson disease.
4. Wilson disease affects both motor and sensory central nervous systems.

CHOOSE THE BEST ANSWER:

5. Conditions associated with Kaiser-Fleischer rings include all of the following except:
    a. Primary biliary cirrhosis.
    b. Cryptogenic cirrhosis.
    c. Intrahepatic cholestasis with cirrhosis.
    d. Wilson disease.
    e. Hepatitis C infection.

6. Conditions associated with elevated hepatic copper include all of the following except:
    a. Extrahepatic biliary atresia.
    b. Sclerosing cholangitis.
    c. Normal in infant < 9 months old.
    d. Primary hepatic tumors.
    e. Indian childhood cirrhosis.

7. The following are associated with decreased ceruloplasmin levels except:
    a. Malnutrition.
    b. Protein losing enteropathy.
    c. Nephrotic syndrome.
    d. Infection.
    e. Menkes syndrome.
    f. Neonates.

8. Elevated urinary copper is seen in all of the following except:
   a. Wilson disease.
   b. Sclerosing cholangitis.
   c. Fulminant hepatic failure.
   d. Chronic active hepatitis.
   e. Neonate.

9. The following are true of penicillamine except:
   a. Increases excretion of copper in urine.
   b. Associated with abnormalities in connective tissue.
   c. Once side effects occur, unable to use penicillamine again.
   d. Sudden discontinuation associated with death.

10. The following are true of zinc therapy for Wilson disease except:
    a. Interferes with absorption.
    b. Increases enteral copper losses.
    c. Can be used as initial therapy in symptomatic patients.
    d. Induces metallothionein.
    e. All of the above are true.

11. The following are indications for liver transplant in Wilson disease except:
    a. Fulminant hepatic failure.
    b. Cirrhosis with decompensation.
    c. Exacerbation after discontinuation of therapy.
    d. Progressive neurologic disease.
    e. All of the above.

SYSTEMIC CONDITIONS AFFECTING THE LIVER

SYNOPSIS

CARDIAC DISEASE

1. Acute circulatory failure:
   a. Liver uniformly enlarged.
   b. Jaundice usually is a later manifestation (3–5 d); liver transaminitis 200 times normal. Aspartate transaminase (AST) > alanine aminotransferase (ALT). Usually mild jaundice relative to elevation in transaminases. Peak transaminitis in first 3 d; enzymes return to normal in 5–7 d. Lactate dehydrogenase (LDH) elevated (mainly hepatic origin)—usually not seen in viral hepatitis.
   c. Also accompanied by renal hypoperfusion and rising blood urea nitrogen (BUN) and creatinine.
   d. Notable coagulopathy: not correctable by Vitamin K
   e. Clinically ill.
   f. Prognosis depends on correction of original insult.
   g. Ischemia > 24 h can lead to liver failure.
   h. Most common cardiac lesions: hypoplastic left heart syndrome and coarctation of aorta.

2. Chronic heart disease: chronic congestion leads to sinusoidal dilatation, engorgement, fibrosis, and ultimately cirrhosis.
   a. Clinically, liver enlarged and hard.
   b. Liver function tests (LFTs) demonstrate minimal or nonexistent elevation. Hyperbilirubinemia fluctuates.
   c. Histology: sinusoidal enlargement, inhomogeneous fibrosis. With chronic congestion, hepatocyte atrophy in zone 3. Liver has nutmeg appearance owing to variable engorgement and atrophy. In fetal hydrops, liver congestion is accompanied by hemosiderosis in zone 1.
   d. Correction of underlying cause often therapeutic.

SEPSIS

1. Organisms implicated in hepatic dysfunction include gram-negative enteric pathogens, streptococci, and staphylococci.
2. Jaundice from septicemia occurs infrequently. Onset of jaundice 2–5 d after infection. Direct hyperbilirubinemia varies from 5–60 mg/dL. Elevation in bilirubin is greater than that seen in liver and biliary tree enzymes.
3. Hepatomegaly in 50%. Need to exclude abscess or cholangitis.
4. Cholestasis of septicemia is result of abnormal regulation of multidrug resistance (MDR) protein 2, responsible for secretion of bilirubin at canalicular membrane (Figures 1 and 2).
5. Characteristic features of certain infections:
   a. Hepatic abscesses complicate appendiceal infections.
   b. In pneumococcal pneumonia, right lobe most commonly affected; male-to-female ratio 10:1; swelling of hepatocytes with focal necrosis. Moderate elevation of LFTs, with AST > ALT. Streptococcal infections can be associated with jaundice.
   c. Ehrlichiosis: hepatitis with jaundice, hepatomegaly, and typical rash. Resolution with antibiotic therapy.
   d. Mild hepatitis with varicella-zoster virus infection; usually benign course.
6. Liver histology may show suppurative cholangitis with intrahepatic cholestasis.
7. Treatment of underlying problem curative.
8. Cephalosporins can contribute to cholestasis.

CONNECTIVE TISSUE DISEASE

1. Juvenile rheumatoid arthritis (JRA):
   a. Hepatosplenomegaly (HSM) not uncommon. Splenomegaly is more common than hepatomegaly. Felty syndrome: splenomegaly, neutropenia, and active systemic JRA.
   b. Hepatomegaly histology: nonspecific, Kupffer hyperplasia, and focal hepatitis.
   c. Long-standing JRA (usually > 8 yr) associated with amyloidosis.
   d. Elevation with transaminases associated with aspirin therapy. Patient with JRA on aspirin is more susceptible to Reye syndrome.
   e. Gold toxicity manifests as cholestasis; deposits of gold in Kupffer cells.

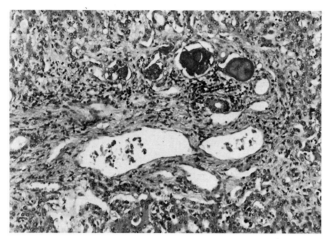

FIGURE 1   Cholangitis lente in the context of prolonged septicemia. Note severe cholestasis (hematoxylin and eosin; ×40 original magnification). Courtesy of Dr. L. Burgart, Mayo Clinic and Foundation.

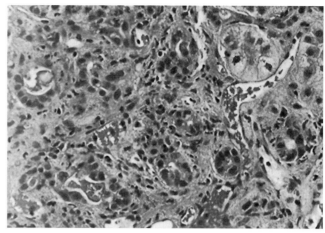

FIGURE 2   Cholangiolar cholestasis in the context of septicemia (hematoxylin and eosin; ×40 original magnification). Courtesy of Dr. L. Burgart, Mayo Clinic and Foundation.

   f. Methotrexate causes either a mild increase in liver enzymes (15%) or progressive fibrosis, especially with a cumulative methotrexate dose > 1.5 g.

2. Systemic lupus erythematosus (SLE):
   a. Involved in 40% of SLE patients.
   b. Hepatomegaly in one-third of patients.
   c. Liver enzyme elevations occur in association with hepatotoxic medications, especially aspirin.
   d. Association of SLE and autoimmune hepatitis (AIH) well-described. Liver lesion indistinguishable from AIH. Improves with immunosuppression.
   e. Hypercoagulable state may lead to veno-occlusive disease (VOD) of liver or Budd-Chiari syndrome.
   f. Liver may be involved with transient abnormalities in neonatal SLE. Neonatal SLE shows a cholestatic picture that resolves by 6 mo, described by portal fibrosis, bile duct obstruction, and inflammation.

3. Juvenile dermatomyositis:
   a. Liver seldom involved in this condition.
   b. Elevation of AST may be from muscle.
   c. HSM seen in severe disease.

4. Miscellaneous connective tissue disease:
     Liver and spleen can be involved. Involvement secondary to generalized vasculitis at medium size vessels.

5. Kawasaki disease:
     Hydrops of gallbladder, hepatomegaly, and elevation of liver enzymes seen. High dose aspirin can lead to dose-dependent liver toxicity. Hydrops may respond to low dose nonsteroidal anti-inflammatory drugs.

HEMATOLOGIC DISORDERS

1. Sickle cell (SC) disease:
   a. Acute hepatitis crisis: 10–15% of patients have SC disease. Right upper quadrant pain, tender hepatomegaly, elevated transaminases, conjugated hyperbilirubinemia, and fever. Coagulation studies normal. Elevated LDH secondary to hemolysis. Imaging of intrahepatic and extrahepatic ducts can help differentiate from acute cholecystitis. Biopsy reveals sinusoidal congestion, sickling, Kupffer cell hyperplasia, and erythrophagocytosis.
   b. Acute and chronic cholecystitis: triad right upper quadrant pain, tenderness, fever, and elevated biliary markers. Imaging important: ductal dilation. Chronic pigment gallstones in 70–80% SC patients. Incidence increases with age.
   c. Chronic iron overload: condition not as common as in patients with thalassemia. Associated with congestive heart failure, bronzed skin, hepatosplenomegaly, diabetes, and increased susceptibility to *Yersinia* infection.
   d. Chronic viral hepatitis occurs in 25–30% of SC patients.

2. Thalassemia
   a. High transfusion requirement leads to iron overload, fibrosis, and cirrhosis.
   b. Risk of viral infection high.

3. Coagulation disorders:
     Contaminated blood products before 1990 led to high incidence of hepatitis C virus in hemophilia.

BUDD-CHIARI SYNDROME

1. Most common cause worldwide of Budd-Chiari syndrome: membranous obstruction of hepatic veins.

2. Acute form: sudden onset right upper quadrant pain, tender hepatomegaly, and ascites. Mild LFT elevations and cardiac congestion. Zone 3 involvement. Prothrombin time (PT) prolongation common. Etiologies: protein C deficiency, antithrombin 3 deficiency, factor V Leiden, thrombin mutations, polycythemia vera, primary lymphoproliferative disorder, contraceptive use, inflammatory bowel disease, paroxysmal nocturnal hemoglobinuria, Behçet syndrome, collagen vascular disease, and acute obstruction (tumor invasion).

3. Chronic form: usually due to membranous obstruction of hepatic veins (common in developing countries). Can be congenital or due to thrombosis. Liver enzymes mildly elevated. Coagulation normal. Pro-

gression of disease leads to portal hypertension, liver failure. Treat by invasive radiologic techniques.
4. Diagnosis: based on imaging, ultrasonograpy to magnetic resonance imaging. Hypertrophy of caudate lobe on technetium uptake due to differential drainage of this lobe (caudate lobe drains directly into inferior vena cava and thus enlarges due to hypertrophy in the context of portal hypertension in Budd-Chiari syndrome).
5. Management depends on etiology. If liver shows only congestion, and response to diuretic therapy is good, try anticoagulation. If severe necrosis: surgical shunting. If fibrosis: medical therapy and evaluation for liver transplant.

VASCULAR DISEASES
1. Development of liver infarct requires both arterial and venous occlusion to occur simultaneously given dual blood supply of the liver.
2. Once atrophy occurs, compensatory hypertrophy occurs in remaining liver tissue with reactive nodular hyperplasia.
3. In cases where vascular supply severely impaired, particularly with venous injury, cirrhosis is the end result.
4. Involvement of hepatic arteries in systemic conditions not uncommon. Arterial compromise affects large intrahepatic bile ducts. Stricture formation at biliary tree is a well-recognized complication of hepatic artery injury.
5. Normally, endothelial cells make both endothelin and nitric oxide to control microvasculature; play important role in ischemic liver injury.

MALIGNANCIES
1. Leukemia:
   a. HSM common.
   b. One rare presentation of neonatal leukemia is liver failure (histology: leukemic infiltration) (Figure 3).
   c. Transient elevation of enzymes occurs often, especially during therapy.
   d. Fungal infection can present with hepatomegaly, elevated liver enzymes, and fever.

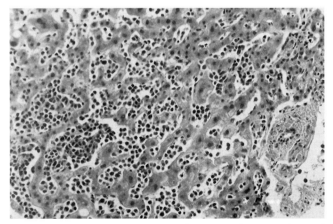

FIGURE 3   Liver involvement by leukemia (hematoxylin and eosin; ×40 original magnification). Courtesy of Dr. L. Burgart, Mayo Clinic and Foundation.

2. Hodgkin lymphoma:
   a. Direct involvement of liver (25%) or nonspecific inflammation and noncaseating granulomas (50%).
   b. Reed-Sternberg lesion (25%).
   c. Jaundice occurs with direct liver involvement. Obstructive lesion of biliary tree less common.
3. Langerhans cell histiocytosis (LCH):
   a. Diaper dermatitis, drainage from external auditory canal, and HSM.
   b. Liver involved in up to 30%. Wide spectrum of liver disease encompassing acute hepatitis, severe cholestatic disease, and silent hepatomegaly. Progression to biliary cirrhosis rapid despite successful treatment of skin and bone lesions.
   c. Definitive diagnosis: presence of Birbeck granules on election microscopy. T6 antigen on cells also gives diagnosis.
   d. Liver transplant has been successful but increased risk of lymphoproliferative disease. Recurrence of LCH in 33%.
4. Hemophagocytic syndrome:
   a. Sporadic form: reactive proliferation of lymphohistiocytic lineage in reaction to viral infection particularly Epstein-Barr virus, bacteria, or fungus. Activated lymphocytes are benign. Fever and hepatomegaly present. Liver enzymes abnormal in 80%. Uncontrolled inflammatory response. Resolves with resolution of original insult.
   b. Familial: autosomal recessive. Liver and other organs are infiltrated with malignant histiocytes; best demonstrated on bone marrow biopsy. Gene mapped to 10q22 (perforin) is mutated. Occurs in first 3 months of life with poor prognosis. HSM, fever, and weight loss. Anemia, thrombocytopenia, hyperlipidemia, and low fibrinogen. Hyperlipidemia is important feature.

AFTER BONE MARROW TRANSPLANTATION
1. Liver involvement can be secondary to original condition.
2. Liver is often the site of opportunistic infection.
3. Medications can lead to liver injury.
4. Prolonged fasting can lead to liver disease.
5. Total parenteral nutrition (TPN)–induced liver disease.
6. VOD:
   a. Triad of hepatomegaly, elevated liver enzymes, and ascites.
   b. Due to obstruction of terminal hepatic venules.
   c. Occurs in 20–25% of patients undergoing bone marrow transplantaion (BMT).
   d. More likely in allogeneic than in autologous transplantation.
   e. More common in patients transplanted for malignancies rather than aplastic anemia.
   f. Preexisting liver disease, total body radiation therapy, and intensity of condition regimen contributes to endothelial injury and development of VOD.

g. Criteria: onset within 20 d of transplant, weight gain 2–10%, hepatomegaly, ascites, and serum bilirubin > 2 mg/dL.

h. Poor outcome correlated with severity of hyperbilirubinemia and presence of multiorgan failure.

i. Pathophysiology: direct injury to endothelium of central hepatic veins. Injury often associated with zone 3 necrosis from radiation therapy. The endothelium initiates local thrombosis potentiating congestion and hypoxia. Eventually, significant fibrosis and collagen deposition around occluded central veins lead to clinical triad of weight gain, jaundice, and hepatomegaly.

j. Characterized by fibrous intimal thickening or occlusion of hepatic venules (< 0.3 mm).

k. Treatment: infusion of tissue plasminogen activator (t-PA) and transjugular intrahepatic portosystemic shunt (TIPS) may be beneficial in early stages. Heparin has shown some efficacy.

l. 50% resolve over time.

7. Graft-versus-host disease (GVDH):

a. Chronic GVHD in 70% after bone marrow transplantation. Disease most commonly affects skin, liver, and gastrointestinal tract. Chronic GVHD occurs by definition after 100 d after transplant (Acute GVHD is within the first 100 d after transplant). Predisposing factors include acute GVHD and degree of human leukocyte antigen mismatch. Portal tracts enlarged, variable lymphocytic infiltration. Long-standing GVHD is associated with vanishing bile ducts. Treatment: immunosuppressive agents, ursodeoxycholic acid, and thalidomide.

b. Acute GVHD can occur when immunocompromised host receives immunocompetent T cells. Occurs 3–6 wk after transplant: anorexia, nausea, emesis, and occasional profuse diarrhea. Maculopapular rash common. Liver injury and cholestasis common but severe insufficiency rare. Rectal and skin biopsies can help diagnosis. Immunosuppression is treatment of choice.

NUTRITIONAL DISEASE

1. Malnutrition:

a. Liver affected in all forms of malnutrition

b. Chronic malnutrition leads to mobilization of free fatty acids from periphery, which are not oxidized effectively in liver. This leads to accumulation of fat in hepatocyte with macrovesicular steatosis.

c. Kwashiorkor associated with severe steatosis.

d. Livers of patients in prolonged starvation have decreased peroxisomes and depleted carnitine stores.

e. Deficiencies of trace metals may contribute to liver injury.

2. Fatty liver, obesity, and nonalcoholic steatohepatitis (NASH):

a. Excluding metabolic causes of fatty liver, NASH is the most severe form of nonalcoholic fatty liver.

b. During excessive food intake, the liver stores fats; steatosis may develop (Table 1).

TABLE 1   CAUSES OF STEATOSIS

Malnutrition
Essential fatty acid deficiency
Celiac disease
Diabetes mellitus
Galactosemia
Hereditary fructose intolerance
Glycogen storage disease
Tyrosinemia
Homocystinuria
Mitochondrial oxidation and respiratory chain defects
Carnitine deficiency
Cholesterol ester storage disease
Abetalipoproteinemia
Cystic fibrosis
Drugs
Total parenteral nutrition
Obesity
Reye syndrome

c. Pure macrovesicular steatosis without increases in liver enzymes common in obesity. 15% of obese children have elevated liver enzymes associated with inflammation and bridging fibrosis.

3. Short bowel syndrome; liver involvement owing to the following:

a. Malnutrition.

b. Vitamin and trace element deficiencies.

c. TPN

d. Intra-abdominal infections.

e. Small bowel bacterial overgrowth.

f. Early institution of enteral feeds decreases incidence of liver injury.

4. TPN:

a. Cholestatic liver disease predominates in premature and young infants. Steatohepatitis predominates in older children and adolescents.

b. Cholestasis resolves after cessation of TPN.

c. Earliest biochemical abnormality is rise in serum bile acids. Hyperbilirubinemia, elevated alkaline phosphatase, elevated γ-glutamyltransferase occurs later. Associated hepatomegaly. Ultrasonography shows evidence of steatosis.

d. Development of sludge in 100% infants on TPN > 6 wk. Small proportion develop gallstones.

e. Increased risk of sepsis (especially with bacterial overgrowth), leading to dysregulation of MDR2 and worsening cholestasis.

f. Early pathology: lobular cholestasis. Portal inflammation, bile duct proliferation, and giant cell transformation can be present. Steatosis occurs with increased caloric intake in form of glucose.

5. Herbal therapy: Table 2

6. Celiac disease:

a. Chronic malnutrition may lead to hepatic steatosis indistinguishable from kwashiorkor.

b. Histology shows nonspecific hepatitis, chronic active hepatitis, and cryptogenic cirrhosis.

c. 5% of patients with type I diabetes have celiac disease. Steatosis can result from diabetes or chronic malnutrition.

TABLE 2   HERBAL MEDICINES ASSOCIATED WITH
DOCUMENTED CASES OF HEPATOTOXICITY

Soy phytoestrogens
Green tea leaf
Pyrrolizidine alkaloids and Jamaican tea preparations
Anthronoids
Protoberberine alkaloids
Germander (*Teucrium* spp)
Herbs rich in coumarin
Herbs rich in podophyllotoxin
Impila (*Callilepis laureola*) root
Kava (*Piper methysticum*) rhizome
Kombucha
Ma huang (*Ephedra* spp)
Skullcap (*Scutellaria* spp)

Adapted from Bauer BA. Herbal therapy: what a clinician needs to know to coun-
sel patients effectively. Mayo Clin Proc 2000;75:835–41.

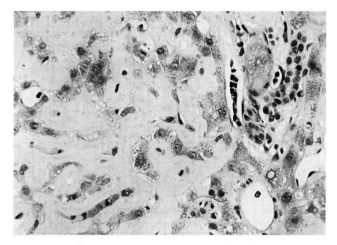

FIGURE 4   Amyloidosis (hematoxylin and eosin; ×100 original magnification). Courtesy of Dr. L. Burgart, Mayo Clinic and
Foundation.

d. Granulomatous changes may also occur as celiac
disease has been associated with sarcoidosis.

ENDOCRINE DISEASE

1. Hypopituitarism:
   a. Constellation of hypoglycemia, nystagmus, and
      cholestasis should prompt evaluation for hypopitu-
      itarism. Associated with absence of septum pal-
      lidum and septo-optic dysplasia.
   b. Lack of thyroid hormones and cortisol affects bile-
      independent bile flow in liver with resulting
      cholestasis.
   c. Histology: cholestasis and neonatal hepatitis associ-
      ated with hypopituitarism.
   d. Treatment: aimed at underlying disorder. Rapid cor-
      rection with thyroid hormone and adrenal hormone
      replacement therapy.
2. Hypothyroidism:
   a. Association of neonatal hypothyroidism and jaun-
      dice well-described. 20% hypothyroid infants will
      be jaundiced due to indirect hyperbilirubinemia
      and immature conjugation enzymes.
   b. Older children and adolescents: association of liver
      and thyroid disease occurs in context of autoim-
      mune disease.
3. Diabetes mellitus (DM):
   a. Poor glycemic control results in glycogen accumu-
      lation in liver and hepatomegaly.
   b. Association between DM and cholelithiasis.
4. Autoimmune polyglandular syndrome (APS) type I:
   a. Association of autoimmune disease and effect on
      parathyroid, adrenals, and ovaries constitutes APS
      type I. Also includes mucocutaneous candidiasis
      and AIH.
   b. AIH is type II (ALKM1 positive).
   c. Screening for AIH with yearly liver enzymes essential.

RENAL DISEASE

1. Diseases affecting both kidney and liver includes:
   autosomal recessive polycystic kidney and congenital
   hepatic fibrosis.

2. In dialysis or renal transplant patient, hepatopathy
   attributed to viral infections, immunosuppressive
   medications, opportunistic infections, and iron
   overload.

AMYLOIDOSIS

1. Primary amyloid (AL) composed of light chain of
   immunoglobulin. Secondary amyloid (AA) associated
   with chronic inflammation (secreted by liver as acute
   phase reactant) (Figure 4).
2. Rare in children age < 15 yr.
3. Cystic fibrosis most common association, with one-
   third having amyloid at autopsy.
4. Reported in familial Mediterranean fever, JRA, and
   tuberculosis.
5. Hepatomegaly and proteinuria in a chronic inflammatory condition should prompt search for amyloid in
   rectal and renal tissue.
6. Liver biopsy helpful in hepatomegaly. No correlation
   between degree of amyloidosis and elevation of liver
   enzymes.

SARCOIDOSIS

1. Multisystem chronic granulomatous disease.
2. Associated with Crohn disease, celiac disease, lymphoma, Addison disease, thyroiditis, and drugs.
3. Lung: most commonly affected organ.
4. Hepatomegaly is late phenomenon in one-third of
   patients.
5. Long-standing sarcoidosis leads to portal hypertension.
6. Treatment: steroids and methotrexate.

QUESTIONS

TRUE OR FALSE:
1. Ischemia over 24 h is associated with hepatic failure.
2. Cholestatic liver disease predominates in older children on total parenteral nutrition.

CHOOSE THE BEST ANSWER:

3. You are asked to evaluate a young girl with pneumococcal pneumonia with elevated transaminases. Which of the following are true?
   a. Boys are more commonly affected in regards to hepatitis in the setting of pneumococcal pneumonia.
   b. The left lobe of the liver is more commonly affected.
   c. Alanine aminotransferase (ALT) is moderately elevated and greater than aspartate transaminase (AST).
   d. Liver biopsy often reveals cholestasis.
   e. All of the above.

4. You are called to see a neonate with cardiac arrhythmias and cholestasis. What test will most likely give you the diagnosis?
   a. Transaminase evaluation.
   b. Total and direct bilirubin.
   c. Ultrasonography.
   d. Anti-Ro and Anti-La antibodies.
   e. Electrocardiography.

5. What is the most common cause of Budd-Chiari syndrome worldwide?
   a. Antithrombin 3 deficiency
   b. Factor V Leiden deficiency.
   c. Protein S deficiency.
   d. Contraceptive use.
   e. Membranous obstruction of hepatic vein.

6. What is the finding on technetium scan of Budd-Chiari syndrome?
   a. Increased uptake throughout liver.
   b. Decreased uptake throughout liver.
   c. Increased uptake at the caudate lobe.
   d. Decreased uptake at the caudate lobe.
   e. None of the above.

7. What is associated with hepatic artery injury?
   a. Biliary tree strictures.
   b. Ischemic hepatopathy.
   c. Cirrhosis.
   d. Cholelithiasis.
   e. None of the above.

8. The following are risk factors for the development of veno-occlusive disease except:
   a. Preexisting liver disease.
   b. Total body radiation therapy.
   c. Intensity of conditioning chemotherapy.
   d. Allogeneic bone marrow transplantation.
   e. Bone marrow transplantation for aplastic anemia.

9. Which of the following are criteria for veno-occlusive disease?
   a. Onset within 3 months post-transplant.
   b. Weight gain of 2–10%.
   c. Serum bilirubin < 2 mg/dL.
   d. Splenomegaly.
   e. All of the above.

10. What is the cut-off time for differentiating between acute and chronic graft-versus-host disease?
    a. 30 d post-transplant.
    b. 60 d post-transplant.
    c. 100 d post-transplant.
    d. 120 d post-transplant.
    e. >120 d post-transplant.

11. Steatosis is associated with all of the following except:
    a. Malnutrition.
    b. Celiac disease.
    c. Diabetes mellitus.
    d. Abetalipoproteinemia.
    e. Ischemia.

MATCH THE CONDITIONS:
   a. Familial hemophagocytic syndrome.
   b. Septo-optic dysplasia.
   c. Autoimmune polyglandular syndrome type I.
   d. Sarcoidosis.
   e. Kwashiorkor.
   f. Amyloidosis.

12. Hyperlipidemia.
13. Mucocutaneous candidiasis.
14. Hypoglycemia.
15. Celiac disease.
16. Hypopituitarism.
17. Cystic fibrosis.
18. Autoimmune hepatitis type II.
19. Severe steatosis at the liver.

ACUTE LIVER FAILURE

SYNOPSIS

DEFINITION
In pediatric population, characterized by severe impairment of liver function with or without encephalopathy in association with hepatocellular necrosis in persons without recognized underlying chronic liver disease.

ETIOLOGY
Refer to Tables 1 and 2.

CLINICAL SYNDROME
1. Encephalopathy: multifactorial:
   a. Hyperammonemia.
   b. Increased γ-aminobutyric acid (GABA).
   c. Intestinal decarboxylation of amino acids in the colon leads to formation of products inhibiting dopamine- and catecholamine-mediated transmission, acting as false neurotransmitters.
   d. Imbalance of branched-chain and aromatic amino acids.
   e. Other toxins.

2. Stages of encephalopathy in children:
   a. Stage I: Mild confusion or anxiety, disturbed sleep, and irritability.
   b. Stage II: Drowsiness, confusion, mood swings, and inappropriate behavior.
   c. Stage III: Pronounced confusion and hyperreflexia.
   d. Stage IV: Comatose with or without decerebrate or decorticate posturing, with or without pain response. Intracranial hypertension and cerebral edema invariably present in stage IV encephalopathy. Raised intracerebral pressure can lead to brainstem herniation.
3. Renal failure: occurs in 55% of acute liver failure (ALF) patients. In children, incidence lower (10–15%). Functional renal failure (hepatorenal syndrome) progresses to tubular damage. Avid sodium retention (urinary sodium < 20 mmol/L) and normal urine sediment can differentiate functional renal failure from tubular damage. In hepatorenal syndrome, decrease in renal perfusion leads to increased vasoactive mediators leading to vasoconstriction and decreased glomerular filtration rate.
4. Metabolic derangements: hypoglycemia seen in 40%. Acid–base imbalance common with metabolic acidosis and lactic acidosis. Respiratory alkalosis can occur when there is hyperventilation. Hypokalemia common as well as hyponatremia, hypocalcemia, hypomagnesemia, and hypophosphatemia (in acetaminophen-induced ALF).
5. Hemodynamic changes seen owing to decreased systemic peripheral vascular resistance and increased cardiac output. Cardiac arrhythmias can occur and are usually caused by electrolyte disturbances.
6. Pulmonary complications common (50%): aspiration, atelectasis, infection, respiratory depression, and pulmonary edema.
7. Coagulopathy seen secondary to decreased synthesis of coagulation factors by the liver. Factors V and VII have shortest half-lives and are more sensitive than international normalized ratio (INR) for hepatic synthetic function. Disseminated intravascular coagulation unusual. Thrombocytopenia also seen owing to increased platelet destruction and decreased hepatic synthesis of factors necessary for platelet maturation and release into blood.
8. Infections: common owing to poor host defenses. Also, infection can lead to development and progression of multiorgan failure.

TABLE 1 CAUSES OF ACUTE LIVER FAILURE

INFECTIVE
Viral
  Viral hepatitis
  A, B, B + D, E
  Non-A–E hepatitis (seronegative hepatitis)
  Adenovirus, Epstein-Barr virus, cytomegalovirus
  Echovirus
  Varicella, measles
  Yellow fever
  Rarely, Lassa, Ebola, Marburg virus, dengue, Toga virus
Bacterial
  Salmonellosis
  Tuberculosis
  Septicemia
Others
  Malaria
  Bartonella
  Leptospirosis

DRUGS
Dose dependent
  Acetaminophen
  Halothane
Idiosyncratic reaction
  Isoniazid
  Nonsteroidal anti-inflammatory drugs
  Phenytoin
  Sodium valproate
  Carbamazepine
  Ecstasy
  Troglitazone
  Antibiotics (penicillin, erythromycin, tetracyclines, sulfonamides, quinolones)
  Allopurinol
  Propylthiouracil
  Amiodarone
  Ketoconazole
  Antiretroviral drugs

Synergistic drug interactions
  Isoniazid + rifampicin
  Trimethoprim + sulfamethoxazole
  Barbiturates + acetaminophen
  Amoxycillin + clavulinic acid

TOXINS
Amanita phalloides (mushroom poisoning)
Herbal medicines
Carbon tetrachloride
Yellow phosphorus
Industrial solvents
Chlorobenzenes

METABOLIC
Galactosemia
Tyrosinemia
Hereditary fructose intolerance
Neonatal hemochromatosis
Niemann-Pick disease type C
Wilson disease
Mitochondrial cytopathies
Congenital disorders of glycosylation
Acute fatty liver of pregnancy

AUTOIMMUNE
Type 1 autoimmune hepatitis
Type 2 autoimmune hepatitis
Giant cell hepatitis with Coombs-positive hemolytic anemia

VASCULAR/ISCHEMIC
Budd-Chiari syndrome
Acute circulatory failure
Heat stroke
Acute cardiac failure
Cardiomyopathies

INFILTRATIVE
Leukemia
Lymphoma
Hemophagocytic lymphohistiocytosis

TABLE 2   CAUSES OF NEONATAL LIVER FAILURE

Perinatal herpes simplex virus infection
Neonatal hemochromatosis
Galactosemia
Tyrosinemia
Hemophagocytic lymphohistiocytosis
Septicemia
Mitochondrial cytopathies
Congenital disorders of glycosylation
Severe birth asphyxia

9. Mild elevation of serum amylase not uncommon, but clinical pancreatitis unusual.
10. Adrenal hyporesponsiveness has been seen.

PROGNOSIS

1. Variable. Prothrombin time is best indicator of survival. In children, factor V concentration < 25% suggests poor outcome. Liver biopsy rarely helpful and usually is contraindicated because of coagulopathy unless done by transjugular approach.
2. Fulminant Wilson disease invariably fatal; liver transplant only effective therapy.
3. Survival depends on ability of liver to recover from insult; difficult to predict potential of recovery.

MANAGEMENT

1. If child with encephalopathy or INR > 4, admit to intensive care unit.
2. No sedation unless mechanically ventilated.
3. Monitoring: oxygen saturation monitoring, hourly urine output, vital signs (every 6 h), neurologic evaluation and glucose estimation (every 6 h); electrolyte and coagulation studies (every 12 h); daily complete blood count and surveillance of blood and urine cultures.
4. Fluid intake should be restricted to two-thirds of maintenance if no dehydration present to decrease possibility of developing cerebral edema.
5. Neurologic complications:
    a. Hyperammonemia: dietary protein restriction, bowel decontamination, and lactulose (limited value in rapid encephalopathy).
    b. Cerebral edema: intracranial pressure (ICP) monitoring debated (may allow early and accurate detection of ICP changes, but high risk of intracranial hemorrhage). If used, ICP should be maintained < 50 mm Hg. Avoid excessive hyperventilation, which compromises cerebral perfusion pressure. Mannitol remains mainstay of therapy with rapid bolus of 0.5 g/kg 20% solution over 15 min, which can be repeated if serum osmolarity < 320 mosm/L.
6. Infections: respiratory tract most common site followed by urinary tract. Topical antifungal and intravenous antibiotic prophylaxis used. Efficacy of systemic antifungals for prophylaxis not studied.
7. Hemodynamic instability: vasopressors may be helpful.
8. Renal failure: low-dose dopamine may be harmful. Hemodialysis may be necessary when urine output < 1 cc/kg/h.

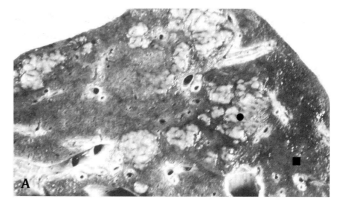

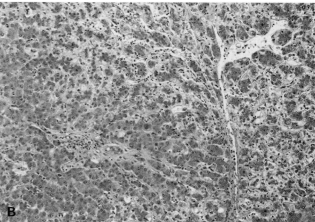

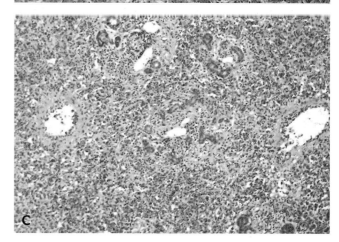

FIGURE 1 *A*, Macroscopic appearance of areas of collapse (■) and regeneration (●) in an explanted liver. Microscopic appearances from these areas show regenerating hepatic parenchyma (*B*) or collapse (*C*) (hematoxylin and eosin; ×100 original magnification). Courtesy of Professor Bernard Portmann, King's College Hospital.

9. Coagulopathy: correction only if listed for transplant or prior to invasive procedure since it is a good tool for assessment of prognosis and monitoring of disease. Maintain platelet count > 50,000. Most common site of bleeding is gastrointestinal tract, thus prophylactic antacids recommended.
10. Ventilation: support when grade 3 encephalopathy or when requires sedation. N-acetylcysteine may improve parameters of oxygen metabolism.

11. Liver transplant: only proven therapy for ALF. Contraindications: fixed or dilated pupils, uncontrolled sepsis, severe respiratory failure. Relative contraindications: accelerating inotropic requirements, infection under therapy, cerebral perfusion pressure < 40 mm Hg for > 2 h, or history of progressive or severe neurologic problems.

12. Auxiliary liver transplant may be useful while awaiting the native liver to regenerate. No universally accepted indications in the setting of ALF.

13. Liver assist devices: pediatric experience limited. Hepatocyte transplant: experimental.

QUESTIONS

CHOOSE THE BEST ANSWER:

1. Which of the following has not been postulated to play a role in hepatic encephalopathy?
   a. Hyperammonemia.
   b. Decreased γ-aminobutyric acid (GABA).
   c. Imbalance of branched-chain to aromatic amino acid ratio.
   d. False neurotransmitters
   e. All of the above have been postulated to play a role.

2. You are asked to manage a child with acute liver failure. Your recommendations include all of the following except:
   a. Pulse oximetry monitoring.
   b. Urine output measurement.
   c. Intravenous fluids at 1.5 times maintenance.
   d. Broad-spectrum antibiotics.
   e. All of the above should be prescribed in the setting of acute liver failure.

3. What is the most common site of bleeding in liver failure?
   a. Lung.
   b. Intestines.
   c. Brain.
   d. Muscle.
   e. Bone.

4. Which is the best indicator of survival of acute liver failure?
   a. Aspartate transaminase.
   b. Alanine aminotransferase.
   c. Serum bilirubin.
   d. Prothrombin time.
   e. Factor VIII level.

END-STAGE LIVER DISEASE

SYNOPSIS

MALNUTRITION

1. Fat malabsorption occurs owing to requirement of micellar action of bile acids for absorption of long-chain fatty acids.

2. Oral intake decreased owing to increased abdominal girth with ascites, organomegaly, and anorexia of chronic disease.

3. Subcutaneous tissue depleted (decreased triceps skinfold), followed by loss of muscle mass (decreased mid-arm circumference). Fall-off in linear growth.

4. Peripheral insulin resistance.

5. Branched chain amino acids (BCAA) decrease as utilized by peripheral muscles.

6. Caloric requirement increased to 1.5–2.0 times caloric requirement for age. Catabolic rate can also be increased with increased rate of infection.

7. In children with cholestatic disease, growth hormone (GH) elevated and low insulin-like growth factor (IGF)-1. Additional doses of GH do not help, suggesting GH resistance.

8. Interventions: supplemental medium-chain triglyceride (MCT) oil, fat-soluble vitamins given fat malabsorption, low sodium diet owing to hyperaldosteronism, supplemental enteral feeds (nasogastric or nasojejunal), increased caloric-density formulas, and total parenteral nutrition (TPN) if enteral supplements not successful.

FAT-SOLUBLE VITAMINS

1. Vitamin D: measure 25-hydroxy (OH) vitamin D levels to determine deficiency. Supplement orally 25-OH vitamin D 5–7 μg/kg/d.

2. Vitamin A: Deficiency (< 100–200 mg/L) results in xerosis and night blindness. Supplement with aqueous form (5,000–15,000 IU/d). Monitor levels to avoid toxicity.

3. Vitamin K: Prothrombin time best measure of deficiency. Treat with oral vitamin K_1 5–10 mg/d. If not absorbed, deliver intramuscularly.

4. Vitamin E: first sign of deficiency: symmetric decrease in peripheral stretch reflexes. Then, cerebellar ataxia, posterior column, and peripheral neuropathy. Most accurate assessment: ratio of vitamin E levels to total serum lipids. In children age < 12 yr, ratio should be > 0.6. Oral alpha-tocopheryl polyethylene glycol-1,000 succinate doses 15–25 IU/kg/d.

PORTAL HYPERTENSION

1. Presinusoidal causes: extrahepatic (usually secondary to umbilical vein catheterization, omphalitis, congenital malformation, trauma, and intra-abdominal infections) or intrahepatic (congenital hepatic fibrosis, and schistosomiasis). Presinusoidal obstruction cases usually have normal liver function (good functional reserve).

2. Cirrhosis is most common cause of portal hypertension.
3. Sinusoidal portal hypertension diagnosed by intrahepatic wedge pressure.
4. Postsinusoidal causes: Budd-Chiari syndrome, webs in suprahepatic vena cava, veno-occlusive disease (VOD), and cardiac disease.
5. Definition: portal vein (PV) pressure > 5 mm Hg or PV-to-hepatic vein (HV) gradient of > 10 mm Hg.
6. Palpable spleen, ascites, caput medusa, and hemorrhoids. Ultrasonography with Doppler: hepatofugal flow associated with severe portal hypertension.
7. Variceal bleeding rarely occurs if PV-to-HV gradient < 12 mm Hg. Greatest likelihood of variceal bleed if extrahepatic PV obstruction. Budd-Chiari syndrome: low incidence of variceal bleed. Variceal rebleeding predicted by endoscopy appearance: most likely bleed if large, tense, red, wale marks.

MANAGEMENT OF VARICEAL BLEED

1. Sclerotherapy is first line of therapy to control variceal bleeding in children, can eradicate varices in up to 90%. Ligation may be more effective in preventing a first variceal bleed than sclerotherapy but requires minimum esophageal diameter of 10 mm for safe passage of instrument.
2. Pharmacologic therapy: vasopressin; no survival benefit. Side effects: myocardial infarction, cerebral vascular accident (stroke), and mesenteric ischemia. Octreotide: current preferred agent. Dosing: 1 µcg/kg bolus then 1 µcg/kg/h up to 5 µcg/kg/h. Effective in 86% within 40 h. Both propranolol and nadolol prevent variceal bleeding. Nadolol advantage: not metabolized by liver; given once a day.
3. Portosystemic shunts and transjugular intrahepatic portosystemic shunts (TIPS) also used if refractory to endoscopic and pharmacologic management.
4. In the case of uncontrollable bleeding, balloon tamponade may be used. The Linton tube is used for smaller children or a gastric bleed; Sengstaken-Blakemore tube is used in larger children (> 40 kg). Correct position of tube necessary to avoid inflating gastric balloon in esophagus. Inflation only for 12–24 h.
5. Transection and devascularization procedures are infrequently necessary to control acute variceal bleeding. Three techniques. High mortality.
   a. Staple-gun transection of esophagus
   b. Sugiura procedure (devascularization lower esophagus, upper gastrium then splenectomy, pyloromyotomy, vagotomy, and esophageal transection)
   c. Esophagogastric devascularization with staple-gun transection.

ASCITES

1. Underfill theory: decreased plasma volume increases activity of renin-angiotensin-aldosterone pathway causing sodium retention.
2. Overfill theory: renal sodium retention is initiating event leading to increased plasma volume.

3. Peripheral arterial vasodilation theory: primary event splanchnic arteriolar vasodilation secondary to portal hypertension, which causes sequestration of blood into splanchnic bed, decrease in circulating blood volume, and subsequent sodium and water retention.
4. 50% of patients die within 2 yr of developing ascites.
5. Pathophysiologic intra-abdominal factors: decreased plasma colloid osmotic pressure, increased capillary pressure, increased ascitic colloid osmotic fluid pressure, and decreased ascitic fluid hydrostatic pressure. When rate of hepatic lymph formation exceeds drainage, accumulates in space of Disse then escapes as ascites.
6. Ascites in liver disease without complications: clear, straw-colored or bile-tinged; protein < 2.5 g/L, cell count < 250 cells/mm^3 (mostly lymphocytes). Glucose and lactate dehydrogenase (LDH) levels similar to plasma.

MANAGEMENT OF ASCITES

Medical

1. Monitoring 24 h urine Na is a helpful guide to therapy. With appropriate sodium restriction and diuresis, urine Na should be > 15 meq/d. Once urine Na excretion falls below 15 meq/24 h, diuresis required. Spironolactone (counteracts secondary hyperaldosteronism) is rapidly, almost completely absorbed from gastrointestinal (GI) tract. If no result, start Lasix. Water restriction to 50–75% of normal daily requirement may be required if inadequate diuresis and if serum sodium < 120 meq/mL (also requires suspension of diuretic therapy).
2. In hypoalbuminemia, intravenous albumin rapidly increases colloid osmotic pressure, mobilize fluid into the intravascular space. Combine with diuretic to allow diuresis.
3. Most important, serious complication of aggressive diuresis: hypovolemia and precipitation of renal failure. Vigorous diuresis can precipitate encephalopathy.
4. In cases where ascites is medically refractory, large-volume paracentesis may be required.

Surgical

1. Leveen shunt: creates ascites drainage path from intraperitoneal cavity to jugular vein.
2. Portal systemic shunts: major disadvantages: reduced portal blood flow and precipitation of encephalopathy. Splenorenal shunt preferred since preserves forward portal flow. Good candidates: patients with extrahepatic PV obstruction. In orthotopic liver transplant (OLT) candidates, mesocaval may be better for shunting since distant from porta hepatis. Size of shunt increased until PV-to-HV gradient < 18 mm Hg.
3. TIPS (Figure 2): once placed, monitor size every 3 mo via ultrasonography with Doppler. Use in children who have failed sclerotherapy and are awaiting OLT. Reserve for patients in whom OLT will occur in 6–12 mo. Shunt patency decreases markedly with time. Contraindicated in cholangitis and hepatic infection or abscess. Polycystic liver disease, hepatic neoplasm,

right-sided heart failure, and severe hepatic failure with uncorrectable coagulopathy are also contraindications. Mortality rates 40–67% at 1 year, and incidence of encephalopathy 50% after TIPS.

SPONTANEOUS BACTERIAL PERITONITIS

1. Infection of ascites without bowel perforation or intra-abdominal abscess: *Escherichia coli* cultured in 50% of infections, *Streptococcus* in 25%.
2. High index of suspicion needed since clinical signs subtle or patients can be asymptomatic. Fever present, but abdominal pain and rebound tenderness often absent.
3. Paracentesis (incidence of bowel perforation and hematoma rare: < 1%) and ascites culture essential for diagnosis. Preferred site: linea alba below umbilicus.
4. Examine cell count. If polymorphonuclear neutrophil leukocytes (PMN) > 500/mm^3, start empiric antibiotics. Cell counts > 250/mm^3: start empiric antibiotics if clinical suspicion high, or wait and retap. PMN > 10,000/mm^3: consistent with bowel perforation or intra-abdominal abscess (multiple organisms in culture, low glucose, and high LDH).
5. Cefotaxime 85% success. Add ampicillin to cover *Enterococcus*. Avoid aminoglycosides because of renal toxicity.
6. First occurrence portends accelerated risk of death and urgency for OLT. 79% first-year mortality in adults. Recurrence common. No evidence basis for prophylaxis.

HEPATORENAL SYNDROME

1. Characteristic pattern (Table 1): urine Na < 10 meq/L, fractional excretion Na < 1%, urine–plasma creatinine ratio < 10.
2. Hallmark: intense renal vasoconstriction with coexistent systemic vasodilation. Ascites often present.

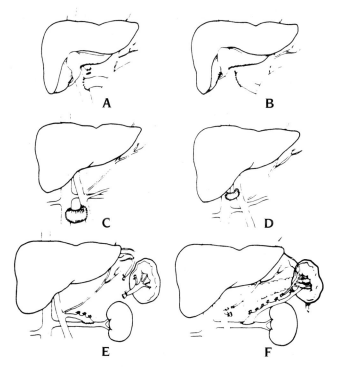

FIGURE 1 Portosystemic shunts used for emergency treatment of variceal bleeding: end-to-side portocaval shunt (A), side-to-side portocaval shunt (B), mesocaval interpositional H-graft (C), portocaval interpositional H-graft (D), central splenorenal shunt (E), and selective distal splenorenal shunt (Warren Shunt; F). Reproduced with permission from Terblanche J, Burroughs AK, Hobbs KE. Controversies in the management of bleeding esophageal varices (1). N Engl J Med 1989;320:1393.

3. Best treat with OLT. Hepatorenal syndrome associated with increased mortality before transplant, but after OLT no effect on survival.

FIGURE 2 Anatomic location of the transjugular intrahepatic portosystemic shunt. Reproduced with permission from Vargas HE, Gerber D, Abu-Elmagd K. Management of portal hypertension-related bleeding. Surg Clin North Am 1999;79:1.

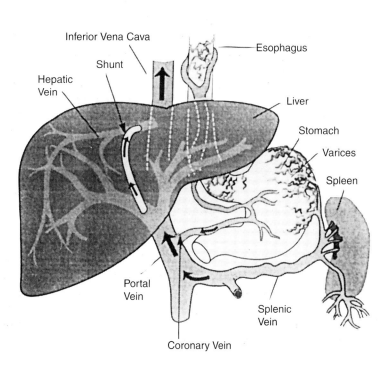

TABLE 1   HEPATORENAL SYNDROME:
           DIAGNOSTIC CRITERIA

Oliguria: < 1 mL/kg/d
Fractorial excretion sodium < 1%
Urine-to-plasma creatinine ratio < 10
↓ Glomerular filtration rate, ↑ creatinine
Absence of hypovolemia
Other kidney pathology excluded

PULMONARY INVOLVEMENT IN LIVER DISEASE

PORTOPULMONARY HYPERTENSION

1. Characterized by pulmonary artery vasoconstriction (Table 2). Rarely described in children.
2. Defined as mean pulmonary artery pressure > 25 mm Hg with pulmonary capillary wedge pressure < 15 mm Hg in absence of secondary cases of pulmonary hypertension.
3. Pathology: concentric medial hypertrophy and intimal fibrosis.
4. Diagnosis: electrocardiogram (ECG) abnormality: right ventricular hypertrophy, right atrium deviation, right bundle branch block. Right heart catheterization to document pressures, for trial of vasodilator therapy (NO, calcium channel blockers, or prostaglandins). Mean pulmonary artery pressure > 40–45 mm Hg contraindication to OLT. If pulmonary pressures < 40 mm Hg, resolution after OLT.

HEPATOPULMONARY SYNDROME

1. Triad of hypoxemia, intrapulmonary vascular dilations, and liver disease. Defined as arterial oxygen pressure (PaO_2) < 70 mm Hg in room air with alveolar to arterial (Aa) gradient of > 20 mm Hg.
2. Two types: both characterized by right to left shunt within lungs.
   a. Type 1: more common. Extensive dilation of pulmonary precapillary circulation. Able to increase PaO_2 somewhat with 100% O_2.
   b. Type 2: anatomic arteriovenous (AV) shunts within pulmonary circulation. Not able to increase PaO_2 with 100% O_2. Prognosis very poor.
3. Diagnosis: suspect if cyanosis and digital clubbing. Many with plethora of spider nevi and platypnea (increased dyspnea with standing).

4. Arterial blood gases: obtain with patient standing. Fall in PaO_2 from recumbent to standing characteristic.
5. Best method to evaluate the shunting in hepatopulmonary syndrome: contrast-enhanced echocardiogram. Normally, microbubbles trapped in lungs. In intracardiac shunt, microbubbles found immediately and opacity left ventricle; in intrapulmonary shunt, 3–6 ventricular contractions occur before microbubbles found at left heart.
6. Only definitive therapy is OLT. If unable to increase PaO_2 over 100 mm Hg on 100% O_2, not suitable candidate for OLT.
7. Sequelae in severe hepatopulmonary syndrome status-post-transplant: prolonged ventilator requirement, hypoxic graft injury, portal vein thrombosis, and intracranial thrombosis.

CENTRAL NERVOUS SYSTEM INVOLVEMENT

1. Irritability and lethargy: two most common signs in children. Mental status changes should prompt investigation for occult gastrointestinal (GI) bleeding or intracranial hemorrhage secondary to coagulopathy. Aggressive diuresis, spontaneous bacterial peritonitis, and portosystemic shunt may precipitate encephalopathy.
2. Management: restrict dietary protein and evacuate blood from GI tract, administering oral lactulose and neomycin to reduce bacterial flora.

CHOLESTATIC DISEASES: SPECIAL ISSUES

CHOLANGITIS

1. Presents with fever and elevated bilirubin, alkaline phosphatase/ gamma glutamyl transferase or serum transaminases from baseline. Common organisms: gram-negative enteric organisms. Blood cultures frequently negative. Important to initiate appropriate antibiotic treatment if clinical suspicion high.
2. Major risk factors: biliary system stasis and status-post portoenterostomy.
3. If fails to defervesce after 72 h or recurs, liver biopsy helpful. Common regimen: ampicillin or cefotaxime for 10–14 d. Prophylaxis of variable efficacy.

PRURITUS

Treatment often poorly effective. Cholestyramine usually not helpful because already low concentration of bile acids.

TABLE 2   COMPARISON AND CONTRAST: HEPATOPULMONARY SYNDROME
           AND PORTOPULMONARY HYPERTENSION

HEPATOPULMONARY SYNDROME	PORTOPULMONARY HYPERTENSION
Intrapulmonary vasodilation	Intrapulmonary vasoconstriction
Alveolar arterial gradient > 20 mm Hg	Alveolar arterial gradient usually normal
Normal mean PA pressure	Mean PA pressure > 25 mm Hg
Perform shunt fraction study	Perform right heart catheterization
Trial of 100% O_2	Vasodilator therapy trial
Often reversible with liver treatment	May not reverse with liver transplant
Poor prognosis: PaO_2 < 300 mm Hg on 100% O_2	Poor prognosis: PA pressure > 45 mm Hg
Histology: PA normal	Histology: PA abnormal; concentric medial hypertrophy

PA = pulmonary artery; PaO_2 = arterial oxygen pressure.

Try choleretics such as phenobarbital. Antihistamines seldom useful. Ursodeoxycholine (25–30 mg/kg/d in divided doses) helps reduce pruritus. Rifampin 10 mg/kg/d also successful. Naloxone (opiate antagonist) efficacious but limited by poor oral bioavailability and short half-life. Partial biliary diversion successful in treating some children.

QUESTIONS

CHOOSE THE BEST ANSWER:

1. Which of the following is not true in end-stage liver disease?
   a. Loss of muscle mass.
   b. Low insulin-like growth factor (IGF)-1.
   c. Increased aromatic amino acids.
   d. Insulin resistance.
   e. Subcutaneous tissue depletion.

2. What is the most accurate way to assess vitamin E levels?
   a. Peripheral stretch reflex examination.
   b. Serum Vitamin E levels.
   c. Peripheral nerve conduction testing.
   d. Cerebellar function testing.
   e. Ratio of vitamin E levels to serum lipid levels.

3. The following are etiologies of extrahepatic presinusoidal portal hypertension except:
   a. Umbilical vein catheterization.
   b. Schistosomiasis.
   c. Trauma.
   d. Omphalitis.
   e. Intra-abdominal infections.

4. The following are true about spontaneous bacterial peritonitis except:
   a. Most common infectious organism identified is *Escherichia coli*.
   b. Second most common infectious organism is *Streptococcus*.
   c. Diagnostic if cell count > 500/mm^3.
   d. Can be asymptomatic.
   e. Accompanied by bowel perforation.

5. The following are true about hepatorenal syndrome except:
   a. Urine Na < 10 meq/L.
   b. Fractional excretion Na < 1%.
   c. Urine–plasma creatinine ratio > 10.
   d. Not responsive to volume bolus.
   e. No urinary sediment.

TRUE OR FALSE:

6. The only definitive therapy for hepatopulmonary syndrome is liver transplantation.

7. A fall in PaO$_2$ from recumbent to standing is characteristic of hepatopulmonary syndrome.

8. Hepatopulmonary syndrome has no effect on post-transplant course.

9. Portopulmonary hypertension is always reversible with liver transplantation.

10. Portopulmonary hypertension has an abnormal alveolar arterial gradient.

LIVER TRANSPLANTATION

SYNOPSIS

1. Child survival rates: 1 yr 90%, 5–10 yr 80%.
2. Chronic liver failure second to cholestatic disease is most common indication for liver transplantation in children.

FULMINANT HEPATITIS: FACTORS ASSOCIATED WITH POOR OUTCOME

1. Non viral A–G hepatitis.
2. Development of Grade 3–4 hepatic coma.
3. Reduction in hepatic size with increasing bilirubin and decreasing transaminases.
4. Persistent severe coagulopathy internationalized normalized ration (INR) > 4.
5. In acetaminophen overdose, poor outcome if taken with another drug (ecstasy or alcohol), INR > 4, pH < 7.3, and rapid progression to hepatic coma grade 3.

CONTRAINDICATIONS TO ORTHOTOPIC LIVER TRANSPLANTATION

1. Severe systemic sepsis at time of operation.
2. Malignant hepatic tumors with extrahepatic metastases.
3. Severe irreversible extrahepatic disease.
4. Multiorgan failure: especially secondary to mitochondrial defects.
5. Alpers disease and sodium valproate toxicity (defects in respiratory chain): progression of neurodegeneration despite orthotopic liver transplantaion (OLT).
6. Recurrent disease: hepatitis B and C virus recur 90–100% post-OLT; reduced with antiviral agents before and after OLT. Autoimmune hemolytic anemia in association with giant cell hepatitis recurs in 100% post-transplant; thus, OLT not recommended.

PREPARATION FOR OLT

1. Immunization: complete series prior to OLT since contraindicated (especially live vaccines) after immunosuppression; if older than 6 mo, offer vaccines for measles, mumps, and rubella; hepatitis A virus, and hepatitis B virus (HBV).
2. Recurrent variceal bleeding should be managed with sclerotherapy or variceal ligation.
3. Treat sepsis with broad-spectrum antibiotics. Children awaiting liver transplantation for acute liver failure should be on antifungal prophylaxis.
4. Ascites should be managed with diuretics and salt restriction. Intervention with hemodialysis and hemofiltration should be considered if acute renal or hepatorenal failure develops.

5. Nutrition should be provided to prevent or reverse malnutrition and to minimize fat malabsorption and ongoing catabolism.

6. Psychological counseling and preparation of child and family is important.

LIVER TRANSPLANTATION SURGERY

1. Organ procurement: liver grafts matched by size, donor blood group, and cytomegalovirus (CMV) status. Malignancy (except localized brain tumors), uncontrolled bacterial sepsis, and HIV-positive: absolute contraindications for donors (Table 1).

2. Recipient operation: 1st venous, 2nd arterial, and 3rd biliary (duct-to-duct) anastomoses. Choledocho-jejunostomy for extrahepatic biliary atresia (EHBA) and those < 40 kg.

5. Auxiliary liver transplant (Figure 1). Native liver retained in event of graft failure. Advisable for patients with metabolic liver disease secondary to hepatic enzyme deficiency in whom liver transplant is considered owing to severe extrahepatic disease (Crigler-Najjar syndrome type 1, propionicacidemia, and OTC deficiency).

POST-TRANSPLANT MANAGEMENT

1. Ensure urine output 1 cc/kg/h, central venous pressure > 5–6 mm Hg.

2. Maintain hemoglobin (Hgb) 8–10 mg/dL to prevent hepatic artery thrombosis.

3. Immunosuppression started immediately postoperatively.

4. Broad-spectrum antibiotics for 48 h. Fluconazole and amphotericin in children with acute liver failure, or in those with second laparotomy. Low-dose trimethoprim-sulfamethoxazole (TMP-SFX) for *Pneumocystis carinii* pneumonia prophylaxis; oral nystatin and amphotericin used to prevent *Candida* for 6–12 mo. Cytomegalovirus

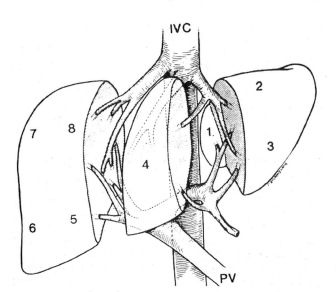

FIGURE 1   Schematic diagram of liver demonstrating eight segments. The left lateral segments 2 and 3 are most commonly used for reduction hepatectomy, split livers, living-related transplant, or auxiliary transplant.

(CMV) prophylaxis if recipient receives CMV-positive graft via acyclovir (ACV) or ganciclovir (GCV).

5. Zantac, Prilosec, or sucralfate to prevent stress gastritis.

6. Antihypertensive medications usually required owing to immunosuppression treatment.

7. Vascular thrombosis higher in children: aspirin and dipyridamole may be useful.

8. Some may require total parenteral nutrition postoperatively, but majority will begin enteral feeds between days 3–5.

POSTOPERATIVE COMPLICATIONS

EARLY

1. Infection: most common complication after transplant. Bacterial infections most common.

2. Primary graft nonfunction : occurs within 48 h. Cause unknown. Presentation: prolonged coagulopathy INR > 3, raised transaminases, rising bilirubin, and rise in serum potassium. Occasionally secondary to hyperacute rejection (diagnosed by biopsy or by identification of elevated immunoglobulins). Only appropriate therapy: retransplant.

3. Hepatic artery thrombosis: in 10%; reduced with microsurgical techniques and living related or split livers owing to increased vessel size. Ultrasonography diagnosis. Treatment: emergency thrombectomy and use of anticoagulants or thrombolytics.

4. Portal vein thrombosis: less common. Ultrasonography diagnosis. Treatment: emergency thrombectomy and use of anticoagulants or thrombolytics.

5. Acute cellular rejection: occurs 7–10 d postoperatively. Less common in infants (20%); increases in children and adults (50–60%). Laboratory results: elevated bilirubin, γ-glutamyltransferase, alkaline phosphatase, and transaminases. Histology essential: mixed inflammatory infiltrate including eosinophils at portal tract with endotheliitis (lymphoid infiltration) and bile duct inflammation. Usually treat with intravenous (IV) solumedrol in doses 20 mg/kg/d for 3 d to 45 mg/kg in total with additional increase in baseline suppression (Table 2). If insufficient improvement, may repeat;if failure, usually convert to more potent agents such as OKT3 or FK506.

6. Cyclosporine (Neoral): partially water-soluble; good absorption with peak at 2 h (half-life 8–10 h). Neoral with similar side effects to Sandimmune, especially gingival hyperplasia and hirsutism, but incidence of nephrotoxicity and hypertension less.

7. FK506: associated with serious neurologic side effects, lymphoproliferative disease, and hypertrophic cardiomyopathy.

8. Chronic rejection: < 10%. Clinical presentation: gradual onset jaundice, pruritus, pale stools (indications of biliary obstruction). Histology: damage and disappearing bile ducts (arterial obliteration and fibrosis). Nonresponse to increased immunosuppression requires retransplantation.

TABLE 1   TRANSPLANT INDICATIONS ACCORDING TO DISEASE

DISEASE	TREATMENT	TRANSPLANT INDICATION
EHBA	Kasai (success rate 60%)	Immediately unsuccessful Kasai or nutrition or hepatic complications
Alagille syndrome; PFIC; nonsyndromic biliary hypoplasia	Supportive	Cirrhosis, portal HTN, malnutrition, failure to thrive, and intractable pruritus nonresponsive to medical therapy or biliary diversion
Neonatal hepatitis	Supportive	Persistent cholestasis, rapid cirrhosis progression, and portal HTN
A1AT deficiency	Supportive	20–30% require OLT
Tyrosinemia I	NTBC with frequent AFP check, with US, MRI, or CT to monitor for HCC	Poor quality of life, no response to NTBC or hepatic ca
Wilson disease	Penicillamine and chelation	Established cirrhosis or FHF or progressive disease despite penicillamine
Cystic fibrosis	Enzymes and pulmonary therapy. Liver disease in 20%; management of portal HTN	Hepatic decompensation (falling albumin and prolonged coagulopathy unresponsive to vitamin K), severe malnutrition unresponsive to increased calories, and portal HTN unresponsive to medical therapy. < 70% lung function may indicate need for heart, lung, and liver transplant.
GSD type I	Medical or nutritional treatment	Patients with multiple hepatic adenomas or in whom metabolic control affect quality of life
GSD type III or IV		More likely to require OLT than type I owing to cirrhosis and portal HTN
Bile acid metabolism	Oral bile acid supplementation	May avoid OLT
Autoimmune hepatitis	Immunosuppression	No response to immunosuppression despite CyA, FK506, and mycophenylate and for those presenting with fulminant hepatic failure.
Chronic HBV and HCV	Usually no symptoms of disease in childhood	Recurrence likely 90% after OLT
Fibropolycystic liver disease	Rare indication for OLT	Patients with hepatic decompensation with portal HTN or in whom hepatomegal affects quality of life
Primary immunodeficiency	Most common: CD40 ligand deficiency (hyper-IgM syndrome) where recurrent *Cryptosporidium* in gut and biliary tree leads to sclerosing cholangitis	Consider bone marrow transplant before liver disease develops or combined BMT/liver transplant.
Inborn errors of metabolism	Selection based on quality of life, medical management, and morbidity and mortality of primary disease and outcome of OLT	Crigler-Najjar syndrome type 1: select for OLT prior to irreversible brain damage and when phototherapy affects quality of life. Good candidate for auxiliary OLT. Also true for OTC deficiency
Familial hypercholesterolemia		Perform prior to irreversible coronary artery disease. Possible auxiliary OLT.
Organic acidemias (propionic acidemia and methylmalonic acidemia)	Palliative treatment since affects all parts of body.	Propionic acidemia: auxiliary OLT is accepted treatment.
Urea cycle defects (eg OTC deficiency)	Withdraw dietary protein and treat with oral sodium benzoate or phenylbutyrate	Consider for patients in whom dietary management ineffective. OLT corrects hyperammonemia but not completely and does not reverse prior brain damage (so need to do prior irreversible neurotoxicity).
Primary oxalosis: deficiency in hepatic enzyme alanine glycoxylate aminotransferase		OLT prior to renal stone development or severe systemic oxalosis. If patients present in renal failure, combine renal and liver transplant. Auxiliary liver transplant not suitable since systemic oxalosis deposition.
Benign liver tumors (hemangiomas, adenomas, focal nodular hyperplasia, and hemangio-endotheliomas)		Consider if liver function affected or unacceptable increase in size without capability for resection
Malignant hepatocellular carcinoma; hepatoblastoma		Unresectable or refractory to chemotherapy. Only if no extrahepatic metastases: check with CT of chest and abdomen and AFP levels. Rhabdomyosarcoma: do not transplant since extent of tumor is large and usually early extrahepatic metastases.

A1AT = α_1-antitrypsin; AFP = α-fetoprotein; CT = computed tomography; EHBA = extrahepatic biliary atresia; FHF = fulminant hepatic failure; GSD = glycogen storage disease; HBV = hepatitis B virus; HCC = hepatocellular carcinoma; HCV = hepatitis C virus; HTN = hypertension; IgM = immunoglobulin M; MRI = magnetic resonance imaging; NTBC = 2(2-nitro4-trifluoromethylbenzoyl)-1,3-cyclohexanedione; OLT = orthotopic liver transplant; OTC = ornithine transcarbamylase; PFIC = progressive familial intrahepatic cholestasis; US = ultrasonography.

TABLE 2   POSTOPERATIVE IMMUNOSUPPRESSION

| TIME OF INTRODUCTION (MO) | TROUGH LEVELS* | |
	CYCLOSPORIN A (MICROEMULSION) (5 MG/KG BD)	TACROLIMUS (0.15 MG/KG)
0–1	180–230 ng/L	10–15 ng/mL
1–3	100–160 ng/L	8–12 ng/mL
3–12	70–110 ng/L	5–8 ng/mL
>12	60–90 ng/L	3–5 ng/mL

TIME OF INTRODUCTION	IMMUNOSUPPRESSANT
3–12	Prednisolone 2 mg/kg
12	Azathioprine 2 mg/kg
—	Mycophenolate mofetil 1–3 g/d

*Whole-blood monoclonal assay.

9. Biliary complications:
   a. Biliary strictures: secondary to anastomotic stricture owing to edema or to hepatic artery ischemia. Management: ursodeoxycholate, which allows edema to settle. If persists, manage radiologically with percutaneous cholangiography and dilatation. If failure, then surgery.
   b. Biliary leaks: secondary to leaks from cut edge of liver or to hepatic artery ischemia. Majority settle with conservative management; if persist, peritonitis, abscesses, and sepsis require surgical reconstruction.

LATE

1. CMV infection occurs 5–6 wk post-transplant; highest risk if CMV-positive graft in CMV recipient. Treat with GCV. Prophylaxis with ACV and IV immunoglobulin (Ig) better than GCV alone.
2. Posttransplant lymphoproliferative disease (PTLD): diarrhea, weight loss, and gastrointestinal (GI) bleed. Associated with Epstein-Barr virus (EBV) infection and reactivation. Diagnose via tissue biopsy (B-cell proliferation and lymphomatous features). First line of treatment: reduction of immunosuppression. ACV or GCV may be used. Chemotherapy may be required.
3. Late biliary strictures may be due to hepatic artery ischemia or thrombosis and can lead to recurrent cholangitis, hepatic abscess, and secondary biliary cirrhosis.
4. Portal vein stenosis secondary to anastomotic stricture can lead to varices, splenomegaly, and portal hypertension. Initial treatment is venoplasty through interventional radiology, but surgical reconstruction with mesoportal shunt may be required.
5. GI perforation: infrequent complication after liver transplant.

PROGNOSIS

1. In children receiving one graft, 1 yr survival > 90%; 5–10 yr survival 60–80%. In children receiving more than one graft, 1 yr survival 50%.

2. Protein malnutrition at time of liver transplant has significant influence on morbidity and mortality.

QUALITY OF LIFE AFTER TRANSPLANTATION

1. Nutritional rehabilitation: 80% will achieve normal growth and body habitus.
2. Normal puberty.
3. Nephrotoxicity with CyA/FK506 inevitable, but only 5% develop chronic renal failure requiring renal transplant as adults.
4. Normal psychosocial development within 1–2 yr but toll on family: 20% of marriages with transplantation in child dissolve.

QUESTIONS

CHOOSE THE BEST ANSWER:

1. The most common cause for liver transplantation in children is:
   a. Acute liver failure.
   b. Metabolic disease.
   c. Cancers.
   d. Cholestatic liver disease.
   e. Cirrhosis.

2. What is the usual success rate of a Kasai portoenterostomy for extrahepatic biliary atresia?
   a. 15%.
   b. 30%.
   c. 50%.
   d. 60%.
   e. 80%.

MATCH THE DISEASE WITH ITS INDICATION(S) FOR LIVER TRANSPLANT (MAY BE MORE THAN ONE ANSWER):

a. Failure to respond to chelation therapy.
b. Fulminant hepatic failure.
c. Cirrhosis.
d. Severe malnutrition unresponsive to nutritional therapies.
e. Multiple hepatic adenomas.
f. Not responding to immunosuppressive therapy.
g. Hepatomegaly affecting quality of life.
h. When phototherapy affects quality of life.
i. Intractable pruritus.
j. Before irreversible neurologic consequences.
k. Hepatocellular carcinoma.
l. Before irreversible coronary artery disease.
m. Ineffective dietary management.
n. Unresectable and nonresponsive to chemotherapy.
o. Not responding to NTBC.
p. Do not transplant.
q. Prior to renal stone development.

3. Primary oxalosis.
4. Autoimmune hemolytic anemia with giant cell hepatitis.

5. Wilson disease.
6. Autoimmune hepatitis.
7. Glycogen storage disease I.
8. Hemangiomas.
9. Hepatoblastoma.
10. Crigler-Najjar type I.
11. Tyrosinemia I.
12. Familial hypercholesterolemia.
13. Rhabdomyosarcomas.
14. Fibropolycystic liver disease.
15. Ornithine transcarbamylase deficiency.
16. Cystic fibrosis.
17. Glycogen storage disease III and IV.

CHOOSE THE BEST ANSWER:

18. The following are associated with poor outcome in acetaminophen overdose except:
    a. Arterial pH < 7.3.
    b. Obesity.
    c. International normalized ratio > 4.
    d. Rapid progression to Grade 3 hepatic coma.
    e. Taken with another drug.

19. The following are absolute contraindications to liver transplant except:
    a. Human immunodeficiency virus infection.
    b. Severe systemic sepsis at time of operation.
    c. Severe extrahepatic disease irreversible by orthotopic liver transplant.
    d. Multiorgan failure.
    e. Hepatitis B or C infection.
    f. Valproic acid toxicity.

20. Which segments of the liver are used in auxiliary transplantation?
    a. 1,4.
    b. 2,3.
    c. 3,5.
    d. 5,6.
    e. None of the above.

21. What is the order in which re-anastomosis occurs in the recipient during liver transplant?
    a. Arterial, venous, biliary.
    b. Venous, arterial, biliary.
    c. Biliary, arterial, venous.
    d. Biliary, venous, arterial.
    e. Arterial, biliary, venous.
    f. Venous, biliary, arterial.

22. When do Cytomegalovirus (CMV) infections occur in the posttransplant period in the recipient of a CMV-positive graft?
    a. Immediately.
    b. 1–2 weeks.
    c. 3–4 weeks.
    d. 5–6 weeks.
    e. 6–12 months.

MATCH THE COMPLICATIONS WITH THE DRUG:
a. Salt and water retention.
b. Nephrotoxicity.
c. Cardiomyopathy.

23. Tacrolimus.
24. Cyclosporin A.
25. Steroids.

GALLBLADDER DISEASE

SYNOPSIS

1. In the United States, highest rate of cholesterol gallstones is in Native Americans, especially in women after puberty. Bile cholesterol saturation increases in both genders after puberty, but the rate of occurrence is higher in females. In males, the bile acid pool increases postpuberty, but not in women.
2. Medical conditions associated with gallstones in children: cystic fibrosis and hemolytic disease.

TYPES OF GALLSTONES

1. Cholesterol: gallstone formation requires the following:
   a. Hypersecretion of cholesterol into bile (via adenosine triphophate [ATP] transporters ABCG5 and ABCG8).
   b. Decreased gallbladder motility.
   c. Increased mucin production.
   d. Increased conversion of primary bile salts to more hydrophobic bile secondary bile salts.
   e. Increased rate of formation of cholesterol crystals.
   f. Associated with female gender and positive family history; parity in female adolescents.
2. Black pigment: excess conjugated bilirubin in the bile:
   a. Hemolysis and disorders of dysfunctional erythropoiesis.
   b. Diseases increasing bilirubin enterohepatic circulation (eg, Crohn disease, distal small intestinal resection, cystic fibrosis, and bile salt malabsorption).
   c. Medications are also risk factors, especially furosemide and cyclosporine.
   d. Deconjugation of conjugated bilirubin in bile occurs with resulting unconjugated bilirubin, which then precipitates as an insoluble calcium salt.
3. Brown pigment:
   a. Occurs in the presence of cholesterol or black pigment stones, which cause obstruction and then infection.
   b. Intrahepatic brown pigment stones associated with decreased multidrug resistant protein (MDR)3 and phosphatidylcholine transfer protein expression, and increased 3-hydroxy-3-methyl-glutaryl coenzyme A reductase (HMG CoA) reductase activity.

CLINICAL FEATURES

1. Congenital anomalies: generally asymptomatic.
2. Acute disease:
   a. Biliary colic: steady, intense pain at right upper quadrant and epigastrium. Pain may radiate to the shoulder. Often emesis occurs.
   b. Acute cholecystitis: fever, right upper quadrant pain, Murphy sign, and leukocytosis. If no gallstones present but inflammation exists: acute acalculous cholecystitis (usually occurs in setting of major medical problems and infections).
3. Chronic disease:
   a. Chronic gallstone disease: usually with biliary colic but short durations.
   b. Chronic acalculous cholecystitis: associated with gallbladder dyskinesia.
   c. Sphincter of Oddi dysfunction: similar complaints to those with gallbladder dyskinesia, but cholecystectomy will not provide relief. Associated with acute recurrent pancreatitis. Obstruction at level of sphincter. Endoscopic retrograde cholangiopancreatography (ERCP) with manometry provides diagnosis. Treatment of choice: sphincterotomy.
4. Gallstones can also lead to pancreatitis.

ASSESSMENT OF FUNCTION AND IMAGING OF THE GALLBLADDER

1. Radiograph: radiopaque stones seen in 10–15%. Rare condition of "milk of calcium cholelithiasis"; bile formed of calcium carbonate; multiple calculi on radiograph.
2. Ultrasonography: investigation of choice. Best in patient fasted for ≥ 4 h. Can measure gallbladder length, diameter of common bile duct (normal: < 1 mm in neonates, < 2 mm in infants, < 4 mm in children, < 7 mm in adolescents), and gallbladder wall thickness (when inflamed > 3 mm) and evaluate for stones > 1 mm. Polyps may appear as stones on ultrasonography.
3. Computed tomography (CT) and magnetic resonance imaging (MRI): CT not as reliable as ultrasonography for gallstones. Magnetic resonance cholangiopancreatography (MRCP) more reliable than CT for investigation of hepatobiliary tree and pancreatic duct.
4. ERCP: investigation of choice to define extrahepatic pancreatic duct systems. Allows for performance of manometry at the sphincter of Oddi to diagnose sphincter of Oddi dysfunction and interventions. However, children undergoing ERCP have more complications than adults.
5. Hepatobiliary scintigraphy (HBS): biliary disease assessment and function assessment. Lack of gallbladder visualization in cholecystitis by HBS (radioactively labeled iminodiacetic acid is secreted from the liver but unable to enter the gallbladder owing to obstruction of the cystic duct). Perforation of the gallbladder can be seen by spillage of the radionuclide into the peritoneal cavity. Useful for chronic acalculous cholecystitis (gallbladder ejection fraction < 35%).

SURGICAL MANAGEMENT

Laparoscopic cholecystectomy: procedure of choice. Absolute contraindications: acute gallstone pancreatitis, prior upper abdominal surgery, and 2nd–3rd-trimester pregnancy.

MEDICAL MANAGEMENT

Targets cholesterol gallstones only. Nonsurgical therapy consists of bile salt administration or extracorporeal shock wave lithotripsy.

NONGALLSTONE DISEASES OF THE GALLBLADDER

ACALCULOUS CHOLECYSTITIS

1. Uncommon in children: acute < 1 mo, chronic > 1 mo.
2. Acute:
   a. Associated with concurrent systemic infection, recent surgery, and trauma.
   b. Risk factors: prolonged fasting, total parenteral nutrition (TPN), and sepsis.
   c. Present with fever, right upper quadrant pain, and emesis. Leukocytosis and hyperbilirubinemia common.
   d. Ultrasonography shows gallbladder wall > 3.5 mm, hydrops, sludge, and pericholecystic fluid.
   e. Treat with cholecystectomy when deterioration. If managed conservatively (through antibiotics and observation), gallbladder will return to normal function.
3. Chronic:
   a. Usually female, otherwise healthy, with history of right upper quadrant pain; normal white blood count and bilirubin.
   b. Gallbladder normal on ultrasonography. Test of choice: cholecystokinin-stimulated HBS.
   c. Treatment: cholecystectomy.

ACUTE HYDROPS OF THE GALLBLADDER

1. Independent of obstruction or inflammatory disease. Gallstones not present, and gallbladder not acutely inflamed, bile sterile, and extrahepatic bile duct is normal in size. Age: early infancy to adolescence. More boys than girls.
2. Cause not known. One-half have enlarged mesenteric lymph nodes. Temporal relationship to preceding infection, especially streptococcal and staphylococcal. Leptospirosis may also be causal. Acute dilation associated with Kawasaki disease, Sjögren syndrome and systemic sclerosis. Occurs as complication of nephrotic syndrome, familial Mediterranean fever, and leukemia.
3. Onset acute: crampy abdominal pain, nausea, and vomiting. Pain continuous and more intense with time. Frequent preceding history of febrile illness. Examination: upper abdominal tenderness especially on right indicates possible mass. Fever absent or slight; jaundice uncommon.
4. Ultrasonography: massive, echo-free gallbladder with normal bile ducts.

5. Treatment: noninvasive. Prognosis excellent. Spontaneous resolution occurs within few weeks, and gallbladder function returns to normal. Aspiration of gallbladder under ultrasonography or drainage via cholecystostomy occasionally may be considered if rupture appears imminent. Avoid surgery.

GALLBLADDER MASSES
1. Benign: rare in children, usually polyps.
   a. 4 types of polyps: cholesterol, inflammatory, adenomyoma, and lipoma.
   b. Can present with symptoms or biliary colic.
   c. Resect polyps > 1 cm in diameter and solitary polyps. In patients with Peutz-Jeghers syndrome, manage conservatively unless biliary colic present.
2. Malignant:
   a. Carcinoma arises in those with history of acute or chronic cholecystitis.
   b. Poor prognosis 5% survival in 5 years.
   c. 80% are adenocarcinomas, associated with abnormal expression of TP53. Squamous cell adenocanthoma accounts for 20%.
   d. Treatment: radical cholecystectomy, ERCP placement of stents, and palliative radiation therapy.

CONGENITAL ABNORMALITIES
1. Absent gallbladder: can be without symptoms or associated with other conditions (extrahepatic biliary atresia).
2. Double gallbladder: can be true duplication, or just of gallbladder, or consist of bilobed gallbladder. Usually asymptomatic.
3. Phyrgian cap: abnormal folding of gallbladder, but functions normally.
4. Aberrant vascular supply: cystic artery can arise aberrantly from the left hepatic artery instead of the right hepatic artery (important during cholecystectomy).
5. Mirizzi syndrome: rare complication; gallstone impacted at cystic duct or Hartmann pouch (outpouching of the gallbladder wall at junction of the neck of the gallbladder and the cystic duct) and extrinsically compresses common bile duct, resulting in jaundice. Usually in elderly. There are two types: I; hepatic duct stricture by associated inflammation; II; calculus erodes into hepatic duct: cholecystocholedochal fistula.

QUESTIONS

TRUE OF FALSE:
1. Throughout childhood, girls are more likely than boys to develop gallstones.
2. Black gallstones are more common in women than men.
3. Hydrops of the gallbladder should be treated with cholecystectomy.
4. In the United States, Native Americans have the highest prevalence of gallstone disease.
5. Phyrgian cap anomaly of the gallbladder is associated with normal function.
6. The diameter of the common bile duct in children should be < 4 mm.
7. Medical management is useful for all types of gallstones.

CHOOSE THE BEST ANSWER:
8. The following are associated with acute hydrops of the gallbladder except:
   a. Kawasaki disease.
   b. Sjögren syndrome.
   c. Nephrotic syndrome.
   d. Familial Mediterranean fever.
   e. Gallstones.

MATCH THE CONDITION OR CHARACTERISTIC WITH THE TYPE OF GALLSTONE.
a. Brown pigment stones.
b. Black pigment stones.
c. Cholesterol stones.

9. Infection.
10. Furosemide exposure.
11. Decreased MDR3 expression.
12. Positive family history.
13. Sickle cell disease.
14. Increased HMG CoA reductase activity.
15. Multiparity.
16. Crohn disease.

ANSWERS

NEONATAL CHOLESTASIS
1. True.
2. False. Absence of gallbladder on a fasting ultrasonography is not definitively diagnostic of biliary atresia.
3. False. Suggestive but not diagnostic.
4. True.
5. d. Urine-reducing substances may produce false-negative if not receiving a galactose-containing formula or vomiting in galactosemia (verify instead with measurement of red blood cell count galactose 1-phosphate uridyltransferase provided no recent blood transfusions).
6. e.
7. b. The case is consistent with neonatal hepatitis.

INTRAHEPATIC BILE DUCT DISEASE
1. True.
2. False. Also seen in autosomal dominant polycystic kidney disease and other forms of intrahepatic bile duct disease.

3. b.
4. a.
5. d.
6. c.
7. a.
8. b.
9. c.

EXTRAHEPATIC BILE DUCT DISEASE
1. False. Gallbladder may be present.
2. False. Need to rule out Alagille syndrome.
3. True.
4. True.
5. False. Female-to-male ratio 4:1.
6. False.
7. False.
8. a.
9. e.
10. True.
11. False.

VIRAL HEPATITIS
1. c.
2. d.
3. c.
4. a, c.
5. b, c.
6. e.
7. c.
8. False.
9. True.
10. False. 90%.
11. b.
12. c.
13. d.
14. a.
15. a, b.
16. a, e.
17. c, d.
18. b.
19. f.
20. a.
21. c.
22. d.
23. b.
24. b.
25. b.
26. a.
27. b.
28. c.
29. a.
30. a.
31. a.
32. c.
33. a.
34. False. HIV coinfection with HCV predicts more severe fibrosis in regards to liver disease.
35. True.

BACTERIAL, PARASITIC, AND OTHER INFECTIONS
1. c. Pyogenic liver abscesses should be treated with percutaneous drainage and intravenous antibiotics.
2. b. Suggestive history and physical and isolation of causative organisms from cervical or urethral culture confirm the diagnosis of Fitz-Hugh–Curtis syndrome.
3. d. Human schistosomiasis occurs when schistosoma penetrate human skin.
4. f.
5. a.
6. e.
7. d.
8. b.
9. c.
10. False. Most cat scratch disease is self-limited and resolves without therapy.
11. True.
12. False. *P. falciparum* can be chloroquine resistant.
13. True.

THE LIVER, AIDS, AND OTHER IMMUNE DISORDERS
1. True.
2. True.
3. False.
4. True.
5. False. *Cryptosporidium* is.
6. True.
7. True.
8. a.
9. b.
10. c.
11. e.
12. d.

AUTOIMMUNE LIVER DISEASE
1. c.
2. e. If requires too-high steroids for too long; treat with azathioprine.
3. True.
4. True.
5. c.

DRUG-INDUCED LIVER INJURY
1. d.
2. e. Arterial pH < 7.3.
3. b.
4. b.
5. b.
6. c.
7. a.
8. i.
9. f.
10. g.
11. d.
12. e.
13. h.

LIVER TUMORS

1. e.
2. a.
3. e.
4. d.
5. e. Seen in glycogen storage diseases I, III, and IV.
6. a.

CARBOHYDRATE METABOLISM DISORDERS

1. True.
2. h.
3. b.
4. i.
5. e.
6. a.
7. c.
8. g.
9. f.
10. j.

AMINO ACID METABOLISM DISORDERS

1. True. X-linked.
2. False. May require allopurinol or protein load to see laboratory result abnormalities.
3. True.
4. b.
5. c.
6. a.
7. a.
8. c.
9. b.

INHERITED ABNORMALITIES IN MITOCHONDRIAL FATTY ACID OXIDATION

1. a.
2. b.
3. f.
4. d.
5. e.
6. c.
7. g.
8. True.
9. False. Elevated plasma, especially free, carnitine is seen in this disorder.
10. True.
11. False. Only lifesaving in primary carnitine deficiency.

BILE ACID SYNTHESIS AND METABOLISM DISORDERS

1. a.
2. d.
3. e.
4. False. The neutral pathway is.
5. False. Immaturity is present.
6. True.
7. True.
8. a.
9. a.

BILIRUBIN METABOLISM DISORDERS

1. e. Findings of Dubin-Johnson syndrome.
2. d.
3. True. Oral contraceptives increase jaundice, as does pregnancy.
4. False. Although males may have higher total serum bilirubin levels, the ratio of female-to-male prevalence is 1:1.
5. False.
6. True.
7. b.
8. b.
9. b.
10. a.
11. a.
12. c.
13. a.
14. a.
15. a.
16. b.
17. c.

BILIRUBIN TRANSPORT DISORDERS

1. a.
2. c.
3. c.
4. b.
5. c.
6. a.
7. b.
8. b.
9. a.
10. c.
11. b.

α_1-ANTITRYPSIN DEFICIENCY

1. d. α_1-Antitrypsin phenotype level.
2. b.
3. a. Accumulates in endoplasmic reticulum.
4. True.
5. False. Can consider in rare specific clinical situations.
6. True. Similar presentation and PiZZ can also not excrete on HIDA.

ZELLWEGER SYNDROME AND OTHER DISORDERS

1. a.
2. a, b.
3. d.
4. e, f.
5. h.
6. k.
7. i.
8. a, b, j.
9. b.
10. d. X-linked

LYSOSOMAL ACID LIPASE DEFICIENCIES

1. a.
2. b.

3. a.
4. b.
5. b.
6. b.
7. a.
8. b.

WILSON DISEASE

1. False. Most losses via skin (30%); 20% excreted via bile; 50% not absorbed.
2. False. 50% not absorbed.
3. True.
4. False. Sensory central nervous system spared.
5. e.
6. c. Normal in infant age < 6 months.
7. d.
8. e.
9. c. May use if pretreated with prednisone 0.5 mg/kg for 2–3 d; then restart with lower dose of penicillamine.
10. c. Slow effect. Takes 1–2 wk to induce metallo-thionein.
11. e.

SYSTEMIC CONDITIONS AFFECTING THE LIVER

1. True.
2. False. Steatosis.
3. a.
4. d. Neonatal lupus.
5. e.
6. c.
7. a.
8. e.
9. b.
10. c.
11. e.
12. a.
13. c.
14. b.
15. d.
16. b.
17. f. One-third at autopsy.
18. c.
19. e.

ACUTE LIVER FAILURE

1. b. Associated with increased γ-aminobutyric acid.
2. c. IVF should be at two-thirds maintenance to reduce risk of cerebral edema.
3. b.
4. d.

END-STAGE LIVER DISEASE

1. c. Decreased branched chain amino acids. No change in aromatic amino acids
2. e.
3. b. Cause of intrahepatic presinusoidal portal hyper-tension.

4. e. No perforation.
5. c. < 10.
6. True.
7. True.
8. False. Associated with prolonged ventilation, hypoxic injury to graft, portal vein thrombosis, and intracranial thrombosis.
9. False.
10. False. Normal.

LIVER TRANSPLANTATION

1. d.
2. d.
3. q. May perform isolated liver transplant if no significant kidney pathology.
4. p.
5. a, b, c.
6. b, f.
7. e.
8. g.
9. n. Without extrahepatic metastases.
10. h, j.
11. k, o.
12. l.
13. p.
14. c, g.
15. j, m.
16. c, d.
17. c.
18. b.
19. e.
20. b.
21. b.
22. d.
23. c.
24. b.
25. a.

GALLBLADDER DISEASE

1. False. Similar until puberty, then more females than males.
2. False. Equal prevalence.
3. False. Conservative therapy; hold off cholecystectomy as much as possible.
4. True.
5. True.
6. True.
7. False. Only useful for cholesterol stones.
8. e.
9. a.
10. b.
11. a.
12. c.
13. b.
14. a.
15. c.
16. b.

CLINICAL MANIFESTATIONS AND MANAGEMENT:
The Pancreas

CONGENITAL ANOMALIES

SYNOPSIS

EMBRYOLOGY

1. Pancreas forms via fusion of dorsal and ventral foregut buds.
2. Ventral foregut bud: forms dominant pancreatic and bile duct, posterior head of the pancreas, and posterior part of uncinate process.
3. Dorsal foregut bud: forms anterior part of pancreatic head, body of pancreas, and tail of pancreas. Homeobox gene *HLXB9* necessary for dorsal bud formation.
4. Fusion of the ventral and dorsal duct systems in second month of fetal development forms the main pancreatic duct of Wirsung. If the proximal portion of the dorsal duct remains, it forms the accessory duct of Santorini. Failure of fusion of the ventral and dorsal ducts leads to pancreas divisum.
5. Congenital anomalies of pancreas are linked to anomalies in the gene encoding homeodomain protein PDX1.

PANCREATIC TISSUE ANOMALIES

ANNULAR PANCREAS

1. Complete encirclement of the second part of the duodenum by a thin, ring-like flat band of pancreatic tissue. Frequency: 1/20,000 births.
2. Results from failure of atrophy of the left ventral foregut bud. 75% of cases are associated with other congenital malformations.
3. Presentation: duodenal obstruction at any age; one-third of cases symptomatic in neonatal period. Severity of obstruction determines age of presentation.
4. In newborn period, diagnosis based on typical double-bubble sign on radiograph. In older patients, upper gastrointestinal (UGI) series may be useful, or computed tomography. Magnetic resonance cholangiopancreatography (MRCP) can also demonstrate anomaly.
5. Management: surgery. Duodenoduodenostomy recommended as bypass operation. Prognosis excellent.

ECTOPIC PANCREAS

1. Pancreatic tissue lacking anatomic and vascular continuity with the main body of the pancreas. Most common locations: pylorus, duodenum, and Meckel diverticulum.
2. Presentation: in most cases, asymptomatic, usually incidental finding. Can also present with hemorrhage owing to ulcerations, pain secondary to pancreatitis and obstruction and perhaps malignant transformation.
3. Diagnosis: endoscopy or radiography or surgery. Definitive diagnosis histologic.
4. Management: if symptomatic, surgical.

PANCREATIC AGENESIS AND HYPOPLASIA

1. Complete agenesis of the pancreas is a lethal condition.
2. Partial agenesis: endocrine and exocrine functions are normal in general. Agenesis of the dorsal pancreas has been described in diabetes and pancreatitis.
3. Agenesis of the acinar tissue occurs in Shwachman-Diamond syndrome.

DUCTAL ANOMALIES

PANCREAS DIVISUM

1. The ventral and dorsal ducts remain separated and the dorsal pancreas empties into the duodenum via the smaller accessory papilla.
2. Clinical presentation: pancreatitis; causal relationship controversial.
3. Diagnosis: endoscopic retrograde cholangiopancreatography (ERCP) or MRCP.
4. Treatment: endoscopic enlargement of accessory papilla or surgical transduodenal sphincteroplasty.

COMMON CHANNEL SYNDROME

1. Abnormally long common pancreatobiliary channel owing to failure of the junction of the common bile duct and main pancreatic duct to move toward the duodenal wall. The common pancreatobiliary channel usually exceeds 10 mm in length (normal 5 mm) in children, allowing pancreaticobiliary reflux.
2. Presentation: choledochal cyst and pancreatitis. Common channel syndrome identified in 75% of children with choledochal cyst.
3. Diagnosis: ultrasonography, MRCP, or ERCP.
4. Management: excision of choledochal cyst and Roux-en-Y hepaticoenterostomy. Cholangitis and pancreatitis are most frequent complications. Malignancy of the biliary enteric anastomosis reported many years after excision.

CONGENITAL PANCREATIC CYST

1. Uncommon. Unilocular or multiple congenital cysts lined by epithelium.
2. Presentation: asymptomatic, abdominal mass, or pancreatitis. May be associated with other anomalies (polydactyly and anorectal malformations).
3. Multilocular cysts may be an isolated pancreatic lesion or part of von Hippel-Lindau disease.

ENTERIC DUPLICATION CYSTS

1. Gastric or duodenal duplications with pancreatic ductal communications are uncommon.
2. Symptoms: failure to thrive, abdominal pain, and pancreatitis.
3. Diagnosis: UGI, ultrasonography, and MRCP.
4. Management: excision.

QUESTIONS

MATCH THE ANATOMIC STRUCTURE TO ITS ORIGIN:
a. Dorsal bud of the foregut.
b. Ventral bud of the foregut.
c. Dorsal bud of the midgut.
d. Ventral bud of the midgut.

1. Anterior part of the pancreatic head.
2. Posterior part of the pancreatic head.
3. Main pancreatic duct.
4. Extrahepatic bile duct.
5. Pancreatic body.
6. Tail of the pancreas.

CHOOSE THE BEST ANSWER:
7. Annular pancreas:
   a. Occurs at the third portion of the duodenum.
   b. Is histologically normal.
   c. Results from failure of atrophy of the dorsal bud.
   d. Is not associated with congenital malformations.
   e. Should be directly dissected.

8. Pancreas divisum:
   a. Results from lack of fusion of the ventral and dorsal pancreatic ducts.
   b. Is easily diagnosed with ultrasonography.
   c. Is treated by pancreaticoenterostomy.
   d. Is associated with ectopic pancreatic tissue.
   e. All of the above.

9. Common channel syndrome:
   a. Occurs when the common pancreatobiliary channel is ≥ 10 mm in length.
   b. Results from failure of the junction of the common bile duct and main pancreatic duct to move toward the duodenal wall.
   c. Is associated with choledochal cyst and pancreatitis.
   d. All of the above.
   e. None of the above.

TRUE OR FALSE:
10. Complete pancreatic agenesis is a lethal condition.
11. Partial agenesis of the pancreas is often symptomatic.

PANCREATIC TUMORS

SYNOPSIS

Childhood pancreatic cancer: < 5% of all childhood malignancies in children age < 15 yr.

CYSTIC TUMORS

PSEUDOCYSTS
Most common cystic lesions encountered in childhood: 75% of pancreatic cystic lesions. Occurs either secondary to trauma or chronic pancreatitis.

SEROUS CYSTADENOMA
1. Two types: serous microcystic adenoma and serous oligocystic adenoma.
2. Serous microcystic adenoma: female predominance. Benign tumors made of numerous small cysts arranged around a central stellate scar. More commonly found at pancreatic body and tail; One-third of lesions found incidentally; two-thirds present owing to pressure on adjacent structures. After histologic diagnosis confirmed, surgery usually not necessary unless symptomatic.
3. Serous oligocystic adenomas: benign tumors with equal sex predominance. Etiology unknown; possibly cytomegalovirus. Most located at head or body of pancreas with large cysts in tumor. Resection necessary if symptomatic.

MUCINOUS CYSTADENOMA
1. Benign cystic pancreatic tumor. Female preponderance.
2. Usually located at tail of pancreas. Consists of solitary large cyst with mucin-secreting epithelial cells.
3. Malignant potential exists; wide surgical excision recommended.

CYSTADENOCARCINOMA
1. Serous cystadenocarcinoma has not been reported in the pediatric literature.
2. Mucinous cystadenocarcinoma: similar to benign counterpart, but tumor is invasive, spreading locally. Prognosis excellent if resection is complete.

MATURE CYSTIC TERATOMAS
1. Benign extragonadal germ cell cysts derived of all 3 germinal layers.
2. Treatment of choice: excision.

PAPILLARY CYSTIC TUMOR
1. Rare neoplasms in children. Occur most frequently in young females (> 90%), especially Asian and black adolescent girls.

2. Presentation: usually with vague gastrointestinal complaints without endocrine or exocrine pancreatic dysfunction. Tumors slow growing and of low malignant potential with body and tail of pancreas more frequently affected. Tumors are round or oval, encased by capsule with solid and cystic areas. Microscopically, sheets and cords of polygonal cells making pseudopapillary structures or pseudorosettes. No pancreatic hormones present allowing discernment from nonfunctioning endocrine tumors.

3. Treatment: complete excision.

4. Abnormalities in adenomatous polyposis coli (APC) or β-catenin pathways.

APPROACH TO INVESTIGATION OF CYSTIC TUMORS

1. Ultrasonography most useful initial test and can confirm cystic nature.

2. Computed tomography (CT), magnetic resonance imaging (MRI), and magnetic resonance cholangiopancreatography can help determine nature of a cyst and its precise relationship to the pancreatic duct and surrounding tissues.

3. Many require surgery for definitive diagnosis, but intraoperative frozen section may be only 50–60% sensitive. Thus usually resection required, unless diagnosis secure based on both imaging and pathology.

ADENOCARCINOMA

1. Exists in two forms: arises from ductal or acinar tissue, occurring just about equally in children. Genetic and environmental factors play a role.

2. Associated conditions: hamartomatous polyposis syndromes, celiac disease or dermatitis herpetiformis, degreasing agent exposure, smoking, uterine myomas, oophorectomy, higher social class, increased consumption of animal fat or protein and wine consumption, organ allograft recipients, and Down syndrome.

DUCTAL ADENOCARCINOMA

1. Spreads locally.

2. Presentation: abdominal pain and weight loss; > one half present with obstructive jaundice. Tumors usually at head of pancreas, generating a fibrotic reaction.

3. CT demonstrates irregular heterogeneous enhancing lesions without a visible capsule.

4. Histologically: well-differentiated ductal carcinoma cells with mucin but lacking zymogen. Almost all are carcinoembryonic antigen positive.

5. 70% of associated mutations resulted in activation of oncogenes (K-ras, C-erbB12, bax, bcl-2). Studies have also shown role for transforming growth factor (TGF)-β.

6. Only 10–20% amenable to curative surgery (Whipple procedure when confined at head of the pancreas; removal of tumor or en bloc resection of distal stomach, duodenum, and common bile duct). 3-year survival rate 2%. Palliation with chemotherapy and radiation therapy of limited duration value. Celiac plexus neurolysis may help with pain.

ACINAR ADENOCARCINOMA

1. Usually metastasized already by time of presentation. More males than females affected.

2. Symptoms attributable to local expansion and metastases. 15% present with syndrome of polyarthralgia, extrapancreatic fat necrosis, and eosinophilia. Tumor is a well-circumscribed nodular mass occurring evenly throughout pancreas.

3. Ultrasonography shows midrange echogenic mass. CT shows large encapsulated lesions of low attenuation with or without calcification or necrosis.

4. Histologically, tumor cells arranged in a ribbon-like manner with eosinophilic cytoplasm and periodic acid–Schiff stain-positive granules on electron microscopy. Immunostaining of granules for pancreatic enzymes usually positive.

5. Frequent allelic losses at 11p and alterations at APC or β-catenin pathway.

6. Treatment: complete excision (only possible chance of cure). Chemotherapy and radiation therapy used for palliation.

PANCREATOBLASTOMA

1. Most common pancreatic neoplasm in childhood. Usually presents in early childhood (mean age 4 yr). Male-to-female ratio 1.3:1. Asians account for 50% of cases. Association with Beckwith-Wiedemann syndrome.

2. Clinically: incidental abdominal mass.

3. Radiology determines tumor site and extent of disease. Ultrasonography reveals solid, lobulated pancreatic masses with mixed echogenicity. CT reveals large, firm, lobulated masses. MRI shows high signal intensity on T2 weighted images; gadolinium enhancement may help distinguish from other pancreatic tumors. Hemorrhage, cystic change, and necrosis typical. Metastatic spread rare.

4. Serum α-fetoprotein elevated in 80%; follow over course of disease and monitor for recurrence. Yolk sac tumor and hepatoblastoma should also be considered with high levels of α-fetoprotein.

5. Tumor is soft, solid mass, encapsulated in fibrous tissue. Tumor composed of epithelial tissue with acinar differentiation, squamoid cell nests, and occasional endocrine cells.

6. Treat by excision. If complete resection, 80% with complete remission. Chemotherapy provides only transient benefit; need to follow by surgery. Children with better prognosis.

ENDOCRINE TUMORS

INSULINOMA

1. Most common functioning pancreatic endocrine tumors (Table 1). Benign in 90–95% of cases.

2. Presentation: symptoms of hypoglycemia. Symptoms related to catecholamine response (palpitations, tachycardia, and hypertension) also common. Whipple's triad: hypoglycemia symptoms, abnormally low serum

TABLE 1   ENDOCRINE TUMORS OF THE PANCREAS

TUMOR TYPE	MAJOR CLINICAL FEATURE(S)
Insulinoma	Hypoglycemia, altered mental state
Gastrinoma	Gastric acid hypersecretion, peptic ulceration, steatorrhea
GRFoma*	Achromegaly
Glucagonoma*	Hyperglycemia, mild diabetes mellitus, necrolytic erythematous migratory rash
Somatostatinoma*	Hypochlorhydria, weight loss, mild diabetes mellitus, steatorrhea, cholelithiasis
VIPoma	Severe watery diarrhea, achlorhydria, hypokalemia

*These tumors have not yet been reported in the pediatric age group.

glucose, and relief of symptoms with glucose infusion are supportive of diagnosis.

3. Insulin levels > 6 μU/mL despite serum glucose < 40 mg/dL. Hypoglycemia without urinary ketones and elevated free fatty acids supports diagnosis (another cause of hypoketotic hypoglycemia). Hypoglycemia may last for up to 20 days postoperatively. Proinsulin is > 24% of measured insulin in 90% of cases of insulinoma. Check C-peptide to check that insulin is endogenous.

4. > 98% tumors found in pancreas; remainder at duodenum, ileum, or lung. Metastases, when occur, are local. Malignant lesions are usually > 2.5 cm in diameter.

5. 83% are solitary lesions. If > 1 lesion, suspect multiple endocrine neoplasia (MEN) type I.

6. Treatment of choice: surgical removal. However, if cannot localize, medical treatment favored over blind resection. Frequent snacks and prophylactic complex carbohydrates prevent hypoglycemia.

NESIDIOBLASTOSIS OR PERSISTENT HYPERINSULINEMIC HYPOGLYCEMIA OF INFANCY

1. Autosomal recessive form: predominant familial type (Table 2). Most cases (> 95%) sporadic.

2. Mutations in pancreatic K$_{ATP}$ channel genes are responsible for some forms of persistent hyperinsu-

linemic hypoglycemia of infancy (PHHI). Delta F1388 mutation predicts severe disease; H125Q mutation predicts mild disease. N1885 mutation is associated with severe clinical disease despite minimal channel dysfunction.

3. Diagnosis requires establishment of hyperinsulinemia (if glucose < 45 mg/dL, then hyperinsulinemia if insulin > 5 μU/mL). Another test is insulin growth factor (IGF) level at time of hypoglycemia (secretion inhibited by insulin such that PHHI patients have serum levels 10–20% of control subjects). Exogenous glucose requirement > 15–20 mg/kg/min to maintain euglycemia indicates severe hyperinsulinemia.

4. Initial therapy: intravenous glucose at high rates. Diazoxide can maintain patency of the K$_{ATP}$ channel (but require functional K$_{ATP}$ channels, not seen in those with *SUR1* or *Kir6.2* gene mutations). Calcium channel blockers may be helpful.

5. Failure of medical management common. Surgical pancreatectomy may be required to avoid long-term neurologic sequelae of hypoglycemia. If focal lesion, may allow reduction in pancreatic removal. Focal lesion often with focal adenomatous hyperplasia of islet-like cells, while diffuse PHHI shows irregular size islets of Langerhans cells. Also may use transhepatic retrograde pancreatic venous catheterization with measurement of insulin concentration at multiple sites to determine whether lesions are localized or not.

MEN I (WERMER SYNDROME)

1. Autosomal dominant. Syndrome of malignant potential with lesions at parathyroid, pancreas, and anterior pituitary glands.

2. Tumors often multiple, especially gastrinomas, which are typically at duodenum. 80% have one predominant hormone, most commonly insulin.

3. MEN I linked to tumor suppressor gene (*mu*) at 11q13.

TABLE 2   PERSISTENT HYPERINSULINEMIC HYPOGLYCEMIA OF INFANCY: COMPARISON OF CLINICAL PHENOTYPES ASSOCIATED WITH KNOWN MOLECULAR DEFECTS

TYPE (MOLECULAR DEFECTS)	HYPOGLYCEMIA/ HYPERINSULINEMIA	ASSOCIATED CLINICAL, BIOCHEMICAL, OR MOLECULAR FEATURES	RESPONSE TO MEDICAL MANAGEMENT	RECOMMENDED SURGICAL APPROACH	PROGNOSIS
Sporadic (?*SUR1* or *Kir6.2* mutations)	Moderate/severe in first days to weeks of life; macrosomic at birth	Loss of heterozygosity in microadenomatous tissue	Generally poor; may respond to somatostatin better than to diazoxide	Partial pancreatectomy (microadenoma; 30–40% cases)	Excellent
				Subtotal greater than 95% pancreatectomy (diffuse hyperplasia; 60–70% cases)	Guarded; diabetes mellitus develops in 50% of patients; hypoglycemia persists in 33%
Autosomal recessive (*SUR/Kir6.2* mutations)	Severe in first days to weeks of life; macrosomic at birth	Consanguinity a feature in some populations	Poor	Subtotal pancreatectomy	Guarded

Adapted from Sperling MA, Menon RK. Hyperinsulinemic hypoglycemia of infancy. recent insights into ATP-sensitive potassium channels, sulfonylurea receptors, molecular mechanisms, and treatment. Endocrinol Metab Clin North Am 1999;28:vii,695–708i.

4. Screening:
   a. Serum prolactin and insulin (IGF-1) for pituitary lesions
   b. Intact parathyroid hormone and albumin-corrected total serum calcium for parathyroid tumors.
   c. Pancreatoduodenal tumors (serum glucose, insulin, proinsulin, glucagons, gastrin, and plasma chromogranin A)
   d. Standardized meal or secretin stimulation test analyzing serum polypeptides and gastrin recommended.
   e. Radiographic imaging inadequate.

PRIMARY NONEPITHELIAL TUMORS

1. Malignant nonepithelial tumors such as rhabdomyosarcoma and lymphoma have been reported in children. Primitive neuroectodermal tumors may also occur in the pancreas, usually with typical translocation chromosomal abnormalities (t 11;12)(q24; q12) and immunohistochemical staining for O13.
2. A variety of benign nonepithelial pancreatic tumors also reported in children; for example, fibrous histiocytoma, juvenile hemangioendothelioma, lymphangioma, and myofibromatosis.

SECONDARY TUMORS

1. Most commonly from hematogenous spread including melanoma, renal tumors, lung tumors, and leukemia.
2. Tumors directly invading the pancreas include adenocarcinomas of stomach, intestine, and biliary tree.

TUMOR-LIKE EXOCRINE LESIONS

1. Cystic lesions: discussed earlier.
2. Others: chronic pancreatitis, ductal changes, acinar changes, heterotopic pancreas, heterotopic spleen, hamartomas, and inflammatory pseudotumors.
3. Inflammatory pseudotumors are an important group that pose diagnostic and therapeutic challenges owing to resemblance to malignant lesions. Complete excision and radiologic surveillance offers the best chance for successful management.

QUESTIONS

TRUE OR FALSE:

1. Pseudocysts are the most common pancreatic cystic lesion in children.
2. Pancreatoblastomas are mainly seen in early childhood.
3. Insulinomas are more common in Asians.

CHOOSE THE BEST ANSWER:

4. Wermer's syndrome is associated with all of the following except:
   a. Primary hyperparathyroidism.
   b. Pituitary adenomas.
   c. Autosomal recessive inheritance.

   d. *mu* gene mutation at 11q13.
   e. Duodenal gastrinomas.

5. Whipple's triad indicates which of the following:
   a. Hyperinsulinemia.
   b. Ductal adenocarcinoma.
   c. Acinar adenocarcinoma.
   d. Multiple endocrine neoplasias type I.
   e. None of the above.

6. The following describe persistent hyperinsulinemic hypoglycemia of infancy except:
   a. Most cases are inherited genetically.
   b. Focal pancreatic involvement.
   c. Diffuse pancreatic involvement.
   d. Can be treated medically.
   e. Subtotal pancreatectomy can be curative.

7. Insulinoma is associated with all of the following except:
   a. Surgical treatment is preferred over medical therapy.
   b. Hypoketotic hypoglycemia.
   c. Localization of tumor at the pancreas mainly.
   d. Mainly malignant tumors.
   e. > 24% total insulin level is proinsulin fraction.

ACUTE AND CHRONIC PANCREATITIS

SYNOPSIS

PANCREATIC FUNCTIONS

1. Production of a bicarbonate rich fluid by duct cells.
2. Synthesis of digestive enzymes by acinar cells (all enzymes except amylase and lipase are synthesized by proenzymes requiring activation by trypsin).
3. Production of hormones by islet cells to regulate nutrient storage and use.

NORMAL PROTECTIVE MECHANISMS VERSUS PANCREATITIS

1. Most geared toward control of trypsin and preventing trypsinogen activation (synthesized in an inactive form).
2. Inhibiting active trypsin: If activated within acinar cells, inhibited by pancreatic secretory trypsin inhibitor (SPINK1).
3. Destroying trypsin: self-destruct mechanism in trypsin.
4. Sweeping trypsin out of the pancreas (cystic fibrosis transmembrane regulator [CFTR]-dependent mechanism).

ACUTE PANCREATITIS

Clinically defined as sudden onset of abdominal pain associated with a rise in digestive enzymes in the blood and urine. Involves premature activation of trypsinogen. Associated with vigorous immune response.

TABLE 1 ETIOLOGY OF PANCREATITIS IN 1,276 CHILDREN

	STUDY (SETTING)						
	BENIFLA AND WEIZMAN (REVIEW)	DEBANTO ET AL (INPATIENT [MILD])	DEBANTO ET AL (INPATIENT [SEVERE])	LOPEZ (INPATIENT)	WERLIN ET AL (D/C RECORDS)	ALVAREZ CALATAYUD ET AL (INPATIENT)	TOTAL
NUMBER	589	162	40	274	180	31	1,276
Age, mean (median)	9.2	9.4	6.9	NA	(12.5)	7.9	
Male-to-female ratio	1.2	0.9	1	NA	0.9	1.2	
ETIOLOGY							
Systemic (eg, HUS)	14	1.9	20	53	14	6.5	20.8%
Gallstone		7.4	2.5		12	16	3.1%
Structural/divisum	15	2.5	2.5	10	7.7		10.6%
Infectious (eg, viral)	10	2.5	2.5	5	8	19	7.7%
Medications	12	11.1	7.5	5	12	9.7	10.2%
Trauma	22	13	20	19	14	6.5	18.6%
Post-ERCP	3.1	0			5.5		1.2%
Familial	2	6.8	7.5	"A few"	3		2.4%
Cystic fibrosis		3.1	0	0.4	0.6	0.5	0.6%
Hypercalcemia	1	3.1	0		0		0.9%
Hypertriglyceridemia	1	0.6	2.5		1		0.8%
DKA		1.2	0	0.7	4.4		0.9%
Other		3.7	7.5	0.4	10	7	2.4%
Idiopathic	23	40.1	27.5	17	8	35	22.2%

D/C = discharge, DKA = diabetic ketoacidosis and "diabetic"; ERCP = endoscopic retrograde cholangiopancreatography; HUS = hemolytic uremic syndrome; NA = not available. DeBanto JR, Goday PS, Pedroso MR, et al. Acute pancreatitis in children. Am J Gastroenterol 2002;97:1726–31 (from a multicenter (*n* = 6) study in the midwestern United States). Lopez MJ. The changing incidence of acute pancreatitis in children: a single-institution perspective. J Pediatr 2002; 140:622–4 (includes outpatient [Dallas, TX]. Werlin SL, Kugathasan S, Frautschy BC. Pancreatitis in children. J Pediatr Gastroenterol Nutr 2003;37:591–5 (from a referral center in Milwaukee,WI). Alvarez Calatayud G, Bermejo F, Morales JL, et al. Acute pancreatitis in childhood. Rev Esp Enferm Dig 2003;95(1):40–4, 45–8. English, Spanish. (from Madrid, Spain).

ETIOLOGY

Recurrence of acute pancreatitis seen in 10% of children, most commonly in patients with structural abnormalities, idiopathic pancreatitis, and familial pancreatitis (Table 1).

DIAGNOSIS

1. Sudden onset abdominal pain with amylase or lipase elevation at least 3 times the upper limit of normal. Pain epigastric, at the right or left upper quadrant with radiation to the back. Nausea and vomiting common. Jaundice or transaminitis should raise possibility of biliary tract involvement.
2. Computed tomography (CT) and abdominal ultrasonography are used to document pancreatitis, determine severity, or identify complications.
3. Endoscopic retrograde cholangiopancreatography (ERCP) reserved for unexplained recurrent pancreatitis and prolonged pancreatitis when a structural defect or duct disruption is suspected, or for gallstone pancreatitis.

MEDICAL MANAGEMENT

1. Mainstay: analgesia, intravenous fluids, pancreatic rest, and monitoring for complications. Volume expansion early in course important for cardiovascular stability and preventing pancreatic necrosis.
2. Meperidine 1–2 mg/kg intramuscularly or intravenously used for pain control.
3. Jejunal enteral feeds or total parenteral nutrition (TPN) should be considered if a severe or prolonged course is anticipated.

4. Antibiotics usually unnecessary except for most severe cases, especially if pancreatic necrosis present.

SEVERITY

1. Acute pancreatitis can be life threatening. Early death by cardiovascular collapse and respiratory failure. Late complications: infection and multisystem organ failure.
2. Ranson's criteria not applicable to children. A scoring system for children has been developed by the Midwest Multicenter Pancreatic Study Group; in this scoring system: the 7 severity factors include age < 7 yr, weight < 23 kg, admission white blood count > 18.5 thousand cells/mL, admission lactate dehydrogenase

TABLE 2 CAUSES OF HYPERAMYLASEMIA

PANCREATIC	SALIVARY	MIXED OR UNKNOWN
Pancreatitis	Infections (mumps)	Cystic fibrosis
Pancreatic tumors	Trauma	Renal insufficiency
Pancreatic duct obstruction	Salivary duct obstruction	Pregnancy
Biliary obstruction	Lung cancer	Cerebral trauma
Pseudocysts	Ovarian tumors or cysts	Burns
Perforated ulcer	Prostate tumors	Macroamylasemia
Bowel obstruction	DKA	
Acute appendicitis		
Mesenteric infarction/ ischemia		
ERCP		

DKA = diabetic ketoacidosis; ERCP = endoscopic retrograde cholangiopancreatography.

> 2000 U/L, 48 h fluid sequestration > 75 cc/kg/48 h, and a 48 h rise in urea > 5 mg/dL. If each criterion is assigned 1 point, outcome of patients with 5–7 points was 80% severe with 10% death.

COMPLICATIONS

1. Shock, edema, pleural effusions, fat necrosis, phlegmon, acute renal failure, coagulopathy, pancreatic necrosis, pancreatic pseudocysts, pancreatic duct rupture or stricture, bacteremia, sepsis, vascular leak, multiorgan system failure, hemorrhage, hypermetabolic state, and hyperglycemia.

2. Pancreatic necrosis associated with serious complications. Pancreatic pseudocysts can be observed over time for spontaneous resorption or may require drainage. Abscesses can be treated with external drainage and IV antibiotics; rarely surgical drainage necessary. Surgery is necessary for traumatic rupture of the duct.

SURGICAL MANAGEMENT

1. Role of surgery in acute pancreatitis limited to debridement of infected pancreatic necrosis and cholecystectomy to prevent recurrent gallstone pancreatitis.

2. Surgery in severe pancreatitis often deferred for at least 2 weeks to permit demarcation of necrotic areas and to minimize surgery-related loss of vital tissue.

CHRONIC PANCREATITIS

ETIOLOGY

1. Genetic susceptibility factors same as recurrent acute pancreatitis (ie, *PRSS1*, *SPINK1*, and *CFTR* mutations). Trypsinogen mutations responsible for majority of hereditary pancreatitis kindreds (most common mutations include R122H and N29I mutations) (Table 3).

2. Hereditary pancreatitis caused by cationic trypsinogen *PRSS1* mutations usually present as recurrent acute pancreatitis in childhood with median age 10 yr. Most important clinical clue is family history of pancreatitis. Diagnosis confirmed by genetic testing of *PRSS1* gene, but 30–40% with no identifiable mutations.

3. *CFTR*-associated pancreatitis: most important cause of chronic pancreatitis in children.

4. Idiopathic chronic pancreatitis (ICP): age at onset is bimodal. Early onset idiopathic pancreatis: calcification and exocrine and endocrine insufficiency develops more slowly than late-onset idiopathic pancreatitis; pain is severe. Late-onset: pain is absent in 50% of patients. *SPINK1* mutations have been identified in children with ICP.

DIAGNOSIS

1. Imaging: CT, ERCP, endoscopic ultrasonography, and magnetic resonance imaging or magnetic resonance cholangiopancreatography (MRCP).

2. Pancreatic function testing may be used to document chronic pancreatic insufficiency. Two noninvasive pancreatic function tests: fecal elastase 1 and functional MRCP.

TABLE 3   ETIOLOGIC RISK FACTORS ASSOCIATED WITH CHRONIC PANCREATITIS: TIGAR-O CLASSIFICATION SYSTEM (VERSION 1.0)

TOXIC-METABOLIC
Alcoholic
Tobacco smoking
Hypercalcemia
    Hyperparathyroidism
Hyperlipidemia
Chronic renal failure
Medications
    Phenacetin abuse (possibly from chronic renal insufficiency)
Toxins
    Organotin compounds (eg, di-n-butyltin dichloride)

IDIOPATHIC
Early onset
Late onset
Tropical
    Tropical calcific pancreatitis
    Fibrocalculous pancreatic diabetes
Other

GENETIC
Autosomal dominant
    Cationic trypsinogen (codon 29 and 122 mutations)
Autosomal recessive/modifier genes
    CFTR mutations
    SPINK1 mutations
    Cationic trypsinogen (codon A16V, D22G, K23R)
    α_1-Antitrypsin deficiency (possible)

AUTOIMMUNE
Isolated autoimmune chronic pancreatitis
Syndromic autoimmune chronic pancreatitis
    Sjögren syndrome–associated chronic pancreatitis
    Inflammatory bowel disease–associated chronic pancreatitis
    Primary biliary cirrhosis–associated chronic pancreatitis

RECURRENT AND SEVERE ACUTE PANCREATITIS–ASSOCIATED
    CHRONIC PANCREATITIS
Postnecrotic (severe acute pancreatitis)
Recurrent acute pancreatitis
Vascular diseases/ischemic
Postirradiation

OBSTRUCTIVE
Pancreatic divisum
Sphincter of Oddi disorders (controversial)
Duct obstruction (eg, tumor)
Preampullary duodenal wall cysts
Post-traumatic pancreatic duct scars

Adapted from Etemad B, Whitcomb DC. Chronic pancreatitis: diagnosis, classification, and new genetic developments. Gastroenterology 2001;120:682–707.

3. Genetic testing: *PRSS1* and *CFTR* gene testing may be used for diagnosis; *SPINK1* gene analysis for diagnosis is more controversial. Predictive testing not recommended for *PRSS1* mutations unless first-degree relatives with a known *PRSS1* mutation and adequate genetic counseling has been offered. *CFTR* or *SPINK1* predictive genetic testing not indicated.

TREATMENT

Treatment aimed at preventing and treating development of chronic pain syndrome, insulin-dependent diabetes mellitus, and pancreatic insufficiency (treated with enzyme replacement).

QUESTIONS

TRUE OR FALSE:

1. In 50% of late-onset idiopathic chronic pancreatitis, pain is absent.
2. Surgery in severe pancreatitis for removal of necrotic areas should be performed immediately.
3. Pancreatic function testing can be used to diagnose chronic pancreatitis.

CHOOSE THE BEST ANSWER:

4. The following are associated with hyperamylasemia except:
   a. Bowel obstruction.
   b. Head trauma.
   c. Burns.
   d. Lung cancer.
   e. Pregnancy.
   f. All of the above.

5. The following protect against autoactivation of trypsin except:
   a. Enzyme synthesized and stored as inactive precursor.
   b. Trypsin inhibitors.
   c. Autolysis of trypsin.
   d. Quick clearance of trypsin out of the pancreas.
   e. All of the above.

6. The following are mainstays of medical therapy for acute pancreatitis except:
   a. Pancreatic rest.
   b. Pain control.
   c. Fluid management.
   d. Nutrition.
   e. Antibiotics.

7. The following are indications for surgery in acute pancreatitis except:
   a. Gallstone pancreatitis.
   b. Debridement of necrotic tissue.
   c. Abscess refractory to medical management.
   d. Pseudocyst formation.
   e. All of the above.

8. Complications of acute pancreatitis include all except:
   a. Hypocalcemia.
   b. Pulmonary edema.
   c. Coagulopathy.
   d. Fat necrosis.
   e. Hypoglycemia.

9. Hereditary pancreatitis is associated with mutations in what gene?
   a. *SPINK1*.
   b. *CFTR*.
   c. *FAP*.
   d. *PRSS1*.
   e. Lipase.

JUVENILE TROPICAL PANCREATITIS

SYNOPSIS

1. Tropical pancreatitis: chronic pancreatitis characterized by recurrent abdominal pain, pancreatic calculi, and diabetes. Occurs among poor children and young adults in developing nations. Affected individuals are emaciated. Prevalence of this disease restricted to latitude 30° north and south of equator.
2. Size of pancreas: varies inversely with duration and severity of disease. Uneven shrinkage and fibrous adhesions cause displacement of pancreas from normal location. Parenchyma is replaced by fat. Frequent areas of stenosis and dilatation of ducts seen corresponding to solitary calculus or larger stones.
3. Radiologically: multiple calculi; vary in color, size, and shape. Larger stones nearer head; diminish in size towards tail. Composed of 95.5% calcium carbonate, small amount calcium phosphate (mainly in calcite form). Similar to stones in other types of chronic pancreatitis.
4. Histologically: diffuse pancreatic fibrosis. Periductular cellular infiltration: composed of lymphocytes and plasma cells. Fibrous tissue seen adjacent to relatively normal parenchyma. As disease advances, atrophic islets become isolated by dense fibrous tissue (Figure 1). In some instances, islets are hypertrophied.
5. High incidence of pancreatic cancer suggests tropical pancreatitis is a premalignant state.
6. Other organs: liver, and parotid glands show changes indicating uncontrolled diabetes mellitus (DM) or malnutrition. Liver early shows glycogen infiltration of cytoplasm and nuclei and fatty changes. Parotid glands are hypertrophied with varying degrees of round cell infiltration around ducts.

ETIOLOGY

Proposed contributors (not established):

1. Malnutrition.
2. Free-radical injury.
3. Trace element and vitamin deficiencies.
4. Dietary cyanogens: consumption of cassava root.
5. Genetic factors: perhaps similar to hereditary pancreatitis with mutations in tropical pancreatitis found in serine protease inhibitor Kazal type 1 (*SPINK1*).

CLINICAL FEATURES

1. Cardinal manifestations: recurrent upper abdominal pain in childhood (onset age < 13 yr) often lasting for days, followed by DM and pancreatic calculi by puberty, and death in prime of life. In early disease, abdominal pain bouts are severe but often reduce in severity over time. Patients often cannot tolerate food, refusing all food by mouth during episodes. Calculated life expectancy after onset abdominal pain and DM is 35 and 25 yr respectively.

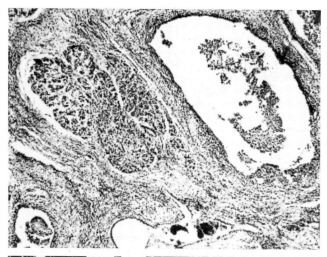

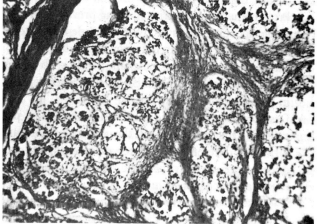

FIGURE 1 The pancreas shows extensive fibrosis, ductular dilatation, and intraductular calcium deposits. The intra- and interacinar fibrosis of the exocrine parenchyma produces the appearance of cirrhosis of the pancreas (hematoxylin and eosin).

2. Diabetes mellitus: pain-free period of 1–2 yr before onset of DM not unusual. Pancreatic DM is brittle with marked fluctuations of blood glucose with or without insulin therapy. Episodes of hypoglycemia may reflect depleted glycogen reserves in liver or decreased glucagon release from pancreas. Ketosis seen in < 5%. C-peptide assay shows partial preservation of beta cells. DM retinopathy and nephropathy occur: related to duration of DM. Autonomic nervous system dysfunction occurs with similar frequency and severity as in non–insulin-dependant DM patients.
3. Exocrine pancreatic insufficiency is the least striking clinical feature; probably secondary to low consumption of fat in diet.
4. Clinical and biochemical obstructive jaundice: well-recognized complication secondary to stenosis and compression of common bile duct (tunneled in head of pancreas).
5. Pancreatic pseudocysts: less common than in alcoholic or biliary pancreatitis.

DIAGNOSIS
1. Early stages: diagnosis rarely made. Endoscopic retrograde cholangiopancreatography (ERCP) or computed tomo-

graphy (CT) help in early detection; ERCP shows markedly dilated main duct with radiopaque and lucent calculi. Ultrasonography and CT identify calculi and dilated ducts.
2. Characteristic picture: can thus diagnose on clinical features alone. Onset of DM with present or past history of recurrent abdominal pain in young individual suggests chronic pancreatitis.
3. Diagnosis established by calculi on plain film (to the right of 1st and 2nd lumbar vertebrae with lateral extension to 2–5 cm to right of vertebrae). Calculi most numerous at head. Calculi may form a cast of the main duct in 30%.
4. Serum amylase not often useful in diagnosis except in acute exacerbations. Amylase below normal in many cases. Steatorrhea manifest only on high-fat diet.

MANAGEMENT
Alleviation of abdominal pain, treatment of DM, prevention of complications, correction of nutritional problems:
1. Meperidine, nothing by mouth, intravenous fluid rehydration (IVF).
2. Role of large doses of pancreatic enzyme not well-studied.
3. Antioxidant therapy: not well proven.
4. Endoscopic papillotomy with removal of stones and clearance of strictures or obstructions. Good results.
5. Surgical treatment: indication: unremitting pain; can include removal of stones and Puestow procedure (pancreatojejunostomy).
6. Dietary manipulation: oral hypoglycemics and insulin.

QUESTIONS

TRUE OR FALSE:
1. Juvenile tropical pancreatitis is a common type chronic pancreatitis in children and young adults in many Afro-Asian countries.
2. The etiology of juvenile tropical pancreatitis has been elucidated.
3. Juvenile tropical pancreatitis is not associated with pancreatic cancer.
4. ERCP and computed tomography are required to diagnose juvenile tropical pancreatitis.
5. Pancreatic diabetes is easily controlled with insulin therapy.

CHOOSE THE BEST ANSWER:
6. The following are clinical features of juvenile tropical pancreatitis except:
   a. Recurrent abdominal pain episodes in childhood.
   b. Brittle diabetes.
   c. Pancreatic calculi.
   d. Steatorrhea.
   e. Emaciation.

7. The following are indicated and efficacious for the treatment of juvenile tropical pancreatitis except:
   a. Meperidine.

b. Bowel rest.
c. Intravenous fluid rehydration.
d. Large doses of pancreatic enzymes.
e. Papillotomy and removal of stones.
f. Dietary manipulation.
g. All of the above are used for treatment.

CYSTIC FIBROSIS

SYNOPSIS

Cystic fibrosis transmembrane regulator (CFTR): cyclic adenosine monophosphate (cAMP)–dependent chloride channel located at apical membrane of epithelial cells (Figure 1).

MUTATIONS OF CFTR

1. Major mutation causing cystic fibrosis (CF): deletion of a single amino acid, phenylalanine, at position 508 (ΔF508); accounts for 66% of cystic fibrosis–associated mutations worldwide. Most frequent in northern Europeans (70–80%); affects only a minority of Ashkenazi Jews (30%). CF is inherited as autosomal recessive disorder: affects 1/2,500 live births in Caucasian communities.
2. Classes I–III are associated with markedly impaired chloride channel function and the pancreatic insufficiency (PI) phenotype. Classes IV and V are associated with the pancreatic sufficiency (PS) phenotype (Figure 3).
3. Phenotype of patients with R117H mutation: most are pancreatic sufficient, some have lung disease, but others have normal lung function. Males with normal lung function may present only with congenital bilateral absence of vas deferens and borderline or normal sweat chloride.
4. Neonatal screening: single measurement of immunoreactive trypsinogen (IRT), followed by mutation screening if IRT is abnormally high.

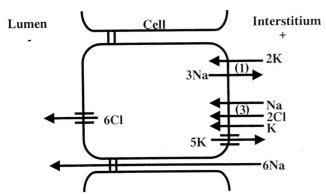

FIGURE 1 Chloride secretion via the cyclic adenosine monophosphate–activated Cl⁻ channel. Cl⁻ accumulates intracellularly via the Na⁺-K⁺-Cl⁻ cotransporter in the basolateral membrane. Na⁺ is recycled via Na⁺-K⁺-adenosine triphosphatase and K⁺ through independent K⁺ channels. Cl⁻ moves down its electrochemical gradient following activation of the Cl⁻ channel and is secreted into the lumen, and Na⁺ follows paracellularly owing to the lumen negative voltage set up by Cl⁻ transport.

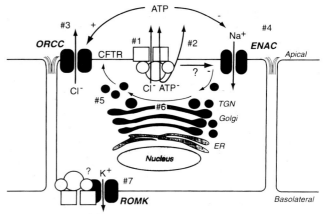

FIGURE 2 Cystic fibrosis transmembrane conductance regulator (CFTR) functions: (1) Cl⁻ channel function, (2) facilitation of adenosine triphosphate (ATP) release, (3) positive regulation of outwardly rectifying Cl⁻ channels (ORCC), (4) negative regulation of epithelial Na⁺ channels (ENAC), (5) regulation of vesicle trafficking, (6) regulation of cell acidification and protein processing, (7) modification of renal outer medullary K⁺ (ROMK) sensitivity to sulfonylureas. Reproduced with permission from Schwiebert EM, et al. CFTR is a conductance regulator as well as a chloride channel. Physiol Rev 1999;79 Suppl 1:S145–66.ER = endoplasmic reticulum; TGN = trans-Golgi network.

5. Classically, diagnosis based on clinical phenotype at presentation (lung disease and PI) and presence of elevated sweat chloride > 60 mmol/L, although affected infants can have sweat chloride 40–60 mmol/L. In cases with normal or borderline sweat chloride, genotyping, nasal potential difference, and quantitative pancreatic stimulation tests measuring HCO_3 secretion are of value.

PANCREATIC CF DISEASE

1. Steatorrhea attributed to lack of lipase or colipase secretion from exocrine pancreas.
2. Diagnosis: fecal fat study reveals > 7% fat excretion in stool on 72 h study.
3. Colipase secretion: correlate with fecal fats.
   a. Pancreatic insufficient: < 100 U/kg/h (< 1% normal), high fecal fats.
   b. Pancreatic sufficient: > 100 U/kg/h, normal fat absorption.

PANCREATIC INSUFFICIENCY

1. In CF infants dying in first 4 months of life, marked lack of pancreatic acinar tissue.
2. Clinical features: steatorrhea. Up to 50% hypoalbuminemic with or without peripheral edema at presentation. Some have hemolysis with vitamin E deficiency, rectal prolapse, coagulopathy with vitamin K deficiency, or raised intracranial pressure or night blindness secondary to vitamin A deficiency.
3. Treatment: oral enzyme replacement therapy. Need to document degree of steatorrhea on enzyme replacement therapy. If stool fat excretion still > 20% in the setting of compliance, assess for liver or biliary tract disease, *Giardia* infection, and celiac disease. Acid suppression also can help enzyme function.

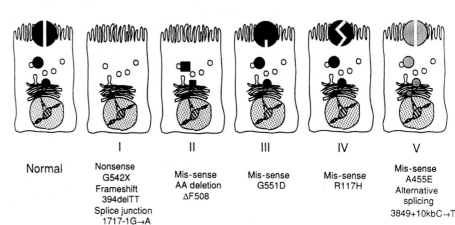

FIGURE 3 Classification of cystic fibrosis transmembrane conductance regulator (CFTR) mutations in relation to properties of CFTR protein. Class I: defective CFTR protein production: nonsense, frameshift, or aberrant splicing of messenger ribonucleic acid (mRNA); class II: defective CFTR processing: CFTR mRNA is formed, but protein fails to traffic to the cell membrane; class III: defective regulation: CFTR reaches membrane but is not stimulated by cyclic adenosine monophosphate; class IV: defective conduction: CFTR functions, but have altered properties; class V: synthesis defect: less synthesis of CFTR, but channel properties are normal.

FIBROSING COLONOPATHY

1. Noninflammatory colonic obstruction associated with marked intramural fibrosis at ascending or transverse colon associated with lipase doses > 50,000 IU/kg/d.
2. Clinically associated with intestinal obstruction and may be preceded by prolonged abdominal pain with or without diarrhea with rectal bleeding. Some may present with chylous ascites.
3. Diagnose by contrast enemas to identify stricture and site of obstruction.
4. Surgery is required to relieve obstruction. Current recommendations are to keep pancreatic enzyme replacement dose < 10,000 U/kg/d.

PANCREATIC SUFFICIENCY

1. Number of PS patients declines from 40–50% of CF cases in the neonatal period to 10–20% in older children.
2. Clinical features: mild disease with minimal pulmonary involvement. Pancreatitis develops, which does not occur in PI patients. Median survival 53 yr. (29 yr for PI).
3. Associated PS mutations: R117H, A455E, and R347P.

TABLE 1   BILIARY TRACT AND LIVER COMPLICATIONS IN CYSTIC FIBROSIS PATIENTS

GALLBLADDER
Microgallbladder
Atretic cystic ducts
Distended gallbladder
Cholelithiasis

BILIARY TRACT
Ductal stones
Common bile duct stenosis
Sclerosing cholangitis
Cholangiocarcinoma

LIVER
Hepatosteatosis
Focal biliary fibrosis (cirrhosis)
Multilobular biliary cirrhosis
  ± Portal hypertension
  + Liver failure

4. Sweat test: impaired chloride transport, but less severe than in PI patients.
5. Treatment: enzyme therapy and fat-soluble vitamin supplements not required; sufficient endogenous enzyme production to prevent malabsorption.

HEPATOBILIARY COMPLICATIONS

1. Two forms of fibrotic liver disease considered pathognomonic of CF: focal and multilobular biliary cirrhosis (Table 1).
2. Presence of liver disease does not correlate with severity of lung or intestinal disease.
3. Diagnosis can be difficult, especially in mild cases. Liver function tests: can be normal even with multilobular biliary cirrhosis and portal hypertension. Ultrasonography: increased echogenicity owing to impacted secretions or steatosis unrelated to fibrosis. Biopsy: subject to sampling error.
4. Clinical: patients with focal biliary cirrhosis relatively asymptomatic. Multilobular disease may have signs of chronic liver disease and portal hypertension or ascites.
5. Treatment: supportive care to provide adequate nutrition, fat-soluble vitamin supplementation, and diuretic therapy for edema and ascites. In case of variceal bleeding, sclerotherapy or banding; if failure, consider lienorenal shunt. Liver transplant is an option; survival rate (70–80%/5 yr). Direct contraindication to liver transplant is severe lung disease and fungal or *Burkhoderia cepacia* lung colonization.

NEONATAL LIVER DISEASE

1. Prolonged neonatal cholestasis occurs in cystic fibrosis but is rare.
2. Some infants present with picture similar to extrahepatic biliary atresia (EHBA) with jaundice and acholic stools. Some have EHBA, but most do not. Jaundice resolves by month 3 or 4 without intervention. Need to exclude EHBA with appropriate evaluations. Finding of elevated sweat chloride should make one circumspect about EHBA diagnosis and delay operative therapy.

GALLBLADDER OR BILIARY TRACT DISEASE

Previously, cholelithiasis was a common biliary tract complication of CF; with oral enzymatic replacement therapy, virtually nonexistent. In patients with right upper quadrant pain, need to rule out cholelithiasis with ultrasonography evaluation and distal common bile duct obstruction with cholangiography.

INTESTINAL DISEASE

ESOPHAGEAL

1. Gastroesophageal reflux is common and multifactorial owing to lung disease and drugs that relax the lower esophageal sphincter (LES) and physiotherapy. Delayed gastric emptying may contribute.
2. Clinical presentation: heartburn, regurgitation, and dysphagia. Can also present with just anorexia.
3. Treatment: medical therapy at least 6 mo before considering surgery (if refractory).

GASTRODUODENAL

Peptic ulcers prevalent.

SMALL INTESTINE DISEASE

Meconium ileus and distal intestinal obstruction syndrome (DIOS) is seen almost exclusively in PI (not PS) patients.

Meconium Ileus

1. Invariably associated with CF. Small bowel obstruction secondary to inspissated meconium at the terminal ileum in 10–20% of CF patients; occurs in utero. 10% of cases suffer perforation in utero and have meconium peritonitis.
2. Distinguish from other causes of gut obstruction by lack of air or fluid levels and ground glass appearance of meconium. Diagnosed best by nonionic contrast radiography (Gastrografin enemas). Avoid contrast radiography in setting of abdominal calcifications and or perforation.
3. If unable to clear obstruction with Gastrografin washout, surgery required to milk out inspissated feces after division of gut followed by washing out with saline or solutions with N-acetylcholine. 50% of cases also have associated malrotation with volvulus or intestinal atresia. Most will have associated microcolon.

DIOS

1. Occurs beyond neonatal period. Inspissation of intestinal contents at the terminal ileum and proximal colon. Etiology unclear. Rare in PS pts.
2. Present with fecal mass at right lower quadrant with or without abdominal pain or with intestinal obstruction.
3. Diagnose by plain erect and supine kidney, ureter, and bladder exam. If obstruction present, suspect concomitant pathology, intussusception, or appendiceal disease. Ultrasonography and CT can diagnose intussusception. If washout fails, try Gastrografin enema to define colonic pathology and relieve impaction. Perform colonoscopy or biopsy if suspect Crohn disease or inflammation.

4. Treatment: if no obstruction, mineral oil 30–60 cc twice daily for 7 d. If condition persists, check ultrasonography to rule out intussusception; try Golytely laxative.

APPENDICEAL DISEASE

Less common than in non-CF community (1 versus 7%).

MISCELLANEOUS SMALL INTESTINE DISEASE

1. Giardiasis, celiac disease, and Crohn disease described.
2. Crohn disease is 11 times more common in CF than non-CF populations.
3. Coexistence of CF and celiac disease rare; consider celiac disease if malabsorption despite compliance with oral enzyme replacement therapy.

LARGE INTESTINE DISEASE

1. Rectal prolapse: occurs in 10–20% patients, usually before age 5 yr. May be initial presentation. More common in PI patients. All children with isolated rectal prolapse need sweat test. In most cases self-resolving; requires no therapy other than oral enzyme replacement and laxatives if constipated. If recurrent, can treat with pararectal triple saline injections under anesthesia.
2. Fibrosing colonopathy: see above.
3. Gastrointestinal malignancy: need to consider in older CF patients. The majority are intestinal adenocarcinoma, but esophageal, gastric, biliary, and pancreatic cancers described.

NUTRITIONAL PROBLEMS

1. Toronto study showed improved prognosis and pulmonary function if nutritionally replete. Boston cohort with improved median survival with nutritional repletion (Table 2).
2. Encourage high-fat diet (40% dietary fat) to replace stool losses with 110% recommended daily calories. Improvement in intake reverses growth failure.
3. Resting energy expenditure can be elevated, especially in PI patients in the setting of infection.

NUTRITIONAL ASSESSMENT

1. 3–5 d fat balance study: fecal fat value > 10% in infants or > 7% in children age > 1 yr indicates need for oral enzyme replacement therapy. Need to also assess serum fat-soluble vitamin levels and albumin at diagnosis and annually. Anthropometry should be performed every 2–3 mo.
2. Osteopenia is reported in CF population. Bone density analyses in patients with suboptimal growth should be performed annually.
3. Large proportion of CF patients age > 10 yr are glucose-intolerant. Consider annual fasting glucose check to screen for diabetes.
4. Note: there appears to be no advantage to semi-elemental formulas over breast milk if appropriate enzyme replacement is delivered.
5. In adults or adolescents with growth failure unable to supplement enteral feeds orally, consider nasogastric and gastrostomy tube placement for supplemental feeds.

TABLE 2   MALNUTRITION IN PATIENTS WITH
CYSTIC FIBROSIS

MACRONUTRIENT DEFICIENCY
Protein deficiency with hypoalbuminemia
Edema
Linear growth failure
Loss of bone matrix (osteopenia with associated low calcium intake)
Energy deficiency with weight loss
Wasting of fat and lean mass
Wasting of shoulder girdle and buttocks
Stunting of growth
Delayed puberty

MICRONUTRIENT DEFICIENCY
Fat-soluble vitamin deficiency

Vitamin A	Benign intracranial hypertension (distention of fontanel in infants)
	Night blindness
	Xerophthalmia: Bitôt spots
Vitamin D	Rickets (rare in sunny climates)
Vitamin E	Hemolytic anemia (infants)
	Peripheral neuropathy
	Ataxia with spinocerebellar tract degeneration
	External ophthalmoplegia
Vitamin K	Coagulopathy
Water-soluble vitamins	Vitamin B_{12} deficiency (rare)
Essential fatty acid deficiency	Seborrheic dermatitis
Salt depletion (hot climates)	Hyponatremia
	If severe, associated with hypochloremia, hypokalemia, and metabolic alkalosis

QUESTIONS

CHOOSE THE BEST ANSWER:

1. Cystic fibrosis transmembrane regulator is:
    a. Located at the basolateral membrane of epithelial cells.
    b. Located at the apical membrane of epithelial cells.
    c. Cyclic adenosine monophosphate–independent.
    d. Adenosine triphosphate–dependent.
    e. Causes chloride to accumulate intracellularly.
    f. None of the above.

2. Neonatal screening for cystic fibrosis is all of the following except:
    a. Based on a single measurement of immunoreactive trypsinogen.
    b. Followed by mutation analysis if immunoreactive trypsinogen is low.
    c. All of the above.
    d. None of the above.

MATCH THE CFTR MUTATIONS TO THEIR EFFECTS (MAY BE MORE THAN ONE ANSWER):

a. ΔF508.
b. R117H.
c. A455E.

3. Affects 66% of cystic fibrosis chromosomes worldwide.
4. Associated with pancreatic sufficiency.
5. May present in males with only congenital bilateral absence of vas deferens and a normal sweat chloride.
6. Causes deletion of phenylalanine at position 508.

MATCH THE CYSTIC FIBROSIS PANCREATIC SUBTYPE WITH ITS CHARACTERISTICS:

a. Cystic fibrosis with pancreatic sufficiency.
b. Cystic fibrosis with pancreatic insufficiency.

7. Associated with colipase secretion > 100U/kg/h.
8. Develop pancreatitis.
9. Associated with Class IV and V CFTR mutations.

MATCH THE FOLLOWING SYMPTOMS AND SIGNS WITH THEIR ASSOCIATED CYSTIC FIBROSIS CONDITIONS:

a. Night blindness.
b. Hemolysis.
c. Rickets.
d. Coagulopathy.
e. Fontanelle distention in infants.
f. Peripheral neuropathy.
g. Seborrheic dermatitis.
h. Salt depletion.

10. Vitamin D deficiency.
11. Vitamin K deficiency.
12. Cystic fibrosis patients in hot climates.
13. Vitamin E deficiency.
14. Vitamin A deficiency.
15. Essential fatty-acid depletion.

TRUE OR FALSE:

16. If pancreatic sufficient at birth, cystic fibrosis patients will remain pancreatic sufficient throughout their lives.
17. Pancreatic sufficient patients do not require fat-soluble vitamin supplements.
18. One-half of meconium ileus cases are associated with malrotation or intestinal atresia.
19. Crohn disease is more common in cystic fibrosis patients than in persons without cystic fibrosis.
20. Focal biliary cirrhosis is easily diagnosed by usual examinations (liver function test, ultrasonography, and biopsy).
21. In cystic fibrosis, liver disease correlates with pulmonary disease.
22. Neonates with cystic fibrosis and jaundice, acholic stools are most likely to also have extrahepatic biliary atresia.
23. Contrast enemas are indicated to diagnose meconium ileus in the setting of intraabdominal calcifications.
24. Fibrosing colonopathy mainly occurs at the distal colon.

SHWACHMAN-DIAMOND SYNDROME

SYNOPSIS

1. After cystic fibrosis, Shwachman-Diamond syndrome (SDS) is the most common inherited cause of exocrine pancreatic dysfunction.
2. Autosomal recessive inheritance. *SBDS* gene (Shwachman-Bodian-Diamond syndrome) contains disease-associated mutations. Most common *SBDS* mutations

TABLE 1   SPECTRUM OF CLINICAL FEATURES OF SHWACHMAN-DIAMOND SYNDROME

EXOCRINE PANCREAS	HEMATOLOGIC	SKELETAL/ DENTAL	GROWTH/ NUTRITION	LIVER	PSYCHOLOGICAL/ NEUROLOGIC
Acinar cell: dysfunction, pancreatic insufficiency, pancreatic sufficiency	Cytopenias: neutropenia, anemia, thrombocytopenia, pancytopenia ↑ Hemoglobin F Marrow aplasia Myelodysplasia Acute myelogenous leukemia	Long bones: delayed maturation, metaphyseal, dysplasia, tubulation Thorax: thoracic dystrophy, short flared rib, costochondral thickening, clinodactyly, osteopenia Teeth: caries, dysplasia, mouth ulcer	Malnutrition (at diagnosis) Short stature	Hepatomegaly ↑ Aminotransferases Histology: portal inflammation, portal fibrosis	Low intelligence Learning difficulties Pontine leukoencephalopathy

Other: dermatologic; eczema, ichthyosis; renal: anatomic anomalies, tubular dysfunction; cardiac: endocardial fibrosis.

are derived from gene conversion events between *SBDS* and an adjacent *SBDS* pseudogene.

3. Exocrine pancreas dysfunction: universal manifestation (Table 1). The pancreatic defect arises from a failure of pancreatic acini to develop. Histologically, normal ductular architecture and islets, sparse or absent acinar cells, and extensive fatty replacement. 50% of affected patients will show sufficient improvement in pancreatic acinar capacity, particularly in trypsinogen concentrations (other pancreatic enzymes still low) with advancing age and may no longer require enzyme supplements.

4. Bone marrow failure: all patients, varying degrees. Persistent or intermittent neutropenia is virtually universal. Some patients have a variety of isolated cytopenias involving one or more bone marrow elements. The bone marrow of SDS shows reduced precursors, suggesting a stem cell defect. SDS patients carry a high risk of developing leukemia.

5. Infections: risk of severe life-threatening infections. Recurrent fevers of unknown origin also observed in SDS.

6. Nutrition and growth: short stature common (primary manifestation of syndrome). Malnutrition may be present at diagnosis.

7. Skeleton and dentition: typically, infants show delayed appearance of secondary ossification centers. Varying degrees of widening and irregular metaphyses common at ribs and proximal or distal femurs. SDS patients may have oral and dental anomalies.

8. Liver: hepatomegaly common in infancy; usually resolves by age 5 yr. Aminotransferases also elevated in infants. Histology reveals mild abnormalities. Progressive liver disease not reported.

9. Psychological, behavioral, and neurologic features: learning and behavioral difficulties common.

CLINICAL DIAGNOSIS
1. No single disease characteristic or biochemical test is capable of establishing or excluding a diagnosis of SDS.

2. Two clinical features of disease are consistently observed: exocrine pancreatic and bone marrow dysfunction. Other common primary features are used to provide supportive evidence (short stature, skeletal abnormalities, and hepatomegaly).

3. Exocrine pancreatic dysfunction as demonstrated by:
   a. Deficit of pancreatic enzyme secretion with stimulation testing.
   b. Abnormal 72 h fat balance study plus pancreatic imaging demonstrating a small or lipomatous pancreas.
   c. Low serum trypsinogen in patients age < 3 yr; low serum trypsinogen or pancreatic isoamylase if age > 3yr.

4. Bone marrow dysfunction as manifested by:
   a. Neutropenia.
   b. Anemia.
   c. Persistent thrombocytopenia.
   d. Persistent pancytopenia.
   e. Myelodysplasia with or without clonal abnormalities.

5. Genetic testing may be used for diagnostic confirmation.

6. Clinical assessment should be performed every 6–12 mo: anthropometric measures, bone age, pubertal development, and review of development. Complete blood count should be performed every 6 mo, as well as serum fat-soluble vitamin concentrations, prothrombin time, and partial thromboplastin time (Table 2).

7. Steatorrhea may resolve with advancing age, despite the fact that pancreatic enzyme secretion remains well below normal. If nutrient maldigestion identified, enzyme replacement therapy required.

8. No recommended therapy for short stature. Growth velocity usually normal, as are growth hormone levels. Puberty may be delayed.

9. Bone marrow aspirates, biopsies, and cytogenetic studies suggested annually.

10. If repeated infections with severe neutropenia, treat with prophylactic antibiotics and granulocyte–colony stimulating factor (G-CSF). However, may need to be concerned that long-term G-CSF may increase leukemogenic risk.

TABLE 2   ASSESSMENT AT DIAGNOSIS

DIAGNOSIS*
Clinical confirmation of SDS by excluding other causes of pancreatic
   dysfunction and bone marrow failure
          PLUS
Objective confirmation of pancreatic dysfunction
          AND
Bone marrow failure

BASELINE ASSESSMENT
Imaging
   Imaging of liver and pancreas (ultrasonography, CT, or MRI)
   Skeletal survey
   Bone age (older patients only)
Blood
   CBC, differential, platelets; hemoglobin electrophoresis
   Total and direct bilirubin, aminotransferases, alkaline phosphatase
   Serum vitamins A, E, D (25-hydroxyvitamin D)
   Prothrombin time, partial thromboplastin time
   Serum trypsinogen and pancreatic isoamylase
Bone marrow
   Aspirate
   Biopsy
   Cytogenetic analysis
Stool
   72-Hour fecal fat balance study

CBC = complete blood count; CT = computed tomography; MRI = magnetic resonance imaging; SDS = Shwachman-Diamond syndrome.
*Genotyping may be considered for confirming the diagnosis.

QUESTIONS

TRUE OR FALSE:

1. Exocrine pancreatic insufficiency is a universal manifestation in Shwachman-Diamond syndrome.
2. Exocrine pancreatic insufficiency in Shwachman-
   Diamond syndrome arises from ductular inflammation.
3. Shwachman-Diamond syndrome patients almost universally exhibit intermittent or persistent neutropenia.
4. Shwachman-Diamond syndrome adolescents commonly have hepatomegaly.
5. Shwachman-Diamond syndrome is diagnosed based
   on clinical characteristics.

CHOOSE THE BEST ANSWER:

6. Short stature in Shwachman-Diamond patients is:
   a. Always associated with growth hormone deficiency.
   b. Correctable with pancreatic enzyme replacement.
   c. Correctable with growth hormone replacement.
   d. Necessary to diagnose Shwachman-Diamond syn-
      drome.
   e. All of the above.
   f. None of the above.

7. Steatorrhea in Shwachman-Diamond syndrome:
   a. Is a persistent characteristic.
   b. Correlates well with measurement of pancreatic
      enzyme secretion.
   c. Results from recurrent pancreatitis.
   d. Tends to improve with age.

OTHER HEREDITARY AND ACQUIRED DISORDERS

SYNOPSIS

PEARSON MARROW-PANCREAS SYNDROME

1. Bone marrow changes: cell vacuolization and ringed
   sideroblasts mark distinction from Shwachman-
   Diamond syndrome.
2. Exocrine pancreatic insufficiency with pancreatic
   fibrosis.
3. Results from defective oxidative phosphorylation;
   associated with mitochondrial deoxyribonucleic acid
   (DNA) deletions (complex I of respiratory chain
   enzymes most severely affected). Oxidation of reduced
   nicotinamide adenine dinucleotide is abnormal in
   lymphocytes.

JOHANSON-BLIZZARD SYNDROME

1. Pancreatic exocrine deficiency, aplasia or hypoplasia of
   alae nasi, congenital deafness, hypothyroidism, developmental delay, short stature, ectodermal scalp
   defects, absence of permanent teeth, urogenital malformations, and imperforate anus. Hypopituitarism,
   diabetes, growth hormone deficiency, and congenital
   heart disease also described.
2. Primary failure of pancreatic acinar development (similar to Shwachman-Diamond syndrome but no bone
   marrow or skeletal abnormalities).

JEUNE SYNDROME

1. Rare, autosomal recessive disorder characterized by
   skeletal abnormalities of the thorax and extremities
   and nephronophthisis.
2. Associated with respiratory distress in infancy.
3. Associated with exocrine pancreatic insufficiency.

ISOLATED ENZYME DEFICIENCIES

1. Lipase deficiency: present with severe steatorrhea in
   infancy; failure to thrive (FTT) is not a feature. Duodenal juice reveals absent or low lipase and occasional
   low amylase and trypsin. Responds well to pancreatic
   enzyme supplements.
2. Colipase deficiency: colipase cofactor overcomes the
   inhibitory effects of bile salts on pancreatic lipase;
   deficiency not associated with FTT.
3. Combined lipase-colipase deficiency.
4. Amylase deficiency: abnormally low pancreatic amylase at age 1 yr is physiologic. Otherwise, true deficiency. Also, low pancreatic isoamylase observed in
   patients with Shwachman-Diamond syndrome who
   have normal fat digestion.
5. Trypsinogen deficiency: deficiency leads to disruption of
   pancreatic enzyme activation cascade; severe malabsorption beginning neonatally. Gene found on chromosome 7.

6. Enterokinase deficiency: enterokinase initiates the activation of pancreatic proteolytic proenzymes by converting trypsinogen to trypsin, which activates other proenzymes. Presents in neonatal period with diarrhea, failure to thrive, edema, and hypoproteinemia. Responds to pancreatic enzyme replacement. Gene located at 21q21.

ACQUIRED DISORDERS

Malnutrition

Protein calorie malnutrition causes significant reduction in pancreatic exocrine function via acinar atrophy and reduction in enzyme output. Acute malnutrition in children associated with elevated trypsinogen levels, which correlate with severity of malnutrition. In chronic malnutrition, low trypsinogen levels seen with extensive acinar cell atrophy and diffuse fibrosis.

Surgical Resection

Malabsorption occurs when values of pancreatic lipase and colipase fall < 1–2% of normal.

Celiac Disease

1. Exocrine pancreas dysfunction recognized in celiac disease. Degree of impairment variable. Those with low fecal chymotrypsin may represent a subset of patients who may benefit from pancreatic enzyme supplementation for a few months.
2. Profound, irreversible pancreatic insufficiency with acinar atrophy and fibrosis is rare.

QUESTIONS

MATCH THE CONDITION TO THE CHARACTERISTICS (MAY BE MORE THAN ONE ANSWER):

a. Jeune syndrome.
b. Pearson syndrome.
c. Shwachman-Diamond syndrome.
d. Johanson-Blizzard syndrome.

1. Asphyxiating thoracic cavity.
2. Metaphyseal abnormalities.
3. Sideroblasts.
4. Aplasia of the alae nasi.
5. Congenital deafness.
6. Neutropenia.
7. Mitochondrial DNA deletions.
8. Ectodermal scalp defects.

a. Trypsinogen deficiency.
b. Lipase deficiency.
c. Enterokinase deficiency.
d. Amylase deficiency.

9. Severe steatorrhea in infancy.
10. Failure to thrive.
11. Hypoproteinemia.
12. Can be normal.

ANSWERS

CONGENITAL ANOMALIES

1. a.
2. b.
3. b.
4. b.
5. a.
6. a.
7. b.
8. a. Diagnosed by magnetic resonance cholangiopancreatography or ERCP, treated by sphincteroplasty or papillary enlargement; is not associated with ectopic pancreatic tissue.
9. d.
10. True.
11. False. Usually asymptomatic since exocrine and endocrine functions are normal.

PANCREATIC TUMORS

1. True.
2. True.
3. False. 50% pancreatoblastomas seen in Asians; majority of papillary cystic neoplasms in Asian and black girls.
4. c. Autosomal dominant.
5. a.
6. a. Usually sporadic (> 95%).
7. d. 90% benign.

ACUTE AND CHRONIC PANCREATITIS

1. True.
2. False. Surgery in severe pancreatitis deferred often for at least 2 weeks to permit demarcation of necrotic areas and minimizes surgery-related loss of vital tissue.
3. False. Pancreatic function testing allows documentation of exocrine pancreatic insufficiency.
4. f.
5. e.
6. e.
7. d.
8. e. Hyperglycemia is a complication of acute pancreatitis.
9. d.

JUVENILE TROPICAL PANCREATITIS

1. True.
2. False.

3. False.
4. False. Radiography can be used to diagnose with calculi on plain film to the right of 1st and 2nd lumbar vertebrae (calculi most numerous at head); also can diagnose on clinical characteristics given typical picture.
5. False. Pancreatic diabetes is brittle with or without insulin.
6. d. Usually not manifest owing to low-fat diet.
7. d. Not well proven.

CYSTIC FIBROSIS
1. b.
2. a.
3. a.
4. b, c.
5. b.
6. a.
7. a.
8. a.
9. a.
10. c.
11. d.
12. h.
13. b, f.
14. a, e.
15. g.
16. False. At birth 40–50% are pancreatic sufficient; in older children, 10–20%.
17. True.
18. True.
19. True.
20. False. Difficult to diagnose.

21. False. No correlation.
22. False. Most are not extrahepatic biliary atresia; most resolve by 3–4 mo, but usual investigations required.
23. False. Calcifications indicative of perforation; thus, Gastrografin enemas are contraindicated.
24. False. Occurs at proximal, ascending, and transverse colon.

SHWACHMAN-DIAMOND SYNDROME
1. True.
2. False. Arises from a failure of pancreatic acini to develop.
3. True
4. False. Seen in infants; usually resolves by age 5 yr.
5. True.
6. f.
7. d.

OTHER HEREDITARY AND ACQUIRED DISORDERS
1. a.
2. c.
3. b.
4. d.
5. d.
6. c.
7. b.
8. d.
9. a, b, c.
10. a, c.
11. a, c.
12. d. Especially in age ≤ 1 yr.

RESEARCH METHODOLOGY

OUTCOMES RESEARCH

SYNOPSIS

OUTCOMES RESEARCH
The systematic study of clinical practice with a focus on clinical effectiveness and patient-centered outcomes (Table 1).

EVALUATION OF STUDY TYPES
See Table 2.

PATIENT-CENTERED STUDIES
Quantitative measures:

1. Functional status: measure of the impact of health or disease condition on the ability of patients to function in various roles in society.
2. Patient satisfaction: patients' satisfaction with health care or with their state of health or disease condition.

TABLE 1   DEFINITION OF TERMS USED IN THE EVALUATION OF MEDICAL CARE QUALITY

Efficacy	*Can* it work? (eg, in controlled trials)
Effectiveness	*Does* it work? (eg, in the real world)
Efficiency	Is it *worth* doing?
Safety	Does it *reduce risk* to patients?
Equity	Is it *nonvarying* in quality?
Patient centered	Is it *respectful* of individual patient preferences?

TABLE 2   PROS AND CONS OF DIFFERENT STUDY DESIGNS

STUDY TYPE	MERITS	PROBLEMS
EXPERIMENTAL		
Randomized controlled trial: outcome comparison of intervention group and control group	Randomization removes potential for bias. Evenly matched groups with randomization.	If outcome rare, may require enormous population to detect differences. Requires specific clinical question in well-defined patient populations.
OBSERVATIONAL		
Cohort studies: follow group of interest who do not have outcome of interest at time of enrollment over time. Often prospective.	Useful for studying the incidence and natural history of disease. Do not occur in tightly controlled research settings but in real-world arena.	Members of the cohort may need to be followed for a lengthy period of time before a significant number develop the outcome of interest (cost limitation). Impractical study design for investigating risk factors for rare diseases.
Case-control studies: people who have the disease (cases) compared with similar people without the disease (controls). Retrospective.	Performed relatively quickly and inexpensively, even for rare diseases or those that take lengthy periods of time to appear.	Subject to bias (recall bias). Relies on studying already identified cases: misses those who are asymptomatic or misdiagnosed or already dead, and depends on the identification of an appropriate control group.
Cross-sectional studies: single examination of an entire population at a particular point in time	Important for generating hypotheses for experimental designs.	Since identify existing cases and do not capture new cases, likely to overrepresent chronic illness and underrepresent acute illness. May be limited by lead-time bias (ie, those with disease change behaviors owing to symptoms, resulting in misclassification by reported current exposures). Caution with interpretation: an observed association does not mean that a causal relationship exists.
Case series: describe the presentation and often the clinical management of a disease in more than one patient; generally not followed prospectively; not compared with a control group.	Present information about patients with rare diseases. May be important for stimulating new hypothesis.	May be prone to reporting bias. Validity may be difficult to establish.
Large database review studies: utilize large administrative databases maintained by health care providers, payers, or government agencies	Electronically maintained, computer-ready for analysis, and inexpensive.	Limited in quality, type of information available. Data may be incorrect or incomplete. Inconsistencies in diagnostic coding may limit usefulness.
Meta-analysis: employs statistical methodologies to retrospectively review and integrate quantitative data across multiple studies	Useful method for assimilating data from multiple small studies with conflicting answers or statistically insignificant results.	Positive publication bias. Inequality of study designs and endpoints measured.

3. Health-related quality of life: general physical and mental health status of individuals, including psychosocial well-being as it is affected by illness, injury, and health care interventions or policies. Consists of five domains: state of disease, associated physical symptoms, functional status, psychological functioning, and social functioning.

STUDIES OF MEDICAL EFFICIENCY

1. Determine clinical efficiency or value of medical intervention.
2. Types of cost analyses:
   a. Cost-identification analysis (CIA): simplest means of determining health care costs; cost per unit of treatment or service provided.
   b. Cost-benefit analysis (CBA): compares the cost of a given medical intervention with the cost of its benefit. Limitation: how to express the dollar worth of benefit.
   c. Cost-effectiveness analysis (CEA): all costs in CEA expressed with outcome as the denominator. Most often used to compare two different treatment options with variable or unequal endpoints. Options that offer less cost with same or better outcomes are dominant.
   d. Cost-utility analysis: CEA analysis where outcomes are ranked in regards to value or importance. Employs the following components:
      • Quality-adjusted life-year (QALY): estimation of people's personal preferences of different health states.
      • Decision analysis: analyzing decision making under conditions of uncertainty; requires knowledge of all possible choices, all outcomes, probabilities of outcomes, and utilities and values assigned to each outcome. Utilities often defined as a relative preference for the outcome (1 = perfect outcome; 0 = worst outcome). Best choice is that with the highest expected utility.
3. Types of cost:
   a. Direct: financial expenses.
   b. Indirect: lost opportunities in a patient's life because of illness.
   c. Intangible: pain, suffering, and grief.
4. Perspectives of cost:
   a. Patient.
   b. Provider.
   c. Payer.
   d. Society.

QUESTIONS

MATCH THE STUDY DESIGN TO THE OBJECTIVE:
a. Randomized, controlled trial.
b. Case-control study.
c. Cohort study.
d. Meta-analysis.

1. Study to follow the natural history of children with a rare pancreatic tumor.
2. Study to determine whether erythropoietin is effective in increasing blood count in parvovirus-induced anemia.
3. Study to evaluate prior studies looking at the efficacy of probiotics in the treatment of acute diarrhea.
4. Study to determine the predisposing risk factors for a very rare illness in children.

MATCH THE BIAS TO THE STUDY DESIGN.
a. Recall bias.
b. Lead-time bias.
c. Positive publication bias.

5. Meta-analysis.
6. Case-control study.
7. Cross-sectional study.

METHODOLOGY

SYNOPSIS

SCREENING TESTS
1. Screening involves the testing of apparently healthy persons to identify those who are at increased risk for having a disease.
2. The most useful screening tests are for those diseases that result in substantial morbidity or mortality, diseases that have a presymptomatic phase during which the test is positive, and diseases for which treatment and prevention strategies are available and cost-effective.

DIAGNOSTIC TESTS
1. Test outcome in relationship to the truth (ie, whether or not a disease is present) (Table 1).
   a. Sensitivity: number of true-positive (TP)/number with disease: TP/(TP + false-negative [FN]).
   b. Specificity: number of true-negatives (TN)/number without disease: TN/(TN + false-positive [FP]).
   c. Positive predictive value: number of true-positives/total positives: TP/(TP + FP).
   d. Negative predictive value: number of true-negatives/total negatives: TN/(TN + FN).
2. Receiver operating characteristic curve (ROC): compares the true-positive rate (sensitivity) with the false-positive rate (specificity). The goal of the diagnostic test is to have the highest true-positive rate and the

TABLE 1   TEST EVALUATION

| TEST EVALUATION | TEST RESULT | |
	POSITIVE	NEGATIVE
Disease status		
Have disease	True-positive (TP)	False-negative (FN)
Healthy	False-positive (FP)	True-negative (TN)

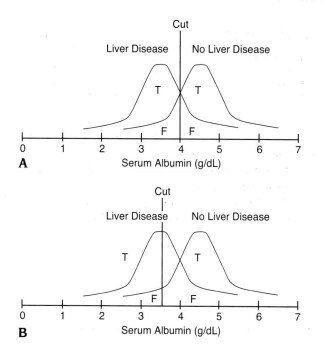

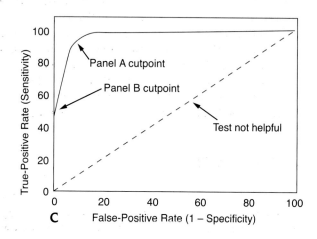

FIGURE 1 Hypothetical distribution of serum albumin levels in normal children and those with end-stage liver disease. F = false; T = true.

TABLE 2 EVALUATING STUDIES OF DIAGNOSTIC TESTS

POTENTIAL THREATS TO STUDY VALIDITY IF ANY OF THE FOLLOWING ARE PRESENT	EFFECT OF THE THREAT	BEST PRACTICES APPROACH TO MINIMIZE THE THREAT OF INVALID RESULTS
POPULATION STUDIED		
Selection of only those patients who are known to have the disease	Cannot estimate diagnostic accuracy of the test	Study population is subjects for whom the test is relevant in clinical practice (eg, all patients presenting with a symptom). Population needs to be described.
Selection of patients known to have the disease and selection of another group known to be healthy normal subjects (case-control study)	Overestimates diagnostic accuracy of the test	
Systematic or unknown reasons for excluding subjects who are part of a relevant clinical population	Over- or underestimates the diagnostic accuracy of the test depending on the reasons for excluding subjects	Consecutive patients in the relevant population are studied
Some patients studied more than once	Over- or underestimates the diagnostic accuracy of the test depending on whether overrepresented subjects have or do not have the disease being studied	Each subject is studied the same number of times (usually once or at first encounter)
COMPARISON WITH A STANDARD		
Gold standard (reference) test is not done in everyone (eg, only those with positive tests have the reference test)	Cannot estimate diagnostic accuracy of the test	Gold standard test is performed on everyone (best practices) or at least a random subset of all subjects
Gold standard test is done for only those patients with positive test and a different test is done for those with negative tests	Cannot estimate diagnostic accuracy of the test	
Gold standard test is read with knowledge of the result of the diagnostic test (or the diagnostic test is read with knowledge of the result of the gold standard test)	Overestimate the accuracy of the test, particularly if either test requires subjective interpretation	The gold standard and diagnostic tests are read independently (blinded) and, if any test requires subjective interpretation, ideally should be read by more than one independent person. Results of agreement of independent reading should be reported.
TESTING		
Way in which the gold standard and diagnostic test were performed is unclear	Cannot interpret diagnostic accuracy	Way in which the gold standard and diagnostic test were performed should be described in sufficient detail to allow reader to replicate the measurements
REPORTING OF RESULTS		
No information on whether indeterminate test results occurred and/or were included or excluded in the analysis	Potential for distortion of diagnostic accuracy	All study results should be reported (positive, negative, indeterminate), and tests of diagnostic accuracy should indicate how indeterminate values were treated and effects on measures of test accuracy

lowest false-positive rate possible (ie, plot as close to the top left of the curve as possible and as far away as possible from the line of equality) (Figure 1).

The ROC can also provide information on the overall accuracy of the test. The area under the ROC curve (AUC) is equal to the probability that a random person with the disease will have a higher test value than a random person without the disease. If the AUC = 0.5, the test has the same accuracy as a coin toss.

QUESTIONS

You are developing a test to screen a population for a new disease called Board phobia. You have run this test in a typical sample population and have come up with the following results:

TEST EVALUATION	TEST RESULT POSITIVE	NEGATIVE
Disease status		
Have disease	65	10
Healthy	5	20

1. What is the sensitivity of this test?
2. What is the specificity of this test?
3. What is the positive predictive value of this test?
4. What is the negative predictive value of this test?
5. What would happen to the positive predictive value if the prevalence of the disease increased?

ANSWERS

OUTCOMES RESEARCH
1. c.
2. a.
3. d.
4. b.
5. c.
6. a.
7. b.

METHODOLOGY
1. 65/75 = 0.87.
2. 20/25 = 0.80.
3. 65/70 = 0.93.
4. 20/30 = 0.67.
5. It would increase.

NUTRITIONAL PRINCIPLES
OF THERAPY

NUTRITIONAL ASSESSMENT AND REQUIREMENTS

SYNOPSIS

ASSESSMENT

METHODS OF DIETARY INTAKE ASSESSMENT

1. 24 h recall sheds light on family eating patterns and food availability. Limited by recall bias.
2. Most reliable: prospective food diary for 3–5 d when child is feeling well; should include at least 1 weekend day. Interpretations requires a qualified dietitian. This method provides average daily intake of energy and macro- and micronutrients.

PHYSICAL EXAM AND ANTHROPOMETRIC DATA

1. Basic anthropometric data includes body weight and height. Children age > 2 yr should be measured with a stadiometer while standing erect with an average of 3 readings obtained for accurate measurements. Raw data plotted on reference curves for age and sex. Criteria for malnutrition are based on Waterlow criteria (Table 1).
2. Body mass index (BMI): an anthropometric index, valid and reliable screening tool for obesity. Children with BMI > 85% are at risk for overweight; those with BMI > 95% are obese.
3. Limitation in anthropometric techniques is their inability to measure body composition (fat mass vs fat-free mass).
4. Available clinical techniques for measurement of body composition in children include skinfold measurements, bioelectrical impedance analysis (BIA), and dual-energy x-ray absorptiometry (DXA):
   a. Skinfold measurements: directly measure body fat. Obtained at four sites: triceps, biceps, subscapular, and suprailiac. Prone to significant inter- and intraobserver variation. Does not measure intra-abdominal fat and poorly correlates with total body fat.
   b. BIA: noninvasive, nonradioactive measure of body composition. Technique relies on principle that fat-free mass conducts an electrical charge better than

fat mass. Because the total body water content of infants and young children is not stable, there are difficulties with using BIA in this age group.
   c. DXA: primary role is to measure bone mineral density, and total body bone mineral content. Also measures body composition.
5. Laboratory tests:
   a. Complete blood count with differential: lymphopenia is a well-known feature of protein-energy malnutrition. Mild malnutrition total lymphocyte count (TLC), 1,200–1,500/mm^3; moderate malnutrition, TLC 800–1,200/mm^3; severe, TLC < 800/mm^3.
   b. Delayed type hypersensitivity testing: cutaneous anergy (delayed response to intradermal antigens) is found in moderate to severe malnutrition.
   c. Nitrogen (N) balance: N intake is compared with N output to calculate net N balance. Negative N balance implies a catabolic state and lean body mass breakdown; positive N balance implies adequate energy intake and an anabolic state.
   d. Blood concentrations of visceral proteins synthesized by the liver are often used to assess nutritional status. Protein levels depend on rates of synthesis, degradation, and escape from the circulatory system and are affected by infectious and catabolic processes. These include albumin, prealbumin, retinol-binding protein, and transferrin. Prealbumin is the best serum marker of nutritional status with a short half-life (2 d) and high ratio of essential to nonessential amino acids.
6. Physical examination can also allow determination of nutritional status (Table 2).

INDIRECT CALORIMETRY AND ENERGY REQUIREMENTS

1. Total energy expenditure is calculated as follows:

$$TEE = BMR + SDA + E_{activity} + E_{growth} + E_{losses}$$

where TEE = total energy expenditure; BMR = basal metabolic rate (energy required at rest and while fasting); SDA = specific dynamic action of food (energy produced as heat during digestion and metabolism of food); $E_{activity}$ = energy required for physical activity; E_{growth} = energy required for somatic growth; E_{losses} = obligatory energy lost in urine and stool.
2. BMR is the largest component of TEE and can be approximated by indirect calorimetry measurement of resting energy expenditure (REE). The difference between BMR and REE is approximately 10%. Indirect calorimetry can also determine whether a patient is being overfed. The ratio of VCO_2 to VO_2 gives the respiratory quotient (RQ). IF RQ > 1, energy intake is in excess of energy requirements.

STABLE ISOTOPES AND ENERGY REQUIREMENTS

1. Two stable isotopes of water, ^2H_2O and $H_2{}^{18}O$, are used to measure total energy expenditure. Relies on the fact that ^2H_2O is excreted solely in body water, but $H_2{}^{18}O$ is excreted via water losses and also via the

---

TABLE 1   WATERLOW CRITERIA FOR CATEGORIZING TYPE AND CHRONICITY OF MALNUTRITION

	ACUTE MALNUTRITION (WEIGHT FOR HEIGHT; % OF MEDIAN)	CHRONIC MALNUTRITION (HEIGHT FOR AGE) (% OF MEDIAN)
Normal	> 90	> 95
Mild	80–90	90–95
Moderate	70–80	85–90
Severe	< 70	< 85

Adapted from Suskind R, Varma R. Assessment of nutritional status of children. Pediatr Rev 1984;5:195–202.
Deficits of weight for height are termed "wasting" and those of height for age are called "stunting."

TABLE 2 CLINICAL SIGNS ASSOCIATED WITH NUTRITIONAL DEFICIENCIES.

ORGAN	CLINICAL SIGN(S)	NUTRIENT DEFICIENCY
Hair	Thin, sparse, easily pluckable	Protein energy, zinc
Face	Diffuse pigmentation	Protein energy
	Moon face	Protein
	Nasolabial seborrhea	Riboflavin, niacin, or pyridoxine
Eyes	Pale conjunctivae	Iron, folate, or vitamin B_{12}
	Bitôt spots, conjunctival or corneal xerosis, or keratomalacia	Vitamin A
	Angular palpebritis	Riboflavin or niacin
Lips	Angular stomatitis or cheilosis	Riboflavin, niacin, iron, or pyridoxine
Mouth	Ageusia, dysgeusia	Zinc
Tongue	Magenta tongue	Riboflavin
	Atrophic filiform papillae	Folate, niacin, riboflavin, iron, or vitamin B_{12}
	Glossitis	Niacin, folate, riboflavin, iron, vitamin B_{12}, pyridoxine, tryptophan
Teeth	Caries	Fluoride
Gums	Swollen, bleeding	Vitamin C
Glands	Thyromegaly	Iodine
	Parotid enlargement	Protein energy
Skin	Xerosis, follicular keratosis	Vitamin A or essential fatty acids
	Perifolliculosis with blood or pigment	Vitamin C
	Petechiae, ecchymoses	Vitamin C or K
	Pellagrous dermatosis	Niacin, tryptophan
	Scrotal or vulval dermatosis	Riboflavin
Nails	Koilonychia	Iron
Subcutaneous tissues	Edema	Protein, thiamine
	Decreased subcutaneous fat	Protein energy
Musculoskeletal system	Muscle wasting	Protein energy
	Craniotabes, frontal bossing, rachitic rosary, epiphyseal enlargement	Vitamin D
	Epiphyseal enlargement, subperiosteal hemorrhage	Vitamin C
Hepatobiliary system	Hepatomegaly	Protein energy
Nervous system	Psychomotor changes, confusion, irritability	Protein
	Sensory loss, motor weakness, calf tenderness	Thiamine
	Loss of vibratory sense, decreased deep tendon reflexes	Vitamin B_{12} or E
Cardiovascular system	Cardiomegaly, tachycardia	Thiamine

Suskind R, Varma R. Assessment of nutritional status of children. Pediatr Rev 1984;5:195–202.

carbonic anhydrase system. This differential decay in rates can be used to measure CO_2 production and calculate TEE.

2. Advantages include the noninvasiveness and safety of the technique and requirement of only serial urine collection. It provides data over 7–14 d.

TABLE 3 DEFINITIONS OF NUTRITIONAL REQUIREMENTS TO SET STANDARDS OF INTAKE (FNB/IOM/NAS)

TERM	ABBREVIATION	YEAR INTRODUCED	DEFINITION/USE
Old			
Recommended Dietary Allowances	RDAs	1943	Average daily dietary intake value sufficient to meet the requirement of nearly all (97–98%) healthy individuals in a group; more recently, the term has been calculated as EAR plus 2 SD of the EAR (see below)
New			
Dietary Reference Intakes	DRIs	1994	Umbrella term including RDA, EAR, AI, and UL (see below)
Estimated Average Requirement	EAR	1994	Nutrient intake value that is estimated to meet the requirement of half the individuals in a group
Adequate Intake	AI	1994	Used when no EAR is available and therefore no RDA can be calculated; nutrient intake value based on observed or experimentally determined approximations of nutrient intakes by a group or groups of healthy people
Tolerable Upper Intake Level	UI	1994	Highest level of a daily nutrient intake that is likely to pose no risks of adverse health effects to almost all individuals in the general population

FNB/IOM/NAS = Food and Nutrition Board of the Institute of Medicine/National Academy of Sciences.

TABLE 4 VITAMINS: FUNCTION, DEFICIENCY STATES, AND LABORATORY ASSESSMENT TECHNIQUES

VITAMIN	FUNCTION	CLINICAL DEFICIENCY STATE	LABORATORY ASSESSMENT
Vitamin A (retinol [β-carotene is dietary precursor])	Retinal in rhodopsin and iodopsin Carbohydrate transfer to glycoprotein Maintains epithelial integrity Required for cell proliferation	Night blindness Xerophthalmia Bitot spots Keratomalacia	Plasma retinol (HPLC) Plasma retinol binding protein Relative dose response Dark adaptation test Liver biopsy concentration
Vitamin D (cholecalciferol D_3 [endogenous], ergocalciferol D_2 [synthetic])	Regulates calcium and phosphate Gut absorption, excretion by kidney, and bone resorption	Rickets/osteomalacia Dental caries Hypocalcemia/hypophosphatemia Increased alkaline phosphatase Phosphaturia, aminoaciduria	Plasma 25-hydroxyvitamin D (HPLC) Serum alkaline phosphatase, calcium, and phosphate Radiography Bone densitometry
Vitamin E (α-tocopherol)	Cell membrane antioxidant Inhibits polyunsaturated fatty acid oxidation	Anemia/hemolysis Neurologic deficit (ocular palsy, wide-based gait, decreased DTRs) Altered prostaglandin synthesis	Plasma tocopherol (HPLC) (corrected for total or LDL cholesterol) Hydrogen peroxide hemolysis
Vitamin K (phylloquinone, menadione [synthetic])	Carboxylation of clotting factors Affects bone formation	Coagulopathy/prolonged PT Abnormal bone matrix synthesis	PT (prolonged) Plasma phylloquinone Clotting factor levels Proteins induced by vitamin K absence or antagonists II
Vitamin B_1 (thiamine)	Oxidative phosphorylation Pentose phosphate shunt Aldehyde transferase Triosephosphate isomerase	Beriberi ("wet" or "dry") Cardiac failure/neuropathy Korsakoff syndrome Wernicke encephalopathy Lactic acidosis	Red cell transketolase activity Whole blood level (HPLC) Urine thiamine-to-creatinine ratio
Vitamin B_2 (riboflavin)	Oxidation/reduction reactions	Seborrheic dermatitis/cheilosis/glossitis Decreased fatty acid oxidation Altered vitamin B_6 activation to coenzyme Decreased tryptophan to niacin conversion	Red cell glutathione reductase activity Red cell flavine adenine dinucleotide Urine riboflavin-to-creatinine ratio
Vitamin B_6 (pyridoxine)	Aminotransferase reactions Irritability/convulsions Decreased tryptophan to niacin conversion	Dermatitis/cheilosis/glossitis Microcytic anemia/weight loss Decreased serum transaminases Peripheral neuritis/irritability/convulsions	Red cell aminotransferase activity Plasma pyridoxal phosphate (HPLC) Tryptophan loading test Urine 4-pyridoxic acid
Vitamin B_{12} (cyanocobalamin)	Methyl group donor Sulfur amino acid conversion Branched-chain amino acid catabolism	Megaloblastic anemia Hypersegmented neutrophils Demyelination/posterior spinal column changes Methylmalonicacidemia Hyperhomocysteinemia	Plasma level (RIA or microbiologic) Schilling test Plasma homocysteine Deoxyuridine suppression test
Vitamin C (ascorbate)	Reducing agent (regenerates vitamin E) Cofactor for hydroxylators Noradrenaline/carnitine synthesis Cholesterol synthesis? Leukocyte function	Scurvy Perifollicular/petechial hemorrhages Hematologic abnormalities Poor wound healing Impaired collagen synthesis Psychological disturbances	Plasma level (enzyme assay/HPLC) Leukocyte concentration (longer term) Whole blood concentration Urine concentration
Folic acid	Methyl group donor DNA/RNA synthesis Amino acid metabolism	Megaloblastic anemia, neutropenia Altered amino acid metabolism Impaired growth Diarrhea	Plasma level (RIA/microbiologic) Red cell level
Biotin	Coenzyme for carboxylases, decarboxylases, and transcarboxylases	Multiple carboxylase deficiency Organic acidemia/acidosis Dermatitis/alopecia CNS: seizures/ataxia/depression	Plasma (microbiologic assay) Plasma lactate Urine organic acids Lymphocyte carboxylase
Niacin	Dehydrogenase activity	Pellagra: diarrhea/dermatitis/dementia Glossitis/stomatitis/vaginitis Impaired absorption of fat, carbohydrate, and vitamin B_{12} Achlorhydria	Urine ratio of metabolites (N-methylnicotinamide: 2-pyridone) Tryptophan load Red cell NAD or NAD:NADP ratio
Pantothenic acid	Pyruvate dehydrogenase cofactor Carrier of acyl groups Acetylation of alcohol/amines	Postural hypotension Anorexia and vomiting Reduced acetylation Neuromuscular defects/hyperreflexia	Urine excretion Whole blood level (RIA/microbiologic)

Adapted from Loughrey C, Duggan C. Assessment of nutritional status: the role of the laboratory. In: Soldin S, Rifai N, Hicks J, editors. Biochemical basis of pediatric disease. Washington (DC): AACC Press; 1998. p. 588–91.
CNS = central nervous system; DNA = deoxyribonucleic acid; DTR = deep tendon reflex; HPLC = high-performance liquid chromatography; LDL = low-density lipoprotein; NAD = nicotinamide adenine dinucleotide; NADP = nicotinamide adenine dinucleotide phosphate; PT = prothrombin time; RIA = radioimmunoassay; RNA = ribonucleic acid.

TABLE 5 MINERALS AND TRACE ELEMENTS: FUNCTION, DEFICIENCY STATES, AND LABORATORY ASSESSMENT TECHNIQUES

MINERAL/ TRACE ELEMENT	FUNCTION	CLINICAL DEFICIENCY STATE	LABORATORY ASSESSMENT
Calcium	Bone structure Cell metabolic regulator Nerve excitation threshold	Bone demineralization Tetany/seizures Cardiac arrhythmias	Plasma total calcium Plasma free calcium in altered protein binding (eg, hypoalbuminemia, acidosis) Radiographs CT and photon densitometry
Chromium	Glucose tolerance factor Metabolism of nucleic acids ? Iodine/thyroid function	Glucose intolerance Neuropathy/encephalopathy Altered nitrogen metabolism Increased free fatty acids	Plasma chromium Glucose tolerance
Copper	Cofactor for several enzymes including superoxide dismutase, tyrosinase, ferrochelatase, cytochrome c oxidase	Hypochromic anemia, neutropenia Skin depigmentation Dyslipidemia CNS problems	Plasma copper Plasma ceruloplasmin (ferrochelatase) Liver biopsy concentration Superoxide dismutase activity
Iodide	Component of thyroid hormones	Goiter Cretinism	Thyroid hormones, TSH Urinary iodide-to-creatinine ratio
Iron	Heme synthesis Component of cytochromes	Hypochromic microcytic anemia Altered oxidative phosphorylation Diminished concentrative ability Decreased exercise tolerance	Plasma iron and ferritin Total iron-binding capacity Hemoglobin/hematocrit, red cell indices RBC zinc protoporphyrin-to-heme ratio Bone marrow aspirate stain
Magnesium	Cofactor for hexokinase and phosphokinase Alters ribosomal aggregation in protein synthesis Increases nerve excitation threshold	Cardiac dysrhythmias Neuromuscular excitability Decreased PTH level/activity Hypocalcemia/hypokalemia Convulsions	Plasma total or free magnesium Magnesium loading test
Manganese	Mucopolysaccharide synthesis Cholesterol synthesis Cartilage/bone formation Pyruvate carboxylase cofactor Superoxide dismutase cofactor	Dermatitis Decreased clotting factors Decreased nail/hair growth ?Hair color change	Plasma level Whole blood level Mitochondrial superoxide dismutase
Phosphorus	Bone structure Cell membrane structure Energy use Glycogen deposition Acid-base balance: buffering Oxygen release (2,3-DPG)	Tissue hypoxia Respiratory failure (ventilatory dependence) Hemolytic anemia Rickets CNS abnormalities	Serum/plasma levels Alkaline phosphatase activity Radiography Densitometry Renal tubular excretion threshold
Selenium	Glutathione peroxidase constituent Thyroid hormone metabolism	Myositis Cardiomyopathy Nail bed changes Macrocytic anemia?	Plasma concentration Glutathione peroxidase acitivity Nail/hair selenium
Zinc	Cofactor for > 70 enzymes Immune function Cell replication Vision	Skin lesions/poor wound healing Immune dysfunction (especially T cell) Anorexia/dysgeusia Growth failure/nitrogen wasting Hypogonadism/delayed puberty Diarrhea	Plasma concentration Alkaline phosphatase activity Urinary excretion Leukocyte concentration

Adapted from Loughrey C, Duggan C. Assessment of nutritional status: the role of the laboratory. In: Soldin S, Rifai N, Hicks J, editors. Biochemical basis of pediatric disease. Washington (DC): AACC Press; 1998. p. 588–91.

CNS = central nervous system; CT = computed tomography; DPG = 2,3-diphosphoglycerate; PTH = parathyroid hormone; RBC = red blood cell; TSH = thyroid-stimulating hormone.

3. Alternatively, labeled bicarbonate can be similarly used to measure energy expenditure over a shorter period of time.

NUTRITIONAL REQUIREMENTS
Recommended daily allowances (RDAs) are still the most appropriate measures to use when reviewing an individual's dietary intake (Tables 3–5).

QUESTIONS

CHOOSE THE BEST ANSWER:
1. Available techniques for the measurement of body composition in children include all of the following except:
   a. Dual energy x-ray absorptiometry.
   b. Bioelectrical impedance analysis.
   c. Skinfold measurements.
   d. Body mass index.
   e. All of the above are used.

2. Protein-energy malnutrition is indicated by all of the following except:
   a. Anergy.
   b. Lymphopenia.
   c. Neutropenia.
   d. Low prealbumin.
   e. Negative nitrogen balance.

3. Basal metabolic rate is best approximated by:
   a. Resting energy expenditure.
   b. Total energy expenditure.
   c. Specific dynamic action of food.
   d. Energy required for physical activity.
   e. Respiratory quotient.

MATCH THE SYMPTOMS WITH THE DEFICIENCY:

a. Glucose intolerance.
b. Myositis and cardiomyopathy.
c. Microcytic anemia.
d. Beriberi.
e. Rickets.
f. Megaloblastic anemia.
g. Diarrhea, dermatitis, and dementia.
h. Postural hypotension.
i. Bitot spots.

4. Vitamin A.
5. Vitamin B_1.
6. Pantothenic acid.
7. Vitamin B_{12}.
8. Iron.
9. Vitamin D.
10. Selenium.
11. Chromium.
12. Niacin.

PARENTERAL NUTRITION

SYNOPSIS

INDICATIONS FOR PARENTERAL NUTRITION

1. Support needed owing to gastrointestinal (GI) non-function or partial function where patient is unable to take in sufficient calories to grow and/or maintain weight and daily living activities.

TABLE 2   ESTIMATES OF PARENTERAL ENERGY REQUIREMENTS

AGE (YR)	ENERGY (KCAL/KG/D)	CARBOHYDRATE (MG/KG/MIN)*
Premature infant	80–120	10–18
Term infant	90–120	11–18
1–3	75–90	9–14
4–6	65–75	8–11
7–10	55–75	7–11
11–18	40–55	7–8.5

Reproduced with permission from Lee PC, Werlin SL. Carbohydrates. In: Baker RD, Baker SS, Davis AM, editors. Pediatric parenteral nutrition. New York: Chapman and Hall; 1997. p. 99–107.
*Estimate based on 60–75% of nonprotein calories as glucose.

2. < 7 d: peripheral nutrition supplement; > 7 d: central nutrition supplement.

CALORIE AND FLUID REQUIREMENTS
Distribution of calories: 7–20% protein, 20–60% carbohydrates, 20–50% lipids (Tables 1 and 2).

PROTEIN REQUIREMENTS
1. Low birth weight: 3–4 g/kg/d; full term–12 mo: 2–3 g/kg/d; age 1–8 yr: 1–1.2 g/kg/d; adolescent boys: 0.9 g/kg/d; adolescent girls: 0.8 g/kg/d; critically ill: 1.5 g/kg/d.
2. Nine essential amino acids: histidine, isoleucine, leucine, lysine, methionine, phenylalanine, threonine, tryptophan, and valine.
3. Body has little in way of protein that can be mobilized during times of insufficient intake. One half of body protein: skeletal muscle, skin, and blood; 10% of body protein: liver and kidney; 15% of body protein: brain, heart, lung, and bone.
4. Immunonutrition: use of specific nutrients to influence nutritional, immunologic, and inflammatory parameters. Use of glutamine in surgical patients associated with reduction in infection rates and shorter hospital stay. Glutamine supplementation associated with reduction in complication and mortality rates.
5. In liver disease: branched-chain enriched parenteral nutrition (PN) solution may offer benefits, particularly those with hepatic encephalopathy.
6. Amino acid solutions specifically designed for infants age < 1 yr contain the following:
   a. Taurine, glutamate, and aspartate.
   b. Increased arginine and leucine.

TABLE 1   FLUID REQUIREMENTS PER DAY IN PEDIATRIC PATIENTS AS DETERMINED BY VARIOUS METHODS

METHOD	BODY WEIGHT (KG)	AMOUNT/D
Volume/weight	0–10	100 mL/kg
	10–20	1,000 + 50 mL/kg over 10 kg
	> 20	1,500 + 20 mL/kg over 20 kg
Volume/surface area	1–70	1,500–1,700 mL/m²
Volume/kcal	0–70	100 mL/100 kcal metabolized

TABLE 3 SUGGESTED PEDIATRIC PARENTERAL SUBSTRATE PROVISION

	NUTRIENT	AMOUNT
INITIATION	Carbohydrate	10% dextrose (6–8 mg/kg/min)
Amino acids	50–100% of goal	
Lipid		0.5–1.0 g/kg/d
ADVANCEMENT	Carbohydrate	5% dextrose per day (2–4 mg/kg/min)
Amino acid	100% of goal	
Lipid		0.5–1.0 g/kg/d
USUAL UPPER LIMIT	Carbohydrate	8–18 mg/kg/min
Peripheral	12.5% dextrose	
Central	25–35% dextrose	
Amino acid		3.0 g/kg/d

TABLE 4 GLUCOSE CONCENTRATION IN PARENTERAL SOLUTIONS

	PREMATURE INFANT (< 1,000 G OR 28 WK GESTATION)	INFANT	CHILD (1–10 YR)	ADOLESCENT (11–18 YR)
Begin infusion	5–7.5% or glucose concentration in current IV solution	5–7.5% or glucose concentration in current IV solution	10% or percent higher than concentration in current IV solution	10% or percent higher than concentration in current IV solution
Advance	2.5% each day as tolerated	2.5% each day as tolerated	5% each day as tolerated	5% each day as tolerated
Usual GIR upper limit (mg/kg/min)	8–12	12–14	8–10	5–6
Peripheral maximum concentration (%)	12	12.5	12.5	12.5
Central glucose concentration (%)	20–25	25	25	25
Monitor at initiation and with every increase	Urine glucose	Urine glucose	Urine glucose	Urine glucose

Adapted from Lee PC, Werlin SL. Carbohydrates. In: Baker RD, Baker SS, Davis AM, editors. Pediatric parenteral nutrition. New York: Chapman and Hall; 1997. p. 99–107.
GIR = glucose infusion rate; IV = intravenous.

c. Reduced methionine, glycine, and alanine.
d. Added cysteine causing reduced pH to allow higher concentration of calcium and phosphorus.

CARBOHYDRATES

1. Glucose is major energy source in PN: safe, economic, and readily available. Glucose solutions > 12.5% must be administered in a central vein (Table 4).
2. Glucose infusion rate (GIR) can be calculated using the following equation:

$$GIR = \frac{g/kg/d \ dextrose \times 1,000}{1,440 \ min/d}$$

3. High glucose levels may not be beneficial and may contribute to hepatosteatosis.
4. Insulin should not be added routinely to PN solutions since infantile responses unpredictable.
5. In critically ill patients, GIR limited to 5–7 mg/kg/min.
6. Glucose results in higher resting energy expenditures and higher metabolic rates, resulting in respiratory quotient > 1. Ratio of calories derived from glucose vs fats in range of 3:1 or 2:1 minimizes CO_2 stress.

INTRAVENOUS FAT ADMINISTRATION

1. Consists of 3 components: aqueous phase, lipid phase, emulsifier. Lipid phase supplies majority of calories and essential fatty acids. Glycerin is in the aqueous phase. Emulsifier is usually egg phospholipids.
2. Caloric density of 10% lipid emulsions equals 1.1 kcal/mL; 20% emulsion, 2 kcal/mL; 30% emulsion, 3 kcal/mL.
3. The essential fats for humans are linoleic ($C_{18:2w-6}$) and linolenic ($C_{18:3w-3}$) acids.
4. Essential fatty acid deficiencies (EFADs) described in children and adults with no exogenous fat source for 3 wk or more. In preterm infants EFAD seen after only 1 wk. Symptoms: scaly skin rash, sparse hair, infection susceptibility, failure to thrive, hypotonia, increased red blood count fragility, electroencephalogram and electrocardiogram changes. EFAD can be prevented by supplying 0.5–1 g/kg/d as intravenous (IV) lipid. In premature infants, 0.6–0.8 g/kg/d IV lipid prevents EFAD.
5. Lipoprotein lipase and lecithin-cholesterol acyltransferase (LCAT) are key proteins involved in clearing infused lipid from circulation. 2–3 g/kg/d can be safely

administered to premature or term infants and older children. Monitor clearance via serum triglycerides.

MINERALS AND TRACE ELEMENTS

1. Calcium: metabolic bone disease is common in premature infants and children receiving long-term PN. Hypocalcemia results from not supplying adequate calcium and from urinary calcium losses. Amino acid solutions for children age < 1 yr have added cysteine, which lowers the pH enough to permit added calcium and phosphorus without precipitation that may meet daily requirements. Aluminum in PN may also contribute to bone disease.

2. Phosphorus and magnesium: must be monitored in malnourished patients receiving nutritional rehabilitation. During rapid renutrition, profound hypomagnesemia, hypokalemia, and hypophosphatemia may result owing to intracellular shifts, precipitating acute respiratory and circulatory collapse (refeeding syndrome).

3. Zinc: essential for growth. Zinc deficiency impairs cell-mediated immunity, results in dermatitis, alopecia, and diarrhea. Severe deficiency resembles acrodermatitis enteropathica. PN administration diminishes plasma zinc by about 30%. Zinc losses occur through urine, sweat, and stool. Acute zinc toxicity has resulted in pancreatitis.

4. Copper: deficiency described in long-term PN patients. Premature infants at special risk because copper accumulates in fetus during third trimester. Deficiency signs: hypochromic or microcystic anemia, depigmentation of skin and hair, hypothermia, and hypotonia. Toxicity should be measured in cholestasis because excretion of copper is via bile.

5. Manganese: two known functions: cofactor for pyruvate carboxylase and part of mitochondrial enzyme superoxide dismutase. Manganese toxicity in long-term PN described, may contribute to cholestasis and basal ganglia damage (Parkinson disease). Toxicity should be measured in those with cholestasis because excretion of manganese is via bile.

6. Chromium: toxicity in children on PN reported; results in skin irritation and carcinogenesis in animals. The trivalent chromium in PN solutions is not highly toxic, so excessive chromium not likely to be harmful.

7. Iodine: 1 μg/kg/d in PN recommended for very low birth weight infant. No toxicity reported; deficiency reported in extremely premature infants.

8. Selenium: deficiency reported in children receiving PN. Parenteral selenium requirements are 2 μg/kg/d for preterm or term infants and children. Selenium toxicity described, especially in those with renal disease (mode of excretion).

9. Iron: deficiency common in children receiving long-term PN. Occurs as result of underlying condition requiring PN. Children should be evaluated for other causes of anemia: anemia of chronic disease, zinc deficiency, vitamin E deficiency, hemolysis, and chronic blood loss. Premature infants at particular risk, since iron transferred to fetus via placenta during last trimester. Iron precipitates as iron phosphate in lipid emulsions and 3 in 1 solutions. Iron dextrans compatible with PN solutions that do not contain lipid. Need to watch for iron overload when administering iron parenterally, as iron homeostasis is regulated at the level of GI absorption.

10. Vitamins: essential nutrients that must be provided by PN to avoid deficiency. Carnitine may need to be provided to the neonate once deficiency confirmed. To avoid toxicity, vitamin preparations designed for preterm infants should not be formulated with propylene glycol or polysorbate.

PN INTRAVENOUS CATHETERS

1. Three categories of central lines:
   a. Tunneled lines: Broviac or Hickman lines.
   b. Subcutaneous port lines: Medi-Port or Hide-a-Port.
   c. Peripheral intravenous central catheter lines.
2. Catheters should be placed into superior vena cava, right atrium.
3. Femoral lines: higher rates of venous thrombosis and catheter-related sepsis. Subclavian access: greater risk of pneumothorax. Internal jugular insertion: higher rates of hematoma formation, arterial injury, and catheter-related infections.

COMPLICATIONS

1. Mechanical: misplaced lines or lines that move, fall out, become occluded, or embolize.
   a. Thrombosis: use of heparin can be associated with thrombocytopenia. Alternatives to heparin include tissue plasminogen activator, streptokinase, and urokinase.
   b. Catheter occlusions resolve with instillation of 0.2–1 cc of 0.1 N HCl for 30 min to 1 h. Alkaline solution (0.1 NaOH) or ethanol 70% may also be used.
2. Metabolic: over- and underhydration are most common. Other complications: hypoglycemia, electrolyte imbalances, inadequate growth, and nutrient deficiencies.
3. Cholestasis: associated factors include lack of enteral feeding; excessive carbohydrate, fat, or calories; inappropriate quality or quantity of amino acids; and deficient trace elements. Only effective treatment of cholestasis is discontinuation of PN.
4. Infections.

CYCLING

1. Sudden discontinuation of high glucose infusion associated with hypoglycemia, especially in children age < 3 yr. PN should be tapered by decreasing to one half the rate for 1 h and to one quarter of the rate for another hour before complete discontinuation.
2. Benefits: reduces persistently high serum insulin levels, which can lead to hepatic lipid deposition and lipogenesis. Essential fatty acid deficiency may occur with continuous PN since insulin inhibits release of free fatty acids from fat.
3. Disadvantages: increases urinary calcium losses.

New!

ProNourish™

At a Glance: FODMAPs and the Low FODMAP Diet

FODMAPs are specific types of carbohydrates that can be poorly absorbed and cause digestive discomfort in some people. FODMAPs are found in a wide variety of food groups.

Fermentable

Examples of High FODMAP Foods and Ingredients

Oligosaccharides

Fructans/GOS: wheat, rye, onions, garlic, artichokes, inulin, baked beans, red kidney beans, cashews

Disaccharides

Lactose: milk, yogurt, ice cream, pudding, custard

Monosaccharides

Excess Fructose: high fructose corn syrup, honey, agave, mango, watermelon

And...

Polyols

Sorbitol/Mannitol: sugar-free products, blackberries, apples, pears, peaches, cauliflower, mushrooms, snow peas

Low FODMAP Diet 101
With the help of a healthcare professional

PHASE 1: Trial elimination Foods high in FODMAPs are removed from your diet (2-6 weeks).

PHASE 2: Reintroduction Reintroduction of specific FODMAPs in a stepwise process to help distinguish individual FODMAP triggers. Once completed, you can then customize a well-balanced diet designed to address your specific dietary needs.

Low FODMAP Diet Resources

lowFODMAPcentral.com

University of Michigan and Cedars-Sinai®— My Nutrition Health: www.myginutrition.com*

Low FODMAP Website: www.med.monash.edu/cecs/gastro/fodmap*

Low FODMAP Diet App: www.med.monash.edu. au/cecs/gastro/fodmap/iphone-app.html*

Kate Scarlata, RDN, LDN The Well-Balanced FODMAPer Blog: blog.katescarlata.com*

*The resources are for educational purposes only and do not constitute endorsement of any product or brand.

ProNourish™

FOOD CATEGORY	HIGH FODMAP FOODS	LOW FODMAP FOOD ALTERNATIVES
Vegetables	Asparagus, artichokes, onions, leeks, garlic, mushrooms, sugar snap peas, snow peas, onion & garlic salts	Alfalfa sprouts, bean sprouts, green beans, bok choy, bell peppers, carrots, chives, cucumber, lettuce, eggplant, kale, spinach, tomato, zucchini
Fruits	Apples, pears, mango, watermelon, nectarines, peaches, plums, prunes, cherries	Bananas, pineapple, oranges, grapes, blueberries, honeydew melon, kiwifruit, strawberries, cantaloupe
Milk and Dairy	Cow's milk, yogurt, buttermilk, cream, custard, ice cream	Lactose-free cow's milk and yogurt, almond milk, feta cheese, Parmesan cheese, Brie cheese, cheddar cheese
Protein	Red kidney beans, black beans, baked beans, soy beans (edamame)	Fish, chicken, pork, beef, eggs, canned tuna, tofu (firm), small portions of canned and drained chick peas and lentils
Nuts and Seeds	Pistachios, cashews	Walnuts, peanuts, pecans, sesame seeds, sunflower seeds, chia seeds
Breads and Grains	Rye, wheat, and barley containing products	Sourdough breads, quinoa, white rice, brown rice, oats, polenta, corn tortillas
Hot Beverages	Chamomile tea, fennel tea, oolong tea	Coffee, green tea, black tea, peppermint tea

This chart is intended to provide examples of foods that are high or low in FODMAPs. It is not meant to be an all-inclusive diet. Check with a healthcare professional to see if the low FODMAP diet is right for you.

Sources:
   Monash University Low FODMAP Diet App. Available at: med.monash.edu/cecs/gastro/fodmap/iphone-app.html.
      Monash University Low FODMAP Diet. Available at: med.monash.edu/cecs/gastro/fodmap/low-high.html.
         Monash University Low FODMAP Diet Book. 2015, Edition 5. Available at: med.monash.edu/cecs/gastro/fodmap/education.html.

ProNourish.com

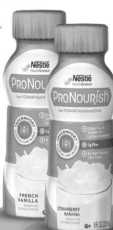

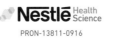 Nestlé Health Science

PRON-13811-0916

CRITICAL CARE

1. Aims of PN: to minimize effects of catabolism and hypermetabolism, to attain a positive nitrogen balance, and to support growth. Danger of overfeeding.
2. Can measure prealbumin and C-reactive protein to determine when anabolic metabolism resumes. If serum C-reactive protein < 2 mg/dL, anabolic metabolism resumed; prealbumin begins to rise once an anabolic state is achieved.
3. Can calculate resting energy expenditure using oxygen consumption and carbon dioxide production. Indirect calorimetry can allow calculation of respiratory quotient (RQ). RQ depends on substrate used: if only fat oxidized RQ = 0.71; if only carbohydrates utilized, RQ = 1.

QUESTIONS

TRUE OR FALSE:

1. Central parenteral nutrition should be provided if suboptimal nutrition exists for more than 1 week.
2. Essential fatty acid deficiencies are seen after 2 weeks of no supplemental dietary fat.
3. Prealbumin decreases in the anabolic state.
4. Electrolyte abnormalities are the most common metabolic complications associated with total parenteral nutrition.
5. Total parenteral nutrition administration itself decreases serum zinc levels.

MATCH THE PARENTERAL NUTRITION TREATMENT TO THE CONDITION:

a. Branched-chain amino acid–enriched parenteral nutrition.
b. Parenteral nutrition with added cysteine.
c. Glutamine supplementation.

6. Infants age < 1 yr.
7. Hepatic encephalopathy
8. Postsurgical patients

CHOOSE THE BEST ANSWER:

9. Metabolic bone disease associated with parenteral nutrition is associated with all of the following except:
   a. Inadequate calcium supplementation.
   b. Urinary calcium losses.
   c. Aluminum contamination of the total parenteral nutrition.
   d. Fecal calcium losses.

10. Essential amino acids include all of the following except:
    a. Isoleucine.
    b. Leucine.
    c. Lysine.
    d. Glutamine.

11. The following are essential fatty acids:
    a. Linoleic acid and phospholipids.
    b. Linoleic and linolenic acid.
    c. Phosphatidyl choline and linolenic acid.
    d. Phosphatidyl choline and phospholipids.

12. The following are true of total parenteral nutrition cycling except:
    a. Sudden discontinuation is associated with hypoglycemia.
    b. Allows for decrease in insulin levels.
    c. Reduces risk of hepatosteatosis.
    d. Increases risk of metabolic bone disease.
    e. All of the above are true.

ENTERAL NUTRITION

SYNOPSIS

1. Enteral nutrition routes: oral, nasogastric (NG), gastrostomy, nasojejunal (NJ), and jejunostomy.
2. Enteral vs parenteral nutrition:
   a. Enteral more physiologic, economic, easier, and safer.
   b. Enteral nutrition is done in the absence of a central venous catheter, decreasing infectious and thrombotic complications.
   c. Delivery of nutrients to the gut in enteral nutrition minimizes gut atrophy and the risk for bacterial translocation.
   d. Enteral nutrition offers more complete nutrient provision.
   e. Enteral nutrition avoids the hepatic complications associated with parenteral nutrition.
   f. Enteral nutrition provides trophic stimulation to the gut.

NUTRITIONAL NEEDS

1. Preterm infant: caloric requirements to support daily weight gain of 15 g/kg estimated at 105–130 kcal/kg/day. Higher energy needs depending on thermal environment, cardiorespiratory status, metabolic stress, and presence of growth retardation. Improved nutrient absorption when fed mixture of medium-chain triglycerides (MCTs), long-chain unsaturated fatty acids, and mixture of lactose and glucose polymers. Owing to high accretion rates for calcium, phosphorus, and trace elements during the last trimester of pregnancy, preterm infants have elevated requirements for these nutrients.
2. Infant and child: recommended daily allowances (RDAs) are for healthy, active children. Overfeeding may result in iatrogenic hepatic, respiratory disease, and decreased survival. In failure to thrive, estimation must be made to account for catch-up growth as follows: required kcal = (RDA kcal/kg for weight age) × [(ideal weight in kg)/(actual weight in kg)].
3. Fluid requirements must also be calculated and specific disease-related factors accounted for.

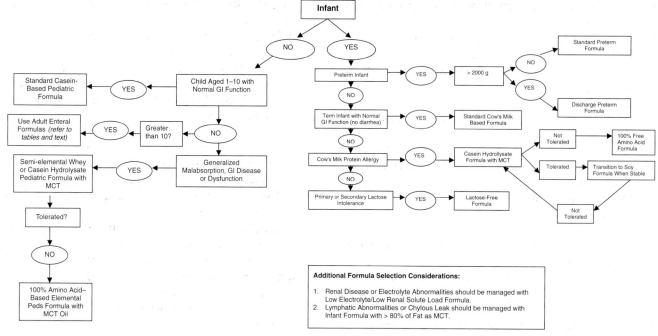

FIGURE 1 Appropriate infant and pediatric formulas based on indication for use. GI = gastrointestinal; MCT = medium-chain triglycerides.

ROUTE OR METHOD OF FEED

1. NG or NJ tubes: when course of therapy not to exceed 3 months. NJ preferred to NG in setting of aspiration risk and reflux.
2. Gastrostomy: long-term tube feeds. In cases where there is neurologic disability, an antireflux procedure may be useful as well.
3. Intermittent bolus feedings: simple; requires minimal supplies. Intolerance indicated by gastric residuals, malabsorption, dumping syndrome, aspiration, and regurgitation. Bolus feeds not well tolerated if delivered distal to the pylorus.
4. Continuous feeds: beneficial for poor absorption, chronic diarrhea, and short-bowel syndrome.

FORMULA SELECTION

1. Preterm infant formulas (< 2,000 g) vs term infant formulas (Figure 1):
   a. Preterm formulas provide combination of lactose and glucose polymers vs lactose only in order to decrease osmolality, improve digestion, and calcium absorption.
   b. Preterm formulas use a fat blend containing long-chain and very-long-chain triglycerides, which promotes improved weight gain, fat, nitrogen, and calcium absorption.
   c. Preterm formulas have elevated protein content and 60:40 whey-to-casein formulation to promote plasma amino acid profiles closer to breast milk.
   d. Preterm formulas provide increased amounts of sodium, calcium, and phosphorous to compensate for urinary sodium losses and promote bone mineralization.
   e. Vitamin concentrations are higher in preterm formulas owing to preterm infants' limited stores.

   f. Iron has been added to preterm formulas owing to lower birth weight and lower initial hemoglobin.
2. Breast milk: preferred enteral nutrition source for preterm and sick neonates owing to numerous trophic peptides. Preterm breast milk higher in protein, sodium, chloride, magnesium, and iron than mature human milk but deficient in calcium and phosphorus. Breast milk fortification recommended for preterm infants who are < 34 weeks' gestation, < 1,500 g, and receiving total parenteral nutrition for > 2 weeks.
3. Children age 1–10 yr: pediatric formulas meet specialized needs of age group. Children age > 10 yr effectively managed with an adult enteral formula.

QUESTIONS

TRUE OR FALSE:

1. Enteral nutrition provides trophic stimulation to the gut.
2. Bolus feeds are well-tolerated when delivered anywhere in the intestine.
3. Preterm formulas have more sodium than do term formulas.
4. Preterm formulas do not have added iron.
5. Critically ill children should receive the recommended daily allowance caloric intake for age.

MATCH THE FEEDING METHOD TO THE CONDITION:

a. Nasogastric tube feeds.
b. Nasojejunal tube feeds.
c. Gastrostomy tube feeds.

6. Infant prematurely born at 34 weeks gestation with difficulty nippling.
7. Neurologically devastated 3-year-old girl.
8. Infant prematurely born at 35 weeks gestation with severe lung disease that is expected to resolve in the next few weeks.

MATCH THE FORMULA TO THE CONDITION:
a. Breast milk fortification.
b. 85% medium-chain triglyceride oil-enriched formula.
c. Casein hydrolysate formula with medium-chain triglycerides.
d. Standard casein-based pediatric formula.
e. Adult enteral formula.

9. Infant prematurely born at 32 weeks gestation who weighs 1,300 g.
10. Healthy 3-month-old infant with mucous and blood streaks in the stool on regular casein-based infant formula
11. Generally healthy 5-year-old girl with poor oral intake.
12. 12-year-old boy with hypoxic encephalopathy.
13. 9-month-old with chylous ascites.

SPECIAL DIETARY THERAPY

SYNOPSIS

1. Dietary reference intakes (DRI): evidenced-based recommendations for healthy US and Canadian populations for nutrient intake for good health.
2. Dietary therapy during chronic illness is directed at providing calories, macronutrients, and micronutrients to support normal growth.
3. In order to meet increased nutritional needs associated with chronic illness, infant formulas can be concentrated. Attention should be given to renal solute load especially for patients with renal dysfunction. Generally, caloric density should only be advanced by 2–4 calories/oz in a 24 h period.

DRI
1. Recommended source of calories:
   a. 45–65% total calories should come from carbohydrates.
   b. 4–35% total calories should come from protein.
   c. 20–40% total calories should come from fat.
2. Fiber: nondigestible carbohydrate and lignin components from the plant cell wall composed of soluble and insoluble fiber. Soluble fiber is fermented by colonic bacteria and converted into short-chain fatty acids, which are absorbed by the colon. Fructo-oligosaccharides are formed in the process and promote growth of probiotic bacteria. Health benefits of fiber include: role in management of diabetes by delaying glucose uptake and reducing the insulin response. Fiber also delays gastric emptying, which may play a role in satiety and weight control. Fiber consumption is important to prevent constipation.
3. Select amino acids may be essential during periods of rapid growth and illness.
   a. Arginine is a precursor of nitric oxide and modulates hepatic protein synthesis, mediates vasodilatory effects of endotoxins, and reduces tumor and bacterial growth.
   b. Glutamine is the precursor for glutathione and has a major role as an energy source for enterocytes, lymphocytes, and macrophages. It may reduce bacterial translocation in the gut.
   c. Taurine is essential for the conjugation of bile acids early in infancy.
   d. Carnitine is important for intracellular fatty acid oxidation and energy production.
4. Docosahexaenoic acid (fish and organ meat) and arachidonic acid (meat, eggs, and fish) are polyunsaturated fatty acids that are important constituents of the brain and retina. Arachidonic acid is essential for growth.

ESSENTIAL FATTY ACID DEFICIENCY
1. Occurs in those receiving long-term parenteral nutrition without enough intravenous fat, with extended use of a formula predominantly containing medium-chain fats or with fat malabsorption.
2. Signs include poor growth, thrombocytopenia, and rough, scaly skin.
3. Diagnosed by a serum triene-to-tetraene ratio > 0.4.

MICRONUTRIENTS
Enhanced outcomes can be related to supplemental micronutrients:
1. Vitamin A: supplementation of extremely low birth weight infants with bronchopulmonary dysplasia associated with improved outcomes. Also used to treat ichthyosis and psoriasis.
2. Vitamin E: decreases atherosclerotic heart disease and lung cancer.
3. Riboflavin: decreases migraine headaches; can clinically improve patients with infantile lactic acidosis, skeletal myopathy, and Leigh disease.
4. Nicotinic acid: treats atherosclerotic heart disease.
5. Folate: benefits megaloblastic anemia but also pregnancy (decreases spontaneous abortion and neural tube defects).
6. Chromium: improves glucose tolerance.
7. Zinc: diarrhea and pneumonia prevention. Zinc supplementation has also demonstrated improvements in growth, neuropsychological performance, fetal growth, and birth outcomes.
8. Iron: improves work capacity, behavior and cognitive function, temperature regulation, immunity, and resistance to infections.

PROBIOTICS
Recognized as being beneficial in normal health for immune modulation and disease prevention. They help control

TABLE 1   SELECTED DISEASE CONDITIONS AND RELATED NUTRITIONAL CONSIDERATIONS

CYSTIC FIBROSIS
High-calorie, high-fat diet
Salt replacement, especially in hot weather
Evaluation of essential fatty acids and bone health
Fat-soluble vitamin supplementation
Enzyme therapy for pancreatic insufficiency
Oral supplements for calories

INFLAMMATORY BOWEL DISEASE
High-calorie diet
Lactose-free diet
Vitamin B_{12} supplementation with ileal disease
Vitamin D, calcium, iron, zinc, folic acid supplementation
Multivitamin supplementation
Elemental diet for inducing remission and providing caloric support
Bone disease evaluation

CONGENITAL HEART DISEASE (in infants)
High-calorie formula in infants
Concentrated formulas
Fortified breast milk in infants
Tube feeds
Sodium restriction
Fluid restriction

CANCER
High-calorie diet
Oral supplements
Tube feeds
Parenteral nutrition for extensive nausea and vomiting
Appetite stimulants
Small, frequent feedings

RENAL DISEASE
Fluid restriction
Fortified breast milk or concentrated formula
Sodium restriction
Provide RDA for protein
Phosphorus restriction
Phosphorus binder
Supplement with vitamin D, calcium
Bone disease evaluation

LIVER DISEASE
Fluid restriction for end-stage disease
Fat-soluble vitamin/multivitamin supplementation
Fat malabsorption may occur with biliary atresia or Alagille syndrome
Evaluation of essential fatty acid status
Evaluation of bone health
Protein restriction with encephalopathy
Adequate calories and protein for growth

METABOLIC DISORDERS
Dietary restriction of the offending nutrients
Adjusted intake of offending amino acids and fats to promote optimal growth and development
Monitor compliance to diet
Replacement of deficient coenzymes

CEREBRAL PALSY
Supplemental tube feeds
Fiber-containing formula
Speech evaluation if chewing/swallowing difficulties
May require modified diet (puree, thickened liquids, etc)
Supplemental multivitamin and minerals
Ketogenic diet (patients with intractable seizures)
Bone disease evaluation

DIABETES MELLITUS
Blood glucose control
Dietary balance with regularly scheduled meals and snacks
Meal planning, carbohydrate counting, insulin education when indicated
Monitor cholesterol and triglycerides and recommend low-fat diet when indicated
Adequate calories for proper growth and development

CELIAC DISEASE
Gluten-free diet
Lactose-free diet may be indicated until complete mucosal healing
Possible infant sensitivity to cow's milk protein
Vitamin and mineral therapy
Adequate calories for catch-up growth
Bone disease evaluation
Monitor compliance to diet

RDA = Recommended Dietary Allowance.

gastrointestinal (GI) inflammation, normalize mucosal function, and down-regulate hypersensitivity reactions.

PREBIOTIC COMPOUNDS

1. Support the growth of probiotic organisms and are found in foods. These compounds are not digested in the small bowel and pass to the colon where they are metabolized into short-chain fatty acids, promote sodium and water absorption, and serve as an energy source for colonocytes. Examples: fructans and soybean oligosaccharides.
2. These substances have a low cariogenic potential, improve lipid metabolism and protect against colorectal cancer and infectious colitis, increase the bioavailability of calcium and magnesium, and may enhance host defenses.

BONE HEALTH

1. Peak bone mass (maximum amount of bone mineral attained in life) is achieved by age 18 yr in 95%. Factors adversely affecting bone development include poor weight and height gain, delayed puberty, immobilization, reduced weight-bearing activity, malnutrition, insufficient calcium intake, vitamin D deficiency, inflammatory conditions, and high levels of cytokines and steroid use.
2. Dual-energy x-ray absorptiometry (DXA) should be obtained for bone density measurement. This is a safe test with about one-twentieth the risk of chest radiograph radiation. Normative data for the lumbar spine scans are available for children age > 4 yr. DXA also can evaluate body composition. Drawbacks include difficulty in interpretation in the setting of delayed puberty and growth.
3. Therapies available to children for low bone density:
   a. Improving nutritional status to normalize weight and height.
   b. Controlling underlying chronic disease and inflammation.
   c. Ensuring adequate or therapeutic intake of calcium, vitamin D, magnesium, and vitamin K.
   d. Monitoring pubertal status.
   e. Increasing weight-bearing physical activity as appropriate.

4. Osteopenia in inflammatory bowel disease: although lower bone mineral density z-scores have been noted, once these results are adjusted for bone age, the difference between control subjects and patients is less.
5. Osteopenia also found in liver disease and celiac disease (gluten-free diet may result in some improvement).

QUESTIONS

TRUE OR FALSE:
1. Peak bone mass is achieved prior to puberty.
2. Docosahexaenoic acid is found in eggs and green vegetables.
3. Prebiotics are the precursors to probiotics.
4. Vitamin E has been shown to decrease atherosclerotic heart disease.
5. Chromium supplementation improves glucose tolerance.

CHOOSE THE BEST ANSWER:
6. The following are associated with essential fatty acid deficiency except:

a. Poor growth.
b. Rough, scaly skin.
c. Thrombocytosis.
d. Serum triene-to-tetraene ratio > 0.4.
e. Extended use of a medium-chain triglyceride oil–based formula.

MATCH THE BENEFITS TO THE MICRONUTRIENT:
a. Improves cognitive function.
b. Treats psoriasis.
c. Helps to prevent pneumonia.
d. Decreases migraine headaches.
e. Decreases incidence of neural tube defects.
f. Treats atherosclerotic disease.

7. Vitamin A.
8. Riboflavin.
9. Nicotinic acid.
10. Folate.
11. Zinc.
12. Iron.

ANSWERS

NUTRITIONAL ASSESSMENT AND REQUIREMENTS
1. d.
2. c.
3. a.
4. i.
5. d.
6. h.
7. f.
8. c.
9. e.
10. b.
11. a.
12. g.

PARENTERAL NUTRITION
1. True.
2. False. Essential fatty acid deficiency described if fat not given for 3 weeks or more.
3. False. Prealbumin rises in the anabolic state.
4. False. Underhydration or overhydration are the most common metabolic problems.
5. True.
6. b.
7. a.
8. c.
9. d.
10. d.
11. b.
12. e.

ENTERAL NUTRITION
1. True.
2. False. Bolus feeds are not well tolerated if delivered distal to the pylorus.
3. True.
4. False. Preterm formulas are iron-enriched.
5. False. Recommended daily allowance is for active children.
6. a.
7. c.
8. b.
9. a.
10. c.
11. d.
12. e.
13. b.

SPECIAL DIETARY THERAPY
1. False. 95% achieved by age18 yr.
2. False. Found in fish and organ meat.
3. False. Prebiotics support the growth of probiotic organisms.
4. True.
5. True.
6. c. Associated with thrombocytopenia.
7. b.
8. d.
9. f.
10. e.
11. c.
12. a.

9021